Hitoshi Sashiwa and David Harding (Eds.)

# Advances in Marine Chitin and Chitosan

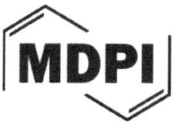

**MDPI**

This book is a reprint of the special issue that appeared in the online open access journal *Marine Drugs* (ISSN 1660-3397) in 2014 (available at: http://www.mdpi.com/journal/marinedrugs/special_issues/advance_chitin).

*Guest Editors*
David Harding
Massey University
New Zealand

Hitoshi Sashiwa
Kaneka Corporation
Japan

*Editorial Office*
MDPI AG
Klybeckstrasse 64
Basel, Switzerland

*Publisher*
Shu-Kun Lin

*Managing Editor*
Tina Yan

**1. Edition 2015**

MDPI • Basel • Beijing • Wuhan

ISBN 978-3-03842-129-0 (PDF)
ISBN 978-3-03842-130-6 (Hbk)

# Table of Contents

## Chapter I: Chemistry

**Priyanka Sahariah, Vivek S. Gaware, Ramona Lieder, Sigríður Jónsdóttir, Martha Á. Hjálmarsdóttir, Olafur E. Sigurjonsson and Már Másson**
The Effect of Substituent, Degree of Acetylation and Positioning of the Cationic Charge
on the Antibacterial Activity of Quaternary Chitosan Derivatives
Reprinted from: *Mar. Drugs* **2014**, *12*(8), 4635-4658

**Syang-Peng Rwei, Yu-Ming Chen, Wen-Yan Lin and Whe-Yi Chiang**
Synthesis and Rheological Characterization of Water-Soluble
Glycidyltrimethylammonium-Chitosan
Reprinted from: *Mar. Drugs* **2014**, *12*(11), 5547-5562

**Inmaculada Aranaz, María C. Gutiérrez, María Luisa Ferrer and Francisco del Monte**
Preparation of Chitosan Nanocompositeswith a Macroporous Structure by
Unidirectional Freezing and Subsequent Freeze-Drying
Reprinted from: *Mar. Drugs* **2014**, *12*(11), 5619-5642

**Sudipta Chatterjee, Fabien Salaün and Christine Campagne**
The Influence of 1-Butanol and Trisodium Citrate Ion on Morphology and Chemical
Properties of Chitosan-Based Microcapsules during Rigidification by Alkali Treatment
Reprinted from: *Mar. Drugs* **2014**, *12*(12), 5801-5816

# Chapter II: Medicinal Biology

# Chapter III: Others

# List of Contributors

**Inmaculada Aranaz:** Instituto de Ciencia de Materiales de Madrid (ICMM), Consejo Superior de Investigaciones Científicas (CSIC), (Materials Science Institute of Madrid, Spanish National Research Counsil), Cantoblanco 28049, Madrid, Spain.

**Toril Andersen:** Drug Transport and Delivery Research Group, Department of Pharmacy, Faculty of Health Sciences, University of Tromsø The Arctic University of Norway, Tromsø 9037, Norway.

**Nawzat Al-Jbour:** The Jordanian Pharmaceutical Manufacturing Company (PLC), Research and Innovation Centre, P.O. Box 94, Naor 11710, Jordan.

**Mayyas A. Al-Remawi:** College of Pharmacy, Taif University, Taif 5700, Saudi Arabia.

**Tawfiq M. Alhussainy:** Department of Pharmacology and Biomedical Sciences, Faculty of Pharmacy and Medical Sciences, University of Petra, P.O. Box 96134, Amman 11196, Jordan.

**Khaldoun A. Al-So'ud:** Department of Chemistry, Faculty of Science, Al al-Bayt University, P.O. Box 130040, Mafraq 25113, Jordan.

**Mahmoud M. H. Al Omari:** The Jordanian Pharmaceutical Manufacturing Company (PLC), Research and Innovation Center (RIC), Suwagh Subsidiary for Drug Delivery Systems, P.O. Box 94, Naor 11710, Jordan.

**Zakieh I. Al-Kurdi:** The Jordanian Pharmaceutical Manufacturing Company (PLC), Suwagh Subsidiary for Drug Delivery Systems, P.O. Box 94, Naor 11710, Jordan; Faculty of Engineering & Science, University of Greenwich, Medway Campus, Chatham Maritime, Kent ME44TB, UK.

**Adnan A. Badwan:** The Jordanian Pharmaceutical Manufacturing Company (PLC), Suwagh Subsidiary for Drug Delivery Systems, P.O. Box 94, Naor 11710, Jordan; Research and Innovation Center (RIC), The Jordanian Pharmaceutical Manufacturing Co., P.O. Box 94, Naor 11710, Jordan.

**Stefan Bleher:** Drug Transport and Delivery Research Group, Department of Pharmacy, Faculty of Health Sciences, University of Tromsø The Arctic University of Norway, Tromsø 9037, Norway.

**Dimitrios N. Bikiaris:** Laboratory of Polymer Chemistry and Technology, Division of Chemical Technology, Department of Chemistry, Aristotle University of Thessaloniki, GR-541 24 Thessaloniki, Greece.

**Yu-Ming Chen:** Institute of Organic and Polymeric Materials, National Taipei University of Technology, 1, Sec. 3, Zhongxiao E. Rd., Taipei 10648, Taiwan.

**Whe-Yi Chiang:** Institute of Organic and Polymeric Materials, National Taipei University of Technology, 1, Sec. 3, Zhongxiao E. Rd., Taipei 10648, Taiwan.

**Yuan-Lu Cui:** Research Center of Traditional Chinese Medicine, Tianjin University of Traditional Chinese Medicine, Tianjin 300193, China.

**Sudipta Chatterjee:** University of Lille Nord de France, F-59000 Lille, France; ENSAIT/GEMTEX, F-59100 Roubaix, France.

**Christine Campagne:** University of Lille Nord de France, F-59000 Lille, France; ENSAIT/GEMTEX, F-59100 Roubaix, France.

**Babur Z. Chowdhry:** Faculty of Engineering & Science, University of Greenwich, Medway Campus, Chatham Maritime, Kent ME44TB, UK.

**Francisco Del Monte:** Instituto de Ciencia de Materiales de Madrid (ICMM), Consejo Superior de Investigaciones Científicas (CSIC), (Materials Science Institute of Madrid, Spanish National Research Counsil), Cantoblanco 28049, Madrid, Spain.

**Trong-Ming Don:** Department of Chemical and Materials Engineering, Tamkang University, New Taipei City 251, Taiwan.

**Nguyen Anh Dzung:** Institute of Biotechnology & Environment, Tay Nguyen University, Buon Ma Thuot 63000, Vietnam.

**Fouad H. Darras:** Research and Innovation Center (RIC), The Jordanian Pharmaceutical Manufacturing Co., P.O. Box 94, Naor 11710, Jordan.

**Nidal Daraghmeh:** The Jordanian Pharmaceutical Manufacturing Co., PO Box 94, Naor 11710, Jordan; Faculty of Engineering & Science, University of Greenwich, Medway Campus, Chatham Maritime Kent ME44TB, UK.

**Gøril Eide Flaten:** Drug Transport and Delivery Research Group, Department of Pharmacy, Faculty of Health Sciences, University of Tromsø The Arctic University of Norway, Tromsø 9037, Norway.

**Moacir Fernandes Queiroz:** Department of Biochemistry, Biosciences Centre, Federal University of Rio Grande do Norte, Salgado Filho avenue 3000, Natal, RN 59078-970, Brazil.

**María Luisa Ferrer:** Instituto de Ciencia de Materiales de Madrid (ICMM), Consejo Superior de Investigaciones Científicas (CSIC), (Materials Science Institute of Madrid, Spanish National Research Counsil), Cantoblanco 28049, Madrid, Spain.

**Vivek S. Gaware:** Faculty of Pharmaceutical Sciences, School of Health Sciences, University of Iceland, Hofsvallagata 53, IS-107 Reykjavík, Iceland; PCI Biotech AS, Strandveien 55, N-1366 Lysaker, Norway.

**María C. Gutiérrez:** Instituto de Ciencia de Materiales de Madrid (ICMM), Consejo Superior de Investigaciones Científicas (CSIC), (Materials Science Institute of Madrid, Spanish National Research Counsil), Cantoblanco 28049, Madrid, Spain.

**Li-Na Gao:** Research Center of Traditional Chinese Medicine, Tianjin University of Traditional Chinese Medicine, Tianjin 300193, China.

**Martha Á. Hjálmarsdóttir:** Department of _Biomedical Science, Faculty of_ Medicine, University of_Iceland, Stapi, Hringbraut 31, 101 Reykjavík, Iceland.

**Jing-Yi Hou:** State Key Laboratory of Earth Surface Processes and Resources Ecology, Beijing Normal University, Haidian District, Beijing 100088, China; State Key Laboratory of Dao-di Herbs, China Academy of Chinese Medical Sciences, Beijing 100700, China.

**Guangshun Hou:** Institute of Resources & Environment, Henan Polytechnic University, Jiaozuo 454000, China.

**Chih-Ting Huang:** Department of Chemistry, Tamkang University, New Taipei City 25137, Taiwan.

**Woo-Jin Jung:** Division of Applied Bioscience & Biotechnology, Institute of Environment-Friendly Agriculture (IEFA), College of Agricultural and Life Sciences, Chonnam National University, Gwangju 500-757, Korea.

**Sigríður Jónsdóttir:** Department of Chemistry, Science Institute, University of Iceland, Dunhagi 3, IS-107 Reykjavik, Iceland.

**George Z. Kyzas:** Laboratory of Polymer Chemistry and Technology, Division of Chemical Technology, Department of Chemistry, Aristotle University of Thessaloniki, GR-541 24 Thessaloniki, Greece.

**Qutuba G. Karwi:** Department of Pharmacology and Biomedical Sciences, Faculty of Pharmacy and Medical Sciences, University of Petra, P.O. Box 96134, Amman 11196, Jordan.

**Ramona Lieder:** The REModeL Lab, The Blood Bank, Landspitali University Hospital, Snorrabraut 60, 105 Reykjavik, Iceland.

**Stephen A. Leharne:** Faculty of Engineering & Science, University of Greenwich, Medway Campus, Chatham Maritime Kent ME44TB, UK.

**Wen-Yan Lin:** Institute of Organic and Polymeric Materials, National Taipei University of Technology, 1, Sec. 3, Zhongxiao E. Rd., Taipei 10648, Taiwan.

**Cheng-Wei Lin:** Department of Biochemistry and Molecular Cell Biology, School of medicine, Taipei Medical University, Taipei City 110, Taiwan; Graduate Institute of Medical Sciences, College of Medicine, Taipei Medical University, Taipei City 110, Taiwan.

**Dong-Qiang Lin:** Key Laboratory of Biomass Chemical Engineering of Ministry of Education, College of Chemical and Biological Engineering, Zhejiang University, Hangzhou 310027, China; Collaborative Innovation Center of Chemical Science and Engineering (Tianjin), Tianjin 300072, China.

**Tzu-Wen Liang:** Life Science Development Center, Tamkang University, No. 151, Yingchuan Rd., Tamsui, New Taipei City 25137, Taiwan; Department of Chemistry, Tamkang University, New Taipei City 25137, Taiwan.

**Aeju Lee:** Biomedical Research Center, Korea Institute of Science and Technology, Seoul 136-791, Korea.

**Riccardo A. A. Muzzarelli:** Faculty of Medicine, Department of Clinical & Molecular Sciences, Polytechnic University of Marche, IT-60100 Ancona, Italy.

**Mohamad El Mehtedi:** Faculty of Engineering, Department of Industrial Engineering & Mathematical Sciences, Polytechnic University of Marche, IT-60100 Ancona, Italy.

**Monica Mattioli-Belmonte:** Faculty of Medicine, Department of Clinical & Molecular Sciences, Polytechnic University of Marche, IT-60100 Ancona, Italy.

**Fwu-Long Mi:** Department of Biochemistry and Molecular Cell Biology, School of Medicine, Taipei Medical University, Taipei City 110, Taiwan; Graduate Institute of Medical Sciences, College of Medicine, Taipei Medical University, Taipei City 110, Taiwan.

**Fan-Yun Meng:** State Key Laboratory of Earth Surface Processes and Resources Ecology, Beijing Normal University, Haidian District, Beijing 100088, China; State Key Laboratory of Dao-di Herbs, China Academy of Chinese Medical Sciences, Beijing 100700, China.

**Karoline Rachel Teodosio Melo:** Department of Biochemistry, Biosciences Centre, Federal University of Rio Grande do Norte, Salgado Filho avenue 3000, Natal, RN 59078-970, Brazil.

**Sofia Mattsson:** Department of Pharmacology and Clinical Neuroscience, Division of Clinical Pharmacology, Umeå University, Umeå SE-90187, Sweden.

**Már Másson:** Faculty of Pharmaceutical Sciences, School of Health Sciences, University of Iceland, Hofsvallagata 53, IS-107 Reykjavík, Iceland.

**Masaaki Nagatsu:** Graduate School of Science and Technology, Shizuoka University, 3-5-1, Johoka-ku, Hamamatsu 432-8561, Japan.

**Ro-Dong Park:** Division of Applied Bioscience & Biotechnology, Institute of Environment-Friendly Agriculture (IEFA), College of Agricultural and Life Sciences, Chonnam National University, Gwangju 500-757, Korea

**Ok Kyu Park:** Division of Bio-imaging, Chuncheon Center, Korea Basic Science Institute, Gangwon-do 200-701, Korea.

**Kyeongsoon Park:** Division of Bio-imaging, Chuncheon Center, Korea Basic Science Institute, Gangwon-do 200-701, Korea.

**Nidal A. Qinna:** Department of Pharmacology and Biomedical Sciences, Faculty of Pharmacy and Medical Sciences, University of Petra, P.O. Box 96134, Amman 11196, Jordan.

**Xuemei Ren:** School of Environment and Chemical Engineering, North China Electric Power University, Beijing 102206, China.

**Syang-Peng Rwei:** Institute of Organic and Polymeric Materials, National Taipei University of Technology, 1, Sec. 3, Zhongxiao E. Rd., Taipei 10648, Taiwan.

**Jin-Kyu Rhee:** Western Seoul Center, Korea Basic Science Institute, Seoul 120-140, Korea.

**Hugo Alexandre Oliveira Rocha:** Department of Biochemistry, Biosciences Centre, Federal University of Rio Grande do Norte, Salgado Filho avenue 3000, Natal, RN 59078-970, Brazil.

**Marguerite Rinaudo:** Biomaterials Applications, 6 rue Lesdiguières, Grenoble 38000, France.

**Iyad Rashid:** Research and Innovation Center (RIC), The Jordanian Pharmaceutical Manufacturing Co., P.O. Box 94, Naor 11710, Jordan.

**Priyanka Sahariah:** Faculty of Pharmaceutical Sciences, School of Health Sciences, University of Iceland, Hofsvallagata 53, IS-107 Reykjavík, Iceland.

**Olafur E. Sigurjonsson:** The REModeL Lab, The Blood Bank, Landspitali University Hospital, Snorrabraut 60, 105 Reykjavik, Iceland;Institute of Biomedical and Neural Engineering, Reykjavik University, Menntavegur 1, 101 Reykjavik, Iceland.

**Fabien Salaün:** University of Lille Nord de France, F-59000 Lille, France; ENSAIT/GEMTEX, F-59100 Roubaix, France.

**Diego Araujo Sabry:** Department of Biochemistry, Biological Sciences Centre, Federal University of Parana, Coronel Francisco H. dos Santos avenue S/N, Curitiba, PR CP 19031, Brazil; Department of Biochemistry, Molecular Biology, Federal University of São Paulo, Três de Maio street 100, São Paulo, SP 04044-020, Brazil.

**Guilherme Lanzi Sassaki:** Department of Biochemistry, Biological Sciences Centre, Federal University of Parana, Coronel Francisco H. dos Santos avenue S/N, Curitiba, PR CP 19031, Brazil.

**Nataša Škalko-Basnet:** Drug Transport and Delivery Research Group, Department of Pharmacy, Faculty of Health Sciences, University of Tromsø The Arctic University of Norway, Tromsø 9037, Norway.

**Dadong Shao:** School of Environment and Chemical Engineering, North China Electric Power University, Beijing 102206, China.

**Ingunn Tho:** PharmaLuxLab Research Group, School of Pharmacy, Faculty of Mathematics and Natural Sciences, University of Oslo, 0316 Oslo, Norway.

**Xiaoli Tan:** School of Environment and Chemical Engineering, North China Electric Power University, Beijing 102206, China.

**Shao-Jung Wu:** Department of Chemical Engineering, Ming Chi University of Technology, New Taipei City 243, Taiwan.

**Qing-Xi Wu:** Integrated Biotechnology Laboratory, School of Life Science, Anhui University, Hefei 230601, China; Key Laboratory of Biomass Chemical Engineering of Ministry of Education, College of Chemical and Biological Engineering, Zhejiang University, Hangzhou 310027, China.

**San-Lang Wang:** Life Science Development Center, Tamkang University, No. 151, Yingchuan Rd., Tamsui, New Taipei City 25137, Taiwan; Department of Chemistry, Tamkang University, New Taipei City 25137, Taiwan.

**Xiangke Wang:** School of Environment and Chemical Engineering, North China Electric Power University, Beijing 102206, China; School for Radiological and Interdisciplinary Sciences, Soochow University, Suzhou 215123, China; Collaborative Innovation Center of Radiation Medicine of Jiangsu Higher Education Institutions, Suzhou 215123, China.

**Dae Hyeok Yang:** Institute of Cell & Tissue Engineering, College of Medicine, The Catholic University of Korea, Seoul 137-701, Korea.

**Shubin Yang:** School of Environment and Chemical Engineering, North China Electric Power University, Beijing 102206, China; Graduate School of Science and Technology, Shizuoka University, 3-5-1, Johoka-ku, Hamamatsu 432-8561, Japan.

**Shan-Jing Yao:** Key Laboratory of Biomass Chemical Engineering of Ministry of Education, College of Chemical and Biological Engineering, Zhejiang University, Hangzhou 310027, China; Collaborative Innovation Center of Chemical Science and Engineering (Tianjin), Tianjin 300072, China.

**Islem Younes:** Laboratory of Enzyme Engineering and Microbiology, University of Sfax, National School of Engineering, PO Box 1173-3038, Sfax, Tunisia.

**Jitao Yu:** Institute of Resources & Environment, Henan Polytechnic University, Jiaozuo 454000, China.

# About the Guest Editors

**David Harding** was born in London, England in 1944. After completing a B.Sc. (Honors) at the University of Canterbury, Christchurch, New Zealand in 1967, he took up a research position with the American drug company, Eli Lilly at their Erl Wood research center in Windlesham, Surrey, England. In 1969, he began a Ph.D. program at the University of Western Ontario, London, Ontario, Canada. On the completion of his PhD study in 1973, he returned to New Zealand to take up a position at Massey University, Palmerston North. His current title is Professor of Separation Science.

He is a synthetic organic chemist with over 100 publications and patents. He has associated interests in analytical chemistry. His association with cellulose in the 1990s led to a commercial product (MEP-cellulose), now sold by the Pall Company for the purification of antibodies using a technique he developed called HCIC (hydrophobic charge induction chromatography). The HCIC program led a special Massey University research award and still returns royalties to the University. His polysaccharide interests in natural polysaccharides have focused on chitosan from the late 1990s. Currently sodium alginate and hyaluronic acid also feature in his research programs. He is a member of the New Zealand Association of Scientists and a Fellow of the New Zealand Institute of Chemistry.

**Hitoshi Sashiwa** was born in Osaka, Japan, in 1963. He received his Ph.D. degree from Hokkaido University (Japan) under the supervision of Professor S. Tokura in 1991. He worked at Tottori University (Japan) as Assistant Associated Professor from 1988 to 2000. He worked with Professor R. Roy at the University of Ottawa (Canada) for two years (1998–2000). He worked at AIST Kansai (Japan) as a postdoctoral scholar during 2000–2004. He has been affiliated with Kaneka Co. Ltd. (Japan) since April 2004. His research interests include chemical modification of chitin and chitosan and their biomedical applications. He is a member of The Society of Polymer Science, Japan, and the Japanese Society for Chitin and Chitosan. He is the sole author of 70 publications and co-author of 30 publications.

# Preface

Recently, biomass-based polymers from renewable resources have received increasing focus owing to the depletion of petroleum resources. Natural polysaccharides such as cellulose, hemicellulose, and starch are among the candidates from natural resources for biomass polysaccharide products including bioplastics. Although several kinds of neutral or anionic polysaccharides such as chitin, alginic acid, hyaluronic acid, heparin, and chondroitin sulfate exist in nature, natural cationic polysaccharides are quite limited. Chitin is second only to cellulose as the most natural abundant polysaccharide in the world. Chitosan, the product from the $N$-deacetylatation of chitin, appears to be the only natural cationic polysaccharide. Therefore, chitin and chitosan due to their unique properties are expected to continue to offer a vast number of possible applications for not only chemical or industrial use, but also biomedicine. The research history on chitins, one of the most major and abundant natural polysaccharides on earth, started around 1970. Since the 1980s, chitin and chitosan research (including D-glucosamine, $N$-acetyl-D-glucosamine, and their oligomers) has progressed significantly over several stages in both fundamental research and industrial fields.

With the opening of this book, we planned to produce a strong, very exciting issue that will encompass breakthroughs in highly valuable, scientific, and industrial research in this field. This book covers recent trends in all aspects of basic and applied scientific research on chitin, chitosan and their derivatives.

Hitoshi Sashiwa and David Harding
*Guest Editors*

# Chapter I:
# Chemistry

# The Effect of Substituent, Degree of Acetylation and Positioning of the Cationic Charge on the Antibacterial Activity of Quaternary Chitosan Derivatives

Priyanka Sahariah, Vivek S. Gaware, Ramona Lieder, Sigríður Jónsdóttir, Martha Á. Hjálmarsdóttir, Olafur E. Sigurjonsson and Már Másson

**Abstract:** A series of water-soluble cationic chitosan derivatives were prepared by chemoselective functionalization at the amino group of five different parent chitosans having varying degrees of acetylation and molecular weight. The quaternary moieties were introduced at different alkyl spacer lengths from the polymer backbone (C-0, C-2 and C-6) with the aid of 3,6-di-*O-tert*-butyldimethylsilyl protection of the chitosan backbone, thus allowing full (100%) substitution of the free amino groups. All of the derivatives were characterized using $^1$H-NMR, $^1$H-$^1$H COSY and FT-IR spectroscopy, while molecular weight was determined by GPC. Antibacterial activity was investigated against Gram positive *S. aureus* and Gram negative *E. coli*. The relationship between structure and activity/toxicity was defined, considering the effect of the cationic group's structure and its distance from the polymer backbone, as well as the degree of acetylation within a molecular weight range of 7–23 kDa for the final compounds. The *N,N,N*-trimethyl chitosan with 100% quaternization showed the highest antibacterial activity with moderate cytotoxicity, while increasing the spacer length reduced the activity. Trimethylammoniumyl quaternary ammonium moieties contributed more to activity than 1-pyridiniumyl moieties. In general, no trend in the antibacterial activity of the compounds with increasing molecular weight or degree of acetylation up to 34% was observed.

Reprinted from *Mar. Drugs*. Cite as: Sahariah, P.; Gaware, V.S.; Lieder, R.; Jónsdóttir, S.; Hjálmarsdóttir, M.Á.; Sigurjonsson, O.E.; Másson, M. The Effect of Substituent, Degree of Acetylation and Positioning of the Cationic Charge on the Antibacterial Activity of Quaternary Chitosan Derivatives. *Mar. Drugs* **2014**, *12*, 4635-4658.

## 1. Introduction

Chitin is a structural polysaccharide that forms the basic constituent of the outer skeleton of insects and crustaceans, including shrimps and crabs. Chitin can be partially or fully deacetylated using strong alkali to give chitosan. Chitosan is therefore a heteropolysaccharide comprised of 2-amino-2-deoxy-D-glucopyranose (glucosamine) and *N*-acetyl glucosamine units linked through (1→4)-β-glycosidic bonds. A number of applications have been found for chitosan in the fields of pharmaceutics [1], biomedicine [2], cosmetics [3] and the food industry [4], due to its unique combination of various properties, like bioactivity, biocompatibility, biodegradability and lack of toxicity [5,6].

Amongst its various properties, the antimicrobial efficacy and applications of chitosan against bacteria have been the focus of many investigations. Chitosan has limited solubility in aqueous media above pH 6. It shows antibacterial properties only in acidic media. This activity is not observed at high pH, due to the absence of the positively charged amino groups and also due to low

4

solubility in aqueous media [7–9]. Chitosan derivatives, in which permanent positive charges were introduced onto the polymer backbone, have been synthesized, which led, in general, to good aqueous solubility and also contributed to significant antibacterial activity at neutral pH [10]. Previously, such derivatives have been prepared by quaternizing the amino group of native chitosan [11,12] or by introducing the quaternized group in one step through an acylation or alkylation reaction [13,14]. This leads to products that are heterogeneous with respect to the degree of substitution (DS) on the amino group and often partially O-modified [15]. Regioselective triphenylmethyl (trityl) protection of the primary (C-6) hydroxyl group of chitosan to give 6-O-trityl chitosan has also been utilized to facilitate the synthesis of N-chloroacyl [16,17], N-betaine [18] and quaternary piperazine derivatives of chitosan [19,20]. Although the use of such selective protection resulted in higher DS, this led to an increase in the number of synthetic steps, and some modification at unprotected hydroxyl groups can also be observed [21]. Recently, we reported on silyl protected 3,6-di-O-tert-butyldimethylsilylchitosan (diTBDMS-CS) [22,23], which has been utilized in various chemoselective modifications to give products like N-(bromoacetyl)-diTBDMS-chitosan, N-(2-(N,N,N-trialkylammoniumyl)-chitosan, N,N,N-trimethyl chitosan and chitosan derivatives modified by covalent linking of the highly lipophilic photosensitizer, meso-tetraphenylporphyrin [24,25]. The TBDMS-protected precursor enabled the synthesis to be carried out in an organic medium, thereby allowing well controlled and regioselective modification, leading to homogenous products that can be fully characterized by spectroscopy with techniques, such as ¹H-NMR, FT-IR, COSY and HSQC.

The role of the cationic charge in the antimicrobial effect is believed to be associated with the binding of the polymer to the bacterial cell wall. Several models have been proposed to explain the antimicrobial activity of chitosan, but the most accepted is electrostatic interaction between the positive charges on the polymer and the negatively charged anionic components of the bacterial surface, which weakens the cell wall and leads to cell lysis [26]. The polycationic structure of chitosan is a pre-requisite for antibacterial activity in spite of the structural differences in Gram positive and Gram negative bacteria [27]. Removal of the cell wall brings the polymer in contact with the cell membrane, thereby affecting membrane permeability and even reversing the surface charge of the bacteria [28]. These reactions finally lead to the leakage of the intracellular components, as evidenced by increased absorption at 260 nm [28], the increased electrical conductivity of the cell suspension [29] and cytoplasmic β-galactosidase release [30–33].

The structure-activity relationship (SAR) for chitosan and chitosan derivatives is not well understood. The relation between molecular weight (Mw) and degree of acetylation (DA) of chitosan to its antibacterial properties has also been explored. While high Mw and degree of quaternization (DQ) of N,N,N-trimethyl chitosan chloride (TMC) derivatives showed high bactericidal activity against both S. aureus and E. coli [34], in another study, it was reported that low Mw chitosan and its derivatives showed better activity [35,36]. A lower DA of acid-soluble chitosan was shown to lead to a greater inhibitory effect against S. aureus and E. coli [37–39], while some other studies have not shown a clear relationship between DA and the antimicrobial effect of unmodified chitosan [40,41].

In the current study, we used five different parent chitosan materials with variations in DA and Mw. These materials were used to synthesize different *N*-modified alkyl quaternary ammoniumyl and pyridiniumyl chitosan derivatives, such as (trimethylammoniumyl)acetyl, (trimethylammoniumyl)hexanoyl, (1-pyridiniumyl)acetyl, (1-pyridiniumyl)hexanoyl and *N,N,N*-trimethyl chitosan. These quaternary chitosan derivatives were then investigated for their antibacterial effects to allow systematic investigation of SAR under conditions where the effect of the functional group and the spacer length, as well as variations in the activity with the Mw and DA of the chitosan could be observed.

## 2. Results and Discussion

The quaternary ammoniumyl and 1-pyridiniumyl derivatives were synthesized from five different chitosan parent materials (denoted in superscript, e.g., **i–v**) (CS$^{i-v}$) varying in their DA from 6% to 34% and from 180 to 308 kDa in their Mw.

The quaternary groups were distanced from the polymer backbone with alkyl chain spacers. Each spacer length required a different approach to the synthesis; the discussion on the synthesized derivatives is therefore divided into four sections in accordance with the length of the alkyl chain (C-spacer) or its absence.

*2.1. Synthesis of N-(2-(N,N,N-Trimethylammoniumyl)acetyl)-chitosan Chloride (TMA-CS) and N-(2-(1-Pyridiniumyl)acetyl)-chitosan Chloride (PyA-CS), the C-2 Spacer Chitosan Derivatives*

The synthetic route to prepare the final TMA-CS (**6**$^{i-v}$) and PyA-CS (**8**$^{i-v}$) is shown in Scheme 1. Initially, all five different chitosan materials (**1**$^{i-v}$) were converted to their corresponding chitosan mesylate salts (Mes-CS) (**2**$^{i-v}$) by careful dropwise addition of methanesulfonic acid to the chitosan suspended in water at 10 °C. The finely powdered materials (**2**$^{i-v}$) were obtained by following our earlier reported protocol. Unlike chitosan starting materials (**1**$^{i-v}$), these mesylates, **2**$^{i-v}$, were completely soluble in H$_2$O, as well as in organic solvents, such as DMSO. The solubility of Mes-CS in DMSO was important, as it facilitated quantitative silyl protection of both hydroxyl groups on the CS under homogeneous conditions. Fully silyl-protected diTBDMS-CS (**3**$^{i-v}$) materials were then obtained by using tert-butyl-dimethylsilyl chloride (TBDMSCl) and imidazole in DMSO at 25 °C. The intermediate *N*-(bromoacetyl)-3,6-di-*O*-TBDMS-chitosan (BrA-diTBDMS-CS) (**4**$^{i-v}$) was prepared by reacting silyl chitosan **3**$^{i-v}$ with four equivalents of bromoacetyl bromide in the presence of five equivalents of triethylamine (Et$_3$N). The reaction temperature was carefully maintained at −20 °C throughout the reaction, and the reaction was quenched after 1 h to avoid any side reactions. The crude material was washed with acetonitrile (CH$_3$CN) to afford the fine powdered material, which was completely soluble in dichloromethane (CH$_2$Cl$_2$). Freshly prepared reactive intermediate **4**$^{i-v}$ was then reacted at 25 °C in CH$_2$Cl$_2$, with an excess of NMe$_3$ or pyridine to afford compounds **5**$^{i-v}$ and **7**$^{i-v}$, respectively. Compounds **5**$^{i-v}$ and **7**$^{i-v}$ were finally deprotected using concentrated (conc) HCl/MeOH to afford the corresponding final quaternized chitosan derivatives, **6**$^{i-v}$ and **8**$^{i-v}$, respectively (Scheme 1).

**Scheme 1.** Synthesis of final *N*-(2-(*N,N,N*-trimethylammoniumyl)acetyl)-chitosan chloride (TMA-CS) (**6**$^{i-v}$) and *N*-(2-(1-pyridiniumyl)acetyl)-chitosan chloride (PyA-CS)(**8**$^{i-v}$) derivatives. Reactions and conditions: (**a**) MeSO₃H/H₂O (1:1), 10 °C, 1 h (90%); (**b**) tert-butyl-dimethylsilyl chloride (TBDMSCl), imidazole, DMSO, 25 °C, 24 h (96%); (**c**) bromoacetyl bromide, Et₃N, CH₂Cl₂, −20 °C, 1 h (92%); (**d**) Me₃N (31%–35% wt in EtOH, 4.2 M), CH₂Cl₂, 25 °C, 12 h; (**e**) pyridine, 25 °C, 24 h; (**f**) conc HCl/MeOH, 25 °C, 24 h, ion exchanged by (8%) acqeos NaCl (w/v), 1 h, dialysed against de-ionised water, 48 h.

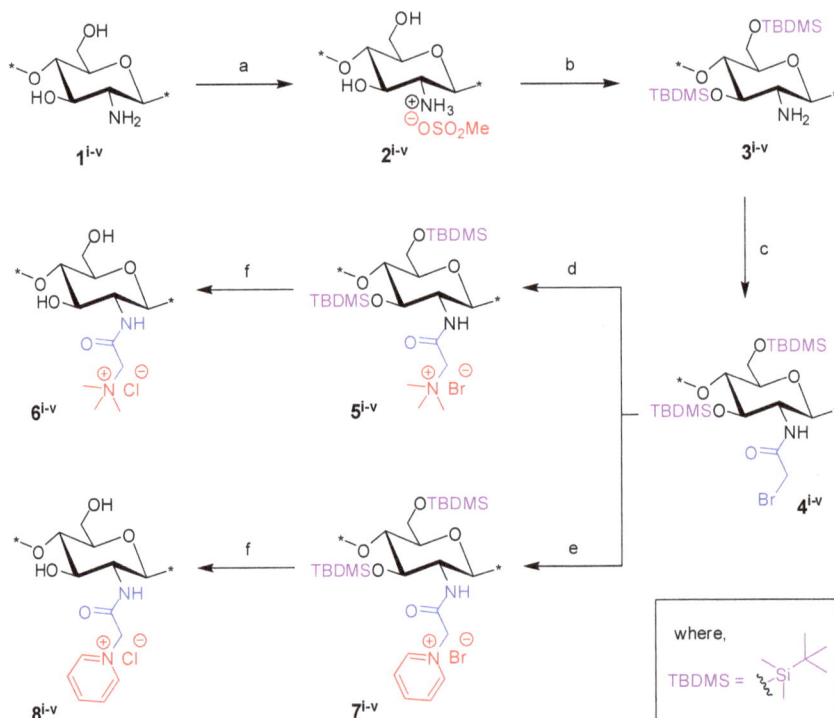

¹H NMR and FT-IR analysis. All of the key intermediates and final TMA-CS and PyA-CS derivatives were thoroughly characterized. The ¹H NMR (Figure 1) and FT-IR (Figure 2) overlay comparison of chitosan derivatives at different stages of synthesis confirmed the *N*-selective covalent modification with 100% substitution at the free amino groups. ¹H NMR and IR spectra of silyl chitosan (**3**$^i$) and the bromoacyl intermediate (**4**$^i$) showed complete silyl protection of both hydroxyls (C-3 and C-6). ¹H NMR (Figure 1B,C) and FT-IR of **4**$^i$ (Figure 2C) showed characteristic amide bond peaks (1676, 1527 cm$^{-1}$) with no sign of ester functionality, as expected for *N*-selective modification. Characteristic TBDMS peaks indicated by red arrows at 1259, 778 and 837 cm$^{-1}$ and C-H peaks at 2858–2956 cm$^{-1}$ remained intact. The final derivatives, TMA-CS (**6**$^i$) and PyA-CS (**8**$^i$), were completely soluble in D₂O (Figure 1D,E) after the removal of the TBDMS peaks, as seen by their absence in the NMR and FT-IR spectra (Figure 2D,E).

**Figure 1.** $^1$H NMR spectra overlay of the main compounds and final C-2 spacer quaternary derivatives of the representative chitosan material (CS-i, 7%_DA): **(A)** chitosan mesylate salts (Mes-CS), **2$^i$**; **(B)** diTBDMS-CS, **3$^i$**; **(C)** N-(bromoacetyl)-3,6-di-O-TBDMS-chitosan (BrA-diTBDMS-CS), **4$^i$**; **(D)** TMA-CS, **6$^i$**; **(E)** PyA-CS, **8$^i$**.

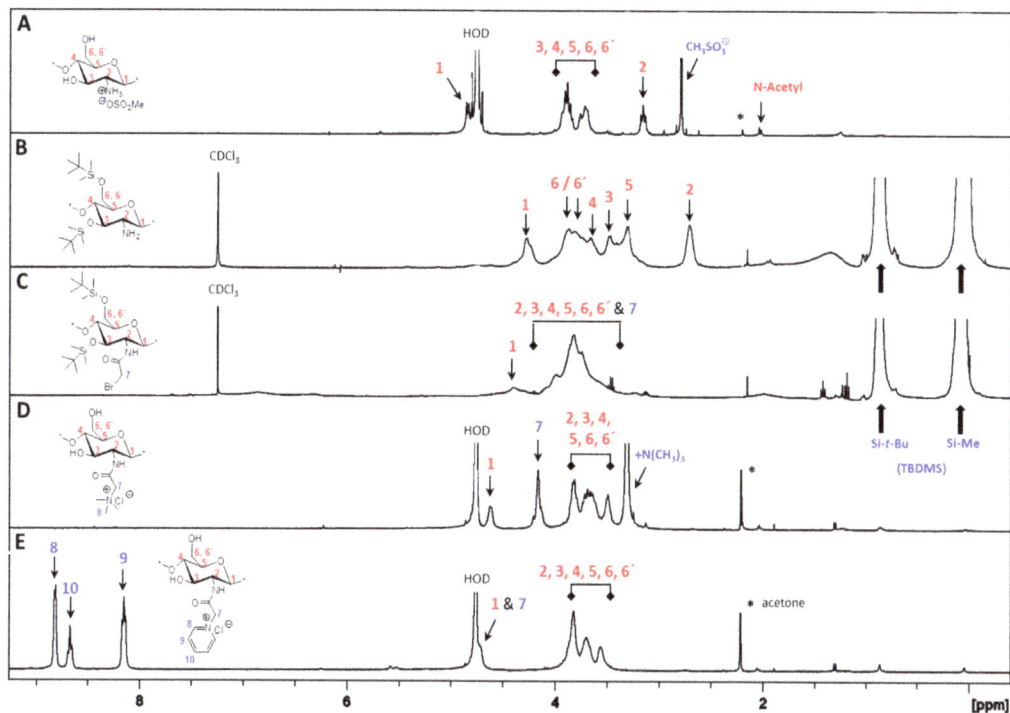

Synthesis of C-3 and C-5 spacer chitosan derivatives: An attempt to synthesize C-3 and C-5 spacer derivatives using 3-chloropropionyl chloride and 5-chlorovaleroyl chloride, respectively, under similar conditions did not succeed. This may be explained by the formation of stable four- or six-membered ring compounds by the intermediate (Figure 3), which will be favored according to Baldwin's rules for favorable ring closure of four-, five- or six-membered rings [42]. Stirling *et al.* (1960) have reported the mechanism of similar intramolecular cyclization of bromo-amides under basic or neutral conditions [43]. The cyclization was indicated in the $^1$H NMR spectra of the chloroacyl-intermediates, where the final deprotected material having the C-3 and C-5 spacer was not soluble in water, indicating that the desired quaternized product was not obtained. The FT-IR analysis (data not shown) of these materials also indicated ring fusion (Figure 3), similar to what was described by Stirling *et al.* [43].

**Figure 2.** FT-IR spectra overlay of the main compounds and final C-2 spacer quaternary derivatives of the representative chitosan material (CS-i, 7%_DA): (**A**) Mes-CS, **2**[i]; (**B**) diTBDMS-CS, **3**[i]; (**C**) BrA-diTBDMS-CS, **4**[i]; (**D**) TMA-CS, **6**[i]; (**E**) PyA-CS, **8**[i].

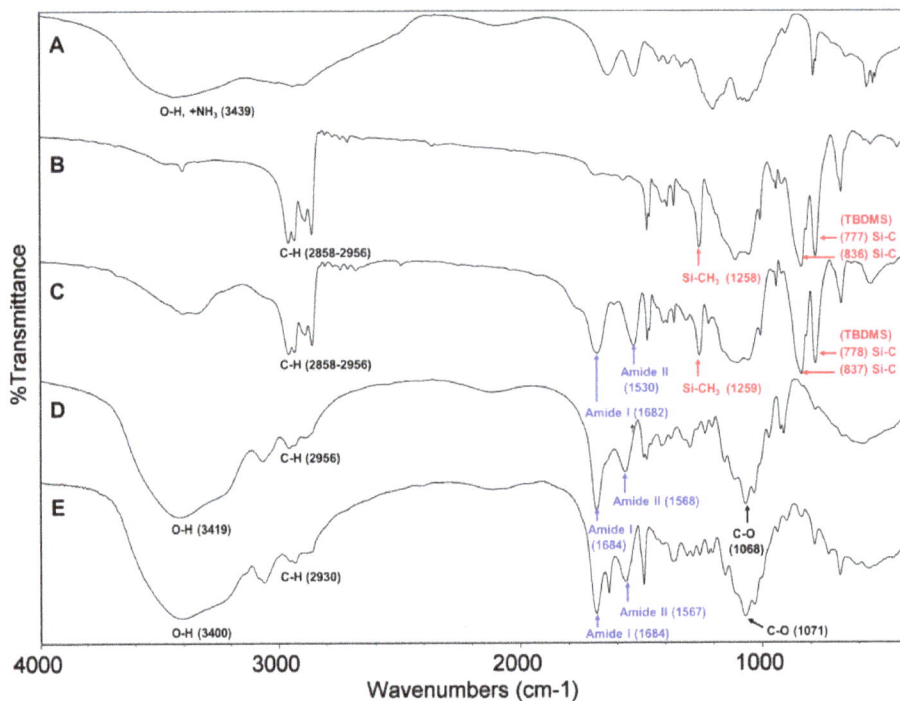

**Figure 3.** Possible intramolecular cyclization of C-3, C-4 and C-5 spacer compounds based on the findings of Stirling *et al.* [43].

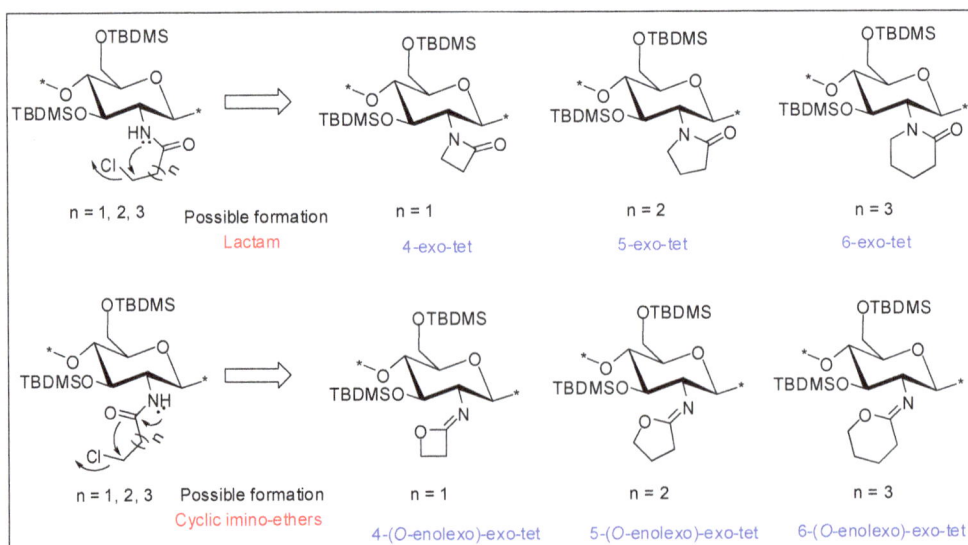

## 2.2. Synthesis of N-(6-(N,N,N-Trimethylammoniumyl)hexanoyl)-chitosan Chloride (TMHA-CS) and N-(6-(1-Pyridiniumyl)hexanoyl)-chitosan Chloride (PyHA-CS), C-6 Spacer Derivatives

The derivatives, *N*-(6-(*N*,*N*,*N*-trimethylammoniumyl)hexanoyl)-chitosan chloride (TMHA-CS) (**11$^{i-v}$**) and PyHA-CS (**13$^{i-v}$**), were synthesized (Scheme 2) under conditions similar to those used for the C-3 spacer compounds, with slight modifications. The key electrophilic intermediate, **9$^{i-v}$**, was prepared by reacting silyl chitosan **3$^{i-v}$** with four equivalents of 6-bromohexanoyl chloride in the presence of five equivalents of Et₃N at −20 °C for 1 h, under almost identical conditions as those described for similar key intermediates with the C-2 spacer, *i.e.*, **4$^{i-v}$**. Intermediate **9$^{i-v}$** was also completely soluble in CH₂Cl₂. However, unlike intermediate **4$^{i-v}$**, **9$^{i-v}$** was found to be more stable and, hence, need not be used immediately after its preparation. The intermediate **9$^{i-v}$** was confirmed by ¹H NMR and FT-IR analysis. Intermediate **9$^{i-v}$** when reacted with an excess of NMe₃ or pyridine, afforded the corresponding compounds **10$^{i-v}$** and **12$^{i-v}$**, respectively. However, the reaction with NMe₃ and/or pyridine appeared to be slower in case of the C-6 spacer as compared to the shorter spacer (C-2), and thus, potassium iodide (KI) was used as a catalyst to assist the reaction along with prolonged reaction time. Crude compounds **10$^{i-v}$** and/or **12$^{i-v}$** were then subjected to final deprotection with conc HCl/MeOH at 25 °C, and the materials were ion-exchanged using aqueous NaCl (5%–8%) (w/v), dialyzed and freeze dried to afford the corresponding final TMHA-CS (**11$^{i-v}$**) and PyHA-CS (**13$^{i-v}$**) derivatives, respectively. The trimethylammoniumyl derivatives solubilized faster in water compared to the pyridinium derivatives.

**Scheme 2.** Synthesis of final *N*-(6-(*N*,*N*,*N*-trimethylammoniumyl)hexanoyl)-chitosan chloride (TMHA-CS) (**11$^{i-v}$**) and PyHA-CS (**13$^{i-v}$**) derivatives. Reactions and conditions: (a) 6-bromohexanoyl chloride, Et₃N, CH₂Cl₂, −20 °C, 1 h (69%); (b) Me₃N (31%–35% wt in EtOH, 4.2 M), KI, CH₂Cl₂, 25 °C, 48 h; (c) pyridine, KI, 25 °C, 48 h; (d) conc HCl/MeOH, 25 °C, 24 h, ion exchange by (5%–8%) NaCl (aqueous) (w/v), 1 h, dialysed against de-ionised water, 48 h.

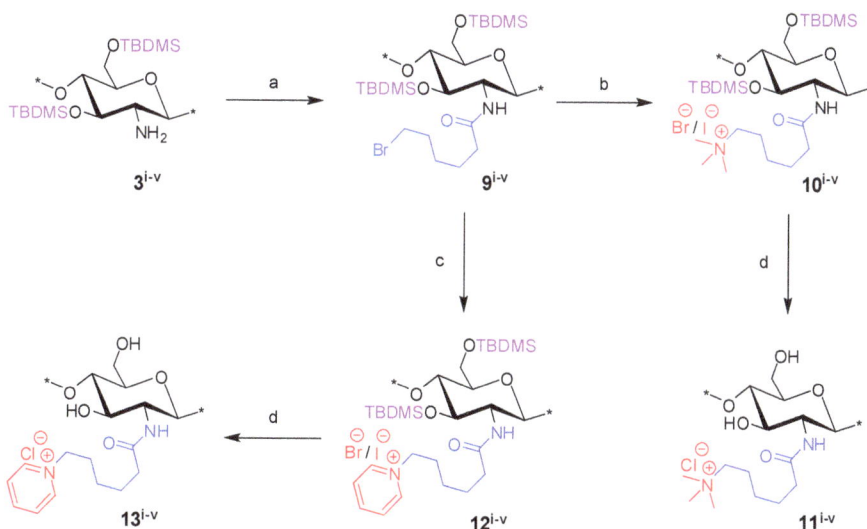

$^1$H NMR and FT-IR analysis: Synthesis of the C-6 spacer compounds was followed by $^1$H NMR (Figure 4) and FT-IR (Figure 5) analysis. In the $^1$H NMR of diTBDMS-CS (3$^{iv}$) in CDCl$_3$ (Figure 4B), the broadening of individual backbone peaks could be seen. This can be attributed to the increased viscosity of the material. The $^1$H NMR spectra of BrHA-diTBDMS-CS (9$^{iv}$) (Figure 4C) showed that the backbone peaks (H-1 to H-6′) appeared together while the CH$_2$ peaks of the alkyl chain, N-acetyl peak and TBDMS peaks could be assigned individually. Furthermore, FT-IR spectra of 3$^{iv}$ (Figure 5B) and 9$^{iv}$ (Figure 5C) confirmed the characteristic TBDMS peaks (shown in red arrows) and amide peaks (in blue arrows). The final C-6 spacer derivatives, TMHA-CS (11$^{iv}$) (Figure 4D) and PyHA-CS (13$^{iv}$) (Figure 4E) could also be confirmed by their individual distinct peaks. The spectra confirmed 100% substitution of the amino groups by either trimethylammoniumyl or 1-pyridiniumyl moieties. The IR spectra (Figure 5D,E) also confirmed the deprotection.

**Figure 4.** $^1$H NMR spectra overlay of the main compounds and final C-6 spacer quaternary derivatives of the representative chitosan material (CS-iv, 19%DA): **(A)** Mes-CS (**2$^{iv}$**); **(B)** diTBDMS-CS (**3$^{iv}$**); **(C)** BrHA-diTBDMS-CS (**9$^{iv}$**); **(D)** TMHA-CS (**11$^{iv}$**); **(E)** PyHA-CS (**13$^{iv}$**).

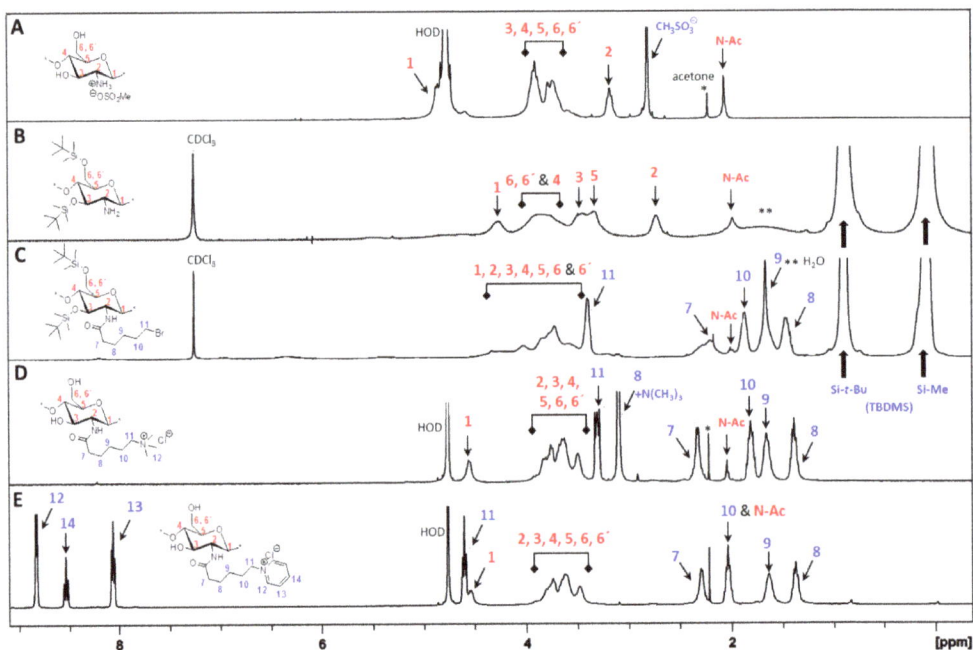

**Figure 5.** FT-IR overlay of the main compounds and final quaternary derivatives of the representative chitosan material (CS-iv, 19%_DA): (**A**) Mes-CS (**2$^{iv}$**); (**B**) diTBDMS-CS (**3$^{iv}$**); (**C**) BrHA-diTBDMS-CS (**9$^{iv}$**); (**D**) TMHA-CS (**11$^{iv}$**); (**E**) PyHA-CS (**13$^{iv}$**).

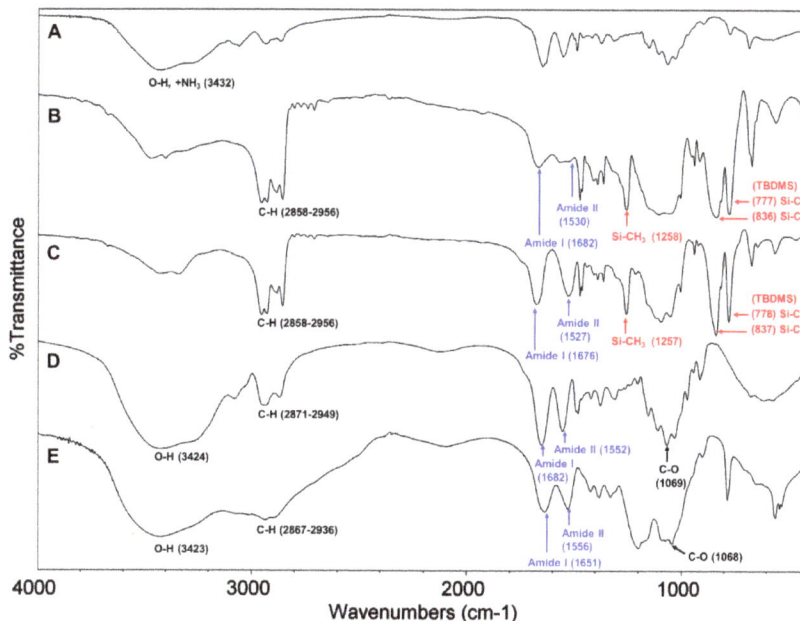

*2.3. Synthesis of C-0 Spacer TMC Derivatives (15$^{i-v}$)*

*N,N,N*-trimethyl-chitosan (TMC) was synthesized according to the procedure developed by Benediktsdottir *et al.* [25] as shown in Scheme 3. Briefly, diTBDMS-CS (**3$^{i-v}$**) was dispersed in *N*-methyl-2-pyrrolidone (NMP), and methylation was carried out using methyl iodide (CH$_3$I) in the presence of cesium carbonate (Cs$_2$CO$_3$) as a base. This method resulted in 100% trimethyl substitution at the amino group without any *O*-methylation. The excess CH$_3$I and NMP used in the reaction were removed by dialyzing the material against deionized water followed by freeze-drying. The *N,N,N*-trimethyl-diTBDMS-CS iodide (**14$^{i-iv}$**) was then subjected to deprotection of the silyl groups under 1M tetrabutyl ammonium fluoride (TBAF)/NMP solution. In cases where traces of the silyl groups still remained in the polymer, the deprotection was repeated under the same conditions. The products were then characterized using $^1$H-NMR, $^1$H-$^1$H COSY and IR spectra. The appearance of a new peak at 3.64 ppm in *N,N,N*-trimethyl-diTBDMS-CS indicated the trimethyl substitution in the polymer. However, due to the presence of the diTBDMS groups, the peaks were broadened and the exact DS was difficult to determine. Only after removal of the silyl groups did the polymer peaks became sharper, so the DS could be calculated from the integrals of H-1 (5.49 ppm) and the trimethyl (3.35 ppm) peak.

**Scheme 3.** Synthetic route for *N,N,N*-trimethyl chitosan chloride (TMC) derivatives (**15^(i-v)**). Reactions and conditions: (**a**) CH$_3$I, Cs$_2$CO$_3$, NMP, 45–50 °C; (**b**) TBAF (1 M), NMP, 50 °C.

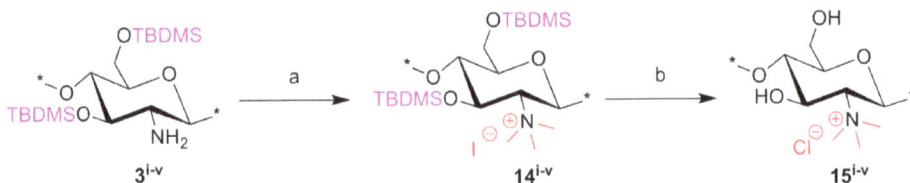

*2.4. Physicochemical Properties of Chitosan-Derivatives*

The DA was calculated by $^1$H NMR analysis of the parent chitosan materials. The weight average molecular weight (Mw) of parent chitosan materials, Mes-CS and the final quaternized derivatives of the chitosan were determined by gel permeation chromatography (GPC) (Table 1).

**Table 1.** Physical properties of chitosan derivatives.

| Parent Chitosan Material | DA (%) | Chitosan (1^(i-v)) | | Mes-CS (2^(i-v)) | | TMA-CS (6^(i-v)) | | PyA-CS (8^(i-v)) | | TMHA-CS (11^(i-v)) | | PyHA-CS (13^(i-v)) | | TMC (15^(i-v)) | |
|---|---|---|---|---|---|---|---|---|---|---|---|---|---|---|---|
| | | Mw | (PDI) | Mw | (PDI) | Mw | (PDI) | Mw | (PDI) | Mw | (PDI) | Mw | (PDI) | Mw | (PDI) |
| CS-i | 7 | 235 | (2.8) | 24.6 | (1.6) | 23.8 | (2.1) | 18.8 | (1.8) | 17.3 | (1.6) | 12.9 | (1.5) | 18.7 | (1.5) |
| CS-ii | 6 | 294 | (2.3) | 20.8 | (1.9) | 17.1 | (1.8) | 17.3 | (2.0) | 15.1 | (1.5) | 9.8 | (1.3) | 15.3 | (1.4) |
| CS-iii | 17.3 | 225 | (2.6) | 19.1 | (1.6) | 16.4 | (1.6) | 12.2 | (1.9) | 13.1 | (1.4) | - | - | 13.2 | (1.4) |
| CS-iv | 19 | 308 | (2.6) | 21.4 | (2.4) | 16.7 | (1.6) | 14.6 | (1.8) | 14.2 | (1.8) | 15.8 | (1.1) | 19.8 | (1.6) |
| CS-v | 34.2 | 180 | (2.9) | 19.5 | (1.5) | 18.9 | (1.7) | 10.8 | (1.4) | 7.4 | (1.4) | - | - | 16.5 | (1.5) |

The average molecular weight (Mw) is in kDa, and the polydispersity index is abbreviated as (PDI). DA = degree of acetylation.

Though the parent chitosan (CS-i to CS-v, **1^(i-v)**) has a higher range of Mw (180–308 kDa), significant degradation of the polymer chain was observed after their conversion to the corresponding mesylate salts (**2^(i-v)**) in all five materials, as this step requires highly acidic conditions, which are known to cause hydrolysis of glycosidic bonds in the polymer backbone [44]. Any further degradation after the first step was limited; so, although the Mw values were reduced, the relative range of Mw (7–23 kDa) for the derivatives was comparable to that of the starting chitosan materials.

*2.5. Antibacterial Properties*

The antibacterial activities of the quaternary chitosan derivatives were determined by measuring the minimum inhibitory concentration (MIC) and minimum lethal concentration (MLC) values against *S. aureus* and *E. coli*. The derivatives varied in their quaternary group, in the length of the spacer bearing the quaternary group, Mw and also in the DA of the chitosan. These parameters were used to observe the influence of the chitosan polymer on the antibacterial properties in order to develop an overall structure-activity relationship. The quaternary derivatives carrying positive charges were highly soluble in water, and hence, their activity could be tested at neutral pH. Table 2 shows that the chitosan derivatives exerted an antibacterial effect against both bacterial strains, with *S. aureus* yielding lower MIC and MLC values compared to *E. coli*. With respect to the variation in the functional group and the length of the spacer carrying the functional group, the following trend in activity was observed: TMC derivatives (**15$^i$–15$^v$**) exhibited the highest antibacterial effect against both strains, with MIC values ranging from 4 to 32 μg/mL against *S. aureus* and 64 to 256 μg/mL against *E. coli*, respectively. These results were consistent with earlier studies where TMC (DS = 0.86) was found to have a MIC of 8 μg/mL and 128 μg/mL against *S. aureus* and *E. coli*, respectively [45]. Thus, the degree of trimethylation does not seem to have a pronounced effect on antibacterial activity, as the DS increased from 0.86 to 0.95. The activity of the series of TMA-CS derivatives (**6$^i$–6$^v$**) was comparable to that of the TMC derivatives against *S. aureus*, but was much lower against *E. coli*. These derivatives showed similar activity as the previously synthesized TMA-CS derivatives (DS = 0.8; MIC = 128 and ≥8192 μg/mL against *S. aureus* and *E. coli*, respectively) [45]. The TMHA-CS derivatives (**11$^i$–11$^v$**) with a C-6 spacer had still lower activity against *S. aureus* (MIC = 1024–2048 μg/mL) compared to the other two series carrying the same quaternary group. However, their activity was found to be higher than that of the TMAC-CS derivatives against *E. coli* (MIC = 128–1024 μg/mL). Thus, in most cases, a decreasing effect on activity could be observed as the spacer between the trimethylammonium group and the polymer increased. The second functional group, *i.e.*, a pyridinium moiety attached to polymers having an acetyl (PyA-CS) or a C-6 spacer (PyHA-CS), also showed bactericidal activity against *S. aureus*; however, they were found to be less effective than their corresponding trimethylammonium derivatives. The acetyl pyridinium moiety exhibited MIC values of 512–1024 μg/mL against *S. aureus*, while the activity against *E. coli* was lower, with the MIC ranging from 128 to 16,384 μg/mL. The C-6 spacer derivative, as expected, showed still less activity than the acetyl pyridinium derivatives against both strains. They were active only against *S. aureus* (MIC = 2048–8192 μg/mL) while remaining almost inactive against the Gram negative *E. coli* within the range of concentrations measured. These results are in agreement with our previous investigations, where our results indicated that antimicrobial action was more efficient when the cationic charge is located at the amino group of the chitosan and not on the quaternary substituent [46].

The effect of the DA and Mw of the chitosan on its antibacterial properties was also investigated. Chitosan derivatives carrying a particular functional group varied in their molecular weight and degree of acetylation. Although the staring chitosan samples had Mw variations from 180 to 308 kDa, due to degradations during the synthesis process, all of the derivatives showed considerably less Mw (7–23 kDa), but the relative range in Mw was not reduced. However, no trend in activity of the derivatives with variation in Mw could be observed. Hence, the difference was mainly based on the DA variation. Earlier studies reported different conclusions regarding the dependency of the antimicrobial activity of chitosan on the DA and Mw. One study of the antibacterial activity of chitosan indicated that low molecular weight chitosan (4.1–5.6 kDa) showed a greater inhibitory effect when the DA, ranging from 0.45–0.52, was reduced to 0.17–0.19 [47]. Again, in another study, the antibacterial activity was found to be independent of variation in the Mw (2–224 kDa) of chitosan, but to decline with increasing DA from 0.16 to 0.48 [48]. Figure 6A,B shows the variation in antibacterial activity (log 1/MIC) of the quaternary derivatives with DA against *S. aureus* and *E. coli*. In contrast, as seen in Figure 6B, only Series **8** showed an apparent increase in antibacterial activity (7–10-fold) against *E. coli* as the DA values increased from 19% to 34.2%. However when the MLC values are considered (Table 2), there is only one dilution difference in this series. For the Series **15** and **6**, the activity seemed to decrease gradually, as the DA changed from 6%–34% with only a 2–3-fold decrease in activity. In contrast, the activity of Series **11** and **13** remained independent of variations in DA against *S. aureus*. In Figure 6B, it can be observed that the activities of the compounds differed by only 1–2 dilutions, and no clear variation in activity with increasing or decreasing DA was observed. Thus, the activity of the complete series against *E. coli* remained independent of variations in DA.

**Table 2.** Antibacterial activity, hemolytic activity and cytotoxicity of the quaternary chitosan derivatives.

| Compounds | Structure | *S. aureus* (ATCC 29213) | | *E. coli* (ATCC 25922) | | $HC_{50}$ | Selectivity ($HC_{50}$/MIC) | | $EC_{50}$ |
|---|---|---|---|---|---|---|---|---|---|
| | | MIC ($\mu$g/mL) | MLC ($\mu$g/mL) | MIC ($\mu$g/mL) | MLC ($\mu$g/mL) | ($\mu$g/mL) | *S. aureus* | *E. coli* | ($\mu$g/mL) |
| TMC (15$^i$) | | 8 | 64 | 256 | 256 | 6114 | 764 | 47.7 | 40 |
| TMC (15$^{ii}$) | | 32 | 32 | 64 | 64 | 6114 | 191 | 95.5 | - |
| TMC (15$^{iii}$) | | 4 | 4 | 64 | 64 | 6114 | 1528 | 95.5 | - |
| TMC (15$^{iv}$) | | 8 | 8 | 256 | 256 | 3072 | 764 | 47.7 | 10 |
| TMC (15$^{v}$) | | 32 | 32 | 256 | 1024 | 640 | 191 | - | - |
| TMA-CS (6$^i$) | | 8 | 8 | 16,384 | ≥32,768 | ≥32,768 | ≥4096 | ≥2 | 26 |
| TMA-CS (6$^{ii}$) | | 8 | 8 | 16,384 | 16,384 | ≥32,768 | ≥4096 | ≥2 | - |
| TMA-CS (6$^{iii}$) | | 32 | 32 | 16,384 | 16,384 | ≥32,768 | ≥1024 | ≥2 | - |
| TMA-CS (6$^{iv}$) | | 32 | 32 | ≥32,768 | ≥32,768 | ≥32,768 | ≥1024 | - | 66 |
| TMA-CS (6$^{v}$) | | 128 | 128 | ≥32,768 | ≥32,768 | ≥32,768 | ≥256 | - | - |
| PyA-CS (8$^i$) | | 8 | 1024 | 16,384 | 16,384 | ≥32,768 | ≥8192 | ≥2 | 38 |
| PyA-CS (8$^{ii}$) | | 8 | 512 | 8192 | 8192 | ≥32,768 | ≥8192 | ≥4 | - |
| PyA-CS (8$^{iii}$) | | 1024 | 1024 | 16,384 | 16,384 | ≥32,768 | ≥8 | ≥2 | - |
| PyA-CS (8$^{iv}$) | | 512 | 1024 | 16,384 | 16,384 | ≥32,768 | ≥16 | ≥2 | 12 |
| PyA-CS (8$^{v}$) | | 512 | 512 | 128 | 8192 | ≥32,768 | ≥64 | ≥256 | - |
| TMHA-CS (11$^i$) | | 1024 | 2048 | 256 | ≥32,768 | ≥32,768 | ≥32 | ≥128 | 644 |
| TMHA-CS (11$^{ii}$) | | 2048 | 2048 | 512 | 16,384 | ≥32,768 | ≥16 | ≥64 | - |
| TMHA-CS (11$^{iii}$) | | 1024 | 2048 | 128 | ≥32,768 | ≥32,768 | ≥4 | ≥256 | - |
| TMHA-CS (11$^{iv}$) | | 2048 | 4096 | 512 | ≥32,768 | ≥32,768 | ≥8 | ≥64 | 108 |
| TMHA-CS (11$^{v}$) | | 1024 | 4096 | 1024 | ≥32,768 | ≥32,768 | ≥32 | ≥32 | - |
| PyHA-CS (13$^i$) | | 4096 | 4096 | ≥32,768 | ≥32,768 | ≥32,768 | ≥8 | - | 4 |
| PyHA-CS (13$^{ii}$) | | 2048 | 2048 | ≥32,768 | ≥32,768 | ≥32,768 | ≥32 | - | - |
| PyHA-CS (13$^{iii}$) | | 8192 | 8192 | ≥32,768 | ≥32,768 | ≥32,768 | ≥4 | - | - |
| PyHA-CS (13$^{iv}$) | | 2048 | 2048 | 16,384 | 16,384 | ≥32,768 | ≥16 | ≥2 | 18 |
| PyHA-CS (13$^{v}$) | | 2048 | 2048 | ≥32,768 | ≥32,768 | ≥32,768 | ≥16 | - | - |

The antibacterial tests was done according the Clinical and Laboratory Standards Institute (CLSI) protocol (see Section 3.4.1). According to this procedure, a single dilution series was done for each compound, and gentamycin was used as a positive control. A difference of 1–2 dilutions is therefore not considered significant. The hemolysis measurements were also done in singlets for each concentration. The cytotoxicity measurements were carried out in triplicate, and the standard deviation varied from 10% to 22%.

**Figure 6.** Variation in the antibacterial activity of chitosan with different DA against (**A**) *S. aureus* and (**B**) *E. coli.*

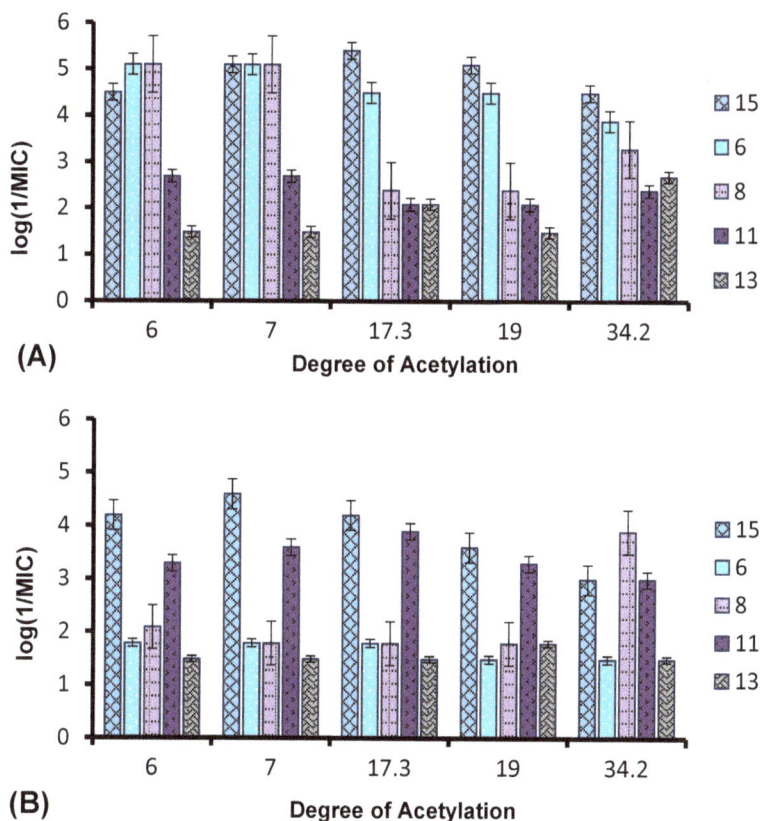

**(A)**

**(B)**

The error bars indicate a deviation equivalent to one dilution.

The screening of the quaternary compounds against the two strains of bacteria and their results led us to the conclusion that the antibacterial activity of the chitosan derivatives decreased as the distance of the positive charge from the polymer backbone increased. This was observed for the trimethylammonium, as well as the pyridinium functional group. Thus, the antibacterial activity of the chitosan polymer not only depended on the number of positive charges present in the polymer, but also on the positioning of the positive charge on the polymer backbone. It has been earlier observed that the activities of other antimicrobial polymers with a synthetic backbone were dependent on the spacer length due to changes in the charge density and conformation of the polymer, which, in turn, affects its interaction with the bacterial membrane [49]. A study of the interaction of chitosan with model membranes has also shown that the mode of action of chitosan is not only related to electrostatic interactions, but also to its specific conformation in solution [50]. This may explain why the TMC derivatives showed the highest activity. In this case the positive charge was located on the polymer backbone, which may be favorable for the conformation required for binding to the bacterial membrane. However, as the spacer length increases, the polymer probably will tend to adopt a

16

conformation that is less favorable for efficient binding with the anionic components of the bacterial membrane, and hence, the activity reduces. All of the quaternary chitosan derivatives showed greater activity, in general, against Gram positive *S. aureus* than Gram negative *E. coli*. This is in agreement with a previous observation where unmodified chitosan was shown to exhibit greater inhibitory effects against Gram positive bacteria as compared to Gram negative bacteria [51] due to differences in the cell wall structure [35]. In the case of Gram positive bacteria, the positive charges on chitosan were thought to bind to the thick peptidoglycan cell wall of the bacteria, resulting in cell wall disruption and leakage of the cellular contents. On the other hand, Gram negative bacteria possess an additional outer membrane composed of lipopolysaccharides, which provide the bacterium with a hydrophilic surface. The anionic units of the lipopolysaccharide form ionic type bonds with the cationic groups of the chitosan, which prevents nutrient flow and ultimately leads to the death of the cell due to depletion of nutrients [31,52]. Since the outer membrane serves as a penetration barrier against macromolecules and hydrophobic substances, overcoming the outer membrane barrier is a pre-requisite to displaying activity against Gram negative bacteria [29].

*2.6. Hemolytic Activity and Cytotoxicity*

To determine their toxicity, the compounds were tested for hemolytic activity against human red blood cells, and cytotoxicity was measured against the Caco-2 cell line. The antibacterial chitosan derivatives were not targeted for a specific organ, and hence, the compounds were evaluated only to get a general overview of potential toxicity. These compounds could be considered for surface treatments or as disinfectants and, therefore, were tested for hemolysis and the effect on a commonly used cell line (Caco-2) derived from mucosal epithelium. As seen in Table 2, the TMC derivatives (**15$^i$–15$^v$**), which showed the highest antibacterial activity, displayed low hemolytic activity ranging from 640 to 6114 µg/mL. The toxicity of the compounds against RBC decreased with decreasing DA of the derivatives within the series. However, no particular trend in HC$_{50}$ values with Mw variations could be observed for the TMC series. Light microscopic images of red blood cells (RBC) treated with different concentrations of one polymer (**15$^{iii}$**) are shown in Figure 7. Figure 7A shows a microscopic image of normal RBC suspended in TBS. When the RBCs were treated with different concentrations (512 µg/mL and 8,192 µg/mL) of the TMC derivative **15$^{iii}$**, no hemolytic effect was observed with the lower concentration (512 µg/mL), as seen in Figure 7B, while the higher concentration (8192 µg/mL) produced the deformation of cell shape, as seen in Figure 7C. In Figure 7D, 100% hemolysis was observed with the release of hemoglobin when the cells were treated with the positive control Triton-X100. TMA-CS and some of the PyA-CS derivatives that showed comparable antibacterial activity to that of TMC did not show any hemolytic activity. The compounds in the other two series with the C-6 spacer also remained non-hemolytic within the measured concentration range. Thus, the ability of the polymers to lyse RBCs diminished as the quaternary group moved away from the polymer backbone.

The cell line cytotoxicity results, on the other hand, differed from those for hemolysis. TMA-CS showed cell toxicity at lower concentrations (10–40 µg/mL) compared to hemolysis. Compounds containing the trimethylammonium group with a spacer, *i.e.*, the TMA-CS (**6$^i$–6$^v$**) and TMHA-CS derivatives (**11$^i$–11$^v$**), were less cytotoxic compared to the TMC derivatives, while compounds containing the pyridinium group, *i.e.*, PyA-CS (**8$^i$–8$^v$**) and PyHA-CS (**13$^i$–13$^v$**), displayed cytotoxicity values comparable to those of TMC derivatives. No trend in the cytotoxicity of the compounds with changes in the length of the spacer could be observed. However, for most of the compounds, within a series, the toxicity was found to be lower in cases having a lower DA. The cytotoxicity was also found to be related to the Mw of the derivatives. Compounds having a lower Mw value within a series were found to exhibit lower cytotoxicity values. In many studies, antibacterial potency and an agent's selectivity for bacteria over mammalian cells are quantified by determining the MIC and hemolytic activity (HC$_{50}$ values) [53]. In our study, we saw that, although the compounds displayed low hemolytic activity, their cellular toxicity was found to be significant. Thus, in order to get a full picture of their potential toxicity, only testing compounds against erythrocytes is not sufficient, and more in-depth studies of potentially toxic effects against various cell types *in vitro* or *in vivo* should be a requirement.

**Figure 7.** Light microscopic images of RBC. (**A**) RBC suspended in TBS; (**B**) RBC treated with Compound **15$^{iii}$** (512 μg/mL); (**C**) RBC treated with Compound **15$^{iii}$** (8192 μg/mL); and (**D**) RBC treated with 1% (v/v) Triton-X100.

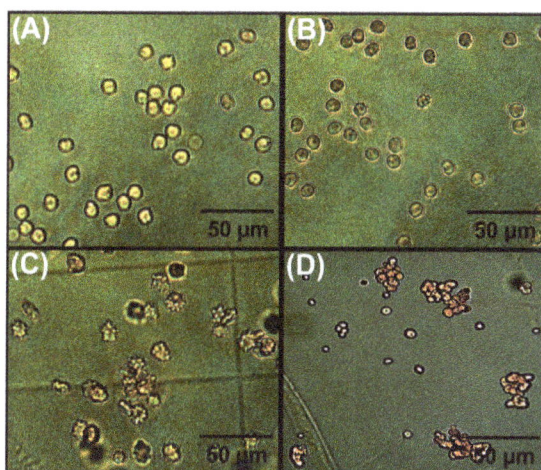

## 3. Experimental Section

### 3.1. Materials

Five different parent chitosan materials provided by Genis ehf (Reykjavik, Iceland): (i) (CS-i (G030626-2) (Mw = 235 kDa, PDI = 2.8, DA = 0.07)); (ii) (CS-ii (S030626-2) (Mw = 294 kDa, PDI = 2.3, DA = 0.06)); (iii) (CS-iii (TM1238) (Mw = 225 kDa, PDI = 2.6, DA = 0.17)); (iv) (CS-iv (TM1534) (Mw = 308 kDa, PDI = 2.6, DA = 0.19)); and (v) (CS-v (S040108-1) (Mw = 180 kDa, PDI = 2.9, DA = 0.34)) were used for synthesis. All chemicals (procured from Sigma-Aldrich®) were used as received, except solvents, like DMSO, CH$_2$Cl$_2$ and NMP, which were stored over molecular sieves before use. Dialysis membranes obtained from Spectrum® Laboratories Inc. (Breda, The Netherlands ,) (RC, Spectra/Por, Mw cutoff 3500 Da) and Float-A-Lyzers

(Spectra/Por, Mw cutoff 3.5–5 kDa, 5-mL sample volume) were used for the dialysis of the final quaternary chitosan derivatives.

## 3.2. Characterization and Calculations

$^1$H NMR, $^1$H-$^1$H COSY samples were recorded with a Bruker AVANCE 400 instrument (Bruker Biospin GmbH, Karlsruhe, Germany) operating at 400.13 MHz at 298 K. NMR samples were prepared in either CDCl$_3$ or D$_2$O in concentrations ranging from 10 to 15 mg/mL. Chemical shifts were reported relative to the deuterated NMR solvents: for CDCl$_3$ (7.26 ppm); whereas in the case of D$_2$O as a solvent, the acetone (2.22 ppm) peak was used as the internal reference. IR measurements were performed with an AVATAR 370 FT-IR instrument (Thermo Nicolet Corporation, Madison, WI, USA) with 32 scans and a resolution of 4 cm$^{-1}$. Samples were mixed thoroughly with KBr and then pressed into pellets with a Specac compressor (Specac Inc., Smyrna, GA, USA). Equivalent quantities of reagents were calculated on the basis of per glucosamine monomer unit. The degree of substitution for acetylation (DA) of CS-(**i–v**) was estimated by following Equation (1) using $^1$H NMR spectra of the corresponding parent chitosans (**1$^{i-v}$**).

$$DA = \left[\frac{\int H1}{\int H1 + 1/3 \int HAc}\right] \times 100 \tag{1}$$

## 3.3. Gel Permeation Chromatography (GPC)

GPC analysis was used for Mw determination of chitosan, chitosan mesylate and the final quaternary alkyl or acyl derivatives of chitosan. GPC measurements were performed using the Polymer Standards Service (PSS) GmbH, Mainz, Germany, WinGPCUnichromon Dionex HPLC system equipped with a series of three columns (Novema 10 μ guard (50 × 8 mm), Novema 10 μ 30 Å (150 × 8 mm) and Novema 10 μ 1000 Å (300 × 8 mm)) (PSS GmbH, Mainz, Germany) and PSS's ETA-2010 viscometer and Shodex RI-101 detectors (Shodex/Showa Denko Europe GmbH, Munich, Germany) using the Dionex Ultimate 3000 HPLC system (Thermo Scientific-Dionex Softron GmbH, Germering, Germany), Dionex Ultimate 3000 HPLC pump and Dionex Ultimate 3000 autosampler (Thermo Scientific-Dionex Softron GmbH, Germering, Germany). WINGPC Unity 7.4 software (PSS GmbH, Mainz, Germany) was used for data collection and processing. The eluent for the CS starting materials and all synthesized materials was 0.1 M NaCl + 0.1% TFA in Millipore water, and the standards used for the universal calibration curve were poly(2-vinylpyridine) (provided by the PSS-kit) (PSS GmbH, Mainz, Germany) with varying average molecular weight. All samples were dissolved in the same eluent as mentioned above, filtered through a 0.45-μL filter (Spartan 13/0.45 RC, Whatman GmBH, Dassel, Germany) before measurement, and the measurements were carried out at 25 °C using a flow rate of 1 mL/min and a 100 μL sample volume.

*3.4. Chemical Synthesis*

3.4.1. General Procedure for *N*-Quaternized-acetyl-chitosan Derivatives

Silyl chitosan $3^{i-v}$ was prepared from chitosan mesylate (Mes-CS) ($2^{i-v}$) using a previously reported procedure [22]. Silyl chitosan $3^{i-v}$ (2.6 mmol) was treated with Et$_3$N (13 mmol) and bromoacetyl bromide (10 mmol) in dry CH$_2$Cl$_2$ (15 mL) under N$_2$ atmosphere at $-20$ °C for 1 h. Concentration *in vacuo* followed by trituration with CH$_3$CN afforded *N*-(bromoacetyl)-3,6-di-*O*-TBDMS-chitosan (BrA-diTBDMS-CS) ($4^{i-v}$). Compound $4^{i-v}$ was then treated with excess of Me$_3$N or pyridine to afford *N*-(2-(*N*,*N*,*N*-trimethylammoniumyl)acetyl)-3,6-di-*O*-TBDMS-chitosan bromide ($5^{i-v}$) and *N*-(2-(*1*-pyridiniumyl)acetyl)-3,6-di-*O*-TBDMS-chitosan bromide ($7^{i-v}$), respectively.

3.4.2. General Procedure for *N*-Quaternized-hexanoyl-chitosan Derivatives

Silyl chitosan $3^{i-v}$ (1.3 mmol) was treated with Et$_3$N (6.5 mmol) and 6-bromohexanoyl chloride (5.2 mmol) in dry CH$_2$Cl$_2$ (15 mL) under N$_2$ atmosphere at $-20$ °C for 1 h. Concentration *in vacuo* followed by trituration with CH$_3$CN afforded *N*-(6-bromohexanoyl)-3,6-di-*O*-TBDMS-chitosan (BrHA-diTBDMS-CS) ($9^{i-v}$). Compound $9^{i-v}$ was then treated with an excess of either Me$_3$N or pyridine to afford *N*-(6-(*N*,*N*,*N*-trimethylammoniumyl)hexanoyl)-3,6-di-*O*-TBDMS-chitosan bromide/iodide ($10^{i-v}$) and *N*-(6-(*1*-pyridiniumyl)hexanoyl)-3,6-di-*O*-TBDMS-chitosan bromide/iodide ($12^{i-v}$), respectively.

3.4.3. General TBDMS Deprotection Procedure to Give the Final Quaternary Ammoniumyl and Pyridiniumyl Derivatives ($6^{i-v}$, $8^{i-v}$, $11^{i-v}$, $13^{i-v}$)

The compounds ($5^{i-v}$, $7^{i-v}$, $10^{i-v}$ or $12^{i-v}$) were stirred in MeOH (4–5 mL) and conc HCl (1–2 mL) for 12 h at 25 °C. Purification was done by dialysis followed by freeze-drying to afford the corresponding quaternized product ($6^{i-v}$, $8^{i-v}$, $11^{i-v}$ or $13^{i-v}$).

3.4.4. General Procedure for *N*-Quaternized-chitosan

Silyl chitosan $3^{i-v}$ (3.6 mmol) was treated with cesium carbonate (Cs$_2$CO$_3$) (14.2 mmol) and CH$_3$I (17.8 mmol) in dry NMP (20 mL) at 50 °C for 48 h. Precipitation in ice-cold water followed by filtration afforded *N*,*N*,*N*-trimethyl-3,6-di-*O*-TBDMS-chitosan iodide ($14^{i-v}$). Compound $14^{i-v}$ (3.30 mmol) was then deprotected by treatment with tetrabutyl ammonium fluoride (TBAF) (1 molar) solution in NMP (10 mL) at 50 °C for 48 h. Purification was done by dialysis followed by freeze-drying to afford *N*,*N*,*N*-trimethyl chitosan chloride (TMC) ($15^{i-v}$).

Note: details of all experimental procedures with assignments of $^1$H NMR spectra are available in the Supplementary Information.

*3.5. Biological Methods*

3.5.1. Bacterial Strains, Media and Culture Conditions

The antibacterial tests were assayed according to standard Clinical and Laboratory Standards Institute (CLSI) methods for antimicrobial dilution susceptibility tests [54]. Minimum inhibitory concentration (MIC) and minimum lethal concentration (MLC) values were measured against *Staphylococcus aureus* (*S. aureus*, ATCC 29213) and *Escherichia coli* (*E. coli*, ATCC 25922) obtained from the American Type Culture Collection, representing Gram positive and Gram negative bacteria that are susceptible to routinely measured antibiotics. The broth microdilution method was used to determine the MIC values using Mueller-Hinton Broth (Oxoid, Hampshire, UK) at pH 7.2 as the medium. Blood agar (heart infusion agar (Oxoid) with 5% (v/v) defibrinated horse blood) was used for the measurement of MLC. The samples were prepared by dissolving chitosan derivatives in sterile water to an initial concentration of 32,768 µg/mL. Fifty microliters of each sample were added to the first two wells on a micro-titer plate, and two-fold dilutions were done in 50 µL of Mueller-Hinton broth from well two on. This gave a final range varying from 16,384 µg/mL to 16 µg/mL, with the option of reporting 32,768 µg/mL as the highest concentration. Gentamicin was used as the positive control during the test. Bacterial solution of 0.5 McFarland suspension ($1–2 \times 10^8$ CFU/mL) was prepared by direct colony suspension in Mueller-Hinton broth and further diluted 100-fold so as to achieve a final test concentration of bacteria of approximately $1 \times 10^6$ CFU/mL (or $5 \times 10^5$ CFU/well in the microtiter plate). The microtiter plates were then incubated at 35 °C for 18 h under moistened conditions. The MIC value was defined as the lowest concentration of the antibacterial agent that completely inhibited visible growth of the microorganism in the microtiter plate. For MLC measurement, 10 µL × 2 of each of the dilutions that showed no visible growth were plated on a blood agar plate and incubated at 35 °C for 18 h. MLC was defined as the lowest concentration that achieved a 99.9% decrease in viable cells.

3.5.2. Hemolytic Activity

Hemolysis assays were performed according to previously published procedures [55,56] with slight modification. Human red blood cell concentrate having an RBC of $6.45 \times 10^{12}$/L, total hemoglobin of 201 g/L and WBC of $0.15 \times 10^9$/L was used for testing the hemolytic activity of the CS derivatives. RBCs (100 µL) were suspended in 10 mL of TBS (pH = 7.2). The polymer solutions were prepared in TBS at an initial concentration of 32,768 µg/mL and serially diluted 2-fold in a 96-well plate, so as to have a minimum concentration of 16 µg/ mL. One hundred microliters of RBC suspension were added to 100 µL of the polymer solutions and incubated at 37 °C with light shaking for 30 min. Cells treated with TBS and 1% Triton-X100 were used as negative and positive controls, respectively. The cell suspensions were centrifuged at 1500 rpm for 10 min, and the supernatant was collected to measure the absorbance of the released hemoglobin at 540 nm on a Thermo Scientific Multiscan Spectrum Photometer. The percentage hemolysis was calculated using the following equation:

$$\text{Hemolysis rate (\%)} = \frac{A - A_0}{(A_{100} - A_0)} \times 100\% \tag{2}$$

where A = absorbance of the polymer solutions, $A_0$ = absorbance of negative control and $A_{100}$ = absorbance of positive control.

## 3.5.3. Cytotoxicity

The cytotoxicity of the compounds were determined on the colorectal adenocarcinoma-derived cell line, Caco-2 (ATCC). Cells were grown in EMEM medium (ATCC) supplemented with L-glutamine, sodium pyruvate, 10% FBS (Invitrogen) and streptomycin/penicillin. Cells were grown until 80% confluent at 37 °C, in 5% $CO_2$ and then seeded at 1000 cells/well in a 96-well plate. After 48 h to allow for attachment and initial proliferation of the cells, the compounds were added at the specified concentrations in full culture media for 24 h. As a positive control, 1% Triton-X100 in PBS was used. After the incubation period, the cell culture medium containing the compounds was removed to prevent media color changes from influencing the spectroscopic measurements. Fresh cell culture medium was added and the cells were left to equilibrate for 30 min. Cytotoxicity was determined using the XTT assay (ATCC) following the manufacturer's instructions. The XTT reagent was incubated for 3 h at 37 °C in the dark before measuring optical density in a Multi Skan spectrometer (Thermo Scientific, Waltham, MA, USA) at 475 nm and 660 nm to account for non-specific absorbance. The compounds were tested in triplicate at each concentration, and the results in each case are presented as the half maximal effective concentration ($EC_{50}$).

## 4. Conclusions

There has been significant interest in the study of antimicrobial chitosan derivatives, as is evident from the many recent original publications [34,57–59] and reviews [27,60,61]. However, taken together, previous studies have not provided a clear picture of the structure-activity relationship. This is possibly due to a lack of uniformity in the products synthesized and also due to insufficient characterization. Reactions performed directly on chitosan are non-selective and usually give rise to heterogeneous products.

In the current study, we used a systematic approach to investigate how certain chemical characteristics can affect the biological activity of chitosan derivatives. The results were validated by synthesizing each type of derivative from five different starting materials. Reproducible synthesis is important for this kind of investigation and, in this case, the series of cationic chitosan derivatives was synthesized using a TBDMS protection strategy (diTBDMS-CS) under homogeneous conditions. This provided full substitution on free amino groups. Two functional groups, trimethylammonium and the pyridinium group, were successfully inserted into the polymer either directly or with the help of C-2 and C-6 spacers and could be well characterized by spectroscopic techniques. The MIC values for the compounds revealed that the inhibitory effect was higher against *S. aureus*, as compared to *E. coli*. The MLC values were at most one dilution higher than the MIC values for most of the compounds, showing that many of the compounds were bactericidal within the measured concentration range. Furthermore, the derivatives with trimethylammonium as the quaternary group showed higher activity than the derivatives with the pyridinium group. Amongst all of the derivatives, TMC showed the highest antibacterial activity with MIC values as low as 4 µg/mL. On the other hand, a descending order in activity could be observed with increasing spacer length in the compounds from C-2 to C-6. TMC displayed moderate hemolytic activity, which decreased with a decrease in DA values, while all of the other derivatives remained non-hemolytic within the measured concentration range. Hence, a decrease in activity against RBC was observed with increasing spacer length. A decrease in cytotoxicity with decreasing DA and increasing Mw was also observed in most cases, while no particular trend in cytotoxicity with changes in chain length could be derived. In spite of their cellular cytotoxicity, these highly active TMC, TMAC and PyAC derivatives should be considered as antibacterial agents for topical applications and disinfecting medical equipment. Thus, these results have increased our understanding of the effect of the positioning of the cationic charge, as well as the effects of DA, DS and Mw (for relatively low Mw chitosan derivatives) on the antibacterial properties of this class of agent.

## Acknowledgments

We thank the Icelandic Research Fund (Grant No. 120443023) and Nordforsk Public Private Partnership for financial support; and Genis ehf and Jon M. Einarsson for the generous donation of CS starting material and helpful advice.

## Author Contributions

MM and MH conceived the study, which was planned in collaboration with PS and VSG. The cytotoxicity studies and hemolytic assay were planned in collaboration with OES and RL. VSG synthesized and characterized compounds $1^{i-v}$ to $13^{i-v}$ (Schemes 1 and 2), and PS synthesized and characterized compounds $14^{i-v}$ and $15^{i-v}$ (in Scheme 3). VSG and PS contributed equally to this manuscript. PS and MH preformed the antibacterial study, and PS measured hemolytic activity. RL and OES performed the cytotoxicity studies. SJ did the $^1$H-NMR and $^1$H-$^1$H COSY spectroscopy. The first draft was written by PS, VSG and MM. All authors participated in interpreting the results and preparing the final version of the manuscript.

## Conflicts of Interest

The authors declare no conflict of interest.

## References

1. Xu, X.; Li, L.; Zhou, J.; Lu, S.; Yang, J.; Yin, X.; Ren, J. Preparation and characterization of *N*-succinyl-*N'*-octyl chitosan micelles as doxorubicin carriers for effective anti-tumor activity. *Colloids Surf. B Biointerfaces* **2007**, *55*, 222–228.
2. Sharon, S.; Katanchalee, M.-N. Chitosan based surfactant polymers designed to improve blood compatibility on biomaterials. *Colloids Surf. B Biointerfaces* **2005**, *42*, 147–155.
3. Jimtaisong, A.; Saewan, N. Utilization of carboxymethyl chitosan in cosmetics. *Int. J. Cosmet. Sci.* **2014**, *36*, 12–21.

4.  De Britto, D.; de Assis, O.B.G. Synthesis and mechanical properties of quaternary salts of chitosan-based films for food application. *Int. J. Biol. Macromol.* **2007**, *41*, 198–203.

5.  Rivero, S.G.M.; Garcia, M.A.; Pinotti, A.N. Biodegradable Film, Process for Its Preparation and Uses. Patent AR 80,876A1, 16 May 2012.

6.  Huang, D.; Huang, Y.; Xu, F.; Li, X.; Zhao, Y. Degradable Non-Toxic Seed Dressing Formulation Containing Chitosan, Polyvinyl Alcohol and Plant Extract, and Preparation Method Thereof. Patent CN 101,416,650A, 29 April 2009.

7.  Aiedeh, K.; Taha, M.O. Synthesis of iron-crosslinked chitosan succinate and iron-crosslinked hydroxamated chitosan succinate and their *in vitro* evaluation as potential matrix materials for oral theophylline sustained-release beads. *Eur. J. Pharm. Sci.* **2001**, *13*, 159–168.

8.  Sudarshan, N.R.; Hoover, D.G.; Knorr, D. Antibacterial action of chitosan. *Food Biotechnol.* **1992**, *6*, 257–272.

9.  Papineau, A.M.; Hoover, D.G.; Knorr, D.; Farkas, D.F. Antimicrobial effect of water-soluble chitosans with high hydrostatic pressure. *Food Biotechnol.* **1991**, *5*, 45–57.

10. Sonia, T.A.; Sharma, C.P. Chitosan and Its Derivatives for Drug Delivery Perspective. *Adv. Polym. Sci.* **2011**, *243*, 23–54.

11. Muzzarelli, R.A.A.; Tanfani, F. The *N*-permethylation of chitosan and the preparation of *N*-trimethyl chitosan iodide. *Carbohydr. Polym.* **1985**, *5*, 297–307.

12. Avadi, M.R.; Zohuriaan-Mehr, M.J.; Younessi, P.; Amini, M.; Tehrani, M.R.; Shafiee, A. Optimized synthesis and characterization of *N*-triethyl chitosan. *J. Bioact. Compat. Polym.* **2003**, *18*, 469–479.

13. Seong, H.-S.; Whang, H.S.; Ko, S.-W. Synthesis of a quaternary ammonium derivative of chito-oligosaccharide as antimicrobial agent for cellulosic fibers. *J. Appl. Polym. Sci.* **2000**, *76*, 2009–2015.

14. Xu, Y.; Du, Y.; Huang, R.; Gao, L. Preparation and modification of *N*-(2-hydroxyl) propyl-3-trimethyl ammonium chitosan chloride nanoparticle as a protein carrier. *Biomaterials* **2003**, *24*, 5015–5022.

15. Benediktsdóttir, B.E.; Baldursson, Ó.; Másson, M. Challenges in evaluation of chitosan and trimethylated chitosan (TMC) as mucosal permeation enhancers: From synthesis to *in vitro* application. *J. Control. Release* **2014**, *173*, 18–31.

16. Holappa, J.; Nevalainen, T.; Soininen, P.; Elomaa, M.; Safin, R.; Masson, M.; Jarvinen, T. *N*-chloroacyl-6-*O*-triphenylmethylchitosans: Useful intermediates for synthetic modifications of chitosan. *Biomacromolecules* **2005**, *6*, 858–863.

17. Holappa, J.; Nevalainen, T.; Soininen, P.; Masson, M.; Jarvinen, T. Synthesis of novel quaternary chitosan derivatives via *N*-chloroacyl-6-*O*-triphenylmethylchitosans. *Biomacromolecules* **2006**, *7*, 407–410.

18. Holappa, J.; Nevalainen, T.; Savolainen, J.; Soininen, P.; Elomaa, M.; Safin, R.; Suvanto, S.; Pakkanen, T.; Masson, M.; Loftsson, T.; *et al.* Synthesis and characterization of chitosan *N*-betainates having various degrees of substitution. *Macromolecules* **2004**, *37*, 2784–2789.

19. Holappa, J.; Nevalainen, T.; Safin, R.; Soininen, P.; Asplund, T.; Luttikhedde, T.; Masson, M.; Jarvinen, T. Novel water-soluble quaternary piperazine derivatives of chitosan: Synthesis and characterization. *Macromol. Biosci.* **2006**, *6*, 139–144.

20. Masson, M.; Holappa, J.; Hjalmarsdottir, M.; Runarsson, O.V.; Nevalainen, T.; Jarvinen, T. Antimicrobial activity of piperazine derivatives of chitosan. *Carbohydr. Polym.* **2008**, *74*, 566–571.

21. Rúnarsson, Ö.V.; Holappa, J.; Nevalainen, T.; Hjálmarsdóttir, M.; Järvinen, T.; Loftsson, T.; Einarsson, J.M.; Jónsdóttir, S.; Valdimarsdóttir, M.; Másson, M. Antibacterial activity of methylated chitosan and chitooligomer derivatives: Synthesis and structure activity relationships. *Eur. Polym. J.* **2007**, *43*, 2660–2671.

22. Song, W.L.; Gaware, V.S.; Runarsson, O.V.; Masson, M.; Mano, J.F. Functionalized superhydrophobic biomimetic chitosan-based films. *Carbohydr. Polym.* **2010**, *81*, 140–144.

23. Runarsson, O.V.; Malainer, C.; Holappa, J.; Sigurdsson, S.T.; Masson, M. tert-Butyldimethylsilyl O-protected chitosan and chitooligosaccharides: Useful precursors for N-modifications in common organic solvents. *Carbohydr. Res.* **2008**, *343*, 2576–2582.

24. Gaware, V.S.; Hakerud, M.; Leosson, K.; Jonsdottir, S.; Hogset, A.; Berg, K.; Masson, M. Tetraphenylporphyrin tethered chitosan based carriers for photochemical transfection. *J. Med. Chem.* **2013**, *56*, 807–819.

25. Benediktsdottir, B.E.; Gaware, V.S.; Runarsson, O.V.; Jonsdottir, S.; Jensen, K.J.; Masson, M. Synthesis of *N,N,N*-trimethyl chitosan homopolymer and highly substituted *N*-alkyl-*N,N*-dimethyl chitosan derivatives with the aid of di-tert-butyldimethylsilyl chitosan. *Carbohydr. Polym.* **2011**, *86*, 1451–1460.

26. Eaton, P.; Fernandes, J.C.; Pereira, E.; Pintado, M.E.; Xavier Malcata, F. Atomic force microscopy study of the antibacterial effects of chitosans on Escherichia coli and Staphylococcus aureus. *Ultramicroscopy* **2008**, *108*, 1128–1134.

27. Raafat, D.; Sahl, H.-G. Chitosan and its antimicrobial potential—A critical literature survey. *Microb. Biotechnol.* **2009**, *2*, 186–201.

28. Chen, C.Z.; Cooper, S.L. Interactions between dendrimer biocides and bacterial membranes. *Biomaterials* **2002**, *23*, 3359–3368.

29. Kong, M.; Chen, X.G.; Liu, C.S.; Liu, C.G.; Meng, X.H.; Yu, L.J. Antibacterial mechanism of chitosan microspheres in a solid dispersing system against *E. coli*. *Colloids Surf. B: Biointerfaces* **2008**, *65*, 197–202.

30. Je, J.-Y.; Kim, S.K. Antimicrobial action of novel chitin derivative. *Biochim. Biophys. Acta Gen. Subj.* **2006**, *1760*, 104–109.

31. Je, J.Y.; Kim, S.K. Chitosan Derivatives Killed Bacteria by Disrupting the Outer and Inner Membrane. *J. Agric. Food Chem.* **2006**, *54*, 6629–6633.

32. Liu, H.; Du, Y.; Wang, X.; Sun, L. Chitosan kills bacteria through cell membrane damage. *Int. J. Food Microbiol.* **2004**, *95*, 147–155.

33. Rurián-Henares, J.A.; Morales, F.J. Antimicrobial Activity of Melanoidins against Escherichia coli Is Mediated by a Membrane-Damage Mechanism. *J. Agric. Food Chem.* **2008**, *56*, 2357–2362.

34. Sajomsang, W.; Ruktanonchai, U.R.; Gonil, P.; Warin, C. Quaternization of *N*-(3-pyridylmethyl) chitosan derivatives: Effects of the degree of quaternization, molecular weight and ratio of *N*-methylpyridinium and *N,N,N*-trimethyl ammonium moieties on bactericidal activity. *Carbohydr. Polym.* **2010**, *82*, 1143–1152.

35. Jing, Y.J.; Hao, Y.J.; Qu, H.; Shan, Y.; Li, D.S.; Du, R.Q. Studies on the antibacterial activities and mechanisms of chitosan obtained from cuticles of housefly larvae. *Acta Biol. Hung.* **2007**, *58*, 75–86.

36. Tikhonov, V.E.; Stepnova, E.A.; Babak, V.G.; Yamskov, I.A.; Palma-Guerrero, J.; Jansson, H.-B.; Lopez-Llorca, L.V.; Salinas, J.; Gerasimenko, D.V.; Avdienko, I.D.; *et al.* Bactericidal and antifungal activities of a low molecular weight chitosan and its *N*-/2(3)-(dodec-2-enyl)succinoyl/-derivatives. *Carbohydr. Polym.* **2006**, *64*, 66–72.

37. Liu, N.; Chen, X.G.; Park, H.J.; Liu, C.G.; Liu, C.S.; Meng, X.H.; Yu, L.J. Effect of MW and concentration of chitosan on antibacterial activity of Escherichia coli. *Carbohydr. Polym.* **2006**, *64*, 60–65.

38. Takahashi, T.; Imai, M.; Suzuki, I.; Sawai, J. Growth inhibitory effect on bacteria of chitosan membranes regulated with deacetylation degree. *Biochem. Eng. J.* **2008**, *40*, 485–491.

39. Chung, Y.C.; Wang, H.L.; Chen, Y.M.; Li, S.L. Effect of abiotic factors on the antibacterial activity of chitosan against waterborne pathogens. *Bioresour. Technol.* **2003**, *88*, 179–184.

40. Park, P.J.; Je, J.Y.; Byun, H.G.; Moon, S.H.; Kim, S.-K. Antimicrobial activity of hetero-chitosans and their oligosaccharides with different molecular weights. *J. Microbiol. Biotechnol.* **2004**, *14*, 317–323.

41. Jung, E.J.; Youn, D.K.; Lee, S.H.; No, H.K.; Ha, J.G.; Prinyawiwatkul, W. Antibacterial activity of chitosans with different degrees of deacetylation and viscosities. *Int. J. Food Sci. Technol.* **2010**, *45*, 676–682.

42. Baldwin, J.E. Rules for ring closure. *J. Chem. Soc. Chem. Commun.* **1976**, *18*, 734–736; doi: 10.1039/C39760000734.

43. Stirling, C.J.M. Intramolecular reactions of amides. Part II. Cyclisation of amides of [small omega]-bromo-carboxylic, acids. *J. Chem. Soc. (Resumed)* **1960**, *49*, 255–262; doi:10.1039/JR9600000255.

44. Vårum, K.M.; Ottøy, M.H.; Smidsrød, O. Acid hydrolysis of chitosans. *Carbohydr. Polym.* **2001**, *46*, 89–98.

45. Runarsson, O.V.; Holappa, J.; Malainer, C.; Steinsson, H.; Hjalmarsdottir, M.; Nevalainen, T.; Masson, M. Antibacterial activity of N-quaternary chitosan derivatives: Synthesis, characterization and structure activity relationship (SAR) investigations. *Eur. Polym. J.* **2010**, *46*, 1251–1267.

46. Holappa, J.; Hjalmarsdottir, M.; Masson, M.; Runarsson, O.; Asplund, T.; Soininen, P.; Nevalainen, T.; Jarvinen, T. Antimicrobial activity of chitosan N-betainates. *Carbohydr. Polym.* **2006**, *65*, 114–118.

47. Vishu Kumar, A.B.; Varadaraj, M.C.; Lalitha, R.G.; Tharanathan, R.N. Low molecular weight chitosans: Preparation with the aid of papain and characterization. *Biochim. Biophys. Acta Gen. Subj.* **2004**, *1670*, 137–146.

48. Mellegård, H.; Strand, S.P.; Christensen, B.E.; Granum, P.E.; Hardy, S.P. Antibacterial activity of chemically defined chitosans: Influence of molecular weight, degree of acetylation and test organism. *Int. J. Food Microbiol.* **2011**, *148*, 48–54.

49. Kenawy, E.R.; Worley, S.D.; Broughton, R. The Chemistry and Applications of Antimicrobial Polymers: A State-of-the-Art Review. *Biomacromolecules* **2007**, *8*, 1359–1384.

50. Pavinatto, A.; Pavinatto, F.J.; Barros-Timmons, A.; Oliveira, O.N. Electrostatic Interactions Are Not Sufficient to Account for Chitosan Bioactivity. *ACS Appl. Mater. Interfaces* **2009**, *2*, 246–251.

51. Jeon, Y.J.; Park, P.J.; Kim, S.K. Antimicrobial effect of chitooligosaccharides produced by bioreactor. *Carbohydr. Polym.* **2001**, *44*, 71–76.

52. Helander, I.M.; Nurmiaho-Lassila, E.L.; Ahvenainen, R.; Rhoades, J.; Roller, S. Chitosan disrupts the barrier properties of the outer membrane of Gram-negative bacteria. *Int. J. Food Microbiol.* **2001**, *71*, 235–244.

53. Lienkamp, K.; Madkour, A.; Tew, G. Antibacterial Peptidomimetics: Polymeric Synthetic Mimics of Antimicrobial Peptides. In *Polymer Composites—Polyolefin Fractionation—Polymeric Peptidomimetics—Collagens*; Abe, A., Kausch, H.H., Möller, M., Pasch, H., Eds.; Springer: Berlin/Heidelberg, Germany, 2013; Volume 251, pp. 141–172.

54. CLSI. *Methods for Dilution Antimicrobial Susceptibility Tests for Bacteria That Grow Aerobically*, 8th ed.; Approved Standard. CLSI document M07-A8; Clinical Laboratory Standards Instiute: Wayne, PA, USA, 2009; Volume 29.

55. Ilker, M.F.; Nusslein, K.; Tew, G.N.; Coughlin, E.B. Tuning the hemolytic and antibacterial activities of amphiphilic polynorbornene derivatives. *J. Am. Chem. Soc.* **2004**, *126*, 15870–15875.

56. Zhou, C.; Qi, X.; Li, P.; Chen, W.N.; Mouad, L.; Chang, M.W.; Leong, S.S.; Chan-Park, M.B. High potency and broad-spectrum antimicrobial peptides synthesized via ring-opening polymerization of alpha-aminoacid-*N*-carboxyanhydrides. *Biomacromolecules* **2010**, *11*, 60–67.

57. Liang, Z.; Zhu, M.; Yang, Y.W.; Gao, H. Antimicrobial activities of polymeric quaternary ammonium salts from poly(glycidyl methacrylate)s. *Polym. Adv. Technol.* **2014**, *25*, 117–122.

58. Yalinca, Z.; Yilmaz, E.; Taneri, B.; Bullici, F.T. A comparative study on antibacterial activities of chitosan based products and their combinations with gentamicin against *S. epidermidis* and *E. coli. Polym. Bull.* **2013**, *70*, 3407–3423.

59. Mohamed, N.A.; Sabaa, M.W.; El-Ghandour, A.H.; Abdel-Aziz, M.M.; Abdel-Gawad, O.F. Quaternized N-substituted carboxymethyl chitosan derivatives as antimicrobial agents. *Int. J. Biol. Macromol.* **2013**, *60*, 156–164.

60. Kong, M.; Chen, X.G.; Xing, K.; Park, H.J. Antimicrobial properties of chitosan and mode of action: A state of the art review. *Int. J. Food Microbiol.* **2010**, *144*, 51–63.

61. Goy, R.C.; de Britto, D.; Assis, O.B.G. A review of the antimicrobial activity of chitosan. *Polímeros* **2009**, *19*, 241–247.

# Synthesis and Rheological Characterization of Water-Soluble Glycidyltrimethylammonium-Chitosan

Syang-Peng Rwei, Yu-Ming Chen, Wen-Yan Lin and Whe-Yi Chiang

**Abstract:** In this study, chitosan (CS) grafted by glycidyltrimethylammonium chloride (GTMAC) to form GTMAC-CS was synthesized, chemically identified, and rheologically characterized. The Maxwell Model can be applied to closely simulate the dynamic rheological performance of the chitosan and the GTMAC-CS solutions, revealing a single relaxation time pertains to both systems. The crossover point of G′ and G″ shifted toward lower frequencies as the CS concentration increased but remained almost constant frequencies as the GTMAC-CS concentration increased, indicating the solubility of GTMAC-CS in water is good enough to diminish influence from the interaction among polymer chains so as to ensure the relaxation time is independent of the concentration. A frequency–concentration superposition master curve of the CS and GTMAC-CS solutions was subsequently proposed and well fitted with the experimental results. Finally, the sol-gel transition of CS is 8.5 weight % (wt %), while that of GTMAC-CS is 20 wt %, reconfirming the excellent water solubility of the latter.

Reprinted from *Mar. Drugs*. Cite as: Rwei, S.-P.; Chen, Y.-M.; Lin, W.-Y.; Chiang, W.-Y. Synthesis and Rheological Characterization of Water-Soluble Glycidyltrimethylammonium-Chitosan. *Mar. Drugs* **2014**, *12*, 5547-5562.

## 1. Introduction

Chitin, as the only source of chitosan (CS) and their derivatives, is the second-most abundant natural polymer next to cellulose. Chitin, as a universal template for biomineralized skeletal structures in a broad variety of invertebrates [1], is industrially produced mostly from seashell materials. Chitin has been seen as one of the most important resources from marine natural products to be applied in bio-related fields. However, it is hard to dissolve in any kind of solvent due to high crystallinity. Chitosan, a deacetylation form of chitin, can dissolve in a low pH solution to form a gel owing to the free amine group easily interacting with acid. CS is therefore firstly used in the field of wastewater treatment. Moreover, CS possesses antimicrobial and biocompatible characteristics which underlie its primary use in medicine, including wound dressing and some other medical related areas [2,3]. For example, chitosan has played a leading role in advanced biomaterial applications, including non-viral vectors for DNA-gene and drug delivery because it is non-toxic, stable, biodegradable, and easily sterilized [4,5]. However, CS is not soluble in pure water that limits the use in some daily life areas such as the cosmetic industry and food industry [6,7]. Accordingly, the solubility of CS in pure water must be improved and such an issue has drawn great attention to many scholars [8,9].

Rwei *et al.* have modified chitosan with "1, 3-propane sultone" to produce a novel sulfonated chitosan (SCS) which has great water-solubility [10]. However, the reacting monomer 1, 3-propane sultone is known as a potent human carcinogen [11]. To remove the unreacted sultone, performing a complete reaction followed by additional purification thus becomes crucial and costly for the SCS preparation. In this study, another water-soluble CS-related compound, GTMAC-CS, of which CS is modified by glycidyltrimethylammonium chloride (GTMAC) in order to gain good aqueous solubility, was prepared.

GTMAC is known to be a widely used chemical for starch modification in food and paper industries. Low-substituted cationic starch is commonly prepared by reacting starch with GTMAC [12]. Regarding its medical application, Giammona [13] has been reported to successfully react poly(asparthylhydrazide) (PAHy) with GTMAC for application in the systemic gene delivery. The biocompatibility of PAHy-GTA derivatives with different degrees of positive charge substitution were found to be neither haemolytic nor cytotoxicity. Moreover, Xiao *et al.* [14] and Lim *et al.* [15] have demonstrated the synthesization of chitosan with GTMAC to form 2-hydroxyl-propyl-3-trimethylammonium chitosan chloride, abbreviated as HTCC in their work and denoted as GTMAC-CS herein, for better water solubility and application as a drug delivery carrier. The GTMAC-CS has been reported thereafter to successfully load Parathyroid Hormone-Related Protein 1–34 [16], BSA [17], and insulin [18]. *In vitro* study showed the protein/GTMAC-CS/TPP nanoparticles demonstrate an initial burst then a slow and continuous release [19].

The synthesized compounds of GTMAC-CS in this work were chemically identified by FTIR and NMR. The viscoelastic characterization of GTMAC-CS under various concentrations at a wide range of frequencies (0.01 to 100 Hz) was performed. The frequency–concentration superposition relationship was built and the sol-gel transition was then investigated. It is our goal to understand the rheological properties of GTMAC-CS aqueous solutions from a dilute state to a gel state and to explore the feasibility of applying it to daily life.

## 2. Experimental Method

Chitosan used in this study was obtained from VA7G Bioscience (Taipei, Taiwan). It possessed a molecular weight (Mn, number average) of about $5 \times 10^4$ and had a deacetylation degree (DD) of 90%. A regular CS solution was prepared using deionized water with 5 wt % of acetic acid as a solvent. The acetic acid used herein was purchased from Acros (Pittsburgh, PA, USA) and was used as received.

The GTMAC-CS was prepared by reacting chitosan with glycidyltrimethylammonium chloride (GTMAC). Five grams of chitosan was completely dissolved in 191 mL of deionized water to which 2 wt % acetic acid was added. In total, 27.6 mL of GTMAC was then injected into the CS solution under a nitrogen environment [11,20]. The reaction proceeded at 50 °C for 18 h. After the reaction, the reacted solution was poured into cold acetone, causing the precipitation of product. The crude solid was washed using methanol to remove the excess glycidyltrimethylammonium chloride. After drying for 6 h in a vacuum oven, the GTMAC-CS was obtained as a white powder at a yield of approximately 80% (Scheme 1).

**Scheme 1.** Synthesis procedure of Glycidyltrimethylammonium-chitosan (GTMAC-CS).

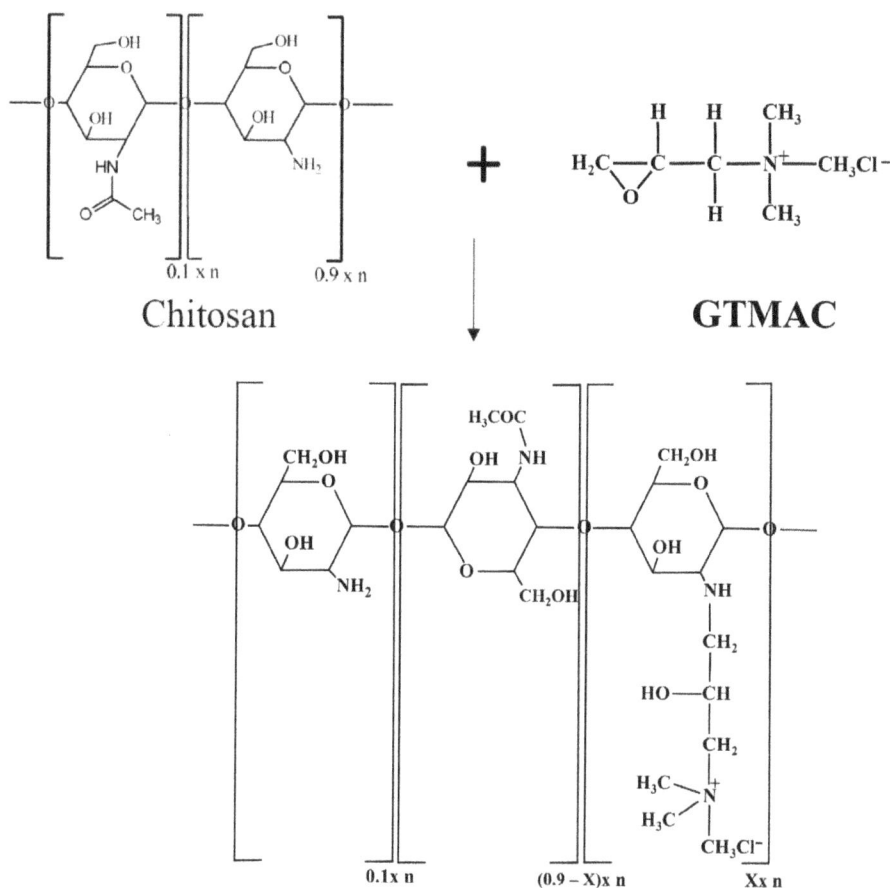

Infrared spectra were performed on the PerkinElmer Spectrum 100 (PerkinElmer, Waltham, MA, USA). $^1$H NMR spectra were measured using a Bruker Avanceat 500 MHz (Bruker, Santa Barbara, CA, USA). D₂O was used as a solvent. GPC analyses were carried out using a GPC/V2000 from Waters Co. (Waters, Milford, MA, USA) and AcOH (Acetic acid) was selected as an eluent. The steady viscosity was measured for pure solvent and polymer solution by the rheometer of Brookfield DV-III (Brookfield, Middleboro, MA, USA) plus to obtain the specific viscosity. Dynamic rheology was examined using a strain-controlled rheometer, Vilastic (Vilastic Scientific, Austin, TX, USA), which produced an oscillatory flow using a vibratile membrane, and detected the instantaneous pressure variation as a stress-response. The samples were examined under dynamic shear of constant but low amplitude within the linear viscoelastic range. The frequency was swept over the range $10^{-2}$ Hz $< \omega < 10^2$ Hz, the real part and the imaginary part of the shear moduli, representing the storage modulus G′ and loss modulus G″, respectively, were obtained. A detailed description of the instrument and measurement can be found in the authors' other work [10,21,22].

## 3. Results and Discussion

The FT-IR spectrum to verify the GTMAC-CS synthesis was shown in Figure 1. The spectrum included strong adsorption at 1607 cm$^{-1}$, corresponding to the C-N-C bending vibration of the GTMAC-CS branch. The C = O stretching vibration of the amide group from the chitin segment, occurring at 1731 cm$^{-1}$, can be considered as an invariant peak which should be the same for both CS and GTMAC-CS polymers. The adsorption centered at 2938 cm$^{-1}$ was attributed to the C-H stretching vibration of the CH$_2$ or CH$_3$ groups. Finally, a broad peak centered at 3317 cm$^{-1}$ represented the combined O-H stretching vibration and N-H stretching vibration.

**Figure 1.** The IR spectra of CS and GTMAC-CS.

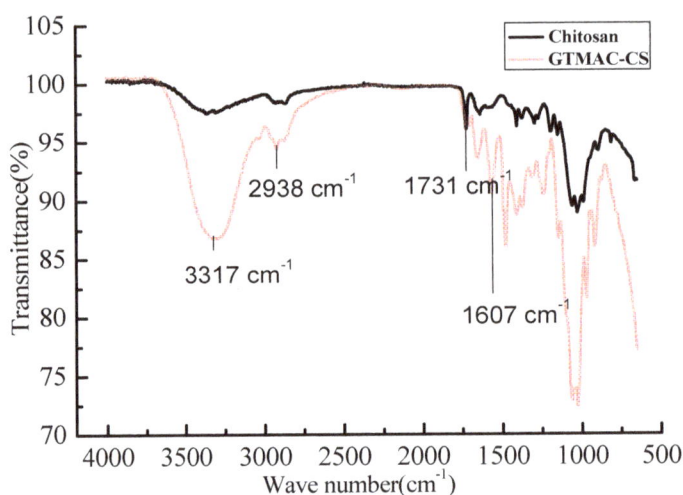

To further identify the synthesized product of GTMAC-CS, the $^1$H NMR spectrum was performed and IS shown in Figure 2. From the obtained NMR spectrum, peaks at $\delta$ = 2.02–2.24 ppm (a), $\delta$ = 3.71 ppm (c), and $\delta$ = 3.98 ppm (d) were assigned to -COCH$_3$ (from chitin), -N-CH-, and -NH, respectively. Notably, peaks at $\delta$ = 3.41 ppm (b) and $\delta$ = 4.42 ppm (e) were found only for the GTMAC-CS, which represent the existence of the groups of N(CH$_3$)$_3$ and -N-CH$_2$-, respectively. Based on the result of NMR analyses shown in Figure 2, the ratio of grafted segments, X, to the total segments of GTMAC-CS is approximately 63 mole %.

**Figure 2.** The $^1$H NMR spectra of GTMAC-CS. N(CH$_3$)$_3$ area/total area = 14.608/51.648 = 9X/(13 * 0.1 + 11 * (0.9 − X) + 25X); X = 63%.

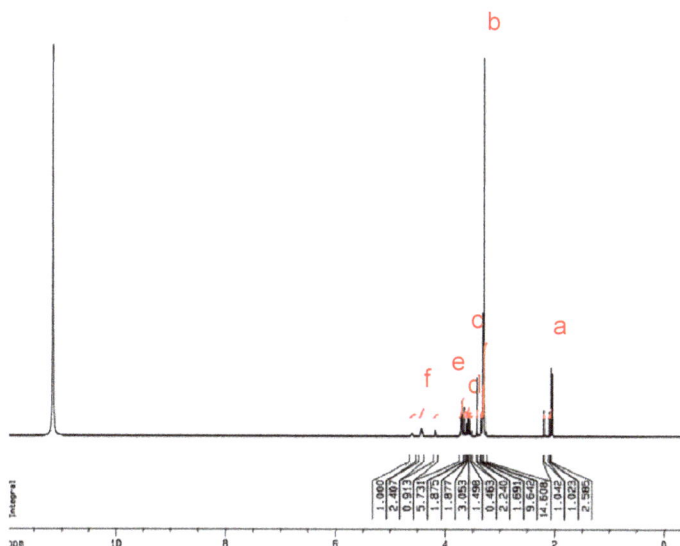

Figure 3a,b show the complex viscosity as a function of oscillation frequency at different concentrations for CS and GTMAC-CS, respectively. The complex viscosities of both solutions increase with the polymer concentration as usual. Moreover, all the viscosity curves display two regions, a Newtonian plateau region followed by a shear thinning region. The Newtonian behavior indicates that little deformation by the shearing on the chain conformation was created, while the shear thinning phenomena suggests that the chain deformation induced by the stress is too strong to be relaxed and the chain orientation along the flow direction may occur. The inverse of the turning point between the two regions, therefore, can be treated as the relaxation time, λ, representing the longest period of polymer-chains to recover to its original conformation under shearing. A distinguished difference between Figure 3a,b was that the turning points of CS solutions shift to the low frequency region as the concentration increases while those of GTMAC-CS solutions remained the same. In general, a given shearing stress would generate greater torque for a linear polymer with a higher molecular weight, which would thus orientate the polymer easier to yield a turning point at the lower-frequency region. In a highly concentrated environment, the CS polymers might be entangled together to have a bigger conformation and exhibit longer relaxation time. However, good water solubility of GTMAC-CS would cause some lubrication effect to prevent the entanglement. The inverse of the turning point, namely, the relaxation time, therefore was independent of the concentration.

**Figure 3.** Complex viscosity as function of frequency for (**a**) CS; (**b**) GTMAC-CS solutions at different concentrations (1 wt %~3 wt %).

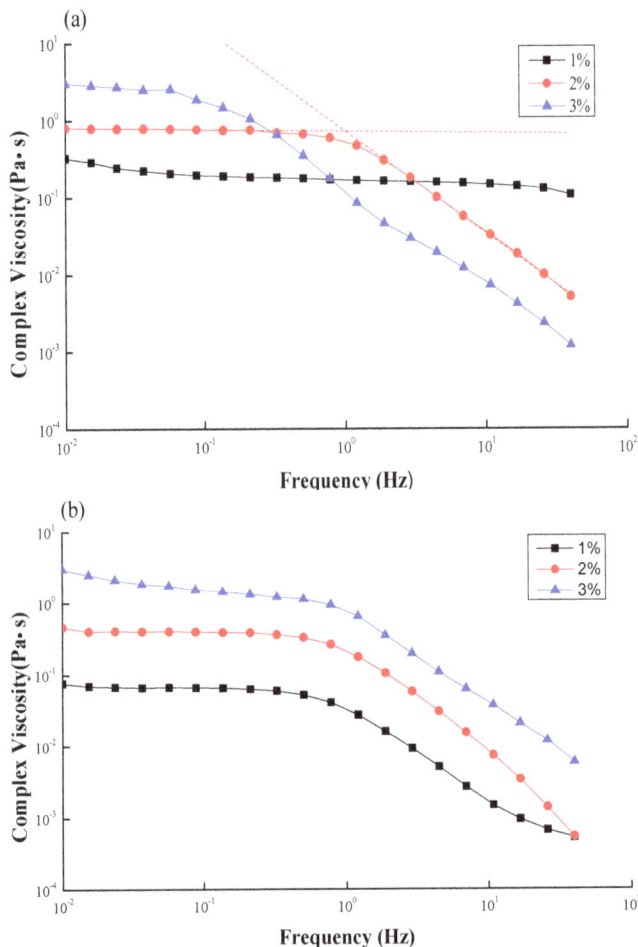

Figure 4a,b depict the plots of specific viscosity against polymer concentration in a log scale; a critical concentration point, Ce, can be found at 1.7 wt % and 3.8 wt % for CS (Figure 4a) and GTMAC-CS (Figure 4b), respectively. Moreover, the slopes at the concentration range lower and higher than Ce are 1.1 and 4.2, respectively, for CS (Figure 4a) and 0.9 and 1.2, respectively, for GTMAC-CS (Figure 4b). Increasing polymer concentration enhances the interaction among the polymer chains. If the polymer concentration exceeds a threshold value, usually symbolized as Ce, the response of the polymer to the oscillation is no longer merely affected by the individual molecular size of dissolved polymer; it will also depend on the chain–chain interactions in the conformation-overlapped zone, usually called "chain-entanglement" among polymers. When the polymer concentration is increased from a dilute to a concentrated condition over such a critical threshold, Ce, the individual chains have chances to be in contact with each other. Further increasing the polymer concentration (C > Ce), the crowded molecular chains would be entangled and act as if they were in a molten state. For random-coil polymer solutions, the dependence of specific viscosity at zero shear rate on the concentration C therefore yields an increasing trend with concentration, *i.e.*, from a linear to an exponential dependence. The exponent of C usually equals to 1 for C < Ce and 3~5 for C > Ce. The viscosity data presented in Figure 4a,b show a regular behavior of random-coil polymer solutions [23–26]. Interestingly, Figure 4a,b exhibit CS has lower Ce and higher exponent values at the concentrated region than GTMAC-CS does, indicating the solubility of GTMAC-CS in pure water is much better than that of CS in an aqueous solution mixed with 5% acetic acid. Good water solubility can prevent GTMAC-CS from entanglement because water molecules persistently attaching to polymer chains function as lubricants to prevent polymer chains from entanglement. Such a character can be confirmed by the constant relaxation time of GTMAC-CS with respect to various concentrations investigated in this work.

**Figure 4.** The overlap concentration Ce of (**a**) CS; (**b**) GTMAC-CS solutions.

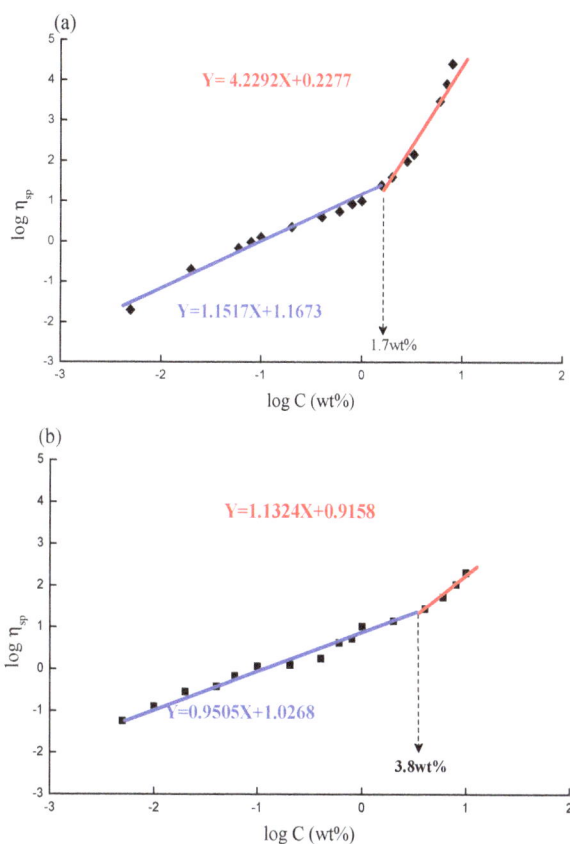

Figure 5a,b show typical plots of a dynamic rheological measurement on CS and GTMAC-CS solutions, respectively. The storage (G′) and loss (G″) moduli increase with frequency. The storage modulus G′ generally symbolizes the elastic behavior while the loss modulus G″ symbolizes the viscous behavior; both of them can be obtained by a small amplitude oscillation shearing test

(SAOS) within a linear viscoelastic range. However, as the frequency keeps increasing, G″ decreases beyond the crossover point, while G′ increases toward a plateau region. Notably, the inverse of frequency at the cross-over point of G′ and G″ can also yield a relaxation time, λ, which reveals the longest time required for the polymer structures in the fluid to relax. As mentioned earlier about the turning point in Figure 3, the results shown from Figure 5 can offer another way to obtain the relaxation time of polymer under a SAOS test [27,28].

**Figure 5.** Typical plots of a dynamic rheological measurement on (**a**) 2 wt % CS; and (**b**) 2 wt % GTMAC-CS solutions. The data was simulated by the Maxwell model (solid line).

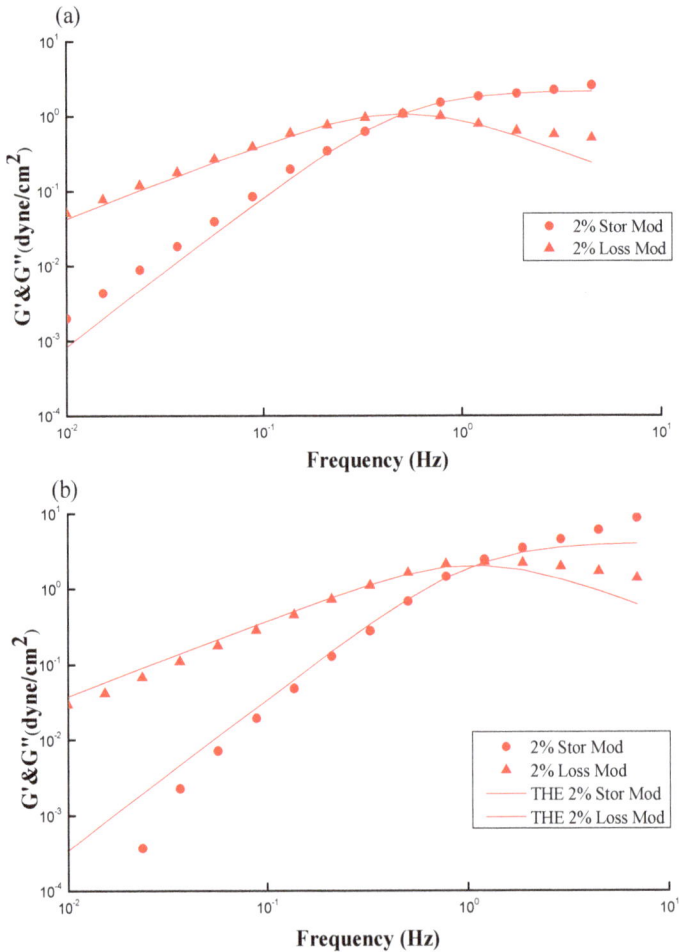

A Maxwell model (Equations (1) and (2)), consisting of a dashpot (viscosity element) connecting with a spring (elasticity element) in series, was used to describe the rheological behavior of Figure 5 [29–33].

$$G' = G_\infty(\lambda\omega)^2/[1 + (\lambda\omega)^2] \tag{1}$$

$$G'' = G_\infty\lambda\omega/[1 + (\lambda\omega)^2] \qquad (2)$$

where $\omega$ is the oscillation frequency; $G_\infty$ represents a fitting factor, roughly equals double the maximum of the $G''$; and $\lambda$ denotes the relaxation time as mentioned above. Theoretically, the limiting slopes of $\log(G')$ and $\log(G'')$ against $\log(\omega)$ before the crossover point are 2 and 1, respectively. Figure 5a,b show that the simulated results (solid line) are in good agreement with the experimental data (points) at oscillation frequencies from 0.01 to 1 Hz. The limiting slopes of $\log(G')$ *vs.* $\log(G'')$ for CS and GTMAC-CS solutions are 0.9 *vs.* 1.9 and 1.1 *vs.* 2.1, respectively, indicating that both structural buildup $(G')$ and breakdown $(G'')$ log-linearly increase with frequency in the frequency range less than 1 Hz. In general, a Maxwellian behavior observed within a low frequency range ($<10$ Hz) as shown in this study indicates that the chain conformation of dissolved polymers is a random-coiled type with a single relaxation time, namely, a good Gaussian type of polymer chains with narrow distribution [34–36]. Goodwin further illustrated that a good match of the Maxwell model reveals an insignificant or even complete lack of aggregation by the hydrophobes [37,38]. Dissolved polymers with some hydrophobic nature will increase the size of aggregates, reduce the number of aggregates, and thereby decrease both energy storage and energy loss during oscillation. Accordingly, the $G'$ and $G''$ are not sensitive to the frequency and their slopes are less than 2 and 1, respectively. Annable *et al.* [27] gave a similar explanation [22]. In short, the strong fit of Maxwell model in Figure 5a,b reveals a single relaxation time and negligible aggregations for low pH CS solution and regular GTMAC-CS aqueous solution.

Figure 6a,b show the plots similar to Figure 5a,b except two additional conditions with different concentrations, *i.e.*, 1% and 3%. The fitting parameters and simulation deviations were tabulated in Table 1. An interesting fact similar to Figure 3a, Figure 6a shows an increase of concentration results in an increase in both $G'$ and $G''$, and simultaneously a shift in the crossover frequency toward a lower value, revealing an increase of relaxation time with CS concentrations. Notably, the relaxation time of "entangled" CS molecules is increased with concentration once the threshold Ce was passed over, even though all of the chain relaxation is still in a well dissolved state with no occurrence of bulky aggregation, and besides the $G'$ and $G''$ can be described by the Maxwell model. Figure 6a demonstrates that the investigated concentration range of CS solution, 1–3 wt %, is beyond its Ce value of 2 wt %; a longer relaxation time is therefore expected. In contrast, Figure 6b shows that the frequency at which $G'$ and $G''$ of GTMAC-CS are across from each other is independent of concentration, meaning that the relaxation time is constant. The Ce of GTMAC-CS, obtained from Figure 4b, is 4 wt %, which is far beyond the tested range herein, indicating the existence of the non-entangled condition for the GTMAC aqueous solution. Interestingly, the small deviations of $G'$ and $G''$, except the 3 wt % GTMAC-CS condition, shown in Table 1 confirmed the previous statement that the experimental result under SAOS from 0.01 to 1 Hz could be well fitted by a Maxwell model with a single relaxation. Notably, the relatively high deviation of GTMAC-CS 3 wt % might be due to the high intermolecular hydrogen bonds from the hydroxyl groups of GTMAC-CS at a nonacidic environment. The intermolecular hydrogen bonds will prevent the GTMAC-CS polymers from freely random coil behavior which is the basic assumption of applying the Maxwell model.

36

**Figure 6.** Storage modulus (G') and loss modulus (G") for (**a**) CS; (**b**) GTMAC-CS solutions at different concentrations (1 wt %~3 wt %). The data was simulated by the Maxwell model (solid line).

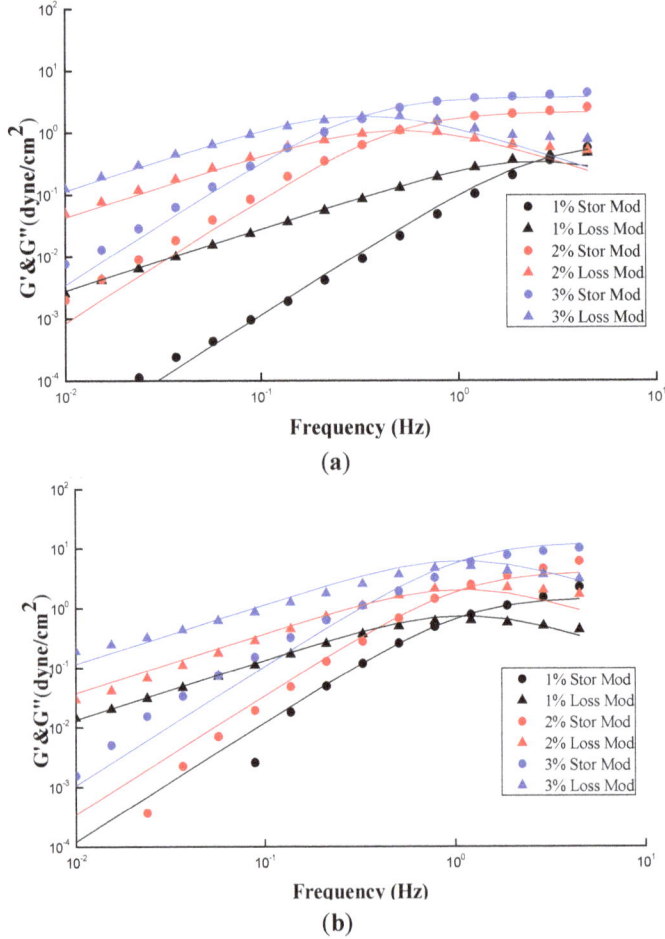

(**a**)

(**b**)

Figure 7a,b show the master curve based on the generalized parameter of G' or G" against the dimensionless frequency of Figure 6. The idea regarding the concentration shifting was adapted from WLF Equations and can be expressed by Equations (3) and (4).

$$G'_p = G'/a_v, \ a_v = (C/C_0), \ a_h = \lambda\omega \tag{3}$$

$$G''_p = G''/a_v, \ a_v = (C/C_0), \ a_h = \lambda\omega \tag{4}$$

where $G'_p$ and $G''_p$ are defined as the "reduced moduli" which is normalized by using concentration ratio, $a_v$, as a vertical shifting factor. The horizontal shifting factor, $a_h$ and the vertical shifting factor, $a_v$, equal to the dimensionless groups "$\lambda\omega$" and "$(C/C_0)$: the ratio of the given concentration to the target concentration which is 2 wt % in this work", respectively. Such a superposing concept is inspired by the derivation of the well-known WLF shifting equation [39–41] and has been thoroughly discussed in our previous paper. Figure 7a,b show that both GTMAC-CS and CS exhibit good shifting into a single curve of G′ and G″, respectively, revealing the absence of a conformational transition or the formation of a supermolecular structure under the selected operating conditions. However, the shift along the y-axis still shows a certain degree of scattering for both CS and GTMAC-CS solutions. The concentration shift based on Equations (3) and (4) actually assumes a linear relationship with the loss modulus as well as the storage modulus, which lacks some theoretical support and requires further verification in the future.

**Table 1.** The fitting parameters and simulation accuracy of CS and GTMAC-CS solutions determined from Figure 6.

|  | Concentration | $\omega_c$ (Hz) | $\lambda$(s) | $G_\infty$(dyne/cm²) | Dev.G′ # | Dev.G″ # |
|---|---|---|---|---|---|---|
|  | 1 wt% | 2.43 | 0.41 | 0.31 | 0.20 | 0.02 |
| CS | 2 wt% | 0.51 | 1.96 | 2.20 | 0.06 | 0.03 |
|  | 3 wt% | 0.33 | 3.03 | 4.52 | 0.04 | 0.02 |
|  | 1 wt% | 1.02 | 0.98 | 0.66 | 0.02 | 0.09 |
| GTMAC-CS | 2 wt% | 1.09 | 0.91 | 2.45 | 0.04 | 0.00 |
|  | 3 wt% | 1.08 | 0.92 | 6.35 | 0.10 | 0.19 |

#: $Dev.G' = \dfrac{\left|G'_{exp} - G'_{the}\right|}{G'_{the}}$; $Dev.G'' = \dfrac{\left|G''_{exp} - G''_{the}\right|}{G''_{the}}$, where $G_{exp}$ and $G_{the}$ represent the average

value of G obtained from experiment and fitting data, respectively. The data of G′ or G″ within the frequency less than $\omega_c$ are used to obtain the averaged values.

**Figure 7.** Master curve of frequency–concentration superposition for (**a**) CS; (**b**) GTMAC-CS solutions at different concentrations (1 wt%~3 wt%) shown in Figure 6.

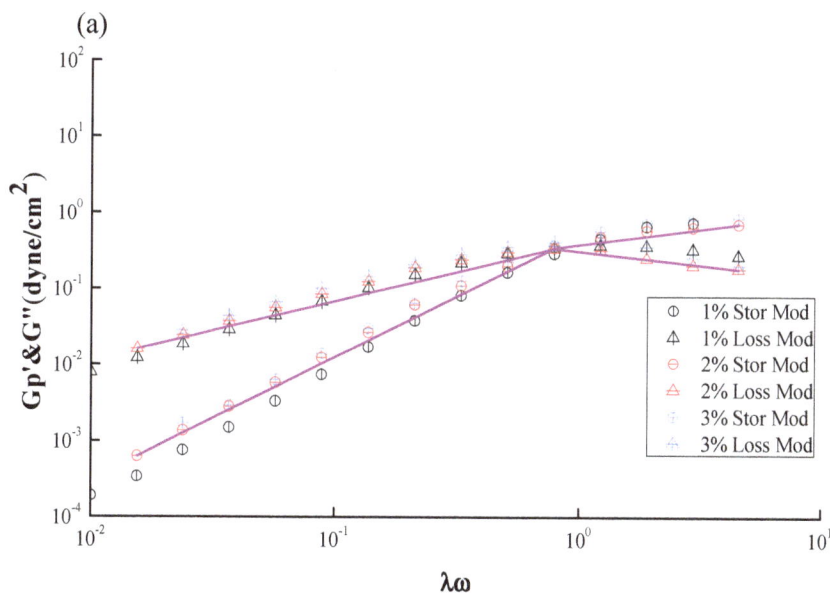

**Figure 7.** *Cont.*

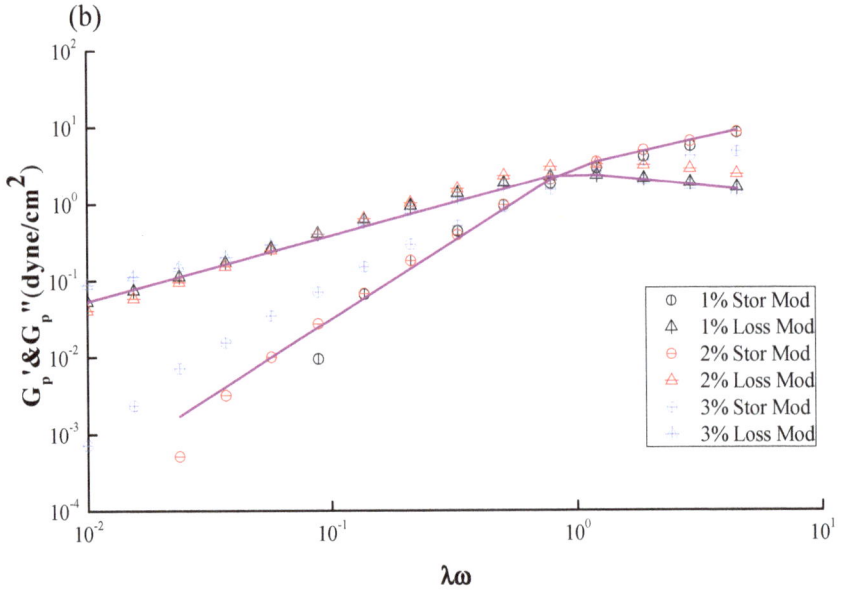

(b)

**Figure 8.** Dynamic moduli (G′, G″) *versus* frequency to obtain the sol–gel transition concentration for (**a**) CS; (**b**) GTMAC-CS solutions.

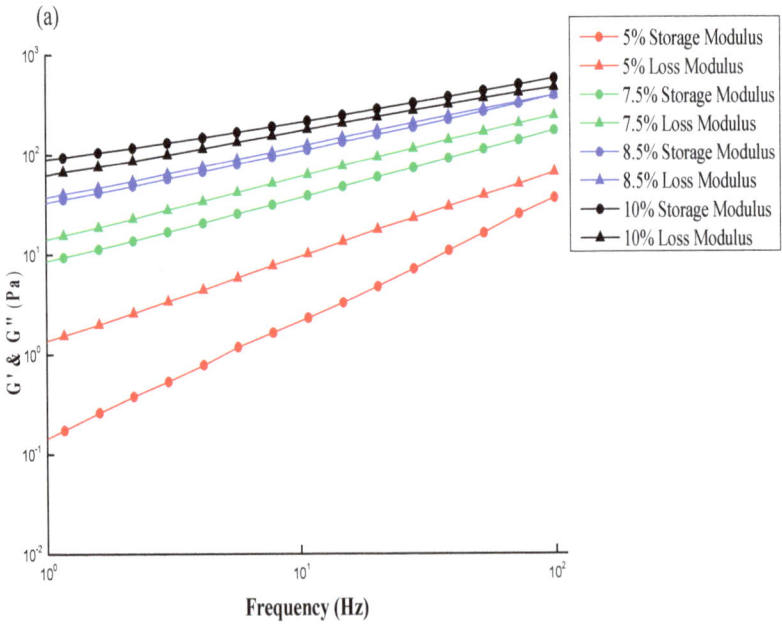

(a)

**Figure 8.** *Cont.*

(b)

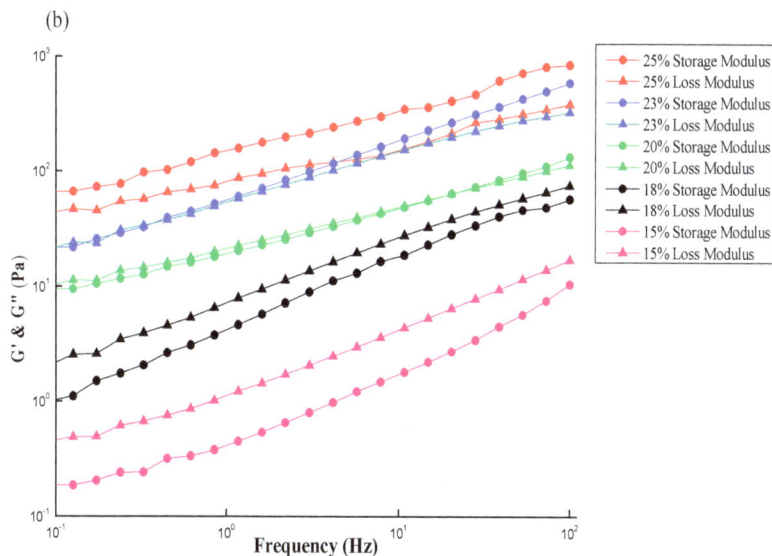

## 4. Conclusions

Chitosan grafted by GTMAC to form GTMAC-CS was successfully produced and rheologically characterized herein. The Maxwell model can be applied to simulate the dynamic rheological performance of the CS and the GTMAC-CS solutions, revealing a single relaxation time exists for both systems. The crossover point of G′ and G″ shifted toward lower frequencies as the CS concentration increased but remained constant as the GTMAC-CS concentration increased, indicating the solubility of GTMAC-CS in water is good enough to eliminate the influence from the interaction among polymer chains so as to make the relaxation time independent of the polymer concentration. A frequency–concentration superposition master curve was subsequently proposed and well fitted with the experimental results for both CS and GTMAC-CS solutions. Finally, the sol–gel transition concentration was investigated, which was 8.5 wt% and 20 wt% for CS and GTMAC-CS, respectively, reconfirming the excellent water solubility of the latter.

## Acknowledgment

The authors would like to thank the National Science Council of the Republic of China, Taiwan, for financially supporting this research under Contract No. NSC_103-2218-E-027-015.

## Author Contributions

Conceived and designed the experiment: SP Rwei. Performed the experiment (Rheology): YM Chen. Performed the experiment (Synthesis): WY Lin. Editted the writing: WY Chiang.

**Conflicts of Interest**

The authors declare no conflict of interest.

**References**

1. Ehrlich, H. Chitin and collagen as universal and alternative templates in biomineralization. *Int. Geol. Rev.* **2010**, *52*, 661–699.
2. Lee, S.Y.; Kim, J.H.; Kuon, I.C.; Jeong, S.Y. Self-aggregates of deoxycholic acid-modified chitosan as a novel carrier of adriamycin. *Colloid Polym. Sci.* **2000**, *278*, 1216–1219.
3. Ávila, A.; Bierbrauer, K.; Pucci, G.; López-González, M.; Strumia, M. Study of optimization of the synthesis and properties of biocomposite films based on grafted chitosan. *J. Food Eng.* **2012**, *109*, 752–761.
4. Bhattarai, N.; Gunn, J.; Zhang M. Chitosan-based hydrogels for controlled, localized drug delivery. *Adv. Drug Deliv. Rev.* **2010**, *62*, 83–99.
5. Casettari, L.; Vllasaliu, D.; Lam J.K.W.; Soliman, M.; Illum, L. Biomedical applications of amino acid-modified chitosans: A review. *Biomaterials* **2012**, *33*, 7565–7583.
6. Cho, J.; Heuzey, M.C.; Bégin, A.; Carreau, P.J. Viscoelastic properties of chitosan solutions: Effect of concentration and ionic strength. *J. Food Eng.* **2006**, *74*, 500–515.
7. Charles, W.P.; Jonathan, J.W.; Gudrun, S. A review on tough and sticky hydrogels. *Colloid Polym. Sci.* **2013**, *291*, 2031–2047.
8. Hamdine, M.; Heuzey, M.C.; Bégin, A. Viscoelastic properties of phosphoric and oxalic acid-based chitosan hydrogels. *Rheol. Acta* **2006**, *45*, 659–675.
9. Seetapan, N.; Maingam, K.; Plucktaveesak, N.; Sirivat, A. Linear viscoelasticity of thermoassociative chitosan-g-poly(*N*-isopropylacrylamide) copolymer. *Rheol. Acta* **2006**, *45*, 1011–1018.
10. Rwei, S.P.; Lien, C.C. Synthesis and Rheological Characterization of Sulfonated Chitosan Solutions. *Colloid Polym. Sci.* **2014**, *292*, 785–795.
11. Hermann, M.B.; Klaus, G. 1,3-Propane sultone, an extremely potent experimental carcinogen: What should be expected in humans. *Toxicol. Lett.* **2004**, *151*, 251–254.
12. Bendoraitiene, J.; Kavaliauskaite, R.; Klimaviciute, R.; Zemaitaitis, A. Peculiarities of Starch Cationization with Glycidyltrimethylammonium Chloride. *Starch/Starke* **2006**, *58*, 623–631.
13. Pedone, E.; Cavallaro, G.; Richardson, S.C.W.; Duncan, R.; Giammona, G. α,β-poly (asparthylhydrazide)–glycidyltrimethylammonium chloride copolymers (PAHy–GTA): Novel polymers with potential for DNA delivery. *J. Controll. Release* **2001**, *77*, 139–153.
14. Xiao, B.; Wan, Y.; Wang, X.Y.; Zha, Q.C.; Liu, H.M.; Qiu, Z.Y.; Zhang, S.M. Synthesis and characterization of *N*-(2-hydroxy)propyl-3-trimethyl ammonium chitosan chloride for potential application in gene delivery. *Colloids Surf. B* **2012**, *91*, 168–174.
15. Lim, S.H.; Hudson, S.M. Synthesis and antimicrobial activity of a watersoluble chitosan derivative with a fiber-reactive group. *Carbohydr. Res.* **2004**, *339*, 313–319.

16. Zhao, S.H.; Wu, X.-T.; Guo, W.-C.; Du, Y.-M.; Yu, L.; Tang, J. *N*-(2-hydroxyl) propyl-3-trimethyl ammonium chitosan chloride nanoparticle as a novel delivery system for Parathyroid Hormone-Related Protein 1–34. *Int. J. Pharm.* **2010**, *393*, 268–272.

17. Xu, Y.M.; Du, Y.M.; Huang, R.H.; Gao, L.P. Preparation and modification of *N*-(2-hydroxyl) propyl-3-trimethyl ammonium chitosan chloride nanoparticle as a protein carrier. *Biomaterials* **2003**, *24*, 5015–5022.

18. Sonia, T.A.; Sharma, C.P. *In vitro* evaluation of *N*-(2-hydroxy)propyl-3-trimethyl ammonium chitosan for oral insulin delivery. *Carbohydr. Polym.* **2011**, *84*, 103–109.

19. Cheng, Y.; Cai, H.; Yin, B.; Yao, P. Cholic acid modified *N*-(2-hydroxy)-propyl-3-trimethylammonium chitosan chloride for superoxide dismutase delivery. *Int. J. Pharm.* **2013**, *454*, 425–434.

20. Van Vlierberghe, S.; Dubruel, P.; Schacht, E. Biopolymer-Based Hydrogels As Scaffolds for Tissue Engineering Applications: A Review. *Biomacromolecules* **2011**, *12*, 1387–1408.

21. Rwei, S.P.; Chen, S.W.; Mao, C.F.; Fang, H.W. Viscoelasticity and wearability of hyaluronate solutions. *Biochem. Eng. J.* **2008**, *40*, 211–217.

22. Rwei, S.P.; Lee, H.Y.; Yoo, S.D.; Wang, L.Y.; Lin, J.G. Magnetorheological characteristics of aqueous suspensions that contain $Fe_3O_4$ nanoparticles. *Colloid Polym. Sci.* **2005**, *283*, 1253–1258.

23. Morris, E.R.; Cutler, A.N.; Ross-Murphy, S.B.; Rees, D.A.; Price, J. Concentration and shear rate dependence of viscosity in random coil polysaccharide solutions. *Carbohydr. Polym.* **1981**, *1*, 5–21.

24. Pereira, M.C.; Wyn-Jones, E.; Morris, E.R.; Ross-Murphy, S.B. Characterisation of interchain association in polysaccharide solutions by ultrasonic relaxation and velocity. *Carbohydr. Polym.* **1982**, *2*, 103–113.

25. Seale, R.; Morris, E.R.; Rees, D.A. Interactions of alginates with univalent cations. *Carbohydr. Res.* **1982**, *110*, 101–112.

26. Calero, N; Muñoz. J.; Ramírez, P.; Guerrero, A. Flow behaviour, linear viscoelasticity and surface properties of chitosan aqueous solutions. *Food Hydrocoll.* **2010**, *24*, 659–666.

27. Annable, T.; Buscall, R.; Ettelaie, R. Network formation and its consequences for the physical behaviour of associating polymers in solution. *Colloids Surf. A* **1996**, *112*, 97–116.

28. Pottier, N. Relaxation time distributions for an anomalously diffusing particle. *Phys. A* **2011**, *390*, 2863–2879.

29. Baig, C.; Mavrantzas, V.G.; Öttinger, H.C. On Maxwell's relations of thermodynamics for polymeric liquids away from equilibrium. *Macromolecules* **2011**, *44*, 640–646.

30. Molchanov, V.S.; Philippova, O.E. Effects of concentration and temperature on viscoelastic properties of aqueous potassium oleate solutions. *Colloid J.* **2009**, *71*, 239–245.

31. Papoulia, K.D.; Panoskaltsis, V.P.; Kurup, N.V.; Korovajchuk, I. Rheological representation of fractional order viscoelastic material models. *Rheol. Acta* **2010**, *49*, 381–400.

32. Van de Manakker, F.; Vermonden, T.; Morabit, N.; van Nostrum, C.F.; Hennink, W.E. Rheological Behavior of Self-Assembling PEG-β-Cyclodextrin/PEG-Cholesterol Hydrogels. *Langmuir* **2008**, *24*, 12559–12567.

33. Steffe, J.F. *Rheological Methods in Food Process Engineering*, 2nd ed.; Freeman Press: East Lansing, MI, USA, 1996; Chapter 5.

34. Likhtman, A.E.; McLeish, T.C.B. Quantitative theory for linear dynamics of linear entangled polymers. *Macromolecules* **2002**, *35*, 6332–6343.

35. Likthman, A.E.; Marques, G.M. First-passage problem for the Rouse polymer chain: An exact solution. *Europhys. Lett.* **2006**, *75*, 971–977.

36. Larson, R.G. *Constitutive Equations for Polymer Melts and Solutions*, 1st ed.; Butterworths: Boston, MA, USA, 1988; Chapter 5.

37. Goodwin, J.W.; Hughes, R.W.; Lam, C.K.; Miles, J.A.; Warren, B.C.H. The rheological properties of a hydrophobically modified cellulose. In *Polymers in Aqueous Media: Performance through Association. Advances in Chemistry*; Glass, J.E., Ed.; American Chemical Society: Washington, DC, USA, 1989; Volume 223, pp. 365–378.

38. Vermonden, T.; van Steenbergen, M.J.; Besseling, N.A.M.; Marcelis, A.T.M.; Hennink, W.E.; Sudhölter, E.J.R.; Cohen Stuart, M.A. Linear rheology of water-soluble reversible neodymium(III) coordination polymers. *J. Am. Chem. Soc.* **2004**, *126*, 15802–15808.

39. Gan, W.; Xiong, W.; Yu Y.; Li, S. Effects of the molecular weight of poly(ether imide) on the viscoelastic phase separation of poly(ether imide)/epoxy blends. *J. Appl. Polym. Sci.* **2009**, *114*, 3158–3167.

40. Kohga, M. Viscoelastic behavior of hydroxyl terminated polybutadiene containing glycerin. *J. Appl. Polym. Sci.* **2011**, *122*, 706–713.

41. Lelli, G.; Terenzi, A.; Kenny, J.M.; Torre, L. Modelling of the chemo-rheological behavior of thermosetting polymer nanocomposites. *Polym. Compos.* **2009**, *30*, 1–12.

# Preparation of Chitosan Nanocompositeswith a Macroporous Structure by Unidirectional Freezing and Subsequent Freeze-Drying

**Inmaculada Aranaz, María C. Gutiérrez, María Luisa Ferrer and Francisco del Monte**

**Abstract:** Chitosan is the *N*-deacetylated derivative of chitin, a naturally abundant mucopolysaccharide that consists of 2-acetamido-2-deoxy-β-D-glucose through a β (1→4) linkage and is found in nature as the supporting material of crustaceans, insects, *etc.* Chitosan has been strongly recommended as a suitable functional material because of its excellent biocompatibility, biodegradability, non-toxicity, and adsorption properties. Boosting all these excellent properties to obtain unprecedented performances requires the core competences of materials chemists to design and develop novel processing strategies that ultimately allow tailoring the structure and/or the composition of the resulting chitosan-based materials. For instance, the preparation of macroporous materials is challenging in catalysis, biocatalysis and biomedicine, because the resulting materials will offer a desirable combination of high internal reactive surface area and straightforward molecular transport through broad "highways" leading to such a surface. Moreover, chitosan-based composites made of two or more distinct components will produce structural or functional properties not present in materials composed of one single component. Our group has been working lately on cryogenic processes based on the unidirectional freezing of water slurries and/or hydrogels, the subsequent freeze-drying of which produce macroporous materials with a well-patterned structure. We have applied this process to different gels and colloidal suspensions of inorganic, organic, and hybrid materials. In this review, we will describe the application of the process to chitosan solutions and gels typically containing a second component (e.g., metal and ceramic nanoparticles, or carbon nanotubes) for the formation of chitosan nanocomposites with a macroporous structure. We will also discuss the role played by this tailored composition and structure in the ultimate performance of these materials.

Reprinted from *Mar. Drugs*. Cite as: Aranaz, I.; Gutiérrez, M.C.; Ferrer, M.L.; del Monte, F. Preparation of Chitosan Nanocompositeswith a Macroporous Structure by Unidirectional Freezing and Subsequent Freeze-Drying. *Mar. Drugs* **2014**, *12*, 5619-5642.

## 1. Introduction

The vast majority of processes devised so far for the achievement of foams and scaffolds (phase emulsion, air bubbling, or use of templates, among others) make use of solvents and templates [1–5]. The complete removal of these chemical compounds is typically required prior to the use of the resulting materials in many applications—e.g., biocatalytical/catalytical or biomedical ones, among others. For instance, the absence of undesired byproducts can be of help in either reducing nanoparticles poisoning in catalytic/biocatalytic reactions or preventing denaturation of biological entities in biomedical applications. Moreover, scaffolds biocompatibility is also improved. Unfortunately, this removal is by no means trivial in most of cases so the search for chemical routes that are template-free or, at least, make use of friendly templates is challenging. Within this context, cryogenic processes offer an interesting alternative. The process consists of the freezing of colloidal aqueous suspensions. The ice formation causes most solutes originally dispersed in the aqueous suspension to be segregated from the ice phase, giving rise to a macroporous structure characterized by "fences" of matter enclosing ice. The scaffolds obtained after subsequent drying (by both simple thawing and freeze-drying) show a macroporosity that corresponds to the empty areas where ice crystals originally resided. Cryogels of polymeric nature were first reported more than 40 years ago, and their properties, rather unusual for polymer gels, soon attracted attention [6,7]. Since then, polymer cryogels of many different compositions (e.g., poly(L-lactic acid) and poly(D,L-lactic-co-glycolic acid), gelatin, g-PGA/chitosan, collagen and elastin, collagen-glycosaminoglycan, or albumin-cross-linked polyvinylpyrrolidone (PVP) hydrogels, among others have been widely used in biomedicine (e.g., for tissue engineering and drug delivery purposes) most likely because of the biocompatible character of the process [8–15]. It is worth noting that the process starts from an aqueous solution/suspension or from a hydrogel and proceeds in the absence of further chemical reactions or purification procedures. Actually, the template is just frozen water, the removal of which can be easily accomplished by freeze-drying, thus avoiding potential complications associated with the presence of byproducts or the use of harsh chemical processes for template removal.

More recently, our group and some other ones have reported the preparation of inorganic, organic, and hybrid materials with well-patterned macroporous structures via the unidirectional freezing of aqueous suspensions and hydrogels in liquid nitrogen—we coined the term ISISA (ice segregation induced self-assembly) to refer to this process [16–26]. This unidirectional freezing allowed for excellent control—by the freezing conditions, such as the freezing temperatures and/or the sample immersion direction (unidirectional) into the cryogenic liquid, among others—of the morphology of the macroporous structure [27–30]. Moreover, we have recently demonstrated that the morphology of polyvinylalcohol (PVA) scaffolds can be tailored—in terms of pore diameter, surface area and thickness of matter accumulated between adjacent microchannels—by the averaged molecular weight of polymer, its concentration in the solution, and the freezing rate of the polymer solution [31]. For instance, SEM micrographs of PVA scaffolds prepared from solutions with a low PVA content (*ca.* 2.5 wt % in water) revealed a morphology consisting of poorly interconnected PVA sheets arranged in parallel layers (Figure 1). The increase of the PVA content (*ca.* 7.8 wt % in water) favored the formation of pillars crossing between layers, fully interconnecting the 3D structure. Besides, the size of the porous channels was scaled down, as a consequence of the increased difficulty for the ice crystals to form in the presence of impurities (in this particular case, PVA). A further increase of the PVA content resulted in structures where the porous channels were almost closed; that is, the PVA content reached values that favor the formation of amorphous (supercooled water) rather than crystalline ice, so that no segregation of matter occurred.

**Figure 1.** SEM (left) and cryo-etch-SEM (right column) images of cross-sectioned (perpendicular to the direction of freezing) monolithic PVA scaffolds. The freezing rate was 5.9 mm/min and the average molecular weight of the PVA was 72,000 (PVA2) for every ISISA-processed sample. All scale bars are 20 μm. Note that, in some cases, the length of the scale bar changes for better visualization of the scaffold macrostructure. Reprinted with permission from [31]. Copyright ©2007 Wiley-VCH.Verlag.

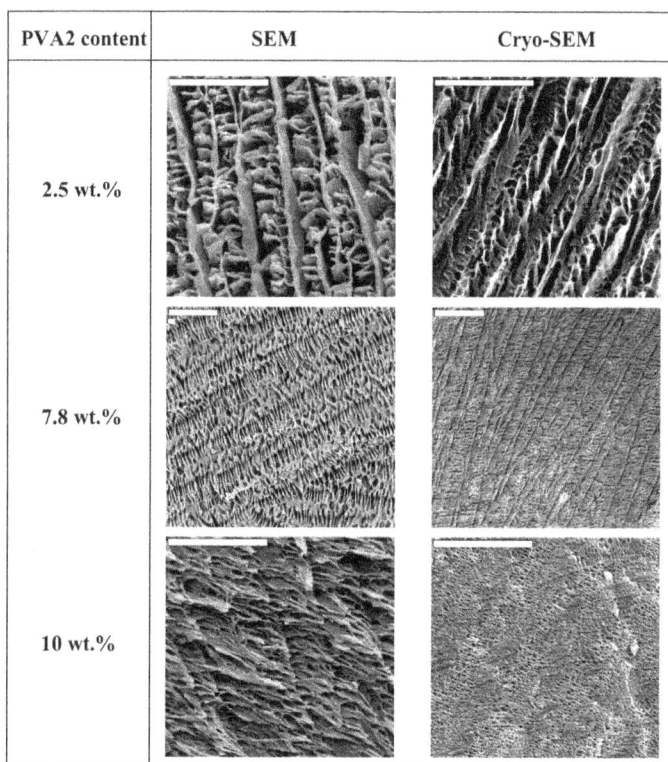

Nonetheless, low PVA contents (e.g., 2.5 wt % in water) resulted in scaffolds with poor mechanical properties. Thus, we fixed the PVA content at 7.8 wt % for the study of the next variables for tailoring of the morphology: the freezing rate (e.g., 0.7, 2.7, 5.9, and 9.1 mm/min) and the molecular weight of the PVA (PVA1: 13,000–23,000, PVA2: 72,000, PVA3: 89,000–98,000, and PVA4: 130,000, respectively). SEM images revealed that for every sample, the macrostructure resulting from ISISA was characterized by well-aligned micrometer-sized pores in the freezing direction (Figure 2). However, the channel size was strongly dependent on the molecular weights and the freezing rate. Figure 2 actually reflects the large variety of morphologies that can be obtained modulating both parameters. These SEM images revealed a clear tendency regarding the influence of the controlled variables on the porous channel size; that is, it decreased with an increase of either the freezing rate or the molecular weight. It is stated that slow freezing rates allow the formation of large ice crystals, which ultimately template the microchanneled structure.

Meanwhile, fast freezing rates favor supercooling and, hence, impede the formation of large ice crystals, so that the microchanneled structure is scaled down.

**Figure 2.** SEM images of cross-sectioned (perpendicular to the direction of freezing) monolithic PVA scaffolds. Tailored morphologies were obtained by using PVA with different weight-average molecular weights (PVA1 = 13,000–23,000, PVA2 = 72,000, PVA3 = 89,000–98,000, and PVA4 = 130,000) and by processing the PVA solution at different freezing rates. All scale bars are 20 μm. Note that, in some cases, the length of the scale bar changes for better visualization of the scaffold macrostructure. The PVA content was 7.8 wt % for every sample. Reprinted with permission from [31]. Copyright ©2007 Wiley-VCH.Verlag.

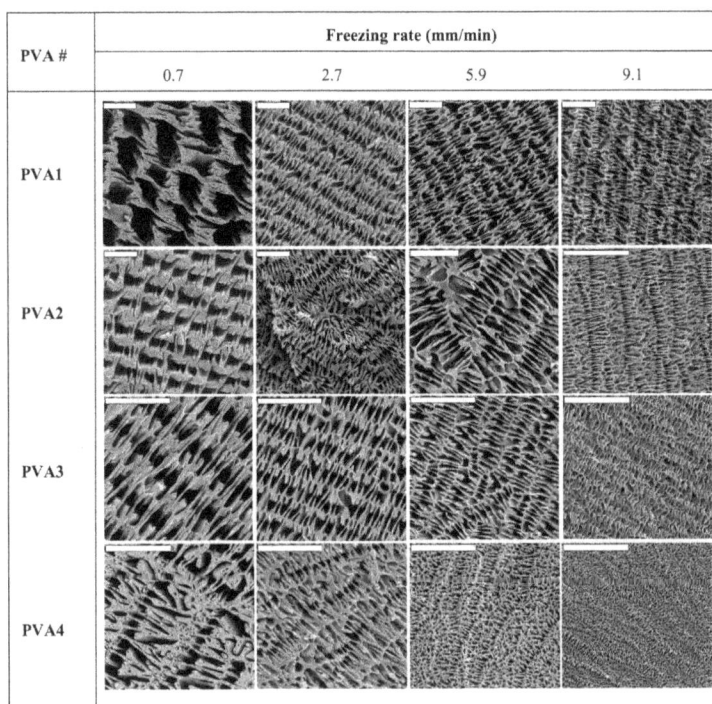

Within the context of this revision, we would like to mention that the ISISA process can also be applied to polymer of marine origin like chitosan. Chitosan (CHI) is actually a quite interesting polymer because its unique properties—in terms of biocompatibility, non-toxicity and biodegradability —made it very interesting for biomedical and biotechnological applications [32]. The chemical structure of chitosan is shown in Figure 3.

**Figure 3.** Chemical structure of chitosan where $n < 40$ and $m > 60$.

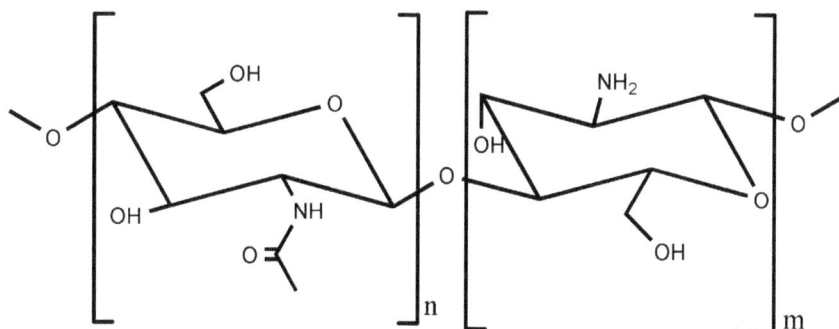

Chitosan is a polycation whose charge density depends on the degree of acetylation and pH. This macromolecule can dissolve in diluted aqueous acidic solvents due to the protonation of $-NH_2$ groups at the C2 position. In acidic conditions, even fully protonated chitosan tends to form aggregates as a result of hydrogen bonds and hydrophobic interactions. This hydrophobic behavior is based on the presence of both the main polysaccharide backbone and the $N$-acetyl groups at C2 position. One can play with the specific pH range where CHI is water-soluble so that its physical gelation can be induced in a controlled fashion. For instance, we may use the urease-assisted hydrolysis of urea to, upon the resulting pH increase, produce CHI gels where the application of the ISISA process creates a homogeneous 3D network structure. Thus, we have applied this process to CHI solutions containing calcium phosphate salts so that we promoted the simultaneous precipitation of calcium phosphate—in form of amorphous calcium phosphate (ACP)—and chitosan gelation to obtain CHI hydrogel nanocomposites [33]. After the application of the ISISA process, the porosity of the hierarchical structure was approximately 85%. The calcination of these materials resulted in the formation of a hierarchical macroporous structure composed of hydroxyapatite nanocrystals (HA-NP). The ISISA process also allowed control of the macroporous size, from 25 up to 90 μm for ACP/chitosan hierarchical structures and from 3 up to 9 μm for HA-NP hierarchical structures. (Figure 4). The mild conditions at which CHI gelation takes place—carried out at biological temperatures of ~37 °C—was critical to obtain microsponge-like morphologies in a homogeneous fashion throughout the whole 3D structure of the resulting scaffolds with superior performances than those of gels obtained by neutralization with alkaline solutions, gaseous $NH_3$, or dialyzing chitosan against alkaline media [34]. This combination of features—mild synthesis conditions and tailored structures—opens interesting perspectives for the use of these materials as substrates in tissue engineering applications.

**Figure 4.** SEM micrographs of different hybrid hierarchical structures resulting from freezing hydrogel nanocomposites, with identical CHI and calcium phosphate composition (93.25 and 6.75 wt %, respectively) at different rates: (**a**) 0.7 mm/min; (**b**) 2.7 mm/min, and (**c**) 5.7 mm/min. Scale bars are 50 μm. TEM (**d**) micrographs of ACP nanoclusters forming the ACP/CHI hierarchical structure. Scale bar is 100 nm. Reprinted with permission from [33]. Copyright ©2008 American Chemical Society.

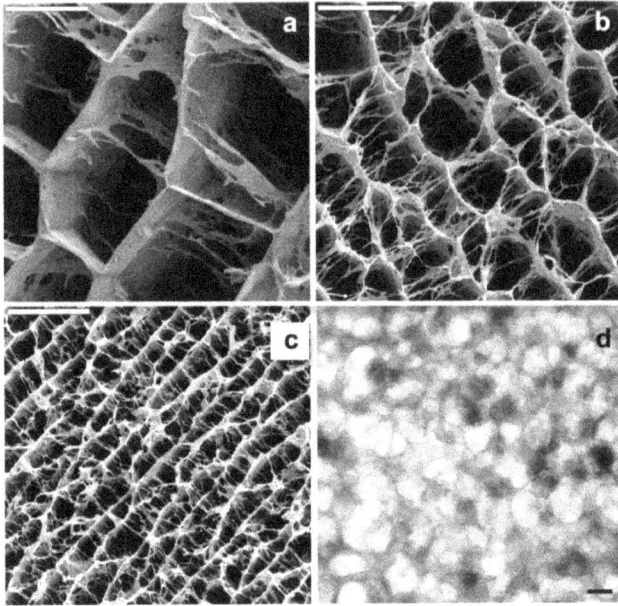

Recently, we have immobilized calcium phosphate salts (CPS) and bone morphogenetic protein 2 (BMP-2)—combined or alone—into chitosan scaffolds using ISISA process [35]. We analyzed whether the immobilized bone morphogenetic protein preserved its osteoinductive capability. We observed that rhBMP2 was not only released in a controlled fashion from CHI scaffolds but also preserved its osteoinductive character after release. Interestingly, we found that this multi-component scaffold exhibited a superior efficacy in bone regeneration than the scaffolds containing only one of the components, either CPS or rhBMP2, separately. This enhanced performance in both osteoconductive and osteoinductive terms opens the path to the future clinical application of these materials in dental surgery and, more specifically, in maxillary sinus augmentation procedure. In this procedure, large area of the maxillary sinus are lifted and replaced with bone, which serves to support future implant placement. It is worth noting that the filling material most used nowadays is porous resorbable hydroxyapatite, which is osteoconductive but not osteoinductive as the rhBMP2-CPS-CHI scaffolds described in this work (Figure 5).

**Figure 5.** Surgery (**A**), gross morphology after euthanasia (**B,C**) and microCT analysis of samples (**D**). Surgery images (A) show scaffold implantation process. After euthanasia gross morphology images were obtained at different angles (B,C) (Dotted circle indicates defect location).Defect area was still observed in CPS-CHI implanted tibias (B), while in rhBMP2-CPS-CHI implanted tibias high amount of newly-formed hard tissue, apparently bone, appeared vertically from the defect (C). MicroCT study (D) confirmed trabecular bone formation in rhBMP2-CPS-CHI implanted tibias, while it seemed no scaffold-resorption in any case. Neither seemed a robust new bone formation in the rest of implanted scaffolds compared to empty controls. Reprinted with permission from [35]. 2014 *PLoS One*. Creative Commons License.

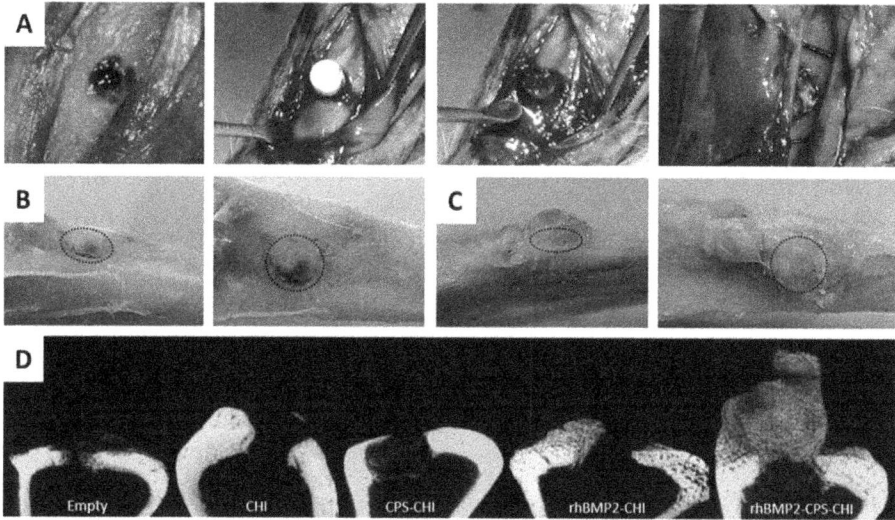

Following the same methodology—this is, the gently pH modification of chitosan solutions by the enzymatic hydrolysis of urea-chitosan scaffolds containing ciprofloxacin (CFX, a synthetic fluoroquinolone antimicrobial agent) were produced for drug delivery purposes [36]. In this case, pH modification resulted in both chitosan gelation and CFX crystallization. Thus, a macroporous CHI scaffold containing anhydrous CFX crystals was obtained after submitting the hydrogel to the ISISA process. Interestingly, the kinetic release of CFX in these chitosan scaffolds was controlled by the peculiarities of the anhydrous form in which CFX crystallizes during the ISISA process as well as by the crystals size rather than by the typical mechanisms based on swelling, hydration and/or erosion of the polymer acting as carrier. It is worth noting that CFX may exist in two different crystalline forms, the hydrated and the anhydrous ones. The hydrated form is hardly soluble in water whereas the anhydrous one is very soluble in water and, unless excipients are used, it transforms readily into the hydrated form upon exposure to water [37]. Thus, when anhydrous CFX crystals were exposed to an aqueous environment, there will be a competition between dissolution and hydration according to Figure 6—*i.e.*, first layers of anhydrous crystals will be readily dissolved, but the internal core of anhydrous CFX crystals will become hydrated before dissolution. This is why two kinetics could be easily observed, one burst type due to the dissolution of the external surface of anhydrous CFX crystals, and a second slower-one due to the poor solubility of hydrous CFX crystals. Interestingly, we were able to tune the percentage of CFX released in a burst type fashion just by tailoring the size of the anhydrous CFX crystals and thus, the external surface to internal core ratio of the crystals.

**Figure 6.** Kinetics release of CFX/CHI scaffolds having different CFX and CHI contents (left). Representation of the solubility (to CFX molecules, light grey)/hydration (to hydrous crystals, dark grey) ratio of anhydrous crystals (light grey) depending on their crystal size (right). Reproduced from [36] with permission from The Royal Society of Chemistry.

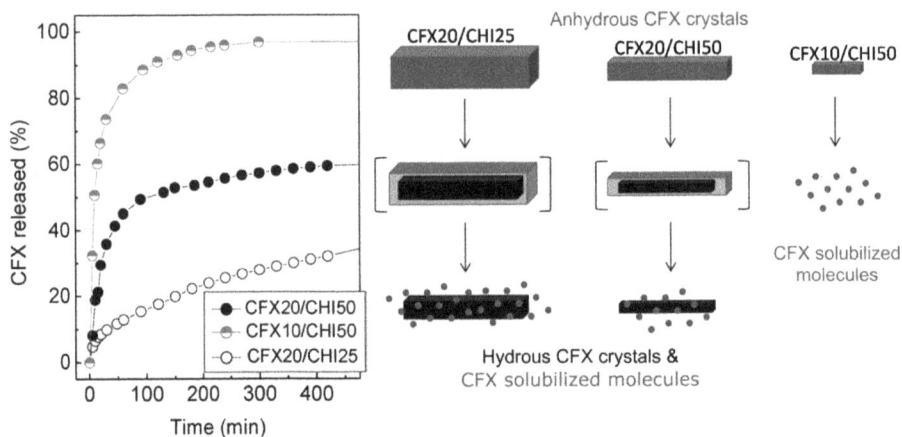

Chitosan gelation could also be induced in presence of gold salts because of the pH increase that results during the transformation of these salts into nanoparticles upon acetic acid consumption [38]. As in the previous cases, the result was the formation of a nanocomposite, in this case composed of a CHI macroporous structure with Au nanoparticles homogeneously distributed throughout the whole 3D structure. In this case, the morphology of the resulting scaffolds was related to either the viscosity or the strength of the solutions or hydrogels subjected to the ISISA process, respectively. Interestingly, both viscosities and strengths increased along with the concentration of the Au salts at the starting solution. Thus, lamellar-type morphologies were obtained in scaffolds prepared from sols, intermediate morphologies were obtained in scaffolds prepared from soft gels, whereas cellular-type morphologies were obtained from strong gels (Figure 7). Interestingly, not only the morphology but also the dissolution and swelling degree of the resulting CHI scaffolds were strongly influenced by the strength of the hydrogels obtained by the *in situ* formation of AuNP.

The capability to, under mild experimental conditions, obtain AuNP-CHI scaffolds with tailored physico-chemical properties without using further chemical additives—this is, the scaffolds were only composed of CHI and AuNPs with neither further reduction nor cross-linking agents–made these materials quite attractive for applications in both catalysis and biomedicine, where the performance of materials can be strongly influenced by the presence of impurities. In particular, we demonstrated the suitability of AuNP-CHI scaffolds for catalytic purposes (e.g., AuNPs assisted reduction of p-nitrophenol by $NaBH_4$) with full preservation of the reaction kinetics for up to four cycles as a result of the structural stability gained in AuNPCHI scaffolds.

**Figure 7.** (Top panel) Picture of AuNP-CHI gels having different $HAuCl_4 \cdot 3H_2O$ concentrations (from left to right; nil, 0.2, 0.5, 1, and 2 mM) obtained after thermal treatment at 40 °C over 150 min. Effect of the viscosities and strength hydrogel on scaffold morphology. (Bottom panel) Examples of sols and gels produced by controlling Au concentration lamellar structure from sols (left) and cellular-type morphology (right). Scale bars are 200 µm. Reprinted with permission from [38]. Copyright ©2011 American Chemical Society.

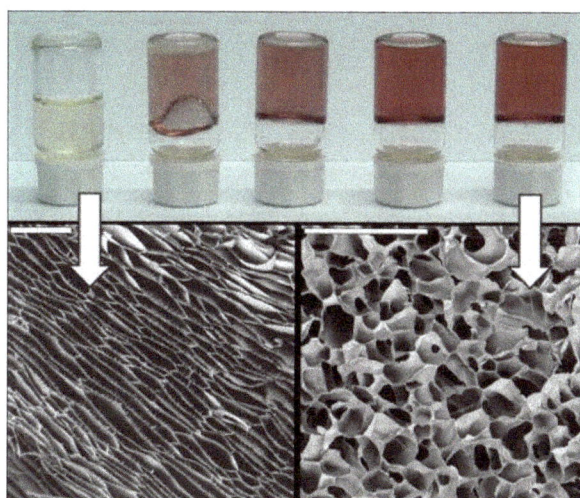

## 2. Carbon Nanotubes Chitosan Based Scaffolds Produced by Ice Segregation Induced Self-Assembly

Within the context of novel CHI nanocomposites processed in form of macroporous structures, we have also studied those based on carbon nanotubes (CNTs).Since their discovery in 1991, CNTs have been the subject of numerous research works given their unique properties, for example, extremely high electrical conductivities, very high thermal conductivities, and outstanding mechanical properties [39]. As a general trend for any catalytic application, the challenge is the preparation of materials with bimodal porous structures because the combination of high internal reactive surface along the nanostructure with facile molecular transport through broad "highways" would contribute to the performance enhancement [40].

Chitosan is an efficient dispersion agent for carbon nanotubes. Thus, we dispersed multi wall carbon nanotubes (MWCNT) homogenously into a CHI aqueous solution and submitted it to the ISISA process [25]. The resulting materials were highly porous monoliths (specific gravity ~$10^{-2}$) with different shapes (both regular and irregular) and sizes, the 3D structure of which was assembled thanks to the gluing features of CHI. The macroporous architecture was chamber-like, in the form of interconnected MWCNT/CHI sheets arranged in parallel layers (Figure 8). The morphology of the resulting structure was strongly dependent on the MWCNTs wt % at the starting aqueous suspension. Thus, the interconnection of MWCNT/CHI sheets was favored for high MWCNTs contents because of the formation of pillars crossing between layers whereas these pillars were scarcer for low MWCNTs contents. Morphology control was also exerted through the freezing rate but further improvement in the regularity of the patterned macrostructure was not achieved in this particular case. In any case, the ISISA process provided well-aligned microchannels in the direction of freezing (Figure 8) and it is worth noting that MWCNTs were not aligned but indeed percolated throughout the 3D structure.

**Figure 8.** SEM micrographs of MWCNT/CHI scaffolds: (**a**) cross-section view; (**b**) longitudinal view according to plane 1 and (**c**) longitudinal view according to plane 2. Scale bars are 200 μm in every case. Reprinted with permission from [41]. Copyright ©2012 Wiley-VCH.Verlag.

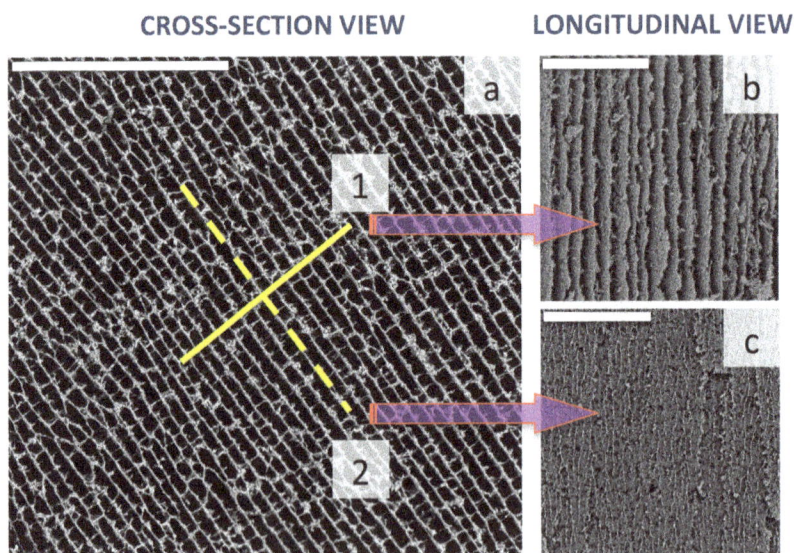

All these morphological features provided interesting properties to these materials. For instance, the electrical conductivity—as measured by the four-probe method—reached values similar to those obtained for pills of densely packed MWCNTs—e.g., 2.5 S/cm was reached with a monolith containing 89% MWCNTs after freeze-drying. This result encouraged us to use these macroporous MWCNT/CHI nanocomposites as 3D electrodes. Thus, we evaluated their performance as anodes in a direct methanol fuel cell. For this purpose, we used MWCNTs that were surface decorated with Pt nanoparticles prior to their suspension in the CHI aqueous solution. The resulting Pt/MWCNT/CHI 3D architectures allowed for a remarkable improvement (e.g., current densities of up to 242 mA/cm) of the catalytic activity toward the methanol oxidation thanks to efficient fuel and product diffusion through the aligned microchannels of the 3D structure.

We further evaluated the suitability of these materials as 3D electrodes in different fuel cells, in particular as anodes in a microbial fuel cell (MFC).The main issue for energy production in MFCs is, first and obvious, the use of bacteria—or of any other microorganisms—capable of electron shuttle electrons to a current collector and, second, the formation of biofilms that will allow this electron transfer in an effective fashion. In this case, we used MWCNT/CHI 3D architectures—Pt nanoparticles were not required—and we promoted the biofilm formation on the internal surface of the microchannels [26]. Bacteria colonization of the internal structure was attempted by different means. We first tried the direct soaking of the MWCNT/CHI 3D architectures into a bacteria culture medium. Unfortunately, cell proliferation throughout the whole scaffold structure was impeded using this procedure [42]. Confocal microscopy taken from the external surface up to a depth of 32 mm of the monolithic structure revealed how bacteria proliferation was indeed limited to just a few bacteria layers in depth (up to *ca.* 24 μm). Beyond those layers (deeper than 24–32 μm, images g and h of Figure 9), bacterial population experienced a significant decrease—up to depletion—because of nutrients and oxygen consumption by the outer bacteria.

**Figure 9.** Confocal fluorescence microscope images showing a MWCNT scaffold soaked for 24 h in a suspension of bacteria in culture medium. The depth of focus was (**a**) the external surface and (**b**) 2; (**c**) 4; (**d**) 8; (**e**) 12; (**f**) 16; (**g**) 24 and (**h**) 32 μm. Scale bar is 20 μm. Inset: MWCNT scaffold, where the arrow indicates the view angle used for confocal fluorescent micrographs. Reproduced from [26] with permission from The Royal Society of Chemistry.

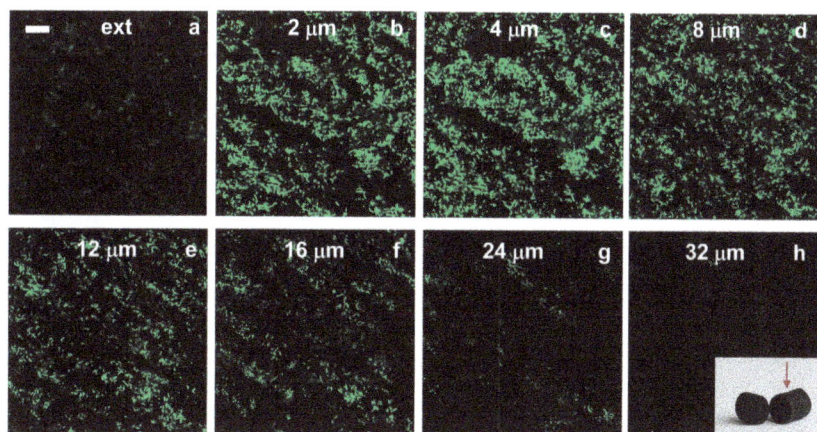

To overcome this partial bacterial colonization of the MWCNT scaffold, we decided to entrap bacteria within beads composed of a natural calcium-alginate polymer (Figure 10a) and add these beads to the MWCNT suspension prior to freezing [24,43]. Unidirectional freezing and subsequent freeze-drying resulted in a monolithic MWCNT scaffold with beads homogeneously immobilized within the three-dimensional macrostructure (Figure 10b,c). The MWCNT scaffolds containing bacteria-glucose-alginate beads were soaked in a culture medium, also containing sodium citrate. Calcium chelation with citrate resulted in dissolution of alginate beads, turning the cavity content to liquid, which allowed for bacterial dispersion and eventual growth within the scaffold. Incubation at 37 °C indeed resulted in bacteria growth and proliferation from the inner to the outer side of the macrostructure up to the culture medium, which became turbid (Figure 10d). Confocal fluorescence microscopy of the scaffold confirmed bacteria proliferation (Figure 10e,f). Unfortunately, the bacterial population per mm$^2$—as obtained from the confocal microscope images—was lower than that found in Figure 9 for the MWCNT scaffold monolith soaked in bacteria culture medium (*ca.* 3000 *versus* 39,000 bacteria mm$^{-2}$) and not sufficient for our purposes. There may be several causes of the viability decrease. As in the previous case, limited diffusion of nutrients and oxygen to the inner sides of the scaffold could still play a role. However, the main issue in this case was most likely the cryogenic process followed for scaffold preparation. It is worth noting that freeze-drying processes will unavoidably damage some of the bacterial cells [44].

**Figure 10. (a)** Three representative bacteria-glucose-alginate beads with diameters around 1 mm; **(b)** A longitudinal section of a monolithic MWCNT scaffold with immobilized bacteria-glucose-alginate beads, where the homogenous allocation of the beads can be visualized; **(c)** SEM image of a longitudinal section of the MWCNT scaffold with a hole left by a bead (bar is 500 μm); **(d)** MWCNT monoliths with immobilized bacteria-glucose-alginate beads right after soaking in culture medium (left) and after incubation at 37 °C for 24 hours (right); **(e,f)** Confocal fluorescence microscope images of the MWCNT monolith with immobilized bacteria-glucose-alginate beads soaked in culture medium before (e) and after (f) incubation at 37 °C for 24 h (bars are 20 μm). Inset: MWCNT scaffold, arrow indicates the view angle used for confocal fluorescent microscopy. In both cases, the focus was at the MWCNT structure and not at the alginate bead. Bacteria visible in (e) most likely corresponded to some minor fraction of bacteria released from alginate. Reproduced from [24] with permission from The Royal Society of Chemistry.

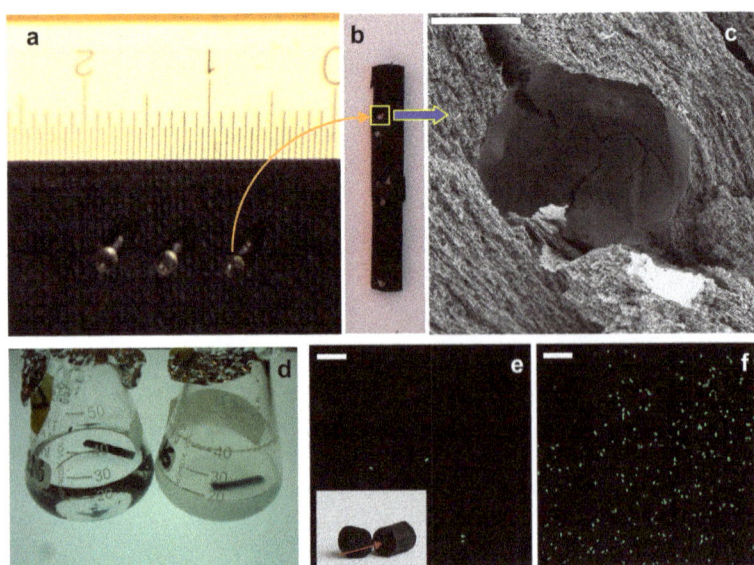

Thus, we explored whether we could force both bacteria and nutrients diffusion through the 3D scaffold [45]. It is worth mentioning that in this case MWCNT scaffolds were submitted to a mild thermal treatment (95 °C over 6 h, similar to that described above for CHI nanocomposites) in order to preserve the integrity of the 3D microchannelled structure during the flow-through experiments. Mass transport was indeed possible in a flow-through configuration thanks to the microchannelled structure of the 3D scaffolds. In this case, we worked with *Geobactersulfurreducens* (*Gs*), a member of the metal-reducing *Geobacteraceae* family, which is capable of complete oxidation of acetate to carbon dioxide with the anode serving as the sole electron acceptor. The scaffold electrode allowed for bacterial colonization of the internal surface area of the 3D structure as well as for mass transport of nutrients and byproducts (Figure 11). Interestingly, the biofilm was capable of providing 19 kA/m, representing the highest volumetric current densities in microbial electrochemical systems reported to date, and a volumetric power density of 2.0 kW/m$^3$ in a non-optimized flow MFC configuration.

**Figure 11.** SEM images (**a–c**) of biofilm at different magnifications taken from the inner part of the 3D scaffold. CLSM images at different magnifications (**d** and **e**), after staining with live/dead (bacLight) kit, of the longitudinal section of Gs biofilm induced to grow in a 3D scaffold, pre-filled with *Gs*, at 0 V *versus* Ag/AgCl, operated under flow of culture medium (10 mM acetate) for ~320 h. Reprinted with permission from [45]. The Royal Society of Chemistry.

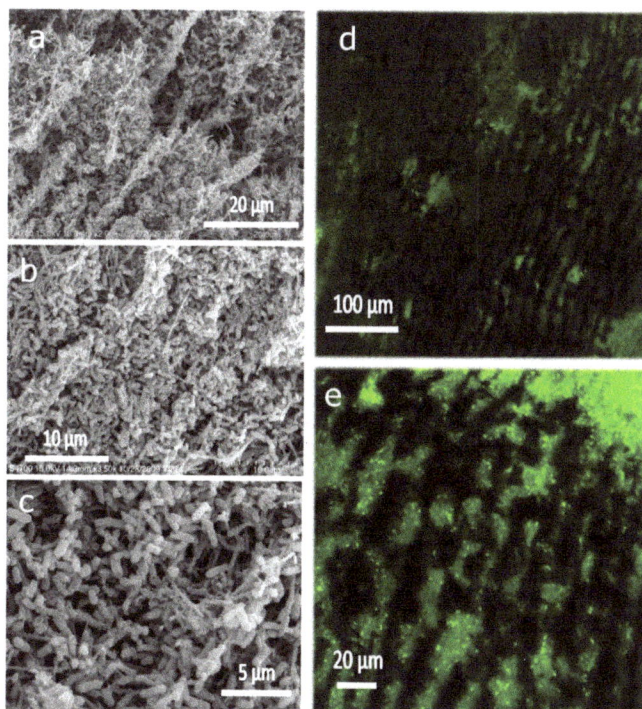

CNTs have also attracted significant attention in the emerging field of nanobiotechnology, thus being already exploited for the preparation of biosensors, molecular transporters for drug, gene and protein delivery, and fuel-powered artificial muscles [46–48]. In the area of tissue engineering, they have been extensively explored for bone regeneration and nerve tissue repair [49–54]. In this context, a wide repertoire of methodologies have been explored and optimized for the preparation of 2D CNT-based composites (e.g., films and fibers) [55]. However, the fabrication of 3D architectures has been more rarely accomplished—with some approaches including chitosan-based matrices, gelatin and/or methacrylate hydrogels collagen scaffolds, poly(lactic-co-glycolic acid) or poly(methylmethacrylates)—despite the obvious potentiality of 3D structures in regenerative medicine and tissue engineering because of their capability to mimic the natural extracellular matrix (ECM) in terms of structure, chemical composition, and mechanical properties [41,56–64].

However, the toxicity of CNTs remains controversial [65]. In order to bring some insights into the still uncertain interaction of 3D structures composed of CNTs with mammalian cells, we explored the interaction of three cell types (*i.e.*, L929 fibroblasts, Saos-2 osteoblasts and porcine endothelial progenitor cells) with MWCNT/CHI 3D scaffolds that showed different architectural and morphological features at the microscale [66]. For this purpose, the scaffold morphology was modified by (1) the incorporation of MWCNTs with two different lengths and (2) the application of the ISISA process at −65 and at −196 °C. In both cases, we found significant changes in the morphology of the resulting scaffolds in terms of porosity and surface roughness (Table 1).

**Table 1.** Scaffold characterization including porosity, surface roughness, mechanical properties, and electrical conductivity. Adapted from [66] with permission from The Royal Society of Chemistry.

| Scaffold | Pore Area per $\mu m^2$ ($A_P$) | Pore Width ($W_P$) ($\mu m$) | RMS Roughness ($R_q$) (nm) | Young's Modulus (MPa) | Conductivity (S/cm) |
|---|---|---|---|---|---|
| LNCHI [a] | 0.60 ± 0.14 | 1.4 ± 2.8 | 220 | 5.2 | 1.70 |
| LNCHI-65 [b] | 0.69 ± 0.05 | 60 ± 40 | 190 | 1.2 | 0.70 |
| SNCHI [c] | 0.69 ± 0.04 | 21 ± 4 | 120 | 4.0 | 0.32 |

[a] LN: MWCNT length 5–9 μm; [b] LNCHI-65: Freezed at −65 °C; [c] SN: MWCNT length 3 μm.

We analyzed the pore area per cross-sectioned area ($A_P$) and the averaged pore width ($W_P$) from SEM micrographs of cross-sectioned scaffolds. The roughness was studied by SEM using a MeX software package for 3D data acquisition and object reconstruction using stereophotogrammetry. Thus, we were capable to obtain the root mean square (RMS) and the roughness (Rq) of the different specimens overa path length of 15 μm. Roughness determination was carried out measuring on the walls that defined the cross-sectioned structures on which cells were cultured (Figure 12).

**Figure 12.** SEM images of LNCHI (**A**) and SNCHI (**B**) scaffolds along with their 3D reconstructed images (**C** and **D**, respectively). Scale bars: 10 mm (A) and 20 mm (B). Red lines in Figure 12 A and B indicate position of measurement. Adapted from [66] with permission from The Royal Society of Chemistry.

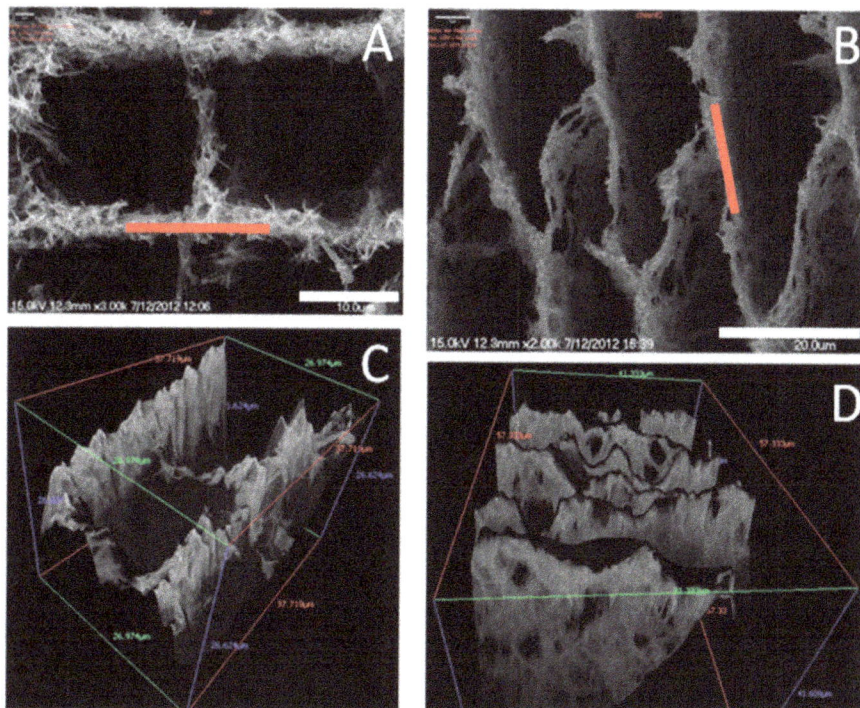

After determination of the most relevant morphological features of the different scaffolds, we studied cell viability for the three cell types mentioned above using a Live/Dead Viability kit that is based on the fluorescent response of two probes: calcein and ethidiumhomodimer-1 (EthD-1). The cell viability was high in every case although some peculiarities were found for each particular case. For instance, L929 fibroblasts and Saos-2 osteoblasts growth on LNCHI scaffolds occupying pore spaces between scaffold walls so they were basically suspended in the air with just few contact points with the substrate. As compared to L929 and Saos-2 cells, the innate adhesion pattern of porcine endothelial progenitor cells led to the increase of their contact surface with the scaffold. With these latter cells, the substrate roughness played a role in the viability so that SNCHI proved more biocompatible than LNCHI (Figure 13).

**Figure 13.** L929 fibroblast cell viability on LNCHI (**A** and **B**), LNCHI-65 (**C** and **D**). Dead cells appear stained in red, while living cells are stained in bright green. Representative culture images at 48 h are shown. Scale bars: 75 mm (**top**) and 25 mm (**bottom**). Reprinted from [66] with permission from The Royal Society of Chemistry.

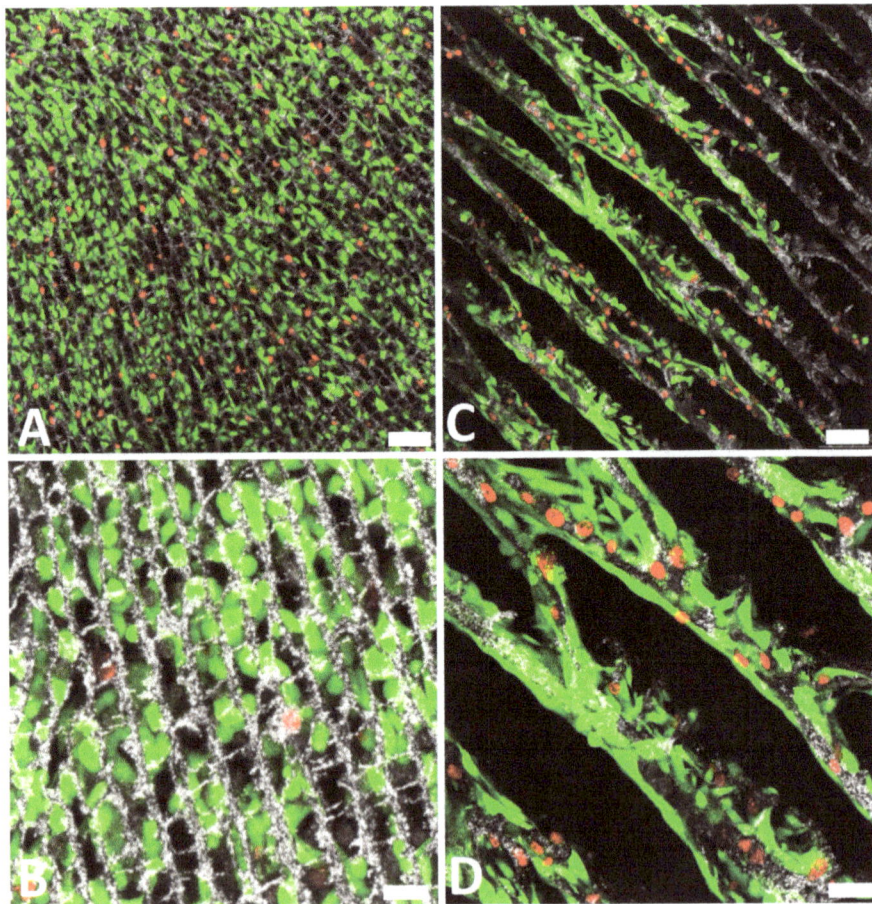

The above-described *in vitro* experiments revealed that a case-by-case study is needed to ascertain the biocompatibility of MCWNT/CHI scaffolds. Moreover, one should consider further requirements for *in vivo* experiments where not only biocompatible but also biodegradable materials are required. For this purpose, we studied the ectopic bone formation in muscle tissue by implantation of MWCNT/CHI scaffolds that contained rhBMP-2 (a potent osseo-inductor protein that promotes the differentiation of differentiated cells into an osteoblastic lineage) adsorbed onto the macrostructure [57]. The excellent biocompatibility found in these experiments was ascribed to the lack of metal traces and amorphous carbon in the scaffolds. It is worth noting that, prior to the formation of the scaffold, MWCNT were submitted to a purification process that eliminated any of the typical byproducts coming from MWCNT preparation procedures. Moreover, biocompatibility also benefited from the presence of chitosan that covers partially the surface of the MWCNTs forming the scaffold structure. Pictures shown in Figure 14 allow further discussion with regard to the mechanism governing scaffold degradation and tissue growth. Thus, one could observe at least three different zones. Zone 1 was mostly occupied by MWCNT/CHI scaffold yet resembling its characteristic well-patterned structure. Meanwhile, partial scaffold disassembly at Zone 2 resulted in the presence of agglomerated MWCNT/CHI in a non-ordered fashion. This second zone also exhibited an abundant presence of blood vessels and some few non-differentiated purple cells (e.g., fibroblasts) between the clusters formed by aggregated MWCNT/CHI (Figure 14d). Finally, Zone 3 was completely occupied by collagen-expressing cells (resulting from fibroblasts differentiation in presence of rh-BMP-2 and visualized as blue-green cells) and MWCNT/CHI—neither as a well-patterned structure nor as agglomerates in a nor-ordered fashion—were not longer visualized (Figure 14f). A close inspection to this tissue and to adjacent muscular tissues allowed the visualization of some few non-aggregated MWCNTs. Based on these pictures and subjected to further experiments to corroborate this hypothesis, we concluded that the implanted MWCNT/CHI scaffold underwent a degradation process—concurrent with cell colonization—based first on structure collapse and then in MWCNT dispersion where the individually dispersed MWCNT were most likely incorporated to the blood circulation system and subsequently eliminated through the renal excretion route.

In view of the good osteoinductive response of MWCNT/CHI scaffolds impregnated with rhBMP, we explored the incorporation of other osteoinductive agents like hydroxyapatite (HA). HA mineralization was achieved by impregnation of MWCNT/CHI scaffolds with calcium and phosphate salts, followed by HA precipitation on the scaffold internal structure [59]. HA precipitation was thermally induced upon urea decomposition that was originally incorporated within the scaffold structure besides the calcium and phosphate salts. This process obviously required of certain reinforcement of the scaffold structure, e.g., glutaraldehyde cross-linking. Otherwise, the scaffold would collapse in the acid aqueous solution of calcium and phosphate salts. We found that thermal treatments of 4 hours resulted in the formation of HA crystalline clusters of *ca.* 1 μm in diameter homogeneously distributed throughout the scaffold macrostructure (Figure 15). Further mineralization was attempted upon prolonged thermal treatments but the enlargement of the crystalline clusters (up to 5 μm) disrupted their originally homogeneous distribution throughout the MWCNT/CHI scaffolds structure so that one could find internal surfaces either fully HA-coated or HA depleted.

This problem was overcome in a subsequent work taking advantage of two particular features, e.g., the electrical conductivity and microchannelled structure—of the MWCNT/CHI scaffolds. Thus, we designed a flow-through system so that the solution containing calcium and phosphate salts was forced to flow throughout the MWCNT/CHI monolithic structure [41] (Figure 16). A layer of crystalline clusters was homogeneously electrodeposited throughout the entire internal surface of the MWCNT/CHI monolithic structure—both longitudinally and radially—by the application of a certain voltage.

**Figure 14.** Picture **A** shows a surgical implantation of MWCNT/CHI scaffolds containing adsorbed rhBMP2 into a mouse subcutaneous muscular pocket. Optical micrograph **B** shows regenerated bone tissue and the small fraction of MWCNT/CHI scaffold remaining three weeks after scaffold implantation. Optical micrographs **C–F** show details of the three main distinguishable zones observed in micrograph B: Zone 1 where the MWCNT/CHI scaffold structure remained basically intact (marked by green circles), Zone 2 where non-differentiated fibroblasts (purple cells) were colonizing the partially disassembled structure of the MWCNT/CHI scaffold (the positions of representative clusters of MWCNT/CHI aggregates are indicated by blue arrows), and Zone 3 where the MWCNT/CHI scaffold was fully disassembled and individual MWCNT/CHI (the locations of some representative MWCNT/CHI are indicated by blue circles) were dispersed within the regenerated bone tissue (collagen expressing cells are colored blue-green). Note the abundance of blood vessels (containing erythrocytes, of which some representative examples are indicated by yellow arrows) in Zone 2. Optical micrograph **F** shows a few individual MWCNT/CHI (also located within blue circles) dispersed within muscle tissue (colored pink) surrounding the implant. Reprinted with permission from [57]. Copyright ©2007 Elsevier.

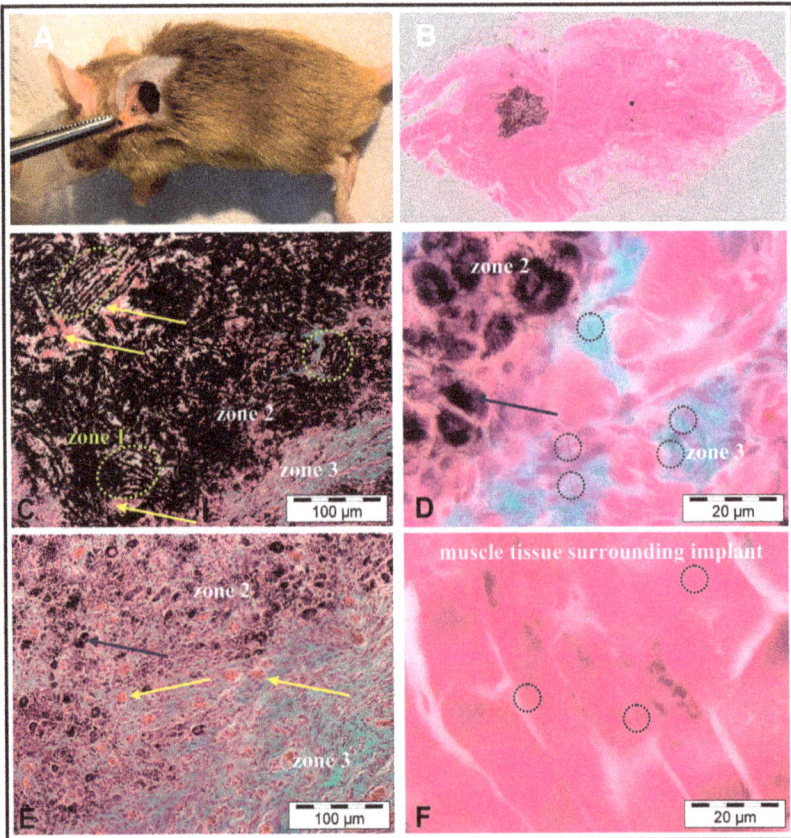

**Figure 15.** Top panel: Schematic representation of the cryogenic process followed for the preparation of MWCNT scaffolds and of the subsequent processes followed for GA architecture reinforcement and HA mineralization (HA crystals are represented as grease open circles). Middle row: SEM micrographs of MWCNT/CHI scaffolds (left) and Hap mineralized MWCNT/CHI scaffolds (right). Bars are 20 mm. Bottom panel: SEM (left) and TEM (right) micrographs show a detail of Hap crystals on the MWCNT forming the scaffold. Scale bars are 10 and 1 μm, respectively Reproduced from [59] with permission from The Royal Society of Chemistry.

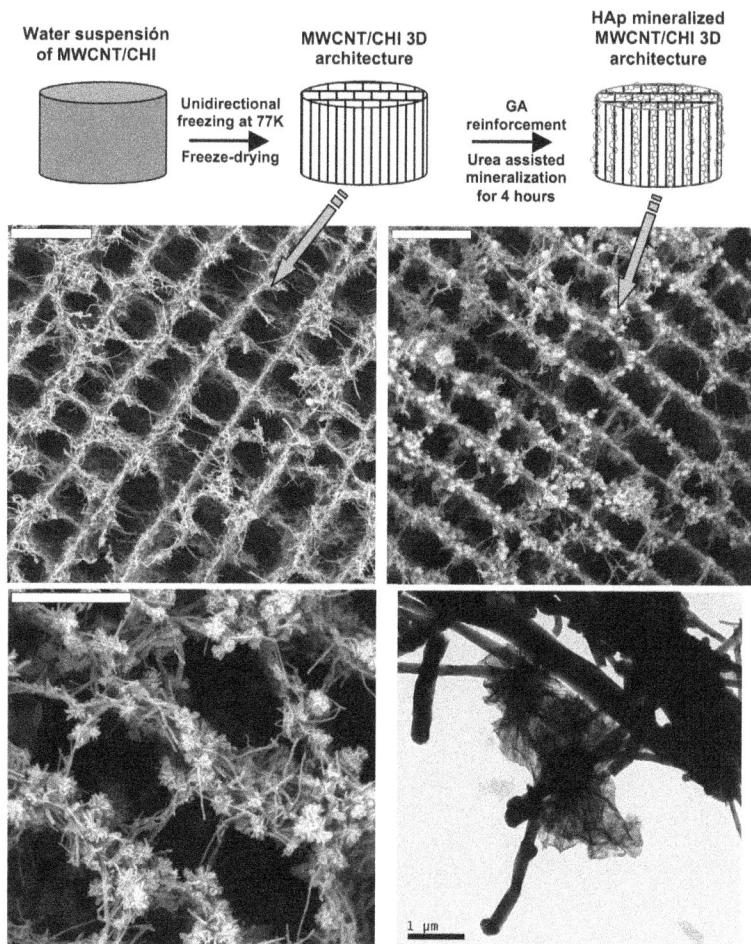

**Figure 16.** SEM micrographs of MWCNT scaffolds mineralized in flow-through conditions revealed the long-range homogeneity of the mineral coating along the entire scaffold structure of the monolith. Electrodeposition was carried out over 30 min at 30 °C and 1.4 V. Top panel: Longitudinal view, scale bars represent 400 μm (**top**) and 20 μm (bottom).Bottom panel: Cross-Section view, scale bars represent 200 μm (**a**); 50 μm (**b**); 20 μm (**c**); and 5 μm (**d**). Reprinted with permission from [41]. Copyright ©2012 WILEY-VCH Verlag.

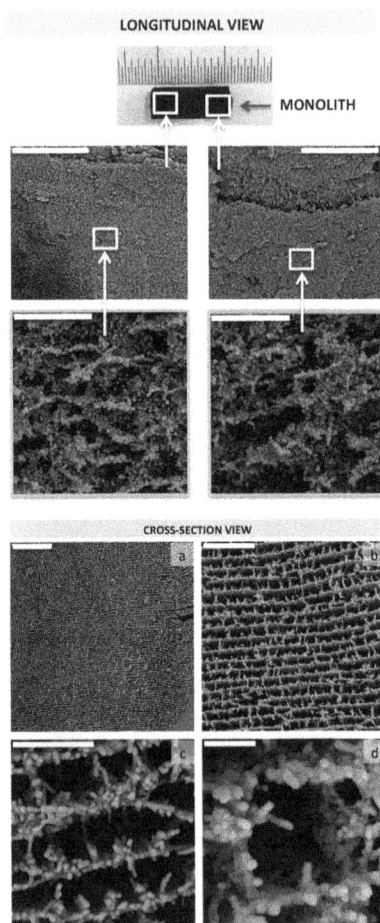

The applied voltage itself, the time the voltage was applied and the temperature at which the voltage was applied determined the nature of the HA crystals, from dicalcium phosphate dehydrate (DCPD) to octacalcium phosphate up to hydroxyapatite (Figure 17). DCPD-mineralized MWCNT/CHI scaffolds showed a remarkable biocompatibility when tested with human osteoblast cells. Interestingly, the initial presence of DCPD on these materials promoted a faster and significant osteoblast terminal differentiation (as early as seven days in calcifying media). Thus, these scaffolds could be considered as attractive multifunctional materials combining a 3D hierarchical structure, biocompatibility and osteoconductive properties.

**Figure 17.** SEM micrographs of MWCNT/CHI scaffolds after mineralization in flow-through conditions that revealed the homogeneity of the mineral coating irrespective of the experimental conditions used for electrodeposition; (**a**) 30 °C-30 min-2.1 V; (**b**) 30 °C-180 min-1.4 V; (**c**) 60 °C-30 min-1.8 V; and (**d**) 60 °C-30 min-2.1 V. Scale bars are 20 μm in every case. Reprinted with permission from [41]. Copyright ©2012 WILEY-VCH. Verlag.

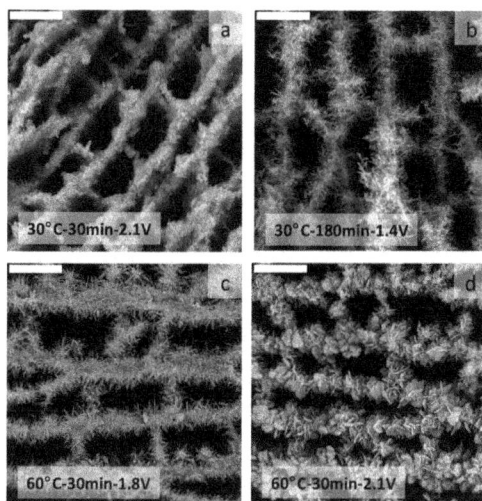

## 3. Conclusions

In this review, we highlight the ability of ice-templating processes for the preparation of chitosan-based macroporous materials—either with bare chitosan or in form of nanocomposites. The ISISA process allowed us to produce highly porous hybrid materials with high surface area and straightforward molecular transport. Besides and with regard to the composition, the combination between the intrinsic properties of chitosan with those coming from the additional components (organic, inorganic, biomolecules and even microorganisms)offered interesting possibilities in number of applications (e.g., tissue engineering, drug delivery, catalytic applications, energy production, among others) as described along this paper.

## Acknowledgments

This work was supported by MINECO (MAT2009-10214 and MAT2012-34811).

## Author Contributions

I.A. and F.M wrote the manuscript: M.L.F and M.C.G contributed with the article with a critical revision. All authors read and approved the final manuscript.

64

## Conflict of Interests

The authors declare no conflict of interest.

## References

1. Barbetta, A.; Dentini, M.; de Vecchis, M.S.; Filippini, P.; Formisano, G.; Caiazza, S. Scaffolds based on biopolymeric foams. *Adv. Funct. Mater.* **2005**, *15*, 118–124.

2. Partap, S.; Rehman, I.; Jones, J.R.; Darr, J.A. "Supercritical carbon dioxide in water" emulsion-templated synthesis of porous calcium alginate hydrogels. *Adv. Mater.* **2006**, *18*, 501–504.

3. Carn, F.; Colin, A.; Achard, M.F.; Deleuze, H.; Saadi, Z.; Backov, R. Rational design of macrocellular silica scaffolds obtained by a tunable sol-gel foaming process. *Adv. Mater.* **2004**, *16*, 140–144.

4. Stachowiak, A.N.; Bershteyn, A.; Tzatzalos, E.; Irvine, D.J. Bioactive hydrogels with an ordered cellular structure combine interconnected macroporosity and robust mechanical properties. *Adv. Mater.* **2005**, *17*, 399–403.

5. Wan, A.C.A.; Tai, B.C.U.; Leck, K.J.; Ying, J.Y. Silica-incorporated polyelectrolyte-complex fibers as tissue-engineering scaffolds. *Adv. Mater.* **2006**, *18*, 641–644.

6. Pate, J.W.; Sawyer, P.N. Freeze-dried aortic grafts. A preliminary report of experimental evaluation. *Am. J. Surg.* **1953**, *86*, 3–13.

7. Ross, D.N. Homograft replacement of the aortic valve. *Lancet* **1962**, *280*, 487.

8. Chen, G.; Ushida, T.; Tateishi, T. Preparation of poly(L-lactic acid) and poly(dl-lactic-co-glycolic acid) foams by use of ice microparticulates. *Biomaterials* **2001**, *22*, 2563–2567.

9. Ho, M.H.; Kuo, P.Y.; Hsieh, H.J.; Hsien, T.Y.; Hou, L.T.; Lai, J.Y.; Wang, D.M. Preparation of porous scaffolds by using freeze-extraction and freeze-gelation methods. *Biomaterials* **2004**, *25*, 129–138.

10. Kang, H.W.; Tabata, Y.; Ikada, Y. Fabrication of porous gelatin scaffolds for tissue engineering. *Biomaterials* **1999**, *20*, 1339–1344.

11. Hsieh, C.Y.; Tsai, S.P.; Wang, D.M.; Chang, Y.N.; Hsieh, H.J. Preparation of γ-PGA/chitosan composite tissue engineering matrices. *Biomaterials* **2005**, *26*, 5617–5623.

12. Hsieh, C.Y.; Tsai, S.P.; Ho, M.H.; Wang, D.M.; Liu, C.E.; Hsieh, C.H.; Tseng, H.C.; Hsieh, H.J. Analysis of freeze-gelation and cross-linking processes for preparing porous chitosan scaffolds. *Carbohydr. Polym.* **2007**, *67*, 124–132.

13. Daamen, W.F.; Van Moerkerk, H.T.B.; Hafmans, T.; Buttafoco, L.; Poot, A.A.; Veerkamp, J.H.; Van Kuppevelt, T.H. Preparation and evaluation of molecularly-defined collagen-elastin-glycosaminoglycan scaffolds for tissue engineering. *Biomaterials* **2003**, *24*, 4001–4009.

14. Dagalakis, N.; Flink, J.; Stasikelis, P.; Burke, J.F.; Yannas, I.V. Design of an artificial skin. Part iii. Control of pore structure. *J. Biomed. Mater. Res.* **1980**, *14*, 511–528.

15. Shalaby, W.S.W.; Peck, G.E.; Park, K. Release of dextromethorphan hydrobromide from freeze-dried enzyme-degradable hydrogels. *J. Control. Release* **1991**, *16*, 355–363.

16. Nishihara, H.; Mukai, S.R.; Tamon, H. Preparation of resorcinol-formaldehyde carbon cryogel microhoneycombs. *Carbon* **2004**, *42*, 899–901.

17. Zhang, H.; Hussain, I.; Brust, M.; Butler, M.F.; Rannard, S.P.; Cooper, A.I. Aligned two- and three-dimensional structures by directional freezing of polymers and nanoparticles. *Nat. Mater.* **2005**, *4*, 787–793.

18. Mukai, S.R.; Nishihara, H.; Shichi, S.; Tamon, H. Preparation of porous $TiO_2$cryogel fibers through unidirectional freezing of hydrogel followed by freeze-drying. *Chem. Mater.* **2004**, *16*, 4987–4991.

19. Deville, S.; Saiz, E.; Nalla, R.K.; Tomsia, A.P. Freezing as a path to build complex composites. *Science* **2006**, *311*, 515–518.

20. Deville, S.; Saiz, E.; Tomsia, A.P. Freeze casting of hydroxyapatite scaffolds for bone tissue engineering. *Biomaterials* **2006**, *27*, 5480–5489.

21. Nishihara, H.; Mukai, S.R.; Fujii, Y.; Tago, T.; Masuda, T.; Tamon, H. Preparation of monolithic $SiO_2$-$Al_2O_3$ cryogels with inter-connected macropores through ice templating. *J. Mater. Chem.* **2006**, *16*, 3231–3236.

22. Ferrer, M.L.; Esquembre, R.; Ortega, I.; Reyes Mateo, C.; Del Monte, F. Freezing of binary colloidal systems for the formation of hierarchy assemblies. *Chem. Mater.* **2006**, *18*, 554–559.

23. Gutiérrez, M.C.; Jobbágy, M.; Rapún, N.; Ferrer, M.L.; Del Monte, F. A biocompatible bottom-up route for the preparation of hierarchical biohybrid materials. *Adv. Mater.* **2006**, *18*, 1137–1140.

24. Gutiérrez, M.C.; García-Carvajal, Z.Y.; Jobbágy, M.; Yuste, L.; Rojo, F.; Abrusci, C.; Catalina, F.; del Monte, F.; Ferrer, M.L. Hydrogel scaffolds with immobilized bacteria for 3D cultures. *Chem. Mater.* **2007**, *19*, 1968–1973.

25. Gutiérrez, M.C.; Hortigüela, M.J.; Manuel Amarilla, J.; Jiménez, R.; Ferrer, M.L.; del Monte, F. Macroporous 3D architectures of self-assembled MWCNT surface decorated with Pt nanoparticles as anodes for a direct methanol fuel cell. *J. Phys. Chem. C* **2007**, *111*, 5557–5560.

26. Gutiérrez, M.C.; García-Carvajal, Z.Y.; Hortigüela, M.J.; Yuste, L.; Rojo, F.; Ferrer, M.L.; del Monte, F. Biocompatible MWCNT scaffolds for immobilization and proliferation of *E. Coli. J. Mater. Chem* .**2007**, *17*, 2992–2995.

27. Fukasawa, T.; Deng, Z.Y.; Ando, M.; Ohji, T.; Goto, Y. Pore structure of porous ceramics synthesized from water-based slurry by freeze-dry process. *J. Mater. Sci.* **2001**, *36*, 2523–2527.

28. Schoof, H.; Bruns, L.; Fischer, A.; Heschel, I.; Rau, G. Dendritic ice morphology in unidirectionally solidified collagen suspensions. *J. Crystal Growth* **2000**, *209*, 122–129.

29. Nishihara, H.; Mukai, S.R.; Yamashita, D.; Tamon, H. Ordered macroporous silica by ice templating. *Chem. Mater.* **2005**, *17*, 683–689.

30. Mukai, S.R.; Nishihara, H.; Tamon, H. Formation of monolithic silica gel microhoneycombs (smhs) using pseudosteady state growth of microstructural ice crystals. *Chem. Commun.* **2004**, *10*, 874–875.

31. Gutiérrez, M.C.; García-Carvajal, Z.Y.; Jobbágy, M.; Rubio, F.; Yuste, L.; Rojo, F.; Ferrer, M.L.; del Monte, F. Poly(vinyl alcohol) scaffolds with tailored morphologies for drug delivery and controlled release. *Adv. Funct. Mater.* **2007**, *17*, 3505–3513.

32. Aranaz, I.; Mengíbar, M.; Harris, R.; Paños, I.; Miralles, B.; Acosta, N.; Galed, G.; Heras, Á. Functional characterization of chitin and chitosan. *Curr. Chem. Biol.* **2009**, *3*, 203–230.

33. Gutiérrez, M.C.; Jobbágy, M.; Ferrer, M.L.; Del Monte, F. Enzymatic synthesis of amorphous calcium phosphate-chitosan nanocomposites and their processing into hierarchical structures. *Chem. Mater.* **2008**, *20*, 11–13.

34. Chenite, A.; Gori, S.; Shive, M.; Desrosiers, E.; Buschmann, M.D. Monolithic gelation of chitosan solutions via enzymatic hydrolysis of urea. *Carbohydr. Polym.* **2006**, *64*, 419–424.

35. Guzmań, R.; Nardecchia, S.; Gutíerrez, M.C.; Ferrer, M.L.; Ramos, V.; del Monte, F.; Abarrategi, A.; López-Lacomba, J.L. Chitosan scaffolds containing calcium phosphate salts and rh-BMP-2: *In vitro* and *in vivo* testing for bone tissue regeneration. *PLoS One* **2014**, *9*, e87149.

36. Aranaz, I.; Gutiérrez, M.C.; Yuste, L.; Rojo, F.; Ferrer, M.L.; del Monte, F. Controlled formation of the anhydrous polymorph of ciprofloxacin crystals embedded within chitosan scaffolds: Study of the kinetic release dependence on crystal size. *J. Mater. Chem.* **2009**, *19*, 1576–1582.

37. Li, X.; Zhi, F.; Hu, Y. Investigation of excipient and processing on solid phase transformation and dissolution of ciprofloxacin. *Int. J. Pharm.* **2007**, *328*, 177–182.

38. Hortigüela, M.J.; Aranaz, I.; Gutiérrez, M.C.; Ferrer, M.L.; Del Monte, F. Chitosan gelation induced by the *in situ* formation of gold nanoparticles and its processing into macroporous scaffolds. *Biomacromolecules* **2011**, *12*, 179–186.

39. Iijima, S. Helical microtubules of graphitic carbon. *Nature* **1991**, *354*, 56–58.

40. Che, G.; Lakshmi, B.B.; Fisher, E.R.; Martin, C.R. Carbon nanotubule membranes for electrochemical energy storage and production. *Nature* **1998**, *393*, 346–349.

41. Nardecchia, S.; Serrano, M.C.; Gutiérrez, M.C.; Portolés, M.T.; Ferrer, M.L.; Del Monte, F. Osteoconductive performance of carbon nanotube scaffolds homogeneously mineralized by flow-through electrodeposition. *Adv. Funct. Mater.* **2012**, *22*, 4411–4420.

42. Hollister, S.J. Porous scaffold design for tissue engineering. *Nature Mater.* **2005**, *4*, 518–524.

43. Green, D.W.; Leveque, I.; Walsh, D.; Howard, D.; Yang, X.; Partridge, K.; Mann, S.; Oreffo, R.O.C. Biomineralized polysaccharide capsules for encapsulation, organization, and delivery of human cell types and growth factors. *Adv. Funct. Mater.* **2005**, *15*, 917–923.

44. Rudge, R.H. *Microorganism and Cultured Cells. A Manual of Laboratory Methods*; Kirsop, B.E., Doyle, A., Eds.; Academic Press: London, UK, 1991; p. 31.

45. Katuri, K.; Ferrer, M.L.; Gutiérrez, M.C.; Jiménez, R.; Del Monte, F.; Leech, D. Three-dimensional microchanelled electrodes in flow-through configuration for bioanode formation and current generation. *Energy Environ. Sci.* **2011**, *4*, 4201–4210.

46. Besteman, K.; Lee, J.O.; Wiertz, F.G.M.; Heering, H.A.; Dekker, C. Enzyme-coated carbon nanotubes as single-molecule biosensors. *Nano Lett.* **2003**, *3*, 727–730.

47. Kam, N.W.S.; O'Connell, M.; Wisdom, J.A.; Dai, H. Carbon nanotubes as multifunctional biological transporters and near-infrared agents for selective cancer cell destruction. *Proc. Natl. Acad. Sci. USA* **2005**, *102*, 11600–11605.

48. Ebron, V.H.; Yang, Z.; Seyer, D.J.; Kozlov, M.E.; Oh, J.; Xie, H.; Razal, J.; Hall, L.J.; Ferraris, J.P.; MacDiarmid, A.G.; *et al.* Fuel-powered artificial muscles. *Science* **2006**, *311*, 1580–1583.

49. Veetil, J.V.; Ye, K. Tailored carbon nanotubes for tissue engineering applications. *Biotechnol. Prog.* **2009**, *25*, 709–721.

50. Tran, P.A.; Zhang, L.; Webster, T.J. Carbon nanofibers and carbon nanotubes in regenerative medicine. *Adv. Drug Deliv. Rev.* **2009**, *61*, 1097–1114.

51. Harrison, B.S.; Atala, A. Carbon nanotube applications for tissue engineering. *Biomaterials* **2007**, *28*, 344–353.

52. Bianco, A.; Kostarelos, K.; Partidos, C.D.; Prato, M. Biomedical applications of functionalised carbon nanotubes. *Chem. Commun.* **2005**, *5*, 571–577.

53. Nayak, T.R.; Jian, L.; Phua, L.C.; Ho, H.K.; Ren, Y.; Pastorin, G. Thin films of functionalized multiwalled carbon nanotubes as suitable scaffold materials for stem cells proliferation and bone formation. *ACS Nano* **2010**, *4*, 7717–7725.

54. Jan, E.; Kotov, N.A. Successful differentiation of mouse neural stem cells on layer-by-layer assembled single-walled carbon nanotube composite. *Nano Lett.* **2007**, *7*, 1123–1128.

55. Byrne, M.T.; Gun'ko, Y.K. Recent advances in research on carbon nanotube-polymer composites. *Adv. Mater.* **2010**, *22*, 1672–1688.

56. Olivas-Armendáriz, I.; García-Casillas, P.; Martínez-Sánchez, R.; Martínez-Villafañe, A.; Martínez-Pérez, C.A. Chitosan/MWCNT composites prepared by thermal induced phase separation. *J. Alloys Compd.* **2010**, *495*, 592–595.

57. Abarrategi, A.; Gutiérrez, M.C.; Moreno-Vicente, C.; Hortigüela, M.J.; Ramos, V.; López-Lacomba, J.L.; Ferrer, M.L.; del Monte, F. Multiwall carbon nanotube scaffolds for tissue engineering purposes. *Biomaterials* **2008**, *29*, 94–102.

58. Lau, C.; Cooney, M.J.; Atanassov, P. Conductive macroporous composite chitosan-carbon nanotube scaffolds. *Langmuir* **2008**, *24*, 7004–7010.

59. Hortigüela, M.J.; Gutiérrez, M.C.; Aranaz, I.; Jobbágy, M.; Abarrategi, A.; Moreno-Vicente, C.; Civantos, A.; Ramos, V.; López-Lacomba, J.L.; Ferrer, M.L.; *et al.* Urea assisted hydroxyapatite mineralization on mwcnt/chi scaffolds. *J. Mater. Chem.* **2008**, *18*, 5933–5940.

60. Shin, S.R.; Bae, H.; Cha, J.M.; Mun, J.Y.; Chen, Y.C.; Tekin, H.; Shin, H.; Farshchi, S.; Dokmeci, M.R.; Tang, S.; *et al.* Carbon nanotube reinforced hybrid microgels as scaffold materials for cell encapsulation. *ACS Nano* **2012**, *6*, 362–372.

61. Zou, J.; Liu, J.; Karakoti, A.S.; Kumar, A.; Joung, D.; Li, Q.; Khondaker, S.I.; Seal, S.; Zhai, L. Ultralight multiwalled carbon nanotube aerogel. *ACS Nano* **2010**, *4*, 7293–7302.

62. Hirata, E.; Uo, M.; Takita, H.; Akasaka, T.; Watari, F.; Yokoyama, A. Multiwalled carbon nanotube-coating of 3d collagen scaffolds for bone tissue engineering. *Carbon* **2011**, *49*, 3284–3291.

63. Zhang, H.; Chen, Z. Fabrication and characterization of electrospun PLGA/MWNTS/ Hydroxyapatite biocomposite scaffolds for bone tissue engineering. *J. Bioact. Compat. Polym.* **2010**, *25*, 241–259.

64. Rege, K.; Raravikar, N.R.; Kim, D.Y.; Schadler, L.S.; Ajayan, P.M.; Dordick, J.S. Enzyme-polymer-single walled carbon nanotube composites as biocatalytic films. *Nano Lett.* **2003**, *3*, 829–832.

65. Cui, H.F.; Vashist, S.K.; Al-Rubeaan, K.; Luong, J.H.T.; Sheu, F.S. Interfacing carbon nanotubes with living mammalian cells and cytotoxicity issues. *Chem. Res. Toxicol.* **2010**, *23*, 1131–1147.

66. Nardecchia, S.; Serrano, M.C.; Gutiérrez, M.C.; Ferrer, M.L.; Del Monte, F. Modulating the cytocompatibility of tridimensional carbon nanotube-based scaffolds. *J. Mater. Chem. B* **2013**, *1*, 3064–3072.

# The Influence of 1-Butanol and Trisodium Citrate Ion on Morphology and Chemical Properties of Chitosan-Based Microcapsules during Rigidification by Alkali Treatment

Sudipta Chatterjee, Fabien Salaün and Christine Campagne

**Abstract:** Linseed oil which has various biomedical applications was encapsulated by chitosan (Chi)-based microcapsules in the development of a suitable carrier. Oil droplets formed in oil-in-water emulsion using sodium dodecyl sulfate (SDS) as emulsifier was stabilized by Chi, and microcapsules with multilayers were formed by alternate additions of SDS and Chi solutions in an emulsion through electrostatic interaction. No chemical cross-linker was used in the study and the multilayer shell membrane was formed by ionic gelation using Chi and SDS. The rigidification of the shell membrane of microcapsules was achieved by alkali treatment in the presence of a small amount of 1-butanol to reduce aggregation. A trisodium citrate solution was used to stabilize the charge of microcapsules by ionic cross-linking. Effects of butanol during alkali treatment and citrate in post alkali treatment were monitored in terms of morphology and the chemical properties of microcapsules. Various characterization techniques revealed that the aggregation was decreased and surface roughness was increased with layer formation.

Reprinted from *Mar. Drugs*. Cite as: Chatterjee, S.; Salaün, F.; Campagne, C. The Influence of 1-Butanol and Trisodium Citrate Ion on Morphology and Chemical Properties of Chitosan-Based Microcapsules during Rigidification by Alkali Treatment. *Mar. Drugs* **2014**, *12*, 5801-5816.

## 1. Introduction

Microencapsulation is a useful and promising technology where biologically active agents such as drugs, functional foods, and probiotics are enclosed within a semi-permeable polymer membrane to assist various pharmaceutical and biomedical processes [1,2]. The striking features of microcapsules include sufficient resistance to environmental conditions, permeability, and release properties [3]. Nowadays, microcapsules are successfully being applied in various biomedical and pharmaceutical processes and, in addition to biomedical applications, encapsulated microcapsules have become very effective materials in food, printing, cosmetics, agriculture, and biotechnology applications [4]. Microcapsules are starting to receive attention in textile applications because various active substances, such as phase change materials, fragrances, flame retardant, cooling agent, essential oils, skin moisturizing agents and probiotic organisms [5] may be protected to achieve new smart functionalities of a textile substrate.

Microcapsules' shell can be made from various polymers, and nanoparticles such as silica and polysiloxane [6]. In particular, natural biodegradable polymers such as chitosan, gelatin, albumin, and alginate are receiving considerable attention due to their biocompatibility and good release properties of the membrane [7,8]. Chitosan (Chi) has been found to be an effective wall material of microcapsules in biomedical fields due to its ability to reside at the target sites within the human body for prolonged periods with controlled release properties [9]. Chi, a natural polycationic compound, is obtained from chitin by alkaline deacetylation, and it shows good solubility in dilute aqueous acid solution because of protonation of the amine groups of glucosamine monomers [10,11]. Chi is also being used as wall materials of microcapsules in food [12], tissue engineering [13], and textile applications [14,15], as it is biodegradable, nontoxic and biocompatible [16]. Chi-based microcapsules obtained by emulsification, precipitation, and spraying methods have single or multilayer membrane structure depending on the microencapsulation method [17,18]. In many scientific literatures, microcapsules are reported to be formed with cationic polyelectrolyte Chi by electrostatic interaction with negatively charged alginate molecules [19], and Chi-alginate microcapsules have been proved to be attractive in multiple fields such as biomedicine, biotechnology, and food [20].

In our earlier study, linseed oil-loaded multilayer microcapsules were developed by oil-in-water emulsification using sodium dodecyl sulfate (SDS) as anionic emulsifier and then, formation of multilayer shell membrane was done through ionic gelation by stepwise addition of the membrane materials Chi and SDS in the emulsion [21]. Linseed oil is obtained from the seed of the flax plant *Linum usitatissimum* and, in comparison with other vegetable oils, linseed oil is distinguished by having the highest content of α-linolenic acid (52% of total fatty acids) which is reported to have a role in decreasing inflammation [22]. Natural polyesters formed from linseed oil have several applications, including biodegradable elastomers and adhesives [23]. The linseed oil-loaded microcapsule formation involved electrostatic interaction between SDS and Chi on the surface of oil droplets stabilized by SDS molecules in the emulsion [24,25]. Biomedical application of SDS is already reported and the vesicles formed with SDS and positively charged azobenzene containing surfactant are used in developing a gene delivery system where photo-triggered release of nucleic acids from the vesicles is achieved [26,27]. Mild alkali treatment of microcapsules was done to solidify the outer shell of microcapsules and charge neutralization of amine groups of Chi on the microcapsules by alkali led to the formation of flocculi in the suspension [21]. However, the post treatment of microencapsules with alkali gave rise to some undesired gel formation by Chi chains and flocculi developed from alkali treatment often produced aggregates in the system, and this is the main drawback for commercial use of this slurry in various applications especially for textiles.

In the present study, linseed oil loaded microcapsule samples obtained from step by step process using Chi and SDS solutions were subject to alkali treatment with a small amount of 1-butanol (butanol) to avoid aggregate formation during alkali treatment. In the study, no chemical cross-linker was used to rigidify the shell membrane and rather ionic gelation between Chi and SDS was applied to develop consecutive shells. Butanol, a primary alcohol with a 4-carbon structure was used in this study to retard gel formation by Chi chains in the system. It was reported in literature that swelling of Chi hydrogel was less in a butanol-water mixture than only in water due to the hydrophobic character of alkyl group (butyl) attached to the hydroxyl group of the alcohol [28]. A small amount of butanol was added in alkali solution to restrict swelling of the outermost shell of microcapsules. In this study, alkali treated microcapsule samples were subject to react with trisodium citrate (citrate) solution for buffering action and ionic cross-linking. Rana *et al.* reported [29] that cationic polyamines like Chi attain ordered microcapsule structure under certain salt solutions, and multivalent counter-ion condensation of Chi in citrate solution leads to rapid formation of ordered microcapsules structure from ionically cross-linked polymer aggregates. Chi ionically cross-linked with citrate shows pH dependent swelling in gastro-intestinal environment [30,31]. The zeta potential and size distribution of alkali-treated samples were investigated to understand the effect of butanol stabilization and citrate treatment on the microcapsules. The changes in morphology and properties of alkali treated microcapsule samples were monitored using FTIR, optical microscopy, scanning electron microscopy (SEM), atomic force microscopy (AFM) combined with surface roughness, and wetting measurements.

## 2. Results and Discussion

### 2.1. Step by Step Microencapsulation Process and Alkali Treatment of Microcapsules

The microcapsules were formed by deposition of Chi on the surface of oil droplets in an oil-in-water emulsion using SDS as anionic emulsifier. Linseed oil was encapsulated by Chi based microcapsules to develop carrier system for this flaxseed oil which has various pharmacological applications [32]. The interaction of positively charged Chi molecules with anionic SDS molecules on the surface of oil droplets led to the microcapsules' shell formation in the emulsion system [21].

The multilayer membrane formation on the microcapsules involved alternate step-by-step addition of SDS and Chi solutions. The rearrangement of the charge groups of wall materials (Chi and SDS) on the surface took place in order to add layers by electrostatic interaction during a step-by-step addition process. However, the electrostatic interaction between SDS and Chi on the surface of microcapsules was partially hindered by the large hydrophobic part of wall materials and this resulted in lowering of interaction between oppositely charged groups of wall materials on the surface of microcapsules [33]. Moreover, unwanted complex formation between Chi and SDS molecules was increased during multilayer microcapsule formation. In our earlier publications, we reported strategies to reduce aggregate formation and enhance interaction of wall materials during formation of microcapsules with a multilayer shell structure [15,33]. The formation of microcapsules by step by step addition of Chi and SDS solutions gave rise to multilayer membrane structure, and positive zeta potential values of microcapsules indicated that microcapsules were formed with a high residual positive charge on their surface [21]. Additionally, positive zeta potential values of microcapsules were found to be increased with layer numbers ($\geq$+30 mV) as microcapsules were becoming overcharged due to the positive charge of Chi molecules. The overcharging of microcapsules' surfaces with positive charge of Chi molecules impeded successive layer formation as SDS addition during multilayer formation could not switch the zeta potential value of microcapsules from positive to negative [21]. So, the calculated amount of SDS and Chi solutions was added during multilayer shell formation in order to avoid overcharging by Chi moieties and maximize the interaction between oppositely charged wall materials [15,33].

The mild alkali treatment of microcapsules was done in order to rigidify the outermost shell of microcapsules. The addition of mild NaOH solution (0.02 N) to microcapsules' suspension led to the development of flocculi by charge neutralization of amine groups of Chi in the microcapsules, and flocculation indicated the phase separation of linseed oil-loaded microcapsules after alkali treatment in the suspension. Nevertheless, alkali treatment of microcapsules was always accompanied by gel formation of Chi molecules and aggregation of microcapsules as charge neutralization took place at protonated amine groups of Chi on the surface of microcapsules by alkali solution. The addition of a small amount of butanol in alkali solution during alkali treatment of microcapsules reduced unwanted gel formation by Chi molecules and impeded aggregate formation by microcapsules in microcapsule suspension.

## 2.2. Influence of Butanol Stabilization on Alkali Treatment of Microcapsules

The property and morphology studies were carried out for a one-layer microcapsule sample to investigate first shell membrane formation over oil droplets in an oil-in-water emulsion, four layers to understand multilayer formation, and 10 layers to study the final product. As shown in Table 1, the mean diameter of alkali treated microcapsules with butanol stabilization varied according to the number of layers of microcapsules. The mean diameter values of alkali-treated microcapsule samples without butanol stabilization were reported earlier, and the mean diameters ± SD of one layer, four layers and 10 layers were 3.6 µm ± 3.4, 5.1 µm ± 5.1, and 5.4 µm ± 4.5, respectively [21]. Table 1 clearly indicates that mean diameter of microcapsules was significantly reduced after butanol treatment up to four layers. The mean diameters of alkali-treated microcapsules after butanol treatment were also measured for six layers (37.5 µm ± 17.0) and eight layers (54.1 µm ± 20.5). The earlier reported mean diameters values of six layers (6.0 µm ± 5.6) and eight layers (6.5 µm ± 4.9) without butanol treatment indicated that mean diameter values of alkali treated microcapsules (four, six and 10 layers) after butanol treatment were higher than samples without butanol treatment. Butanol showed a stabilizing effect during alkali treatment to reduce the aggregation of the microcapsules by controlling their swelling in mild aqueous alkali solution up to four layers [28]. The increased diameter of the sample after four layers might be explained by enhanced swelling of microcapsules in the alkali solution as close packing of the multilayer was somehow relaxed to increase its mean diameter.

The alkali-treated one-layer microcapsules showed negative zeta potential of −12.3 mV, whereas alkali-treated microcapsule samples with higher layer numbers showed positive zeta potential values with butanol treatment (Table 1). The zeta potential values were found to be very similar to the earlier reported values for alkali-treated samples before butanol stabilization [21]. The zeta potential values of alkali-treated microcapsules without butanol treatment were reported to be −20.4, +3.6, and +28.5 mV for one layer, four layers and 10 layers, respectively [21]. The zeta potential results indicated that added alkali amount to the microcapsules suspension was not enough for complete charge neutralization of microcapsules after one layer.

**Table 1.** Mean diameter, zeta potential, and pH values of alkali treated microcapsule samples after butanol stabilization and trisodium citrate treatment.

| Microcapsule Samples | Alkali Treated Samples [a] | | | Alkali Treated Samples [b] | | |
|---|---|---|---|---|---|---|
| | Mean Diameter (µm) | Zeta Potential (mV) | pH | Mean Diameter (µm) | Zeta Potential (mV) | pH |
| 1 layer | 2.3 ± 0.8 | −12.3 | 5.4 | 3.3 ± 1.1 | −1.8 | 7.0 |
| 4 layers | 4.5 ± 2.5 | +7.7 | 5.4 | 5.4 ± 4.2 | −1.7 | 7.0 |
| 10 layers | 61.5 ± 5.2 | +19.5 | 5.4 | 69.7 ± 18.8 | −2.3 | 7.0 |

[a] Butanol stabilization; [b] Butanol stabilization & trisodium citrate treatment ± Standard deviation (SD).

Microcapsules were formed from an oil-in-water emulsion using Chi and SDS as shell materials. FTIR spectra of Chi (Sigma-Aldrich, Saint-Quentin Fallavier, France) and SDS were given in Figure 1. SDS powder (Figure 1A) showed peak near 3450 cm$^{-1}$ representing the bending vibration of adsorbed molecular water. A peak at 2950 cm$^{-1}$ indicated the asymmetric stretching vibration of -CH$_3$, and peaks assigned to asymmetric and symmetric stretching of -CH$_2$- were found at 2920 and 2850 cm$^{-1}$, respectively. The asymmetric and symmetric deformation vibrations of -CH$_3$ were found at 1470 and 1380 cm$^{-1}$, respectively. The peaks for asymmetric and symmetric stretching of the S=O of SDS were found at 1220 and 1108 cm$^{-1}$, respectively. The peak at 995 cm$^{-1}$ was assigned to the asymmetrical stretching vibration of C–O–S. FTIR spectra of low molecular weight Chi powder showed its characteristic peaks: O-H and N-H stretching of Chi powder near 3470 cm$^{-1}$; asymmetric and symmetric stretching of C-H of Chi at 2928 and 2856 cm$^{-1}$, respectively; C-O stretching of amide I at 1652 cm$^{-1}$, and C-O-C stretching of glycosidic linkage at 1146 and 1096 cm$^{-1}$.

**Figure 1.** FTIR spectra of (**A**) sodium dodecyl sulfate (SDS); (**B**) low molecular weight Chi.

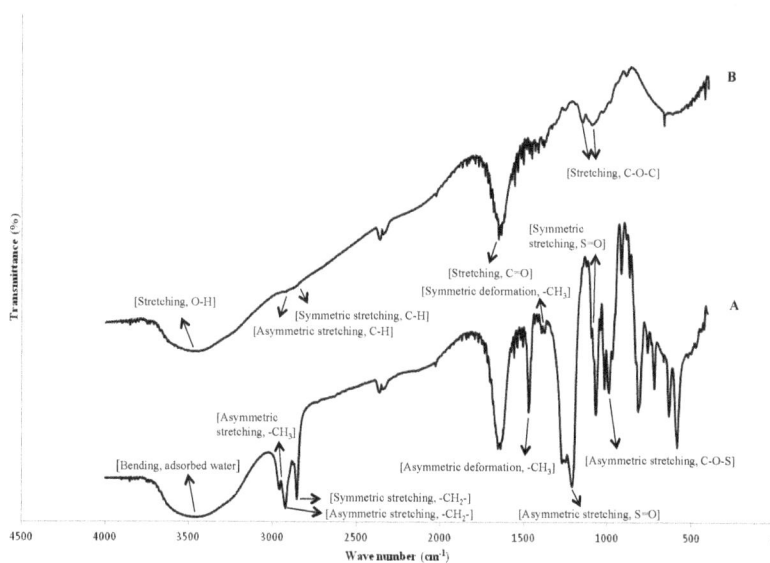

Linseed oil-loaded alkali-treated microcapsule samples after butanol stabilization showed characteristic FTIR peaks of the components (Figure 2), 3476 cm$^{-1}$ representing O-H and N-H stretching of Chi; 2926 and 2857 cm$^{-1}$ representing C-H stretching (asymmetric and symmetric, respectively) of CH$_2$ for linseed oil, Chi, and SDS; and the shoulder on 2926 cm$^{-1}$ at 2956 cm$^{-1}$ represented asymmetric C-H stretching of CH$_3$. The peak at 3014 cm$^{-1}$ represented C-H stretching of aliphatic -CH=CH- which was related to un-conjugated cis-double bonds of linseed oil [34]. The peak at 1648 cm$^{-1}$ was representing C=O stretching of amide I of Chi. The other peaks were at 1556 cm$^{-1}$ (N-H bending of amide II of Chi), 1464 cm$^{-1}$ (C=C ring stretching of linseed oil), and 1106 cm$^{-1}$ (S=O stretching of SDS). FTIR spectra of alkali-treated samples before butanol stabilization were listed in Figure 2 and the spectral characteristics of microcapsules were not noticeably changed after butanol addition during alkali treatment as butanol only acts as a stabilizer in the system.

74

**Figure 2.** FTIR spectra of (**A**) alkali treated microcapsule sample; (**B**) alkali treated microcapsule sample with butanol stabilization; C: alkali treated microcapsules sample with butanol stabilization and citrate treatment.

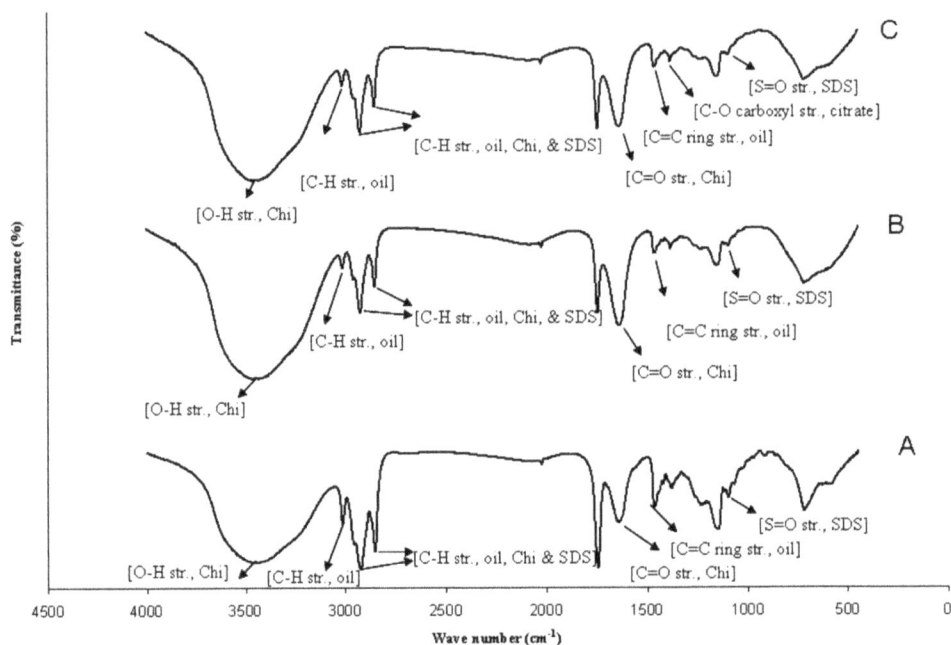

The optical microscopy of alkali-treated microcapsules after butanol treatment (Figure 3) at 40× magnification indicated that microcapsules were well dispersed in the suspension, and sample with 10 layers (Figure 3) showed highly dispersed microcapsules in the micrographs. The optical micrographs exhibited that the unwanted gel formation and aggregation of microcapsules were highly decreased by butanol addition during alkali treatment. Thereby, butanol as a stabilizer during alkali treatment of microcapsules inhibited aggregate formation and acted as dispersant to disperse microcapsules in the system.

The formation of film or functional coating from microcapsule samples over drying on solid support occurred in two consecutive steps: at first, coalescence of the particles occurred followed by a drying step in which the water was released to rigidify or dehydrate the polymer film. It should be taken into account that the shell of microcapsules was not rigidified using any chemical cross-linker and the microcapsule suspension did not produce solid powder after drying on substrate at room temperature. Therefore, the influence of the alkali treatment on the microcapsules could be detected from the surface modification, characterized in this study by roughness, and surface energy of functional coating. The SEM image of functional coating formed from the butanol stabilized one-layer sample (Figure 4A) at 300× magnification showed the presence of microcapsules among a considerable amount of free polymer (Chi). The SEM images of four layers (Figure 4B) and 10 layers (Figure 4C) at 300× indicated the presence of very few microcapsules in a significant amount of polymers, and aggregates were found in their respective functional coatings. Thereby, post treatment of microcapsules caused significant changes on the surface of functional coating, and aggregate formation after post treatment was higher for the microcapsules with a higher number of layers.

**Figure 3.** Optical microscope images at 40× of alkali treated microcapsule samples with butanol stabilization: (**top**) and alkali treated microcapsules samples with butanol stabilization and citrate treatment (**bottom**).

## butanol stabilization

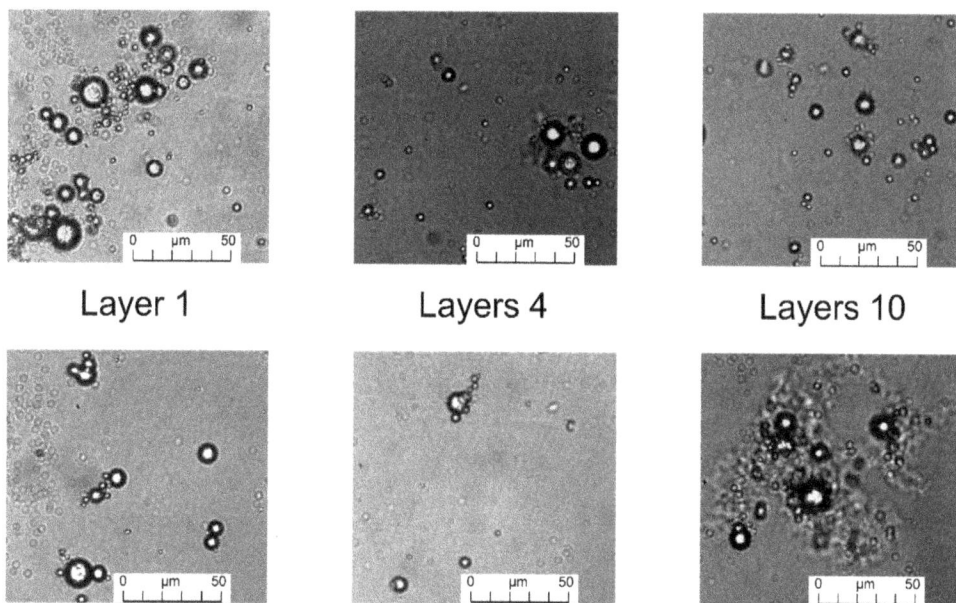

| Layer 1 | Layers 4 | Layers 10 |

## butanol stabilization & citrate treatment

As seen in Table 2, the $\gamma^p$ value of functional coating formed from butanoyl-stabilized alkali-treated microcapsules was increased with an increase in layer numbers, and the $\gamma^p$ value of four layer-(52.2 mN·m$^{-1}$) samples was much higher than that of one layer (21.0 mN·m$^{-1}$) suggesting that polar functional groups of Chi were more exposed on the surface of four layers than that of one layer. Furthermore, a lower $\gamma^d$ value of four layers (15.0 mN·m$^{-1}$) than that of one layer (26.6 mN·m$^{-1}$) was also obtained. These surface energy values suggested that arrangement of polar groups on the surface of microcapsules took place. The lower $\gamma^p$ values of functional coatings for 10 layers (33.9 mN·m$^{-1}$) than that of four layers (52.2 mN·m$^{-1}$), and also, higher $\gamma^d$ values of 10 layers (32.2 mN·m$^{-1}$) than that of four layers (15.0 mN·m$^{-1}$) emphasized that polar groups of Chi were found less on the surface of functional coating with higher layer numbers. During consecutive layer formation on the shell membrane, the hydrophobic non polar groups of SDS and Chi were found more on the surface than that of polar groups of shell materials and that resulted in higher $\gamma^d$ values of 10 layers than that of four layers, and lower $\gamma^p$ values of 10 layers than that of four layers as well. In general, the masking of polar amine groups of Chi was found to be lower in the microcapsule sample with found layers and that gave rise to a maximum polarity value for the four layer sample. So, surface energy values of these microcapsule samples indicated that molecular arrangement on the surface of microcapsules took place due to post treatment of microcapsules by alkali with butanol.

**Figure 4.** SEM images at 300× of alkali treated microcapsule samples with butanol stabilization: (**A**) one layer; (**B**) four layers; (**C**) 10 layers; AFM images of alkali-treated microcapsule samples with butanol stabilization: (**D**) one layer; (**E**) four layers; (**F**) 10 layers.

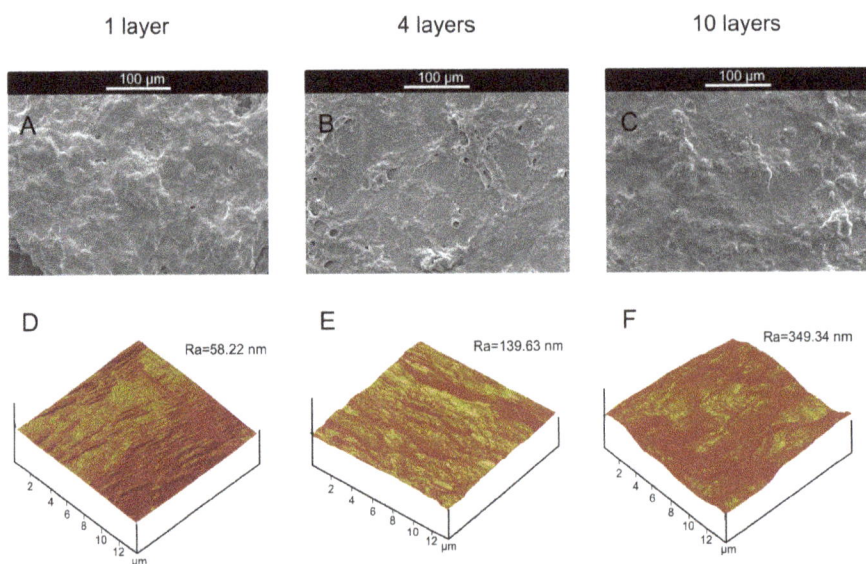

As found in Table 2, average surface roughness of functional coating increased with increasing layer numbers of microcapsules, and surface roughness of functional coating was determined from their respective AFM images (Figure 4D–F). The functional coating (one layer) obtained from post treated microcapsules with butanol showed average surface roughness of 58.22 nm (Figure 4D) and this value was increased to 349.34 nm after increasing layer numbers of microcapsules to 10 layers (Figure 4F). Thereby, post treatment with butanol significantly affected the surface roughness of functional coating, and higher surface roughness resulted from uneven distribution of wall materials on the surface during post treatment.

**Table 2.** Contact angle ($\theta$) and surface energy ($\gamma$) of alkali treated microcapsule samples with butanol stabilization by the Owens and Wendt method, and mean surface roughness of samples in solid state by AFM analysis.

| Alkali Treated Microcapsules Samples (Butanol Stabilization) | $\theta_{water}$ [a] (°) | $\theta_{diiodomethane}$ [a] (°) | $\gamma^p$ (mN/m) | $\gamma^d$ (mN/m) | $\gamma$ (mN/m) | Ra [b] (nm) |
|---|---|---|---|---|---|---|
| 1 layers | 55.8 | 46.6 | 21.0 | 26.6 | 47, 6 | 58.22 |
| 4 layers | 23.6 | 60.5 | 52.2 | 15.0 | 67,2 | 139.63 |
| 10 layers | 29.4 | 25.5 | 33.9 | 32.2 | 66,1 | 349.34 |

[a] Average of contact angle of 5 liquid drops; [b] Average of surface roughness ($R$) obtained at 10 different locations of AFM image.

*2.3. Influence of Citrate Treatment on Butanol Stabilized Alkali-Treated Microcapsules*

Table 1 showed that alkali treated microcapsules after citrate treatment exhibited similar zeta potential values for all the samples namely, one, four, and 10 layers. The negatively charged citrate ions acted as a conjugated base of weak acid (citric acid) in the suspension and caused same extent of charge neutralization for all alkali-treated microcapsule samples. Thereby, buffering action of citrate was exhibited in the system and that created similar negative zeta potential values for all the alkali-treated microcapsule samples. Moreover, Chi chains were ionically cross-linked by citrate ions that led to rapid formation of ordered microcapsule structure in citrate salt solutions by multivalent counter-ion condensation [29]. The mean diameter results of citrate-treated microcapsules indicated that mean diameter was increased with the number of layers of microcapsules.

Microcapsules after butanol stabilization and citrate treatment showed characteristic FTIR peaks which were very similar to those found for the alkali-treated microcapsule samples before citrate treatment as mentioned above (Figure 2). The peak at 1386 cm$^{-1}$ represented C-O symmetric vibration of carboxyl groups of citrate [35].

The optical microscope images of butanol stabilized alkali treated microcapsules (Figure 3) at 40× magnification showed that microcapsules were well dispersed in the suspension after citrate treatment and the images were very similar to the images found for alkali-treated microcapsules with butanol stabilization (Figure 3). Therefore, no significant change was imposed on the structure of microcapsules by citrate treatment of alkali-treated microcapsules stabilized with butanol. However, some aggregates of microcapsules were found in the suspension of 10 layers (Figure 3), due to charge neutralization and the cross-linking effect of citrate ions.

SEM images of alkali-treated microcapsule samples after butanol stabilization and citrate treatment (Figure 5A–C) showed that one layer sample at 300× (Figure 5A) had the presence of few microcapsules among a substantial amount of free polymer. SEM study was done for functional coating which was developed from microcapsule suspension after drying the substrate at room temperature, and the functional coating was formed from free Chi chains due to water evaporation. SEM micrographs showed that some microcapsules were embedded in the functional coating formed by free Chi chains. SEM analysis of functional coating of four layers (Figure 5B) and 10 layers (Figure 5C) after citrate treatment showed the presence of few microcapsules among a significant amount of polymer. Thereby, the morphology obtained from SEM analysis clearly indicated that the citrate treatment of the samples could not impart any significant effect on the morphology of the materials as the samples were more or less the same.

Table 3 showed that $\gamma^p$ value of four layers (36.4 mN·m$^{-1}$) after citrate treatment of butanol stabilized alkali treated microcapsules was higher than that of one layer (20.3 mN·m$^{-1}$), and this trend clearly indicated that microcapsules with four layers possessed more polar functional groups of Chi on the surface that of one layer. However, four layer sample before citrate treatment showed a higher $\gamma^p$ value (52.2 mN·m$^{-1}$) that that of four layer-samples (36.4 mN·m$^{-1}$) after citrate treatment, and this trend clearly indicated that citrate treatment caused some changes in the arrangement of polar groups of Chi on the surface of microcapsules. Furthermore, $\gamma^p$ values of 10 layers (33.9 and 31.9 mN·m$^{-1}$) before and after citrate treatment, respectively, suggested that citrate treatment caused some changes in the arrangement of polar groups of Chi on the surface of functional coating formed after drying the sample at room temperature and polar groups of Chi were less exposed on the surface of the samples. This was also confirmed by $\gamma^d$ values of the samples before and after citrate treatment. Therefore, citrate ions played a role in the arrangement of polar groups of Chi on the surface of microcapsules.

**Figure 5.** SEM images at 300× of alkali treated microcapsule samples with butanol stabilization and citrate treatment: (**A**) one layer; (**B**) four layers; (**C**) 10 layers; AFM images of alkali treated microcapsule samples with butanol stabilization and citrate treatment: (**D**) one layer; (**E**) four layers; (**F**) 10 layers.

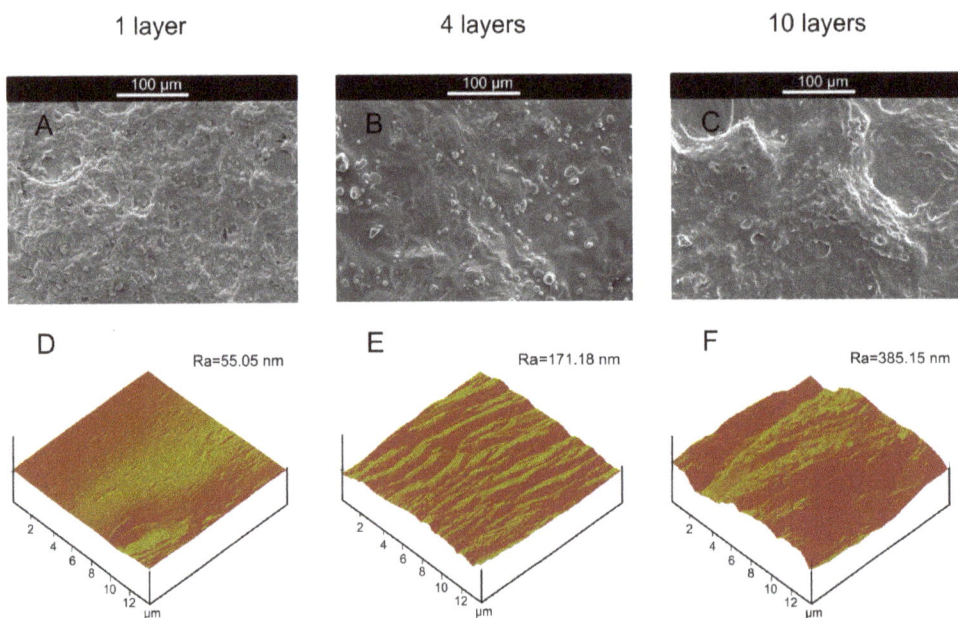

Table 3 clearly indicated that average surface roughness of the samples after citrate treatment was increased by increasing layer numbers and these results were similar to those obtained for the samples before citrate treatment (Table 2). The average surface roughness of the microcapsules with one layer obtained from AFM (Figure 5D) was 55.05 nm, while that of 10 layers (Figure 5F) was 385.15 nm, indicating multilayer formation on the microcapsules enhanced surface roughness of sample. The citrate treatment of butanol stabilized alkali treated microcapsule sample did not impart any additional effect on the surface roughness of functional coating as the values were more or less same for the samples before and after citrate treatment, and these results were highly corroborated by other microscopic observations.

**Table 3.** Contact angle (θ) and surface energy (γ) of alkali-treated microcapsule samples with butanol stabilization and trisodium citrate treatment by the Owens and Wendt method, and mean surface roughness of samples in solid state by AFM analysis.

| Alkali Treated Microcapsules Samples (Butanol Stabilization + Citrate Treatment) | $\theta_{water}$ [a] (°) | $\theta_{diiodomethane}$ [a] (°) | $\gamma^p$ (mN/m) | $\gamma^d$ (mN/m) | $\gamma$ (mN/m) | Ra [b] (nm) |
|---|---|---|---|---|---|---|
| 1 layers | 55.4 | 43.1 | 20.3 | 28.4 | 48.7 | 55.05 |
| 4 layers | 38.9 | 51.3 | 36.4 | 21.3 | 57.7 | 171.78 |
| 10 layers | 37.1 | 33.3 | 31.2 | 30.0 | 61.2 | 385.15 |

[a] Average of contact angle of 5 liquid drops; [b] Average of surface roughness (R) obtained at 10 different locations of AFM image.

## 3. Experimental Section

### 3.1. Materials

Chi having low molecular weight (molecular weight = 50,000–190,000 and deacetylation = 75%–85%), SDS, and linseed oil were purchased from Sigma-Aldrich Co. LLC (Saint-Quentin Fallavier, France). The other analytical grade chemical reagents such as acetic acid, hydrochloric acid, sodium hydroxide, diiodomethane were obtained from Sigma-Aldrich Co. LLC. 1-Butanol and trisodium citrate were purchased from Prolabo, France.

### 3.2. Preparation of Microcapsules

The formulation of microcapsules from oppositely charged Chi and SDS as membrane materials involved step-by-step deposition combined with oil-in-water emulsification process using SDS as an anionic emulsifier. It started with making oil-in-water emulsion by homogenizing 20 wt% linseed oil (Ultra-Turrax, T-25 basic, IKA®WERE, Staufen, Germany) with 80 wt% of aqueous SDS (10 g·L$^{-1}$) solution for 30 min at 16,000 rpm and 50 °C. The first step of the step-by-step formation of microcapsules with Chi and SDS involved addition of 35 mL of Chi solution (3%, w/v in 2%, v/v acetic acid) to 100 mL of emulsion containing 8 g·L$^{-1}$ of SDS, and the reaction was carried out under homogenization condition at 50 °C and 16,000 rpm for 15 min. The measured pH of the prepared microcapsules suspension with one layer was found to be 4.2.

The step-by-step microencapsulation process involved alternate addition of 40 mL of 10 g·L$^{-1}$ SDS solution and 20 mL 3% (w/v) Chi solution (50 °C and 1500 rpm) at 30 min time interval between the additions, and the process was repeated 10 times to develop microcapsules with ten layers. The pH of microcapsules suspension during step-by-step layer formation was maintained at pH 4.2 using 0.1 N HCl or 0.1 N NaOH solution.

### 3.3. Modification of Alkali Treatment Step of Microcapsule Suspension

The alkali treatment of microcapsules was done by mixing 5 mL of microcapsule suspension with 20 mL of 0.02 N NaOH at 30 °C for 10 min under stirring at 1500 rpm [20]. In the present study, 1 mL of butanol was added to the alkaline solution to stabilize microcapsules by impeding gel formation of the Chi molecules during alkali treatment and reducing aggregation of microcapsules. The alkali treatment of microcapsules was accompanied by a pH change of the system from pH 4.2–5.4. The microcapsule samples namely, one layer, and four and ten layers were selected for alkali treatment. The microcapsule samples obtained after alkali treatment were subject to citrate treatment. The citrate treatment of alkali-treated microcapsules was done by reacting 25 mL 0.1 (M) citrate solution with 25 mL of alkali treated microcapsules suspension under stirring at 1500 rpm and 30 °C for 30 min. The citrate treatment helped to increase the pH value of the microcapsule suspension from 5.4–7.2 for one layer, and from pH 5.4–7.0 for four, and ten layers as shown in Table 1. Before freeze drying of the sample, repeated washing and centrifugation were done to remove unreacted materials (Chi, SDS, alkali, citarte) and butanol.

### 3.4. Characterization

#### 3.4.1. Zeta Potential Measurement

The zeta potential of alkali-treated microcapsules suspensions was measured by Zetasizer 2000, Malvern instruments Ltd., Malvern, UK after diluting the samples with de-ionized water 1000 times.

#### 3.4.2. Size Distribution Analysis by Granulometry

The size distribution analysis (granulometry) of microcapsules suspension was performed using Accusizer Particle Sizing Systems (770 Optical Particle Sizer, and 770A Autodiluter), Santa Barbara, CA, USA after diluting the sample 1000 times in de-ionized water to measure the mean diameter of microcapsules.

#### 3.4.3. Chemical Characterization

FTIR spectroscopy of freeze dried microcapsule samples was done using Nicolet Nexus FTIR spectrometer. The optical microscopy of microcapsule samples was done using Axioskos Zeiss equipped with a camera (IVC 800 12S). For FTIR analysis of each sample, 3 scans were assigned for the wave number of 4000–450 cm$^{-1}$.

#### 3.4.4. Scanning Electron Microscopy (SEM) and Atomic Force Microscopy (AFM)

The scanning electron microscopy (SEM) of samples was done by Leica Cambridge S-360 microscope (Leica Cambridge Instrument, Cambridge, UK) operated at an acceleration voltage of 20 kV. The samples for SEM were prepared by depositing single drop of a pre-agitated suspension onto carbon tape, followed by drying at room temperature for 48 h. The drying of microcapsule samples on the solid support at room temperature produces a functional coating.

The surface roughness of microcapsule samples in solid state and PET fabric samples was determined by atomic force microscopy (AFM) at ambient conditions using light tapping mode (TM-AFM), Nanoscope III digital instrument (version 3.2) equipped with image processing software, version 3.2 (Digital Instrument Inc., Digital Instrument Inc., Tonawanda, NY, USA). The set point frequency of the silicon pyramidal cantilever with 4–6 Hz scan speed was about 272 Hz. The microcapsule samples used for AFM in the dry state were prepared by making a film on small and thin glass substrate. The mean roughness (Ra) of surface is expressed by the equation:

$$Ra = \frac{1}{L_x L_y} \int_0^{L_x} \int_0^{L_y} |F(x,y)| dx dy \tag{1}$$

where $L_x$ and $L_y$ are the dimensions of surface, and $F(x, y)$ is the roughness curve relative to the center plane. The mean roughness is the average of Ra obtained at 10 different locations.

### 3.4.5. Wetting Measurement

The surface energy of microcapsule samples was determined from contact angle values of sample with two different probe liquids by the Owens and Wendt method [36]. The contact angles of microcapsule samples in solid state were determined with GBX Digidrop Contact Angle meter (GBX, Bourg de Peage, France) by sessile drop technique. The Owens and Wendt method is based on the following equations:

$$\gamma_L (1 + \cos \theta) = 2\sqrt{\gamma_S^d \gamma_L^d} + 2\sqrt{\gamma_S^p \gamma_L^p} \tag{2}$$

$$\gamma_S = \gamma_S^d + \gamma_S^p \tag{3}$$

where $\theta$ is contact angle, and $\gamma$, $\gamma^p$, and $\gamma^d$ are total, polar component and dispersive component of surface energy, respectively. The two test liquids were water ($\gamma$ = 72.8 mN·m$^{-1}$, $\gamma^p$ = 51.0 mN·m$^{-1}$, and $\gamma^d$ = 21.8 mN·m$^{-1}$) and diiodomethane ($\gamma$ = 50.8 mN·m$^{-1}$, $\gamma^p$ = 2.3 mN·m$^{-1}$, and $\gamma^d$ = 48.5 mN·m$^{-1}$). The subscripts L and S denote liquid and solid, respectively. The samples of microcapsules for surface energy analysis were prepared by uniform deposition of solutions containing microcapsules on thin glass substrate, dried at room temperature conditions for 48 h.

## 4. Conclusions

Linseed oil, a leading source of omega-3 fatty acid α-linolenic acid, was encapsulated by Chi-based microcapsules, and the present study was focused on the development of a suitable carrier system for linseed oil which has various biomedical applications. Multilayer microcapsules were formed from an oil in water emulsification by step wise addition of Chi and SDS solution, and alkali treatment of microcapsules was done to rigidify its outermost shell. In this study, no chemical cross-linker was used to rigidify the shell membrane, and multilayer shell membrane was formed through ionic gelation using SDS and Chi. Rigidification of the shell membrane was finally achieved using a mild alkali solution. However, aggregation of microcapsules and gel formation of Chi molecules in alkali solution were the major drawbacks of the process. The present study was focused on the development of microcapsules with less aggregation during alkali treatment. Here, butanol was used as a stabilizer in alkali solution to minimize the problems of microcapsule aggregation and formation of Chi gel in the system. The changes in morphology and the chemical properties of alkali-treated microcapsules after using butanol were investigated by various microscopic techniques like optical microscopy, SEM and AFM, and analytical techniques like zeta potential, size distribution, FTIR, and wetting measurements. After alkali treatment of microcapsules with butanol, the microcapsules were treated with a citrate solution to stabilize the charge of microcapsules. The citrate ion as a conjugated base of the weak acid (citric acid) caused charge neutralization of protonated amine groups of Chi by buffering action, and all of the microcapsules varieties showed similar zeta potential values. Also, multivalent counter-ion condensation of Chi chains in citrate solutions led to the rapid formation of an ordered microcapsule structure. Citrate treatment did not have any additional stabilizing effect on the structure after butanol but caused some changes in the arrangement of polar groups of Chi on the surface of microcapsules as obtained from wetting experiments. The surface roughness was significantly increased with multilayer formation as the wall materials were not arranged on the surface in the regular manner. The main focus of this study was to develop a carrier system for linseed oil which was formed with better morphological and chemical properties than our earlier reported carrier for linseed oil. In future research, loading and release of linseed oil from the Chi-based carrier and its thermal acid under gastro-intestinal conditions, oxidative (peroxide and anisidine value), and colloidal stability will be reported to give more insight to this carrier for linseed oil.

## Acknowledgments

We gratefully acknowledge financial support from the project ACHILLE (Applied comfort and Health in light leisure equipment)—A crosstexnet ERA-NET project (transnational call 2010—Convention Feder n°11002645). The authors gratefully acknowledge Devan Chemicals and Alexandre Beirão for the SEM images and Ahmida El-Achari for the AFM analyses.

## Author Contributions

Sudipta Chatterjee, Fabien Salaün and Christine Campagne designed the research. Sudipta Chatterjee performed the research. Sudipta Chatterjee, Fabien Salaün and Christine Campagne analyzed and interpreted data. Sudipta Chatterjee, Fabien Salaün and Christine Campagne wrote the paper.

## Conflicts of Interest

The authors declare no conflict of interest.

## References

1. Li, M.; Rouaud, O.; Poncelet, D. Microencapsulation by solvent evaporation: State of the art for process engineering approaches. *Int. J. Pharm.* **2008**, *363*, 26–39.
2. Balazs, A.C. Challenges in polymer science: Controlling vesicle-substrate interactions. *J. Polym. Sci. Part B Polym. Phys.* **2005**, *43*, 3357–3360.
3. Fournier, E.; Passirani, C.; Montero-Menei, C.N.; Benoit, J.P. Biocompatibility of implantable synthetic polymeric drug carriers: Focus on brain biocompatibility. *Biomaterials* **2003**, *24*, 3311–3331.

4.  Lensen, D.; Vriezema, D.M.; Hest, J.C.M.V. Polymeric microcapsules for synthetic applications. *Macromol. Biosci.* **2008**, *8*, 991–1005.
5.  Badulescu, R.; Vivod, V.; Jausovec, D.; Voncina, B. Grafting of ethylcellulose microcapsules onto cotton fibers. *Carbohydr. Polym.* **2008**, *71*, 85–91.
6.  Salaün, F.; Creach, G.; Rault, F.; Giraud, S. Microencapsulation of bisphenol-A bis (diphenyl phosphate) and influence of particle loading on thermal and fire properties of polypropylene and polyethylene terephtalate. *Polym. Degrad. Stab.* **2013**, *98*, 2663–2671.
7.  Wang, C.; Ye, S.; Dai, L.; Liu, X.; Tong, Z. Enzymatic desorption of layer-by-layer assembled multilayer films and effects on the release of encapsulated indomethacin microcrystals. *Carbohydr. Res.* **2007**, *342*, 2237–2243.
8.  Kumar, R.; Nagarwal, R.C.; Dhanawat, M.; Pandit, J.K. *In-vitro* and *in vivo* study of indomethacin loaded gelatin nanoparticles. *J. Biomed. Nanotechnol.* **2011**, *7*, 1–9.
9.  Zhang, J.; Xia, W.; Liu, P.; Cheng, Q.; Tahi, T.; Gu, W.; Li, B. Chitosan modification and pharmaceutical/biomedical applications. *Mar. Drugs* **2010**, *88*, 1962–1987.
10.  Sacco, L.D.; Masotti, A. Chitin and chitosan as multipurpose natural polymers for groundwater arsenic removal and $As_2O_3$ delivery in tumor therapy. *Mar. Drugs* **2010**, *8*, 1518–1525.
11.  Agnihotri, S.A.; Mallikarjuna, N.N.; Aminabhavi, T.M. Recent advances on chitosan based micro- and nanoparticles in drug delivery. *J. Controlled Release* **2004**, *100*, 5–28.
12.  Shi, X.Y.; Tan, T.W. Preparation of chitosan/ethylcellulose complex microcapsule and its application in controlled release of Vitamin D2. *Biomaterials* **2002**, *23*, 4469–4473.
13.  Venkatesan, J.; Kim, S.K. Chitosan composites for bone tissue engineering—An overview. *Mar. Drugs* **2010**, *8*, 2252–2266.
14.  Alonso, D.; Gimeno, M.; Sepúlveda-Sánchez, J.D.; Shirai, K. Chitosan-based microcapsules containing grapefruit seed extract grafted onto cellulose fibers by a non-toxic procedure. *Carbohydr. Res.* **2010**, *345*, 854–859.
15.  Chatterjee, S.; Salaün, F.; Campagne, C. Development of multilayer microcapsules by a phase coacervation method based on ionic interactions for textile applications. *Pharmaceutics* **2014**, *6*, 281–297.
16.  Alves, N.M.; Mano, J.F. Chitosan derivatives obtained by chemical modifications for biomedical and environmental applications. *Int. J. Biol. Macromol.* **2008**, *43*, 401–414.
17.  Yuen, C.W.M.; Yip, J.; Liu, L.; Cheuk, K.; Kan, C.W.; Cheung, H.C.; Cheng, S.Y. Chitosan microcapsules loaded with either miconazole nitrate or clotrimazole, prepared via emulsion technique. *Carbohydr. Polym.* **2012**, *89*, 795–801.
18.  Sinha, V.R.; Singla, A.K.; Wadhawan, S.; Kaushik, R.; Kumria, R.; Bansal, K.; Dhawan, S. Chitosan microspheres as a potential carrier for drugs. *Int. J. Pharm.* **2004**, *274*, 1–33.
19.  Li, X.Y.; Jin, L.J.; Mcallister, T.; Stanford, K.; Xu, J.Y.; Lu, Y.N.; Zhen, Y.H.; Sun, Y.X.; Xu, Y.P. Chitosan–Alginate Microcapsules for Oral Delivery of Egg Yolk Immunoglobulin (IgY). *J. Agric. Food Chem.* **2007**, *55*, 2911–2917.
20.  Wang, X.; Zhu, K.X.; Zhou, H.M. Immobilization of glucose oxidase in alginate-chitosan microcapsules. *Int. J. Mol. Sci.* **2011**, *12*, 3042–3054.

21. Chatterjee, S.; Salaün, F.; Campagne, C.; Vaupre, S.; Beirão, A. Preparation of microcapsules with multi-layers structure stabilized by chitosan and sodium dodecyl sulfate. *Carbohydr. Polym.* **2012**, *90*, 967–975.

22. Simopoulos, A.P. The importance of the ratio of omega-6/omega-3 essential fatty acids. *Biomed. Pharmacother.* **2002**, *56*, 365–379.

23. Ashby, R.D.; Foglia, T.A.; Solaiman, D.K.Y.; Liu, C.K.; Nuñez, A.; Eggink, G. Viscoelastic properties of linseed oil-based medium chain length poly(hydroxyalkanoate) films: Effects of epoxidation and curing. *Int. J. Biol. Macromol.* **2000**, *27*, 355–361.

24. Mun, S.; Decker, E.A.; McClements, D.J. Effect of molecular weight and degree of deacetylation of chitosan on the formation of oil-in-water emulsions stabilized by surfactant–chitosan membranes. *J. Colloid Interface Sci.* **2006**, *296*, 581–590.

25. Aoki, T.; Decker, E.A.; McClements, D. Influence of environmental stresses on stability of O/W emulsions containing droplets stabilized by multilayered membranes produced by a layer-by-layer electrostatic deposition technique. *J. Food Hydrocoll.* **2005**, *19*, 209–220.

26. Liu, Y.C.; Ny, A.L.M.L.; Schmidt, J.; Talmon, Y.; Chmelka, B.F.; Lee, C.T., Jr. Photo-assisted gene delivery using light-responsive catanionic vesicles. *Langmuir* **2009**, *25*, 5713–5724.

27. Shim, M.S.; Kwon, Y.J. Stimuli-responsive polymers and nanomaterials for gene delivery and imaging applications. *Adv. Drug Deliv. Rev.* **2012**, *64*, 1046–1059.

28. Bamgbose, J.T.; Bamigbade, A.A.; Adewuyi, S.; Dare, E.O.; Lasisi, A.A.; Njah, A.N. Equilibrium swelling and kinetic studies of highly swollen chitosan film. *J. Chem. Chem. Eng.* **2012**, *6*, 272–283.

29. Rana, R.K.; Murthy, V.S.; Yu, J.; Wong, M.S. Nanoparticle self-assembly of hierarchically ordered microcapsule structures. *Adv. Mater.* **2005**, *17*, 1145–1150.

30. Shu, X.Z.; Zhu, K.J.; Song W. Novel pH-sensitive citrate cross-linked chitosan film for drug controlled release. *Int. J. Pharm.* **2001**, *212*, 19–28.

31. Rana, V.; Babita, K.; Goyal, D.; Tiwary, A. Sodium citrate cross-linked chitosan films: Optimization as substitute for human/rat/rabbit epidermal sheets. *J. Pharm. Pharm. Sci.* **2005**, *8*, 10–17.

32. Oomah, D. Flaxseed as a functional food source. *J. Sci. Food Agric.* **2001**, *81*, 889–894.

33. Chatterjee, S.; Salaün, F.; Campagne, C.; Vaupre, S.; Beirão, A.; El-Achari, A. Synthesis and characterization of chitosan droplet particles by ionic gelation and phase coacervation. *Polym. Bull.* **2014**, *71*, 1001–1013.

34. Grehk, T.M.; Berger, R.; Bexell, U. Investigation of the drying process of linseed oil using FTIR and ToF-SIMS. *J. Phys. Conf. Ser.* **2008**, *100*, 012019.

35. Rao, C.N.R. *Chemical Application of Infrared Spectroscopy*; Academic Press: New York, NY, USA, 1963.

36. Owens, D.K.; Wendt, R.C. Estimation of the surface free energy of polymers. *J. Appl. Polym. Sci.* **1969**, *13*, 1741–1747.

# Recent Modifications of Chitosan for Adsorption Applications: A Critical and Systematic Review

George Z. Kyzas and Dimitrios N. Bikiaris

**Abstract:** Chitosan is considered to be one of the most promising and applicable materials in adsorption applications. The existence of amino and hydroxyl groups in its molecules contributes to many possible adsorption interactions between chitosan and pollutants (dyes, metals, ions, phenols, pharmaceuticals/drugs, pesticides, herbicides, *etc.*). These functional groups can help in establishing positions for modification. Based on the learning from previously published works in literature, researchers have achieved a modification of chitosan with a number of different functional groups. This work summarizes the published works of the last three years (2012–2014) regarding the modification reactions of chitosans (grafting, cross-linking, *etc.*) and their application to adsorption of different environmental pollutants (in liquid-phase).

Reprinted from *Mar. Drugs*. Cite as: Kyzas, G.Z.; Bikiaris, D.N. Recent Modifications of Chitosan for Adsorption Applications: A Critical and Systematic Review. *Mar. Drugs* **2015**, *13*, 312-337.

## 1. Introduction

Chitosan (poly-β-(1→4)-2-amino-2-deoxy-D-glucose) is a nitrogenous (amino-based) polysaccharide (Figure 1a), which is produced in large quantities by *N*-deacetylation of (its origin compound) chitin [1–3]. Chitin (poly-β-(1→4)-*N*-acetyl-D-glucosamine) can be characterized as one of the most abundant natural biopolymers (Figure 1b) [4,5]. Chitin exists in marine media and especially in the exoskeleton of crustaceans, or cartilages of mollusks, cuticles of insects and cell walls of micro-organisms. Chitosan can be easily characterized as a promising material not only due to its physical properties (macromolecular structure, non-toxicity, biocompatibility, biodegradability, low-cost, *etc.*) [2], and applications to many fields (biotechnology, medicine, membranes, cosmetics, food industry, *etc.* [6–18]), but also its adsorption potential.

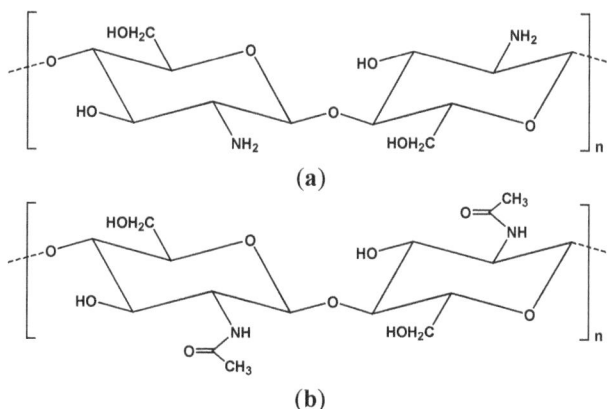

**Figure 1.** Chemical structure of (**a**) chitosan and (**b**) chitin.

Since the primary research work of Muzzarelli in 1969, who described the synthesis and adsorption evaluation of chitosan for the removal of metal ions from organic and sea waters [19], numerous papers have been published regarding the use of chitosan as adsorbent for decontamination of wastewaters (or effluents, sea waters, drinking samples, *etc.*) from various pollutants, either organic (dyes, phenolic and pharmaceutical compounds, herbicides, pesticides, drugs, *etc.*) or inorganic species (metals, ions, *etc.*). In order to obtain a more realistic view of the published works regarding the adsorption use of chitosan during time-periods, the following results were exported after the Scopus database screening (using the terms "chitosan" in combination with "adsorption" or "removal"): (i) 15 papers for 1969–1990; (ii) 116 papers for 1991–2000; (iii) 811 papers for 2001–2010, and (iv) 850 papers for 2011–2014. The results are relative and approximate, because many other papers are not present in the Scopus database or the search is not accurate. However, in any case, the trend is clear.

As it is clearly understood, the major advantage of chitosan is the existence of modifiable positions in its chemical structure. The modification of chitosan molecule with (i) grafting (insert functional groups) or (ii) cross-linking reactions (unite the macromolecular chains each other) leads to the formation of chitosan derivatives with superior properties (enhancement of adsorption capacity and resistance in extreme media conditions, respectively). In the case of grafting reactions, the addition of extra functional groups onto chitosan increases the number of adsorption sites and consequently the adsorption capacity. On the other hand, the cross-linking reactions slightly decrease the adsorption capacity because some functional groups of chitosan (*i.e.*, amino or hydroxyl groups) are bound with the cross-linker and cannot interact with the pollutant. As a general comment, in more recent years (after 1990), researchers have attempted to prepare chitosan-based adsorbent materials modifying the molecules of chitosan.

The scope of this work is to gather and summarize the most recent and updated published works of the last three years (2012–2014) regarding the modification reactions of chitosan derivatives (grafting, cross-linking, *etc.*). However, the present work is related to only chitosan modified materials synthesized for adsorption application (to different environmental pollutants) and not the sum of modified chitosan materials used for other applications (food science, membrane technologies, *etc.*). Scopus database exports 368 review articles for the wide term "chitosan", but only 10 for the combination "chitosan" and "adsorption" or "removal" [20–29]. Therefore, there is a gap in updating the literature published in the last three years emphasizing the modified chitosan adsorbents.

## 2. Modified Chitosans for Dye Adsorption

Auta and Hameed prepared a composite of chitosan and clay for both batch and fixed-bed adsorption experiments [30]. Modified Ball clay (MBC) and chitosan composite (MBC-CH) were the adsorbents used for removal of Methylene blue (MB) from aqueous solutions. For the synthesis of MBC-CH, chitosan was dissolved in acetic acid in order to be mixed and then an amount of MBC was added and stirred for 1 day. The resulted mixture was dropped to NaOH solution in order to form beads. After that, a procedure of freeze-drying was carried out (particle size between 0.5 and 2.0 mm). The effect of pH was tested in the range of 4–10, while the optimum value found was at alkaline conditions. The isotherm curves were fitted to the Langmuir, Freundlich and

Redlich-Peterson models with their non-linear expressions ($Q_m$ = 259.8 mg/g at 30 °C). In the present study, the abbreviation of $Q_m$ corresponds to the maximum theoretical adsorption capacity calculated after fitting to the Langmuir (or Langmuir-Freundlich in some cases) equation. The adsorption columns presented equilibrium capacities (for $C_0$ = 200 mg/L; bed depth = 3.6 cm; flow rate = 5 mL/min) equal to 70 mg/g for MBC and 142 mg/g for MBC-CH.

The same dye (MB) was studied by another research group preparing a magnetic nanocomposite of chitosan/β-cyclodextrin (CDCM) [31]. For its preparation, maleoyl-β-CD was prepared following the method of Binello *et al.* [32]. After SEM (scanning electron microscopy) studies, the shape of the majority of CSCM particles was found to be spherical (~100 nm). The effect-of-pH experiments demonstrated that the highest MB removal was in the range of 4–6 (more protons were available to protonate amino groups to form $NH_3^+$ because the pka of chitosan is 6.0–7.0). The $Q_m$ after fitting (Langmuir, Freundlich equations) was estimated to be 2.78 g/g (30 °C).

A study of Elwakeel *et al.* describes the preparation of a resin based on chitosan and glutaraldehyde [33]. The chemical modification was chemically achieved using $NH_4OH$ for producing the resin, which was then cross-linked with epichlorohydrine. This reaction took place between hydroxyl groups of chitosan molecules. The resultant resin was further modified with 3-amino-1,2,4 triazole,5-thiol to synthesize the final resin (Figure 2). The resin was prepared for binding/removing a cationic dye (BBR250) from aqueous media.

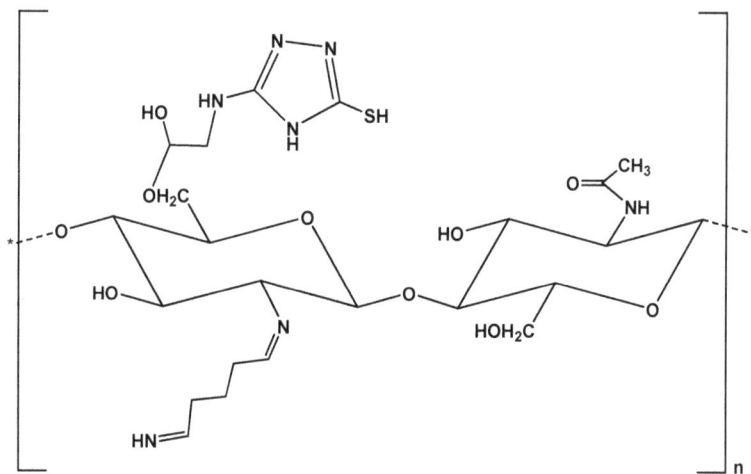

Figure 2. Chemical structure of the modified chitosan resin [33].

The surface area was estimated to be 371.1 $m^2$/g, while the water regain was 17%. The experimental data were fitted to Langmuir and Freundlich model and the adsorption capacity ($Q_m$) was found to be 0.8 mmol/g at 25 °C.

An anionic dye (AR18) was selected to investigate the adsorption properties of chitosan-functionalized with siliceous mesoporous SBA-15 [34]. The final products were SBA-15/CTS(5%), SBA-15/CTS(10%), and SBA-15/CTS(20%). CTS-modified SBA-15 composites were prepared according to rehydrolysis-condensation strategy (Figure 3).

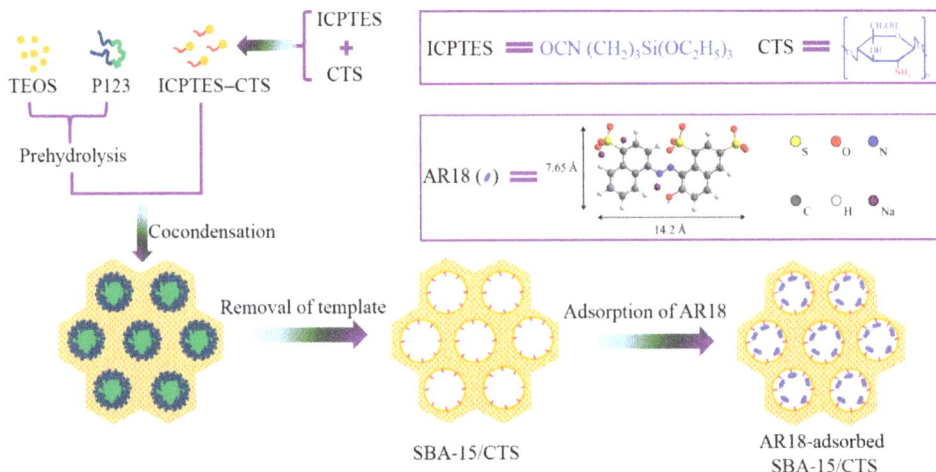

**Figure 3.** Preparation scheme of SBA-15/CTS and its application for the adsorption of AR18. Reprinted with permission from [34], Copyright © 2014 Elsevier Inc.

After characterization, it was observed that the pore sizes of SBA-15, SBA-15/CTS(5%), SBA-15/CTS(10%), and SBA-15/CTS(20%) are 6.6, 6.5, 6.6, and 6.7 nm, respectively, with narrow distributions. The latter demonstrated that the porosity of those materials was not affected by the incorporation of chitosan due to condensation. CTS-modified SBA-15 composites were hydrophilic and the pH-effect experiments (in the range of 4–7) showed a strong dependence of dye uptake on pH (higher adsorption at low pH values; optimum pH value was 2). After fitting with Langmuir model, the highest $Q_m$ was 201.2 mg/g at 30 °C for SBA-15/CTS(20%).

Another anionic dye (RB19) was successfully removed using chitosan grafted with poly(methyl methacrylate) (Figure 4) [35]. The synthesis included two steps: (i) functionalization of chitosan (CTS) with glycidyl methacrylate (GMA) in aqueous solution with pH = 3.8; and (ii) synthesis of the copolymer-(CTS-GMA)-g-PMMA using the mixed solvent of acetic acid and tetrahydrofuran (v/v, 2/1). The molar ratio of CTS/GMA/MMA was 1/1/1. The maximum dye uptake was 1498 mg/g (Langmuir fitting) at 30 °C (pH = 3).

Guo *et al.* modified the chitosan molecule using bentonite [36]. Chitosan modified bentonite (CTS-Bent) and chitosan-hexadecyl trimethyl ammonium bromide modified bentonite (CTS-CTAB-Bent) were the two final products after modifications and were tested for the removal of WASC dye from aqueous solutions. For the synthesis of the materials, a fixed amount of bentonite was added into deionized water and then quaternary ammonium salt solution was added to the above mixture with strong stirring. Chitosan solution was added step by step at a certain temperature. After stirring and cooling down to room temperature, the sample was filtered and washed with deionized water until no bromide ion detected by silver nitrate solution. From the FTIR spectra, a new band at 1564 cm$^{-1}$ was related to the NH$_2$ vibration mode of the chitosan, which indicated that the chitosan molecule was inserted into the interlayer space of the bentonite. The optimum synthesis conditions for the adsorption of 100 mg/L WASC solution were 1%

chitosan and 10% CTAB at 80 °C and 2.5 h. So, the final removal for 1CTS-10CTAB-Bent was higher than 85% ($Q_m = 102$ mg/g) [36].

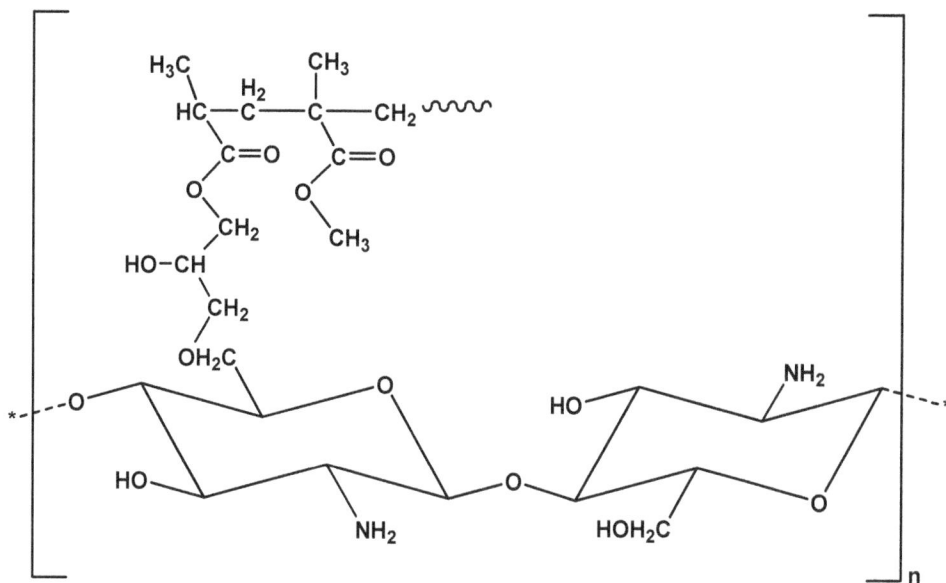

**Figure 4.** Chemical structure of chitosan grafted with poly(methyl methacrylate).

A more complex modification was recently published by Li *et al.* aiming to remove lysozyme using magnetic chitosan, which was previously modified with an affinity dye-ligand (RR120) [37]. The effect of this modification was determined by the increased adsorption amount of lysozyme (116.9 mg/g) on dye-modified microspheres, compared to only absorbing 24.6 mg/g on unmodified magnetic chitosan microspheres. The dye was grafted with covalent bonds onto the surface of magnetic chitosan microspheres via a nucleophilic substitution reaction.

Nezic *et al.* published a research article which presented data about synthesis of chitosan/zeolite composite [38]. In particular, chitosan/zeolite A films were produced after mixing chitosan solutions and dispersions of zeolite A in water. The zeolite A amount in the films was determined to be 40% of chitosan mass. The final films had no color and their thickness was approximately 0.1. The surface of the films was uniform with many agglomerates which were equally distributed all over the surface. An anionic dye used for adsorption evaluation (BO16); the equilibrium data were fitted to Langmuir and Freundlich models, presenting $Q_m = 305.8$ mg/g. This value was taken at pH = 6, which preliminarily was found to be optimum (after pH-effect experiments in the range of 4.0–7.5).

Chitosan-modified palygorskite (CTS-modified PA) was prepared by Peng *et al.* in order to remove an anionic dye (RY3RS) from aqueous media [39]. 3-Aminopropyl triethoxysilane (KH-550) was used as coupling reagent for the synthesis of the grafted derivative. The preparation route is simple; KH-550 was used to add aminopropyl groups onto the plygorskite (PA) surface. Briefly, PA (dried at 105 °C) was dispersed in fixed volume of toluene, and then KH-550 was added and dissolved (continuous stirring). The resulted solution was refluxed and PA was separated by filtration. The KH-550-modified PA was dried at room temperature in vacuum overnight. This product was soaked into glutaraldehyde; chitosan powder was dissolved in acetic acid solution. The two solutions were mixed and the reacted PA was separated using centrifugation and $Na_2CO_3$. CTS-modified PA was finally isolated by centrifugation, then washed with distilled water, and dried in vacuum [39]. For the adsorption experiments, the optimum pH value was found to be 4 and at this value the $Q_m$ was 71.38 mg/g (Langmuir and Freundlich fittings).

Sadeghi-Kiakhani *et al.* synthesized a chitosan grafted polypropylene imine in dendrimer form [40]. As model dye compounds, two anionic dyes were used (RB5 and RR198). The adsorption capacities of the material for both dyes can be characterized as huge (RB5, 6250 mg/g; RR198, 5852 mg/g). The fitting was done with three models (Langmuir, Freundlich, Temkin).

Yan *et al.* studied a more complex adsorption phenomenon, in which two model dyes (AO7 and AG25) were competitively adsorbed onto beads of chitosan grafted with diethylenetriamine [41]. Langmuir and Freundlich equations were run for fitting. $Q_m$ was calculated as 6.02 and 4.37 mmol/g for AO7 and AG25 in single-component solutions, respectively. For binary mixtures, 4.10 and 3.51 mmol/g were the respective values. From this study, characterization techniques do not exist.

Zhu *et al.* prepared chitosan-modified magnetic graphitized multi-walled carbon nanotubes (CS-m-GMCNTs) for removing CR from aqueous media [42]. The surface area of the prepared chitosan modified material was measured (BET analysis) as 39.20 m²/g. The maximum dye uptake was shown at pH = 6.3 and at this value the $Q_m$ was calculated (Langmuir and Freundlich models) as 263.3 mg/g. Authors also made a direct comparison with other chitosan CR adsorbents of recent literature (not those published in 2012–2014); $Q_m$ for CR adsorption on chitosan hydrobeads [43], chitosan [44], and *N,O*-carboxymethyl-chitosan/montmorillonite nanocomposite [45] were 92.59, 81.23, 74.24 mg/g, respectively.

A recent study of our research team [46] investigated the synthesis of a novel composite material (GO-Ch) consisting of cross-linked chitosan (Ch) and graphite oxide (GO) for the removal of RB5. All prepared products (GO, Ch, and GO-Ch) were ground to fine powders, with a size after sieving of 75–125 μm. The capacities found after fitting demonstrated that the functionalization of chitosan enhanced the $Q_m$ (205, 224, and 277 mg/g (pH = 2) for GO, Ch, and GO-Ch).

Travlou *et al.* reveal the use of magnetic chitosan (Chm) instead of pure (Ch) in the functionalization and synthesis of graphite oxide/magnetic chitosan composite (GO-Chm) [47]. It was found that for GO, the $Q_m$ was 221 mg/g (pH = 3) and 391 mg/g for GO-Chm. The possible interactions were illustrated in Figure 5 (found and proposed after characterization techniques).

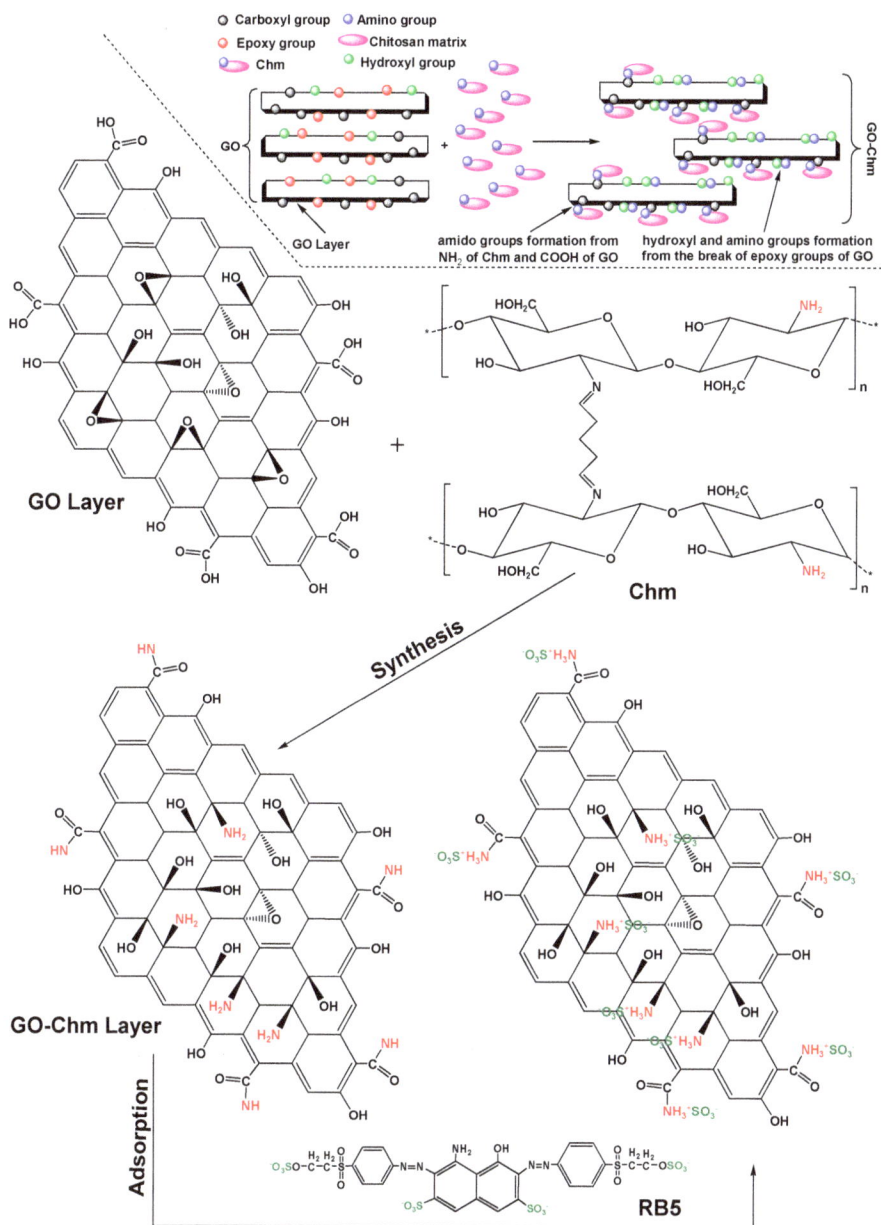

**Figure 5.** Proposed mechanism of synthesis of graphite oxide/magnetic chitosan composite (GO-Chm) after functionalization of magnetic chitosan (Chm) onto graphite oxide (GO). Proposed interactions of the Reactive black 5 (RB5) adsorption onto the prepared GO-Chm. Reprinted with permission from [47], Copyright © 2013 American Chemical Society.

92

Special note should be made of a selective adsorbent synthesized after modification of chitosan. Kyzas *et al.* prepared molecularly imprinted polymers of chitosan (CHI-MIPs) in order to selectively remove RR3BS (anionic dye) for aqueous solutions [48]. $Q_m$ was approximately 35 mg/g and the selectivity very high (in a dye mixture containing other dyes).

Table 1 summarizes all the aforementioned modified chitosans and their respective adsorption application.

**Table 1.** Studies of the adsorption of dyes using modified chitosan adsorbents during 2012–2014.

| Modified Chitosan Adsorbent | Dye | Isotherms | $Q_m$ | Ref. |
|---|---|---|---|---|
| Modified Ball clay/Chitosan composite | MB | L, F, R-P | 259.8 mg/g | [30] |
| β-cyclodextrin/chitosan magnetic nanocomposite | MB | L, F | 2788 mg/g | [31] |
| Chitosan/glutaraldehyde/3-amino-1,2,4 triazole,5-thiol resin | BBR250 | L, F | 0.8 mmol/g | [33] |
| Chitosan/SBA-15 | AR18 | L, F | 201.2 mg/g | [34] |
| Chitosan grafted with poly(methyl methacrylate) | RB19 | L | 1498 mg/g | [35] |
| Chitosan modified bentonite | WASC | H, L, F, T, D-R | 102 mg/g | [36] |
| Chitosan/CTAB modified bentonite | WASC | H, L, F, T, D-R | 175 mg/g | [36] |
| Magnetic chitosan grafted with Reactive red 120 | Lysozyme | L | 116.9 mg/g | [37] |
| Chitosan/Zeolite A | BO16 | L, F | 305.8 mg/g | [38] |
| Chitosan-modified palygorskite | RY3RS | L, F | 71.38 mg/g | [39] |
| Chitosan grafted with polypropylene imine | RB5 | L, F, T | 6250 mg/g | [40] |
| | RR198 | L, F, T | 5855 mg/g | [40] |
| Chitosan grafted with diethylenetriamine | AO7 | L, F | 6.02 mmol/g | [41] |
| | AG25 | L, F | 4.37 mmol/g | [41] |
| Chitosan-modified magnetic graphitized multi-walled carbon nanotubes | CR | L, F | 263.3 mg/g | [42] |
| Chitosan/Graphite oxide composite | RB5 | L-F | 277 mg/g | [46] |
| Magnetic chitosan/Graphite oxide nanocomposite | RB5 | L-F | 391 mg/g | [47] |
| Chitosan-Molecularly Imprinted Polymers | RR3BS | L, F | 35 mg/g | [48] |

L: Langmuir; F: Freundlich; H: Henry; T: Temkin; D-R: Dubinin-Radushkevich; L-F: Langmuir-Freundlich; R-P: Redlich-Peterson.

## 3. Modified Chitosans for Metals/Ions Adsorption

The number of research articles published in literature during these three years regarding the use of chitosan adsorbents for metal/ion removal from aqueous solutions is by far higher than those for dyes removal. A possible explanation is that metals or/and ions cover a wider region of pollutants than dyes which are more toxic. Another reason could be a particular adsorption mechanism dominant in the majority of chitosan-ions systems which is called chelation. Chelation refers to a fixed manner in which ions and molecules bind to metal ions. The International Union of Pure and Applied Chemistry (IUPAC) provides a detailed description of chelation [49]: it involves the creation or even the presence of two or more separate coordinate bonds between a polydentate (multiple bonded) ligand and a single central atom [49]. In the majority of cases, the ligands are organic-based compounds (namely chelants, chelators, chelating agents). Muzzarelli *et al.* have published many works describing the chelation of different ions with chitosan derivatives [50]. In the present work, the papers with metal/ion adsorption onto modified chitosan adsorbents will be described.

Arvand *et al.* prepared a modified with 3,4-dimethoxybenzaldehyde chitosan derivative (Chi/DMB) for the removal and determination of Cd(II) from waters [51]. The successful synthesis of the new material was confirmed with FTIR spectrum before and after modification. Two new bands were recorded in Chi/DMB; A band at 1655 cm$^{-1}$ can be attributed to an imine bond (N=C) and another one at 1562 cm$^{-1}$ is associated with an ethylenic bond (C=C). The characteristic band of free aldehyde groups (1720 cm$^{-1}$) disappeared. After pH-experiments, an increase of metal uptake was observed as the pH increased from 1.0 to 9.0. However, cadmium started to precipitate from solution and therefore the increased capacity at values higher than 7 may be due to a combination of both adsorption and precipitation on the surface. So, the value selected was 6.5. After running the Langmuir isotherm model, $Q_m$ was found to be 217.4 mg/g.

The removal of U(VI) from wastewaters using chitosan-modified multiwalled carbon nanotubes (MWCNT-CS) was proposed by Chen *et al.* [52]. The maximum ion removal was at pH = 7. Using the Langmuir model, the maximum adsorption capacity was found to be 71 mg/g. Chen and Wang synthesized a xanthate-modified magnetic cross-linked chitosan (XMCS) for the removal of Co(II) [53]. The xanthate-modification was based on the treatment of cross-linked magnetic chitosan with NaOH solution and CS$_2$. After stirring at room temperature (24 h) and washing with deionized water, the final derivative was dried at 70 °C. Langmuir and Freundlich isotherms calculated the $Q_m$ for the material (18.5 mg/g).

Chethan and Vishalakshi attempted the selective modification of chitosan by incorporating ethylene-1,2-diamine molecule in a regioselective manner using *N*-phthaloylchitosan and chloro-6-deoxy *N*-phthaloylchitosan as precursors [54]. The derivatives that resulted were ethylene-1,2-diamine-6-deoxy-*N*-phthaloylchitosan (PtCtsEn) and ethylene-1,2-diamine-6-deoxy-chitosan (CtsEn) and were prepared for Cu(II), Pb(II) and Zn(II) removal. The capacities calculated (Langmuir model) for CtsEn were 41.6, 31.8, and 20.0 mg/g, for Cu(II), Pb(II), and Zn(II), respectively, while for PtCtsEn they were 32.3, 28.6 and 28.6 mg/g, respectively. Another study published by Debnath *et al.* presented the removal results of Cr(VI) after adsorption onto magnetically modified graphene oxide-chitosan composite [55]. The graphene oxide was prepared based on Hummers method [56], and the optimum pH found after adsorption experiments was 3.0. Langmuir, Freundlich and Redlich-Peterson models were used for fitting ($Q_m \sim 75$ mg/g, 25 °C).

Elwakeel *et al.* prepared a resin, which was a structure based on magnetic modified chitosan [57]. Chitosan was initially cross-linked with glutaraldehyde in magnetite presence and then chemically modified reacting with tetraethylenepentamine (TEPA). UO$_2$(II) were removed presenting $Q_m = 1.8$ mmol/g (after fitting to Freundlich, Langmuir, and Dubinin-Radushkevich equations) at pH 4 (25 °C). In this study, column experiments were also carried out varying parameters (flow rate, *etc.*). Eser *et al.* chemically modified the raw chitosan with histidine (HIS-ECH-CB) for increasing the Ni(II) uptake [58]. $Q_m$ was calculated with Langmuir (55.6 mg/g) and Freaundlich models. The cross-linking of material was done using epichlorohydrin, while the immobilization of histidine was performed after washing with Na$_2$CO$_3$ solution. The beads forms were placed in a recipient and 10% (w/v) histidine solution and added to a Na$_2$CO$_3$ solution. The mixture was stirred at 60 °C for 1 day and then the beads were washed until excess non-immobilized histidine was removed.

Gandhi *et al.* prepared a series of modified chitosan beads (CB) in order to remove Fe(III) from aqueous solutions [59]. However, the adsorption capacity of the modified forms of chitosan beads (protonated (PCB), carboxylated (CCB) and grafted CB (GCB)) was not high enough (7.042, 9.346, and 14.286 mg/g, respectively). On the other hand, a series of ions (Cu(II), Co(II), Zn(II), Hg(II), Pb(II)) were removed with another grafted chitosan derivative [60]. The modification reaction was based on the reaction of chitosan with 4,4′-diformyl-α-ω-diphenoxy-ethane. The maximum uptake was presented at pH = 5, and the adsorption capacities calculated were 12, 8, 12, 56, 50 mg/g for Cu(II), Co(II), Zn(II), Hg(II), Pb(II), respectively.

Li *et al.* formed an ethylenediamine modified yeast biomass after coating with magnetic chitosan (EYMC) [61]. Interesting morphological properties were exported after characterization (13.2 m$^2$/g as the surface area), but the most interesting property was on the surface of the EYMC material. Numerous, small bumps existed on the surface, forming a large quantity of pores. These pores may significantly contribute to the transfer of Pb(II) ions to the surface of EYMC. After metal adsorption, the pores were adhered by Pb(II) [61]. The maximum uptake of Pb(II) was shown at pH = 4–6 and the Langmuir (both fitting with Freundlich) equation gave Q$_m$ = 121.6 mg/g. The authors propose the following adsorption interactions between lead and chitosan derivative [61]:

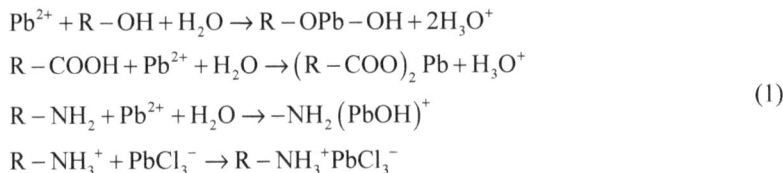

$$Pb^{2+} + R - OH + H_2O \rightarrow R - OPb - OH + 2H_3O^+$$
$$R - COOH + Pb^{2+} + H_2O \rightarrow (R - COO)_2 Pb + H_3O^+$$
$$R - NH_2 + Pb^{2+} + H_2O \rightarrow -NH_2 (PbOH)^+ \tag{1}$$
$$R - NH_3^+ + PbCl_3^- \rightarrow R - NH_3^+ PbCl_3^-$$

Thiocarbohydrazide-modified chitosan (TCHECS) was synthesized for removal of a series of ions (As(V), Ni(II), Cu(II), Cd(II), Pb(II)) [62]. The main application for this study was the evaluation of anti-corrosion ability of TCHECS and not adsorption. For this reason, Q$_m$ was not calculated, but authors observed that the higher uptake was at pH = 9 with 55.6%–99.0% uptake. The same concept was kept in another study by the same research team and two new chitosan grafted materials were prepared [63] and tested just for the same ions (As(V), Ni(II), Cu(II), Cd(II), Pb(II)). Thiosemicarbazide (TSFCS) and thiocarbohydrazide (TCFCS) grafted chitosan were the adsorbents prepared, presenting 66.4%–99.9% and 71.5%–99.9% uptake for the two adsorbents, respectively.

Monier was targeted to the structural modification of chitosan, synthesizing chitosan-thioglyceraldehyde Schiff's base cross-linked magnetic resin (CSTG) [64]. Mercury porosimetry data was used for the characterization of resin, and the average pore size was found to be 795 nm. BET analysis showed that the surface area was 70.5 m$^2$/g. VSM plots indicated that the saturation of magnetization was 29.3 emu/g. This resin was used for the removal of three toxic metals (Hg(II), Cu(II, Zn(II)). The capacities of the resin for Hg(II), Cu(II, Zn(II)) were estimated (Langmuir, Freundlich, Temkin equations) to be 98, 76, 52, mg/g, respectively. Another set of modified chitosan materials (chloroacetic grafted chitosan and glycine grafted chitosan) was produced after equivalent molar amounts of chitosan and glycine/chloroacetic acid in xylene solvent (130 °C for 3 h) [65] were obtained. The key factor of this procedure was the forced stop of this end reaction when the equivalent amount of water was obtained. $Q_m$ was found to be 59.1 (Co(II)), 175.12 (Cu(II)) mg/g for chloroacetic grafted chitosan and 82.9, 165.91 mg/g for glycine grafted chitosan.

Rabelo et al. used only cross-linking reactions for modifying chitosan [66]. The agents used were glutaraldehyde (chitosan-GLA) and epichlorohydrin (chitosan-ECH). The adsorption experiments were done for Cu(II) and Hg(II) removal. Langmuir, Freundlich, Langmuir-Freundlich, Henry, and Toth isotherms fitted the equilibrium results. Chitosan-GLA presented $Q_m$ equal to 2.8 and 3.3 mmol/g for Cu(II) and Hg(II) removal, respectively, while the values for chitosan-ECH were 2.3 and 3.5 mmol/g.

Gandhi and Meenakshi synthesized amino terminated hyperbranched dendritic polyamidoamine 1st generation (1ACB) chitosan beads after the grafting reaction onto the chitosan beads [67]. This modification was done in two stages: (i) Michael addition of methyl acrylate to amino groups on the surface and (ii) amidation of terminal ester groups by ethylene diamine. In this study, the modification reactions are more complex given the synthesis of both 2nd generation chitosan beads (2ACB) and 3rd generation (3ACB) ones. Those were prepared from 1ACB by repeating the above two processes. The authors suggest that for enhancing Cr(VI) adsorption, 3ACB should be further protonated and loaded with Zr(IV). Adsorption results for 3ACB gave $Q_m$ equal to 224.2 mg/g.

Repo et al. investigated the removal of Co(II) by EDTA-modified chitosan [68]. The material prepared has specific surface area of 0.71 $m^2$/g and $1.8 \times 10^{-3}$ $cm^3$/g total pore volume (610 Å average pore size). This adsorbent tested for Co(II) removal and showed $Q_m$ equal to 1.35 mmol/g (Langmuir, Sips equations) Song et al. prepared a novel xanthate carboxymethyl grafted chitosan derivative for removal of Cu(II) and Ni(II) from aqueous solutions (Figure 6) [69]. The effect of pH was tested in the range of 2.0–7.0 and $Q_m$ was calculated using Langmuir and Freundlich models to be 174.2 mg/g and 128.4 mg/g for Cu(II) and Ni(II), respectively.

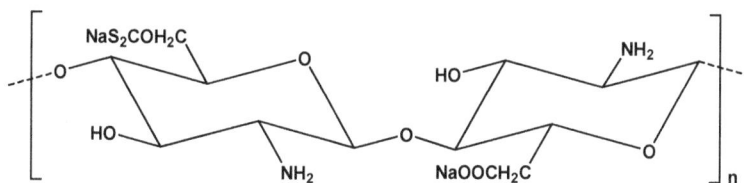

Figure 6. Structure of xanthate carboxymethyl grafted chitosan.

The grafting of n-butylacrylate onto chitosan was studied for use as adsorbent in Cr(VI) uptake [70]. The synthesis procedure was assisted with microwave. FTIR spectrum confirmed the successful preparation of grafted derivative, presenting a peak at 1727 $cm^{-1}$ (ester –C=O group) [70]. For the adsorption experiments, many isotherm models were tested (Langmuir, Freundlich, Dubinin-Radushkevich, Temkin, Elovich and Redlich) and $Q_m$ was found 17.15 mg/g [70]. The authors illustrate a useful scheme for the main interactions (Figure 7).

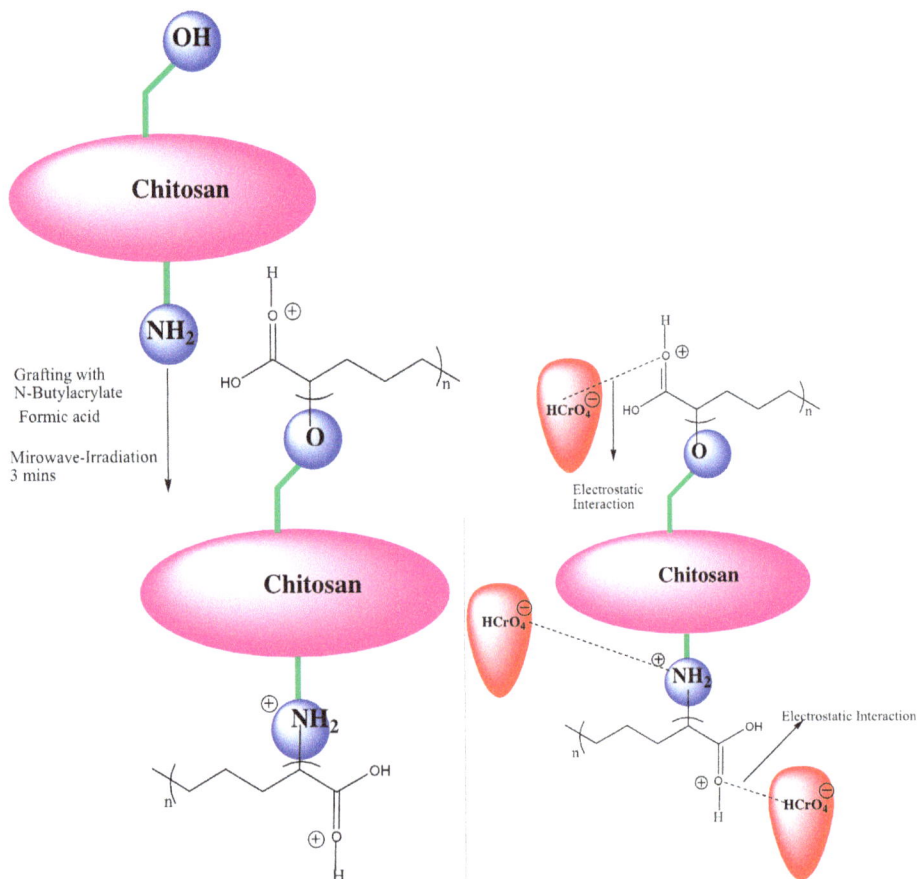

**Figure 7.** Interactions of chitosan, *N*-butylacrylate and chromium(VI). Reprinted with permission from [70], Copyright © 2014 Elsevier B.V.

Suc and Ly achieved the preparation of chitosan flakes which were modified with citric acid and cross-linked with glutaraldehyde [71]. This material was applied to Pb(II) removal, finding that $Q_m$ was 101.7 mg/g (Langmuir, Freundlich, Temkin and Dubinin-Radushkevich models). The authors ran their adsorption experiments at pH = 5 in order to avoid precipitation of Pb(OH)$_2$. Montmorillonite modified with chitosan (CTS-MMT) was another modification achieved by Wang *et al.* for the removal of only Co(II) [72]. 150 mg/g was the $Q_m$ calculated (Langmuir, Freundlich and Temkin equations). Moreover, triethylene-tetramine modified magnetic chitosan (TETA-MCS) was prepared for the removal of Th(IV) from aqueous solutions [73]. Similarly, Langmuir, Freundlich and Temkin models were run for calculation of the maximum adsorption capacity (133.3 mg/g at 25 °C). The same team prepared a similar modified derivative (diethylenetriamine-functionalized magnetic chitosan) for U(VI) removal (65.16 mg/g at 25 °C) [74]. In addition, Yang *et al.* modified magnetic chitosan using α-ketoglutaric acid (α-KA-Fe$_3$O$_4$/CS) for removal of Cd(II) from aqueous solution ($Q_m$ = 201.2 mg/g) [75]. Magnetic chitosan was also prepared by Kyzas and Deliyanni for Hg(II) removal [76]. The optimum pH value for adsorption was 5 and $Q_m$ (fitting with Langmuir and Freundlich model) was 152 mg/g. Furthermore, Kyzas *et al.* used two other modified chitosan adsorbents which were grafted with itaconic acid (CS-g-IA) and cross-linked either with glutaraldehyde (CS-g-IA(G)) or epichlorohydrin (CS-g-IA(E)) (Figure 8). These adsorbents were tested for Cd(II) or Pb(II) uptake. The authors demonstrated that $Q_m$ (Cd(II)) was 405 mg/g and 331 mg/g for CS-g-IA(G) and CS-g-IA(E), respectively, ($Q_m$ were equal to 124 and 92 mg/g before grafting, respectively) [77].

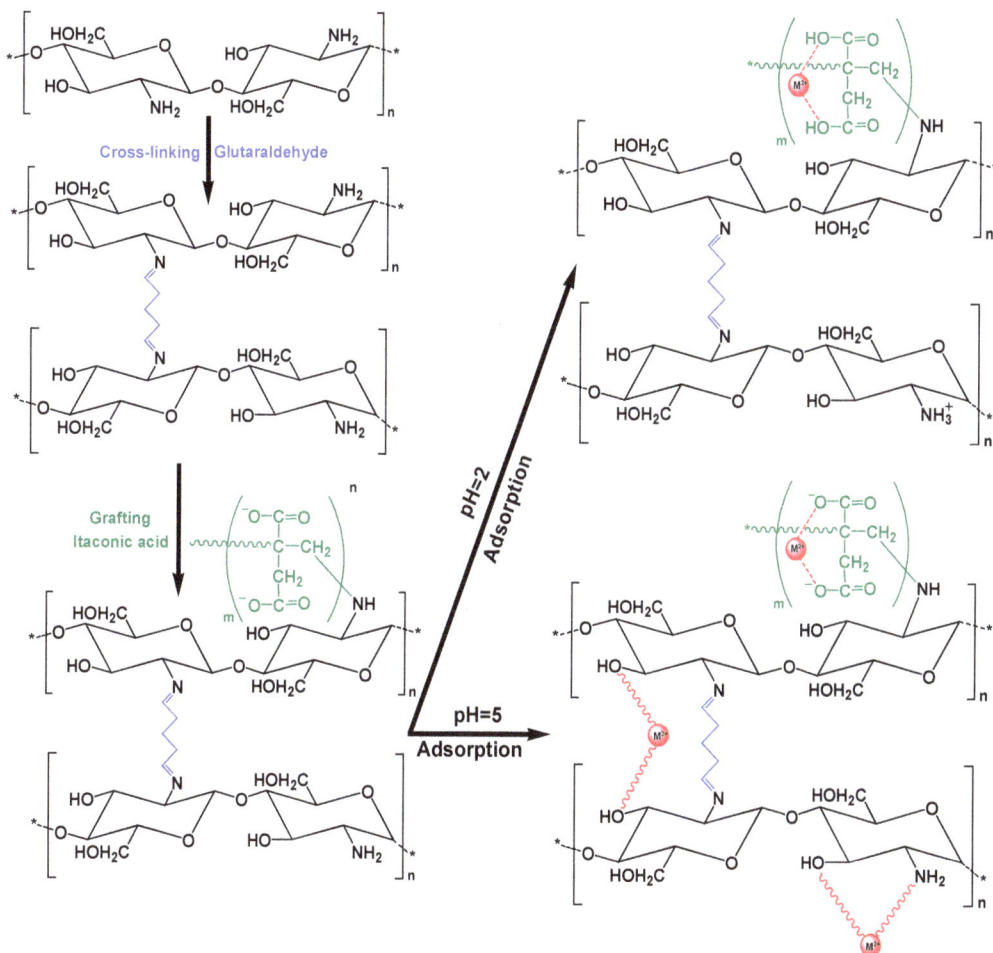

**Figure 8.** Cross-linked and grafted chitosan (CS) with itaconic acid (IA) and interactions between the material cross-linked with glutaraldehyde (CS-g-IA(G)) and metal ions. Reprinted with permission from [77], Copyright © 2014 American Chemical Society.

Table 2 summarizes the aforementioned modified chitosans and their respective adsorption applications to metals/ions.

**Table 2.** Studies of the adsorption of metals/ions using modified chitosan adsorbents during 2012–2014.

| Modified Chitosan Adsorbent | Metals/Ions | Isotherms | Q$_m$ | Ref. |
|---|---|---|---|---|
| Chitosan grafted with with 3,4-dimethoxybenzaldehyde | Cd(II) | L | 217.4 mg/g | [51] |
| Chitosan modified multiwalled carbon nanotubes | U(VI) | L | 71 mg/g | [52] |
| Xanthate-modified magnetic cross-linked chitosan | Co(II) | L, F | 18.5 mg/g | [53] |
| Ethylene-1,2-diamine-6-deoxy-chitosan | Cu(II), Pb(II), Zn(II) | L | 41.6, 31.8, 20.0 mg/g | [54] |
| Ethylene-1,2-diamine-6-deoxy-$N$-phthaloylchitosan | Cu(II), Pb(II), Zn(II) | L | 32.3, 28.6, 18.6 mg/g | [54] |
| Magnetically modified graphene oxide-chitosan composite | Cr(VI) | L, F, R-P | 82 mg/g | [55] |
| Magnetic cross-linked chitosan grafted with tetraethylenepentamine | UO$_2$(II) | L, F, D-R | 486 mg/g | [57] |
| Cross-linked chitosan modified with histidine | Ni(II) | L, F | 55.6 mg/g | [58] |
| Protonated chitosan beads | Fe(III) | L, F | 7.042 mg/g | [59] |
| Carboxymethyl chitosan beads | Fe(III) | L, F | 9.346 mg/g | [59] |
| Grafted chtiosan beads | Fe(III) | L, F, T | 14.286 mg/g | [59] |
| Chitosan grafted with 4,4′-diformyl-α-ω-diphenoxy-ethane | Cu(II), Co(II), Zn(II), | L | 12, 8, 12 mg/g | [60] |
| Chitosan grafted with 4,4′-diformyl-α-ω-diphenoxy-ethane | Hg(II), Pb(II) | L | 56, 50 mg/g | [60] |
| Ethylenediamine-modified yeast biomass coated with magnetic chitosan | Pb(II) | L, F | 121.26 mg/g | [61] |
| Thiocarbohydrazide-modified chitosan | As(V), Ni(II), Cu(II) | | | [62] |
| | Cd(II), Pb(II) | | | [62] |
| Thiosemicarbazide grafted chitosan | As(V), Ni(II), Cu(II) | | | [63] |
| | Cd(II), Pb(II) | | | [63] |
| Thiocarbohydrazide grafted chitosan | As(V), Ni(II), Cu(II) | | | [63] |
| | Cd(II), Pb(II) | | | [63] |
| Chitosan-thioglyceraldehyde Schiff's base cross-linked magnetic resin | Hg(II), Cu(II, Zn(II) | L, F, T | 98, 76, 52 mg/g | [64] |
| Chloroacetic grafted chitosan | Co(II), Cu(II) | L | 59.1, 175.12 mg/g | [65] |
| Glycine grafted chitosan | Co(II), Cu(II) | L | 82.9, 165.91 mg/g | [65] |
| Chitosan cross-linked with glutaraldehyde | Cu(II), Hg(II) | L, F, L-F, H | 177.8, 661.5 mg/g | [66] |

**Table 2.** *Cont.*

| Modified Chitosan Adsorbent | Metals/Ions | Isotherms | $Q_m$ | Ref. |
|---|---|---|---|---|
| Chitosan cross-linked with epichlorohydrin | Cu(II), Hg(II) | L, F, L-F, H | 146.1, 681.7 mg/g | [66] |
| Amino terminated hyperbranched dendritic polyamidoamine 3rd generation chitosan beads | Cr(VI) | L, F, D-R | 224.2 mg/g | [67] |
| EDTA-modified chitosan | Co(II) | L, S | 79.7 mg/g | [68] |
| Chitosan grafted with n-butylacrylate | Cr(VI) | L, F, D-R, T | 17.15 mg/g | [70] |
| Xanthate carboxymethyl grafted chitosan | Cu(II), Ni(II) | L, F | 174.2, 128.4 mg/g | [69] |
| Cross-linked chitosan with citric acid | Pb(II) | L, F, T, D-R | 101.7 mg/g | [71] |
| Montmorillonite modified with chitosan | Co(II) | L, F, T | 150 mg/g | [72] |
| Triethylene-tetramine modified magnetic chitosan | Th(IV) | L, F, T | 133.3 mg/g | [73] |
| Diethylenetriamine-functionalized magnetic chitosan | U(VI) | L, F, S, D-R | 65.16 mg/g | [74] |
| Magnetic chitosan grafted with α-ketoglutaric acid | Cd(II) | L, F, T | 201.2 mg/g | [75] |
| Magnetic chitosan | Hg(II) | L, F | 155 mg/g | [76] |
| Chitosan grafted with itaconic acid | Cd(II), Pb(II) | L-F | 405, 334 mg/g | [77] |

L: Langmuir; F: Freundlich; H: Henry; T: Temkin; D-R: Dubinin-Radushkevich; L-F: Langmuir-Freundlich; R-P: Redlich-Peterson; S: Sips.

## 4. Modified Chitosans for Other Species Adsorption

Apart from the main categories of pollutants (dyes, metals/ions), some other species were recorded in the literature regarding chitosan-modified adsorbents during the last three years. It is important to note that despite the fact there are not many papers on the subject, the under-removal of pollutants is toxic and hazardous for human health and environment; therefore, this subject deserves special attention. Furthermore, PAHs (polycyclic aromatic hydrocarbons) and PCBs (polychlorinated biphenyls) are indeed a serious class of contaminants. However, there were no published studies found in recent literature (as extensively studied in the present review article) regarding the use of chitosan as adsorbent for this type of contaminants.

Poon *et al.* studied the effect of different molar ratios of glutaraldehyde (cross-linkers) on the adsorption capacity of chitosan modified derivatives produced [78]. Three copolymers were synthesized beginning with the same mass of chitosan (6 g), but differentiating the volume of cross-linker in the mixing solution (3.6, 6.3 and 9.0 mL of glutaraldehyde (GLA) solution 50% (w/v) with density 1.106 g/L). Therefore, the calculated GLA/NH$_2$ mole ratios were estimated to be 0.67, 1.17 and 1.68, respectively (samples denoted as CG-1, CG-2, and CG-3, respectively). For the adsorption evaluation, *p*-Nitrophenol was used a model compound, but classical types of isotherms were not exported/given. Only for particular initial phenol concentrations at three fixed values of pH (4.6, 6.6 and 9.0) were the respective adsorption capacities estimated. For CG-1, CG-2, and CG-3, the capacities were calculated as 0.285, 0.327, 0.381 mmol/g (at pH = 4.6). The respective values at pH = 6.6 were 0.289, 0.378, 0.436 mmol/g, while at pH = 9.0 they were 0.306, 0.451, 0.572 mmol/g, respectively. The authors concluded that increasing the cross-linker ratio would result in an increase of the absorption capacity. However, the maximum value occurs at the ration GLA/NH$_2$. This is contrary to what has been published in numerous studies [77,79–81]. Authors also implied that for higher GLA ratio beyond the optimum found above, the result would be because of surface changes and inaccessibility of the sorption sites [78].

Magnetic chitosan derivatives were prepared for the removal of pharmaceutical compounds (diclofenac (DCF), clofibric acid (CA), carbamazepine (CBZ)) from aqueous media [82]. The magnetic chitosan had high sorption affinity for DCF and CA, but for CBZ no sorption was observed. The adsorption capacities of CA and DCF in the single-component solutions were 191.2 and 57.5 mg/g, respectively (Langmuir, Freundlich equations).

Chlorophenols (phenol, 2-chlorophenol (2-CP), 4-chlorophenol (4-CP), 2,4-dichlorophenol (DCP) and 2,4,6-trichlorophenol (TCP)) were also removed with adsorption onto cross-linked chitosan functionalized with β-cyclodextrin [83]. Q$_m$ was calculated for phenol, 2-CP, 4-CP, DCP and TCP on CS-SA-CD and found to be 59.74, 70.52, 96.43, 315.46 and 375.94 mg/g, respectively.

Table 3 summarizes all the aforementioned modified chitosans and their respective adsorption application in other species.

**Table 3.** Studies of the adsorption of other species using modified chitosan adsorbents during 2012–2014.

| Modified Chitosan Adsorbent | Pollutants | Isotherms | Q$_m$ | Ref. |
|---|---|---|---|---|
| Chitosan cross-linked with glutaraldehyde | *p*-nitrophenol | | | [78] |
| Magnetic chitosan | Diclofenac | L, F | 191.2 mg/g | [82] |
| | Clofibric acid | L, F | 57.5mg/g | [82] |
| | Carbamazepine | L, F | - | [82] |
| β-cyclodextrin/cross-linked chitosan | Phenol | L, F | 59.74 mg/g | [83] |
| | 2-chlorophenol | L, F | 70.52 mg/g | [83] |
| | 4-chlorophenol | L, F | 96.43 mg/g | [83] |
| | 2,4-dichlorophenol | L, F | 315.46 mg/g | [83] |
| | 2,4,6-trichlorophenol | L, F | 375.94 mg/g | [83] |
| Chitosan grafted with sulfuric acid | Pramipexole | L-F | 337 mg/g | [84] |
| Chitosan grafted with *N*-(2-carboxybenzyl) | Pramipexole | L-F | 307 mg/g | [84] |
| Graphite oxide/Carboxyl-grafted chitosan | Dorzolamide | L-F | 334 mg/g | [85] |
| Carboxyl-grafted chitosan | Dorzolamide | L-F | 229 mg/g | [85] |

L: Langmuir; F: Freundlich; L-F: Langmuir-Freundlich.

In our previous study, we synthesized two chitosan modified derivatives which were cross-linked with glutaraldehyde and grafted with sulfonate groups (CsSLF) or *N*-(2-carboxybenzyl) groups (CsNCB) [84]. A pharmaceutical compound (pramipexole) was tested for adsorption experiments. After running pH-effect experiments, the optimum pH value was 10. After fitting to the

Langmuir-Freundlich equation, the $Q_m$ values were calculated as 337 and 307 mg/g at 25 °C for CsSLF and CsNCB, respectively. In this work, the most interesting aspect is the adsorption mechanism suggested for both materials. For example, in the case of CsSLF, the proposed mechanism is presented below (Figure 9).

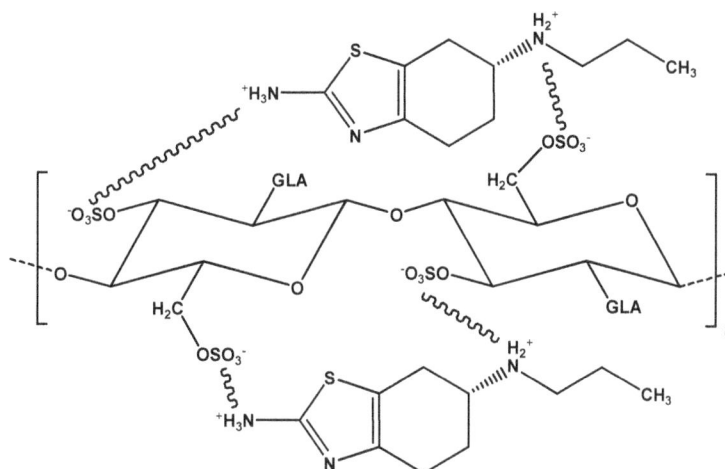

**Figure 9.** Interactions between pramipexole and CsSLF. Reprinted with permission from [84], Copyright © 2013 Elsevier.

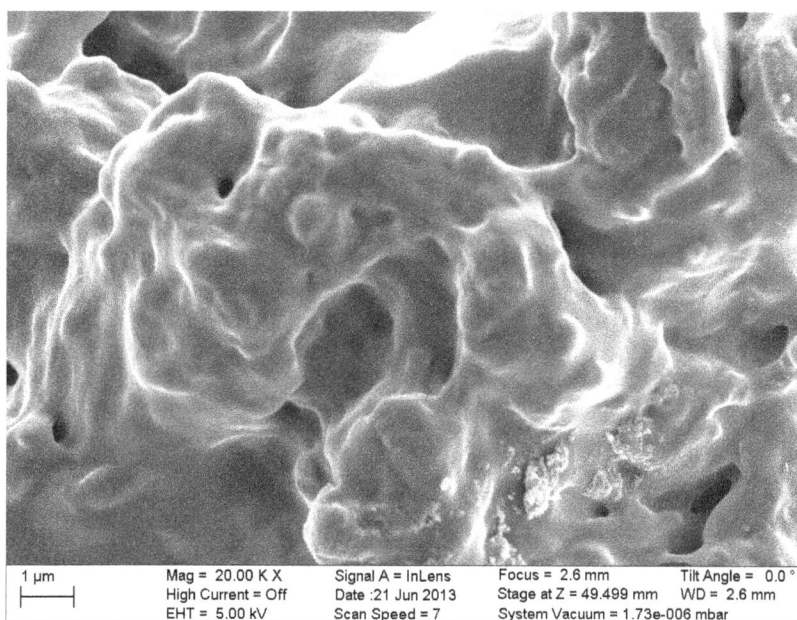

| 1 µm | Mag = 20.00 K X | Signal A = InLens | Focus = 2.6 mm | Tilt Angle = 0.0 ° |
| | High Current = Off | Date :21 Jun 2013 | Stage at Z = 49.499 mm | WD = 2.6 mm |
| | EHT = 5.00 kV | Scan Speed = 7 | System Vacuum = 1.73e-006 mbar | |

(a)

**Figure 10.** *Cont.*

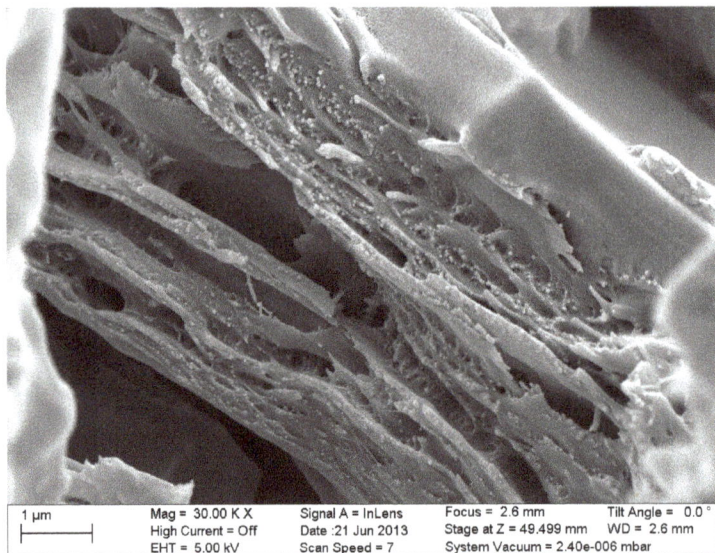

| 1 μm | Mag = 30.00 K X | Signal A = InLens | Focus = 2.6 mm | Tilt Angle = 0.0 ° |
| | High Current = Off | Date :21 Jun 2013 | Stage at Z = 49.499 mm | WD = 2.6 mm |
| | EHT = 5.00 kV | Scan Speed = 7 | System Vacuum = 2.40e-006 mbar | |

**(b)**

**Figure 10.** SEM images of the materials studied **(a)** chitosan cross-linked with glutaraldehyde and grafted with poly(acrylic acid) (CSA); **(b)** composite of cross-linked with glutaraldehyde chitosan which was grafted with poly(acrylic acid) and functionalized with graphite oxide (GO/CSA). Reprinted with permission from [85], Copyright © 2014 Elsevier.

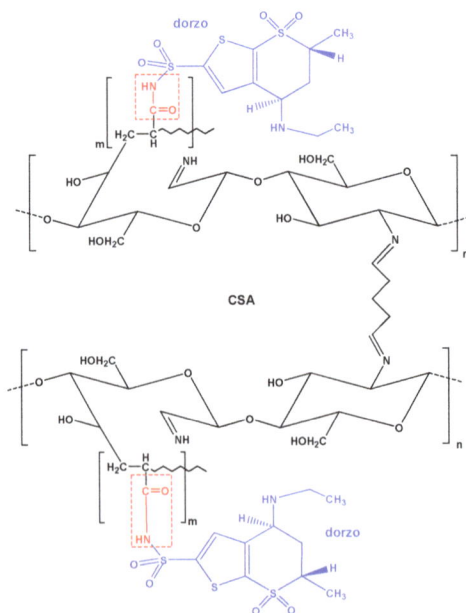

**Figure 11.** Interactions between CSA and dorzo. Reprinted with permission from [85], Copyright © 2014 Elsevier.

The same research team realized another modification in chitosan which was more complex. At first, chitosan was cross-linked with glutaraldehyde and grafted with poly(acrylic acid) to add extra carboxyl groups (denoted as CSA). Then, CSA was functionalized with graphite oxide to produce the final nanocomposite material (GO/CSA) [85]. The surface morphology of the prepared adsorbents is illustrated with SEM images in Figure 10. The latter was used as adsorbent material to remove a particular pharmaceutical compound (dorzolamide) that exists in wastewaters. The optimum pH value was 3. $Q_m$ was calculated with L-F fitting model; for the composite GO/CSA was 334 mg/g, while for the origin materials GO and CSA were 175 and 229 mg/g, respectively.

Similarly, after characterization, the authors proposed an adsorption mechanism between dorzolamide (abbreviated as dorzo) and modified chitosan (CSA) (Figure 11).

## 5. Critical Comparisons

In adsorption technology, it is widely known that two adsorbent materials (even for the same pollutant) cannot be compared without maintaining the same experimental conditions. Some of the basic parameters which strongly influence the whole procedure are (i) the pH solution; (ii) contact time; (iii) initial pollutant's concentration; (iv) temperature; (v) agitation speed; (vi) volume of adsorbate; (viii) ionic strength of solution; (ix) adsorbent's dosage, *etc*. It is clear that if any of the aforementioned conditions vary, the experiment will not be the same and consequently no comparison will be correct. Having the above in mind, the only comparisons that can be realized are those for adsorbent/adsorbate systems of the same study.

Therefore, it is not correct to say that modified ball clay/chitosan composite [30] is a better adsorbent than β-cyclodextrin/chitosan magnetic nanocomposite [31], because the experimental conditions were not the same. The first material presented $Q_m$ equal to 259.8 mg/g for MB adsorption, while the second presented a value of 2788 mg/g for the same dye. The same remark can be concluded for the removal of RB5 with adsorption onto chitosan grafted with polypropylene imine ($Q_m$ = 6250 mg/g) [40], chitosan/graphite oxide composite ($Q_m$ = 277 mg/g) [46] and magnetic chitosan/graphite oxide nanocomposite ($Q_m$ = 391 mg/g) [47]. For those experiments, the adsorption conditions are completely different and therefore an accurate comparison cannot be made.

A similar approach can be takn for the case of metals. As it is clearly shown in Table 2, one of the most studied metals is Cu(II). Many researchers investigated the removal of this metal after modification of chitosan. For example, ethylene-1,2-diamine-6-deoxy-chitosan ($Q_m$ = 41.6 mg/g) and ethylene-1,2-diamine-6-deoxy-$N$-phthaloylchitosan ($Q_m$ = 31.3 mg/g) were synthesized in the literature [54]. However, this synthesis was undertaken with the addition of $N$-phthaloyl groups. The first modified derivative possessed enhanced ability for binding metal ions due to the presence of a flexible ethylenediamine substituent with two nitrogen basic centers in addition to the single bond $NH_2$ at C-2 position. On the other hand, the grafting of $N$-phthaloyl groups renders the material more hydrophobic compared to the former material. Another study employing Cu(II) removal reports the synthesis of chitosan grafted with 4,4′-diformyl-α-ω-diphenoxy-ethane [60], presenting very small adsorption capacity ($Q_m$ = 12 mg/g). It seems that the addition of 4,4′-diformyl-α-ω-diphenoxy-ethane via nucleophilic attack of the amino group of the chitosan on the carbonyl carbon of the aldehyde groups did not improve the adsorption ability of chitosan. Opposite observations were noticed after the adsorption tests on chloroacetic grafted chitosan and glycine grafted chitosan [65]. The grafting of chloroacetic acid on chitosan improved in higher percentages the adsorption capacity ($Q_m$ = 175.12 mg/g) than did the addition of glycine groups ($Q_m$ = 165.91 mg/g). The latter may be due to the structure of functional groups. Another study reported high capacities for modified derivatives which have been only cross-linked (either with glutaraldehyde ($Q_m$ = 177.8 mg/g) or epichlorohydrin ($Q_m$ = 150.4 mg/g)) and not grafted [66]. Obviously, the adsorption conditions were completely different and for this reason the materials prepared showed such high adsorption capacities.

Based on the above, when the grafting reaction of chitosan with various functional groups does not contain nitrogen carriers (for achieving a chelation reaction with metals), the adsorption capacity cannot be enhanced.

## 6. Concluding Remarks

Chitosan is a very promising adsorbent, which can be modified in many ways (grafting, cross-linking, functionalization for forming composites, *etc.*). The potential of chitosan is strong due to its origin product being chitin which can be found in abundance in marine media and especially in the exoskeleton of crustaceans, or cartilages of mollusks, cuticles of insects and cell walls of micro-organisms. However, one serious drawback of using chitosan as adsorbent is its swelling. For this reason, until now industrial use has been limited. However, some international companies purchase industrial grade chitosan for wastewater treatment (Qingdao Develop Chemistry Ltd in China, *etc.*). The recent modifications aim at strengthening the mechanical properties of chitosan in order for it to compete with activated carbon in commercial/industrial applications. A large volume of works has been published during the last three years, presenting results of chitosan-modified adsorbents for removal of various pollutants (dyes, metals/ions, others). It can be concluded that a limited number of works clearly presented novel modifications of the chitosan structure (finding new functional groups for grafting reactions or agents for cross-linking). The majority of works used already published modified materials and tested them for other/different types of pollutants. The latter may be due to the fact that the basic modifications have been completed and extensively published. Another possible reason may be the recent trend for publishing higher quantities of papers and not attempting to find some new modification. In any case, the potential of modified materials is still large and can be significantly developed in the future.

## Acknowledgments

The support for this study was received from the State Scholarships Foundation (IKY) of Greek Ministry of Education and Religious Affairs (in the framework of the Hellenic Republic—Siemens Settlement Agreement) through the research program "IKY Fellowships of Excellence for Postgraduate Studies in Greece—Siemens Program" under the title "Advanced Molecularly Imprinted Polymers (MIPs) as materials for the selective binding and recovery of various high-added value environmental targets with application to industrial-scale adsorption columns", which is gratefully appreciated.

## Nomenclature of Dyes Reported in This Study

| | |
|---|---|
| AG25 | Acid green 25 |
| AO7 | Acid orange 7 |
| AR18 | Acid red 18 |
| BBR250 | Brilliant blue R250 |
| BO16 | Bezactive orange 16 |
| CR | Congo red |
| MB | Methylene blue |
| RB19 | Reactive blue 19 |
| RB5 | Reactive black 5 |
| RR198 | Reactive red 198 |
| RR120 | Reactive red 120 |
| RR3BS | Remazol red 3BS |
| RY3RS | Reactive yellow 3RS |
| WASC | Weak acid scarlet |

## Conflicts of Interest

The authors declare no conflict of interest.

## References

1. Clark, G.L.; Smith, A.F. X-ray diffraction studies of chitin, chitosan, and derivatives. *J. Phys. Chem.* **1936**, *40*, 863–879.
2. Muzzarelli, R.A.A. *Natural Chelating Polymers: Alginic Acid, Chitin, and Chitosan*; Pergamon Press: Oxford, UK, 1973; Volume 55.
3. Rinaudo, M. Chitin and chitosan: Properties and applications. *Prog. Polym. Sci.* **2006**, *31*, 603–632.
4. Lamb, G.F. The chemical constitution of chitin. *Science* **1916**, *44*, 866–868.
5. Irvine, J.C. LXXII.—A polarimetric method of identifying chitin. *J. Chem. Soc. Trans.* **1909**, *95*, 564–570.
6. Zhang, J.; Xia, W.; Liu, P.; Cheng, Q.; Tahirou, T.; Gu, W.; Li, B. Chitosan modification and pharmaceutical/biomedical applications. *Mar. Drugs* **2010**, *8*, 1962–1987.
7. Wen, Z.S.; Xu, Y.L.; Zou, X.T.; Xu, Z.R. Chitosan nanoparticles act as an adjuvant to promote both Th1 and Th2 immune responses induced by ovalbumin in mice. *Mar. Drugs* **2011**, *9*, 1038–1055.
8. Wen, Z.S.; Liu, L.J.; Qu, Y.L.; OuYang, X.K.; Yang, L.Y.; Xu, Z.R. Chitosan nanoparticles attenuate hydrogen peroxide-induced stress injuryin mouse macrophage raw264.7 cells. *Mar. Drugs* **2013**, *11*, 3582–3600.

9. Venkatesan, J.; Kim, S.K. Chitosan composites for bone tissue engineering—An overview. *Mar. Drugs* **2010**, *8*, 2252–2266.

10. Venkatesan, J.; Bhatnagar, I.; Kim, S.K. Chitosan-alginate biocomposite containing fucoidan for bone tissue engineering. *Mar. Drugs* **2014**, *12*, 300–316.

11. Vázquez, J.A.; Rodríguez-Amado, I.; Montemayor, M.I.; Fraguas, J.; del González, M.P.; Murado, M.A. Chondroitin sulfate, hyaluronic acid and chitin/chitosan production using marine waste sources: Characteristics, applications and eco-friendly processes: A review. *Mar. Drugs* **2013**, *11*, 747–774.

12. Tsai, Z.T.; Tsai, F.Y.; Yang, W.C.; Wang, J.F.; Liu, C.L.; Shen, C.R.; Yen, T.C. Preparation and characterization of ferrofluid stabilized with biocompatible chitosan and dextran sulfate hybrid biopolymer as a potential magnetic resonance imaging (MRI) T2 contrast agent. *Mar. Drugs* **2012**, *10*, 2403–2414.

13. Muzzarelli, R.A.A. Biomedical exploitation of chitin and chitosan via mechano-chemical disassembly, electrospinning, dissolution in imidazolium ionic liquids, and supercritical drying. *Mar. Drugs* **2011**, *9*, 1510–1533.

14. Li, B.; Shan, C.L.; Zhou, Q.; Fang, Y.; Wang, Y.L.; Xu, F.; Han, L.R.; Ibrahim, M.; Guo, L.B.; Xie, G.L.; *et al*. Synthesis, characterization, and antibacterial activity of cross-linked chitosan-glutaraldehyde. *Mar. Drugs* **2013**, *11*, 1534–1552.

15. Korkiatithaweechai, S.; Umsarika, P.; Praphairaksit, N.; Muangsin, N. Controlled release of diclofenac from matrix polymer of chitosan and oxidized konjac glucomannan. *Mar. Drugs* **2011**, *9*, 1649–1663.

16. Guo, L.; Liu, G.; Hong, R.Y.; Li, H.Z. Preparation and characterization of chitosan poly(acrylic acid) magnetic microspheres. *Mar. Drugs* **2010**, *8*, 2212–2222.

17. Cheng, M.; Gao, X.; Wang, Y.; Chen, H.; He, B.; Xu, H.; Li, Y.; Han, J.; Zhang, Z. Synthesis of glycyrrhetinic acid-modified chitosan 5-fluorouracil nanoparticles and its inhibition of liver cancer characteristics *in vitro* and *in vivo*. *Mar. Drugs* **2013**, *11*, 3517–3536.

18. Chen, J.K.; Yeh, C.H.; Wang, L.C.; Liou, T.H.; Shen, C.R.; Liu, C.L. Chitosan, the marine functional food, is a potent adsorbent of humic acid. *Mar. Drugs* **2011**, *9*, 2488–2498.

19. Muzzarelli, R.A.A.; Tubertini, O. Chitin and chitosan as chromatographic supports and adsorbents for collection of metal ions from organic and aqueous solutions and sea-water. *Talanta* **1969**, *16*, 1571–1577.

20. No, H.K.; Meyers, S.P. Application of chitosan for treatment of wastewaters. *Rev. Environ. Contam. Toxicol.* **2000**, *163*, 1–27.

21. Varma, A.J.; Deshpande, S.V.; Kennedy, J.F. Metal complexation by chitosan and its derivatives: A review. *Carbohyd. Polym.* **2004**, *55*, 77–93.

22. Guibal, E.; van Vooren, M.; Dempsey, B.A.; Roussy, J. A review of the use of chitosan for the removal of particulate and dissolved contaminants. *Sep. Sci. Technol.* **2006**, *41*, 2487–2514.

23. Gerente, C.; Lee, V.K.C.; Le Cloirec, P.; McKay, G. Application of chitosan for the removal of metals from wastewaters by adsorption—Mechanisms and models review. *Crit. Rev. Environ. Sci. Technol.* **2007**, *37*, 41–127.

24. Crini, G.; Badot, P.M. Application of chitosan, a natural aminopolysaccharide, for dye removal from aqueous solutions by adsorption processes using batch studies: A review of recent literature. *Prog. Polym. Sci.* **2008**, *33*, 399–447.

25. Bhatnagar, A.; Sillanpää, M. Applications of chitin- and chitosan-derivatives for the detoxification of water and wastewater—A short review. *Adv. Colloid Interf. Sci.* **2009**, *152*, 26–38.

26. Miretzky, P.; Cirelli, A.F. Hg(II) removal from water by chitosan and chitosan derivatives: A review. *J. Hazard. Mater.* **2009**, *167*, 10–23.

27. Wu, F.C.; Tseng, R.L.; Juang, R.S. A review and experimental verification of using chitosan and its derivatives as adsorbents for selected heavy metals. *J. Environ. Manag.* **2010**, *91*, 798–806.

28. Wan Ngah, W.S.; Teong, L.C.; Hanafiah, M.A.K.M. Adsorption of dyes and heavy metal ions by chitosan composites: A review. *Carbohyd. Polym.* **2011**, *83*, 1446–1456.

29. Vakili, M.; Rafatullah, M.; Salamatinia, B.; Abdullah, A.Z.; Ibrahim, M.H.; Tan, K.B.; Gholami, Z.; Amouzgar, P. Application of chitosan and its derivatives as adsorbents for dye removal from water and wastewater: A review. *Carbohyd. Polym.* **2014**, *113*, 115–130.

30. Auta, M.; Hameed, B.H. Chitosan-clay composite as highly effective and low-cost adsorbent for batch and fixed-bed adsorption of methylene blue. *Chem. Eng. J.* **2014**, *237*, 352–361.

31. Fan, L.; Zhang, Y.; Luo, C.; Lu, F.; Qiu, H.; Sun, M. Synthesis and characterization of magnetic β-cyclodextrin-chitosan nanoparticles as nano-adsorbents for removal of methyl blue. *Int. J. Biol. Macromol.* **2012**, *50*, 444–450.

32. Binello, A.; Cravotto, G.; Nano, G.M.; Spagliardi, P. Synthesis of chitosan-cyclodextrin adducts and evaluation of their bitter-masking properties. *Flavour Frag. J.* **2004**, *19*, 394–400.

33. Elwakeel, K.Z.; Abd El-Ghaffar, M.A.; El-kousy, S.M.; El-Shorbagy, H.G. Synthesis of new ammonium chitosan derivatives and their application for dye removal from aqueous media. *Chem. Eng. J.* **2012**, *203*, 458–468.

34. Gao, Q.; Zhu, H.; Luo, W.J.; Wang, S.; Zhou, C.G. Preparation, characterization, and adsorption evaluation of chitosan-functionalized mesoporous composites. *Microporous Mesoporous Mater.* **2014**, *193*, 15–26.

35. Jiang, X.; Sun, Y.; Liu, L.; Wang, S.; Tian, X. Adsorption of c.I. Reactive blue 19 from aqueous solutions by porous particles of the grafted chitosan. *Chem. Eng. J.* **2014**, *235*, 151–157.

36. Guo, J.; Chen, S.; Liu, L.; Li, B.; Yang, P.; Zhang, L.; Feng, Y. Adsorption of dye from wastewater using chitosan-ctab modified bentonites. *J. Colloid Interface Sci.* **2012**, *382*, 61–66.

37. Li, Z.; Cao, M.; Zhang, W.; Liu, L.; Wang, J.; Ge, W.; Yuan, Y.; Yue, T.; Li, R.; Yu, W.W. Affinity adsorption of lysozyme with reactive red 120 modified magnetic chitosan microspheres. *Food Chem.* **2014**, *145*, 749–755.

38. Nešić, A.R.; Veličković, S.J.; Antonović, D.G. Modification of chitosan by zeolite a and adsorption of bezactive orange 16 from aqueous solution. *Compos. B: Eng.* **2013**, *53*, 145–151.

39. Peng, Y.; Chen, D.; Ji, J.; Kong, Y.; Wan, H.; Yao, C. Chitosan-modified palygorskite: Preparation, characterization and reactive dye removal. *Appl. Clay Sci.* **2013**, *74*, 81–86.

40. Sadeghi-Kiakhani, M.; Arami, M.; Gharanjig, K. Dye removal from colored-textile wastewater using chitosan-PPI dendrimer hybrid as a biopolymer: Optimization, kinetic, and isotherm studies. *J. Appl. Polym. Sci.* **2013**, *127*, 2607–2619.

41. Yan, Y.; Xiang, B.; Li, Y.; Jia, Q. Preparation and adsorption properties of diethylenetriamine-modified chitosan beads for acid dyes. *J. Appl. Polym. Sci.* **2013**, *130*, 4090–4098.

42. Zhu, H.; Fu, Y.; Jiang, R.; Yao, J.; Liu, L.; Chen, Y.; Xiao, L.; Zeng, G. Preparation, characterization and adsorption properties of chitosan modified magnetic graphitized multi-walled carbon nanotubes for highly effective removal of a carcinogenic dye from aqueous solution. *Appl. Surf. Sci.* **2013**, *285*, 865–873.

43. Chatterjee, S.; Chatterjee, B.P.; Guha, A.K. Adsorptive removal of congo red, a carcinogenic textile dye by chitosan hydrobeads: Binding mechanism, equilibrium and kinetics. *Colloid Surf. A* **2007**, *299*, 146–152.

44. Wang, L.; Wang, A. Adsorption properties of congo red from aqueous solution onto *N,O*-carboxymethyl-chitosan. *Bioresour. Technol.* **2008**, *99*, 1403–1408.

45. Wang, L.; Wang, A. Adsorption behaviors of congo red on the *N,O*-carboxymethyl-chitosan/ montmorillonite nanocomposite. *Chem. Eng. J.* **2008**, *143*, 43–50.

46. Travlou, N.A.; Kyzas, G.Z.; Lazaridis, N.K.; Deliyanni, E.A. Graphite oxide/chitosan composite for reactive dye removal. *Chem. Eng. J.* **2013**, *217*, 256–265.

47. Travlou, N.A.; Kyzas, G.Z.; Lazaridis, N.K.; Deliyanni, E.A. Functionalization of graphite oxide with magnetic chitosan for the preparation of a nanocomposite dye adsorbent. *Langmuir* **2013**, *29*, 1657–1668.

48. Kyzas, G.Z.; Lazaridis, N.K.; Bikiaris, D.N. Optimization of chitosan and β-cyclodextrin molecularly imprinted polymer synthesis for dye adsorption. *Carbohyd. Polym.* **2013**, *91*, 198–208.

49. IUPAC. Available online: http://goldbook.iupac.org/C01012.html (accessed on 5 September 2014).

50. Muzzarelli, R.A.A. Available online: http://www.chitin.it/chelating-capacity-of-chitin-and-chitosan.html (accessed on 5 September 2014).

51. Arvand, M.; Pakseresht, M.A. Cadmium adsorption on modified chitosan-coated bentonite: Batch experimental studies. *J. Chem. Technol. Biot.* **2013**, *88*, 572–578.

52. Chen, J.H.; Lu, D.Q.; Chen, B.; Ouyang, P.K. Removal of U(VI) from aqueous solutions by using MWCNTs and chitosan modified MWCNTs. *J. Radioanal. Nucl. Chem.* **2013**, *295*, 2233–2241.

53. Chen, Y.; Wang, J. The characteristics and mechanism of Co(II) removal from aqueous solution by a novel xanthate-modified magnetic chitosan. *Nucl. Eng. Des.* **2012**, *242*, 452–457.

54. Chethan, P.D.; Vishalakshi, B. Synthesis of ethylenediamine modified chitosan and evaluation for removal of divalent metal ions. *Carbohyd. Polym.* **2013**, *97*, 530–536.

55. Debnath, S.; Maity, A.; Pillay, K. Magnetic chitosan-go nanocomposite: Synthesis, characterization and batch adsorber design for Cr(VI) removal. *J. Environ. Chem. Eng.* **2014**, *2*, 963–973.

56. Hummers, W.S., Jr.; Offeman, R.E. Preparation of graphitic oxide. *J. Am. Chem. Soc.* **1958**, *80*, 1339.

57. Elwakeel, K.Z.; Atia, A.A.; Guibal, E. Fast removal of uranium from aqueous solutions using tetraethylenepentamine modified magnetic chitosan resin. *Bioresour. Technol.* **2014**, *160*, 107–114.
58. Eser, A.; Nüket Tirtom, V.; Aydemir, T.; Becerik, S.; Dinçer, A. Removal of nickel(II) ions by histidine modified chitosan beads. *Chem. Eng. J.* **2012**, *210*, 590–596.
59. Gandhi, M.R.; Kousalya, G.N.; Meenakshi, S. Selective sorption of Fe(III) using modified forms of chitosan beads. *J. Appl. Polym. Sci.* **2012**, *124*, 1858–1865.
60. Kandile, N.G.; Nasr, A.S. New hydrogels based on modified chitosan as metal biosorbent agents. *Int. J. Biol. Macromol.* **2014**, *64*, 328–333.
61. Li, T.T.; Liu, Y.G.; Peng, Q.Q.; Hu, X.J.; Liao, T.; Wang, H.; Lu, M. Removal of lead(II) from aqueous solution with ethylenediamine-modified yeast biomass coated with magnetic chitosan microparticles: Kinetic and equilibrium modeling. *Chem. Eng. J.* **2013**, *214*, 189–197.
62. Li, M.L.; Li, R.H.; Xu, J.; Han, X.; Yao, T.Y.; Wang, J. Thiocarbohydrazide-modified chitosan as anticorrosion and metal ion adsorbent. *J. Appl. Polym. Sci.* **2014**, *131*, 8437–8443.
63. Li, M.; Xu, J.; Li, R.; Wang, D.; Li, T.; Yuan, M.; Wang, J. Simple preparation of aminothiourea-modified chitosan as corrosion inhibitor and heavy metal ion adsorbent. *J. Colloid Interface Sci.* **2014**, *417*, 131–136.
64. Monier, M. Adsorption of Hg$^{2+}$, Cu$^{2+}$ and Zn$^{2+}$ ions from aqueous solution using formaldehyde cross-linked modified chitosan-thioglyceraldehyde schiff's base. *Int. J. Biol. Macromol.* **2012**, *50*, 773–781.
65. Negm, N.A.; El Sheikh, R.; El-Farargy, A.F.; Hefni, H.H.H.; Bekhit, M. Treatment of industrial wastewater containing copper and cobalt ions using modified chitosan. *J. Ind. Eng. Chem.* **2014**, doi:10.1016/j.jiec.2014.03.015.
66. Rabelo, R.; Vieira, R.; Luna, F.; Guibal, E.; Beppu, M. Adsorption of copper(II) and mercury(II) ions onto chemically-modified chitosan membranes: Equilibrium and kinetic properties. *Adsorpt. Sci. Technol.* **2012**, *30*, 1–21.
67. Rajiv Gandhi, M.; Meenakshi, S. Preparation of amino terminated polyamidoamine functionalized chitosan beads and its Cr(VI) uptake studies. *Carbohyd. Polym.* **2013**, *91*, 631–637.
68. Repo, E.; Koivula, R.; Harjula, R.; Sillanpää, M. Effect of edta and some other interfering species on the adsorption of Co(II) by edta-modified chitosan. *Desalination* **2013**, *321*, 93–102.
69. Song, Q.; Wang, C.; Zhang, Z.; Gao, J. Adsorption of Cu(II) and Ni(II) using a novel xanthated carboxymethyl chitosan. *Sep. Sci. Technol.* **2014**, *49*, 1235–1243.
70. Santhana Krishna Kumar, A.; Uday Kumar, C.; Rajesh, V.; Rajesh, N. Microwave assisted preparation of n-butylacrylate grafted chitosan and its application for Cr(VI) adsorption. *Int. J. Biol. Macromol.* **2014**, *66*, 135–143.
71. Suc, N.V.; Ly, H.T.Y. Lead (II) removal from aqueous solution by chitosan flake modified with citric acid via crosslinking with glutaraldehyde. *J. Chem. Technol. Biot.* **2013**, *88*, 1641–1649.
72. Wang, H.; Tang, H.; Liu, Z.; Zhang, X.; Hao, Z.; Liu, Z. Removal of cobalt(II) ion from aqueous solution by chitosan–montmorillonite. *J. Environ. Sci.* **2014**, *26*, 1879–1884.

73. Xu, J.; Zhou, L.; Jia, Y.; Liu, Z.; Adesina, A.A. Adsorption of thorium (IV) ions from aqueous solution by magnetic chitosan resins modified with triethylene-tetramine. *J. Radioanal. Nucl. Chem.* **2014**, doi:10.1007/s10967-014-3227-6.

74. Xu, J.; Chen, M.; Zhang, C.; Yi, Z. Adsorption of uranium(VI) from aqueous solution by diethylenetriamine-functionalized magnetic chitosan. *J. Radioanal. Nucl. Chem.* **2013**, *298*, 1375–1383.

75. Yang, G.; Tang, L.; Lei, X.; Zeng, G.; Cai, Y.; Wei, X.; Zhou, Y.; Li, S.; Fang, Y.; Zhang, Y. Cd(II) removal from aqueous solution by adsorption on α-ketoglutaric acid-modified magnetic chitosan. *Appl. Surf. Sci.* **2014**, *292*, 710–716.

76. Kyzas, G.Z.; Deliyanni, E.A. Mercury(II) removal with modified magnetic chitosan adsorbents. *Molecules* **2013**, *18*, 6193–6214.

77. Kyzas, G.Z.; Siafaka, P.I.; Lambropoulou, D.A.; Lazaridis, N.K.; Bikiaris, D.N. Poly(itaconic acid)-grafted chitosan adsorbents with different cross-linking for Pb(II) and Cd(II) uptake. *Langmuir* **2014**, *40*, 120–131.

78. Poon, L.; Wilson, L.D.; Headley, J.V. Chitosan-glutaraldehyde copolymers and their sorption properties. *Carbohyd. Polym.* **2014**, *109*, 92–101.

79. Kyzas, G.Z.; Bikiaris, D.N.; Lazaridis, N.K. Low-swelling chitosan derivatives as biosorbents for basic dyes. *Langmuir* **2008**, *24*, 4791–4799.

80. Kyzas, G.Z.; Lazaridis, N.K. Reactive and basic dyes removal by sorption onto chitosan derivatives. *J. Colloid Interface Sci.* **2009**, *331*, 32–39.

81. Lazaridis, N.K.; Kyzas, G.Z.; Vassiliou, A.A.; Bikiaris, D.N. Chitosan derivatives as biosorbents for basic dyes. *Langmuir* **2007**, *23*, 7634–7643.

82. Zhang, Y.; Shen, Z.; Dai, C.; Zhou, X. Removal of selected pharmaceuticals from aqueous solution using magnetic chitosan: Sorption behavior and mechanism. *Environ. Sci. Pollut. Res.* **2014**, *21*, 12780–12789.

83. Zhou, L.C.; Meng, X.G.; Fu, J.W.; Yang, Y.C.; Yang, P.; Mi, C. Highly efficient adsorption of chlorophenols onto chemically modified chitosan. *Appl. Surf. Sci.* **2014**, *292*, 735–741.

84. Kyzas, G.Z.; Kostoglou, M.; Lazaridis, N.K.; Lambropoulou, D.A.; Bikiaris, D.N. Environmental friendly technology for the removal of pharmaceutical contaminants from wastewaters using modified chitosan adsorbents. *Chem. Eng. J.* **2013**, *222*, 248–258.

85. Kyzas, G.Z.; Bikiaris, D.N.; Seredych, M.; Bandosz, T.J.; Deliyanni, E.A. Removal of dorzolamide from biomedical wastewaters with adsorption onto graphite oxide/poly(acrylic acid) grafted chitosan nanocomposite. *Bioresour. Technol.* **2014**, *152*, 399–406.

# Co-Processed Chitin-Mannitol as a New Excipient for Oro-Dispersible Tablets

Nidal Daraghmeh, Babur Z. Chowdhry, Stephen A. Leharne, Mahmoud M. H. Al Omari and Adnan A. Badwan

**Abstract:** This study describes the preparation, characterization and performance of a novel excipient for use in oro-dispersible tablets (ODT). The excipient (**Cop–CM**) consists of chitin and mannitol. The excipient with optimal physicochemical properties was obtained at a chitin: mannitol ratio of 2:8 (w/w) and produced by roll compaction (RC). Differential scanning calorimetry (DSC), Fourier transform-Infrared (FT-IR), X-ray powder diffraction (XRPD) and scanning electron microscope (SEM) techniques were used to characterize **Cop–CM**, in addition to characterization of its powder and ODT dosage form. The effect of particle size distribution of **Cop–CM** was investigated and found to have no significant influence on the overall tablet physical properties. The compressibility parameter (a) for **Cop–CM** was calculated from a Kawakita plot and found to be higher (0.661) than that of mannitol (0.576) due to the presence of the highly compressible chitin (0.818). Montelukast sodium and domperidone ODTs produced, using **Cop–CM**, displayed excellent physicochemical properties. The exceptional binding, fast wetting and superdisintegration properties of **Cop–CM**, in comparison with commercially available co-processed ODT excipients, results in a unique multifunctional base which can successfully be used in the formulation of oro-dispersible and fast immediate release tablets.

Reprinted from *Mar. Drugs*. Cite as: Daraghmeh, N.; Chowdhry, B.Z.; Leharne, S.A.; Al Omari, M.M.H.; Badwan, A.A. Co-Processed Chitin-Mannitol as a New Excipient for Oro-Dispersible Tablets. *Mar. Drugs* **2015**, *13*, 1739-1764.

## 1. Introduction

Tablets are widely used as drug delivery system due to their convenience with respect to self-administration and ease of manufacture [1]. Various excipients are used in their preparation [2]. However, pediatric, geriatric and mentally ill patients experience difficulties in swallowing conventional tablets, which leads to poor patient compliance. To overcome this deficiency, ODT formulations have been developed [3,4].

In Ph. Euro., an ODT is defined as a tablet to be placed in the mouth where it disperses rapidly before being swallowed in less than 3 minutes [5], while the FDA considers it as a solid oral preparation that disintegrates rapidly in the oral cavity with an *in vivo* disintegration time of approximately 30 s or less [4]. ODTs are advantageous due to their administration without water, rapid onset of action and improved bioavailability [6,7].

Various ODT patented technologies such as Orasolv/DuraSolv (by direct compression (DC)), Zydis (by freeze drying), FlashTab (Eudragit-microencapsulation and effervescent couple), FlashDose (cotton candy process) and WowTab (compression moulding process) have been commercialized [8,9]. ODTs are highly friable, due to their compaction at lower crushing force compared to conventional tablets, resulting in rapid disintegration; therefore, they are commonly packed in special packaging materials, which add to their cost [10]. A high level of superdisintegrant (up to 20% w/w) is usually needed in ODT preparations in order to enhance their disintegration properties. Additional excipients including a suitable filler, binder, lubricant, sweetener and color may be added to improve product properties [6,11].

Mannitol, in crystalline, granulated, or spray dried form is widely used in ODT tablet formulations due to its sweet, cool taste and compatibility with a wide range of drugs [12–14]. Unlike crystalline mannitol, spray dried mannitol is highly compactible, non-friable, and quick dissolving, which facilitate its use in DC formulations of ODTs. Furthermore, crystalline mannitol is widely used in tablet wet granulation (WG) processes due to its favourable cost [15–17].

Chitin is used as chromatographic supports and adsorbents for industrial pollutants [18,19], for recovery of silver thiosulfate complexes [20], enzyme immobilization [21], wound healing [22], fibers and film formers [23], and binders in the paper making process [15]. Recently, chitin has been used as a starting material to produce pyranoside [24] and furan [25] derivatives. Furthermore, chitin monomer N-acetyl-D-glucosamine has been used as a source of amide/amino substituted sugar alcohols [26].

Chitin is used in tablet formulations because it is non-toxic, non-allergenic, anti-microbial, non-reactive and biodegradable. Its disintegration power is mainly dependent upon a high water uptake rate. Therefore, chitin can be used over a higher concentration range than many commercially available disintegrants without negatively affecting other tablet properties. However, chitin powder shows poor compactibility, which has limited its applications in commercialized dosage forms [27,28]. To overcome this shortcoming, chitin was co-processed with other excipient modifiers in order to facilitate its handling in solid dosage form manufacturing. As with other excipients, co-processing is carried out using different manufacturing techniques such as spray drying or melt extrusion [29]. For example, chitin, a plastic material, has been successfully used to prepare different excipients via co-processing with diverse brittle materials including mannitol, metal silicates and silicon dioxide [30–32]. In all cases co-processing was achieved by incorporating the brittle material (≤30% w/w) inside the pores of chitin (≥70% w/w) using an aqueous vehicle. The result of the foregoing studies showed that the extremely large surface pores of chitin measured by BET analysis [31,33,34] were not fully accommodated by the guest materials and thus chitin preserved its functionality as a disintegrant. Moreover, the co-processed excipients enhanced the physical properties, functionality and performance (e.g., no-hygroscopicity and highly compactable/disintegrable) of tablet preparations [30–32]. A combination of chitin, chitosan-alginate (1:1), and glycine was reported in preparation of a novel superdisintegrant [35]. The forgoing excipient was applied to formulate sulbutamol sulphate ODT by using direct compression. This may offer a valuable practical industrial addition in terms of superdisintegration and mechanical properties of ODT formulations. Furthermore, an article describing the characterization and application of such a novel co-processed excipient in immediate release tablet formulations has been reported in the literature [32]. In the aforementioned study, the tablets prepared by using the co-processed excipient chitin:mannitol (80:20 w/w) and different drugs displayed excellent chemical stability, binding, and disintegration properties. This may extend its application to ODTs [32].

The objective of the work reported herein is to test the possibility of using co-processed chitin-mannitol as a single excipient in producing ODTs. This may help to overcome the problem of low crushing strength inherited from other techniques and to use chitin for the first time as the main excipient allowing the use of conventional industrial machinery for the production and packaging of ODTs.

## 2. Results and Discussion

### 2.1. Selection of Processing Methods and Ratios for Co-Processed Chitin–Mannitol Excipient

In order to select the optimal ratio and process for co-processed excipient preparation, three different ratios of chitin and mannitol (10:90, 20:80 and 30:70 w/w) and three different processing techniques *i.e.*, direct mixing, WG and RC were used. The prepared excipients were lubricated with sodium stearyl fumarate (1.0% w/w) and compressed at different tablet crushing forces (50–150 N). The tablets obtained were tested for friability, disintegration and wetting times *versus* the corresponding crushing forces. The preliminary results of the aforementioned experiments indicated that direct mixing and WG were unsuitable, because the mixtures prepared by direct mixing displayed unacceptable physical properties (e.g., poor flow and powder non-uniformity). The difference in bulk densities of chitin (~0.2 g/cm$^3$) and mannitol (~0.5 g/cm$^3$) is the reason underlying such unacceptable physical properties. In the case of WG, the tablets suffered from capping and high disintegration times due to penetration of the dissolved mannitol into the chitin pores. Such penetration does not allow the pores to act as functional compression and disintegration enhancers. However, RC gave reasonable results. The data in Figure 1 shows the effect of crushing force on the friability, disintegration and wetting times of tablets produced. Up to a crushing force of 90 N, all chitin:mannitol ratios showed acceptable physical properties (low friability and fast disintegration and wetting times). While at crushing forces above 90 N, the excipient prepared by using a chitin:mannitol ratio of 1:9 showed capping upon tablet compression due to an insufficient amount of chitin, responsible for improving the compressibility. Using chitin:mannitol ratios of 2:8 and 3:7 (w/w) over all the investigated range of crushing forces produced tablets with acceptable physical properties. However, a ratio of chitin and mannitol of 2:8 (w/w) was chosen in order to obtain beneficial mannitol taste properties and to reduce the amount of insoluble chitin in ODT preparations.

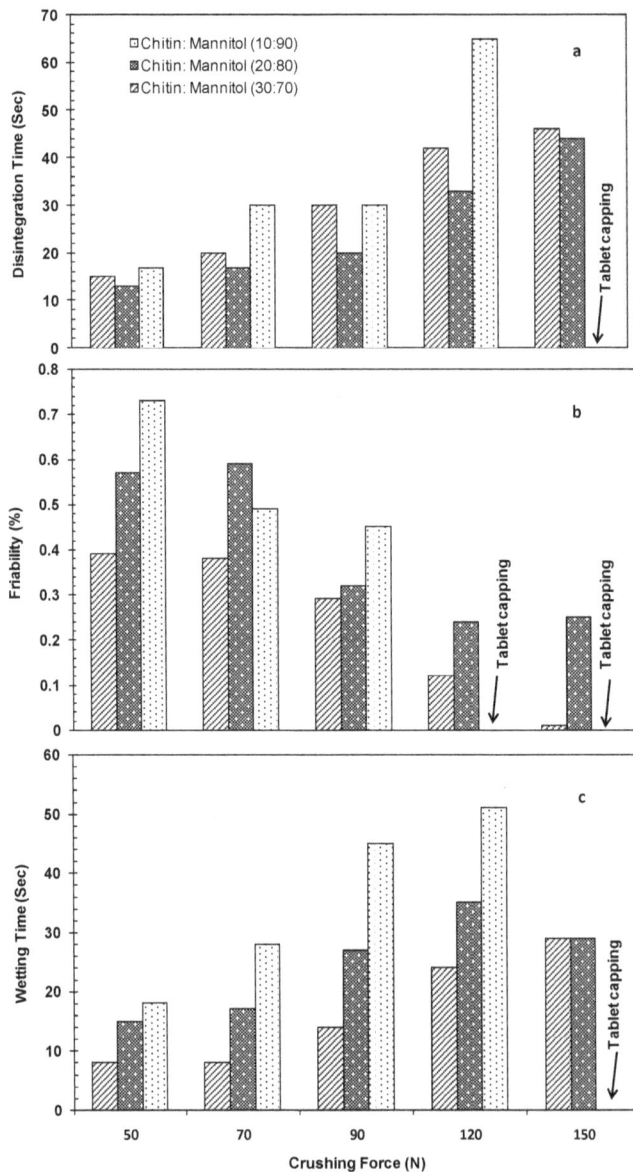

**Figure 1.** Plots of the crushing force (N) *versus* (**a**) disintegration time; (**b**) friability; and (**c**) wetting time for compacted mixtures prepared using different ratios of chitin and mannitol (1:9, 2:8, and 3:7 w/w). Tablets were 10 mm in diameter and 250 mg in weight. All powders were lubricated using 1% (w/w) sodium stearyl fumarate.

## 2.2. Characterization of *Cop–CM* Powder

The FT-IR spectra of chitin, mannitol, the corresponding physical mixtures and **Cop-CM** are presented in Figure 2.

It is clear that the FT-IR spectrum of the physical mixture of chitin and mannitol (Figure 2c) is a superimposition of the vibrational band profiles contributed by chitin and mannitol (Figure 2a,b). The dominance of the principal bands of mannitol in the physical mixture is a result of its high fractional composition in the mixture (80% w/w). The two bands in the 1550–1660 cm$^{-1}$ range, corresponding to the amide I and II vibrational modes of chitin (Figure 2a), persist in the spectra of the physical mixture and **Cop–CM**, while the remaining bands are due to mannitol. The absence of any shift in the FT-IR bands of **Cop–CM** (Figure 2d), in comparison with the bands of the physical mixture (Figure 2c), suggests the absence of chemical interaction due to the use of RC to form **Cop–CM**.

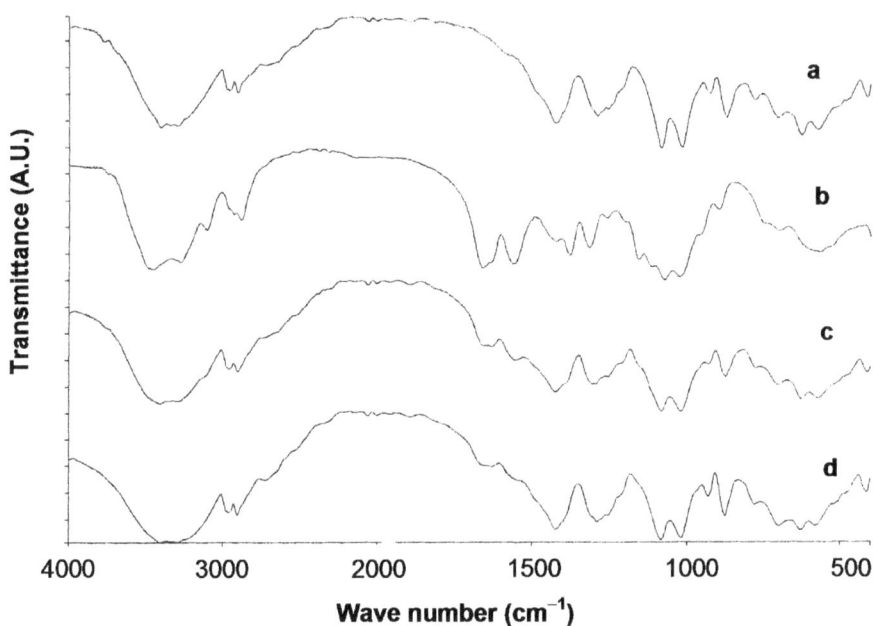

**Figure 2.** FT-IR spectra of (**a**) mannitol; (**b**) chitin; (**c**) physical mixture of chitin-mannitol (2:8, w/w); and (**d**) co-processed chitin-mannitol (2:8 w/w) excipient (**Cop–CM**).

Further analysis of **Cop–CM** by XRPD (Figure 3) and DSC (Figure 4) techniques showed the same results, where the signals corresponding to mannitol are dominant due to its high fractional content and crystallinity. The two broad peaks of chitin appeared at 2θ of around 11 and 22 but not clearly well-defined in both the physical mixture and **Cop–CM** due to the low content of chitin in the mixtures. The absence of new bands or shifts in the patterns indicates the absence of formation of a new crystal form or chemical interaction. This property is essential for such co–processed excipient to work as an excipient.

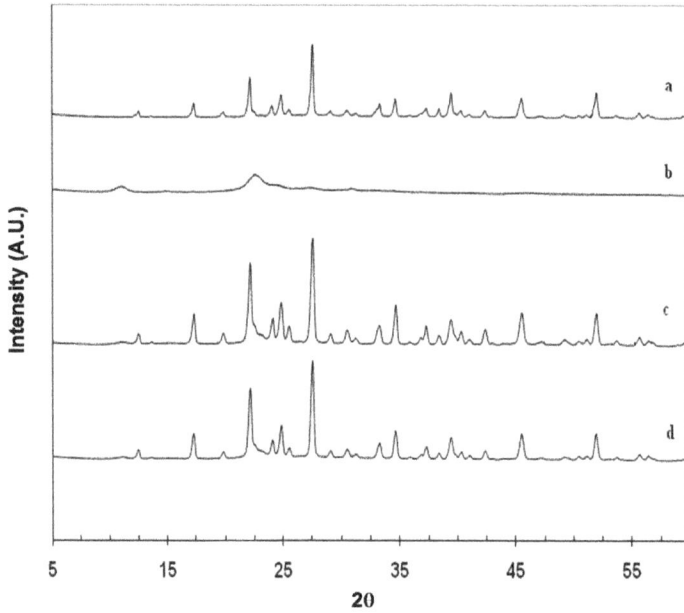

**Figure 3.** XRPD profiles of (**a**) mannitol; (**b**) chitin; (**c**) physical mixture of chitin-mannitol (2:8, w/w); and (**d**) co-processed chitin-mannitol (2:8 w/w) excipient (**Cop–CM**).

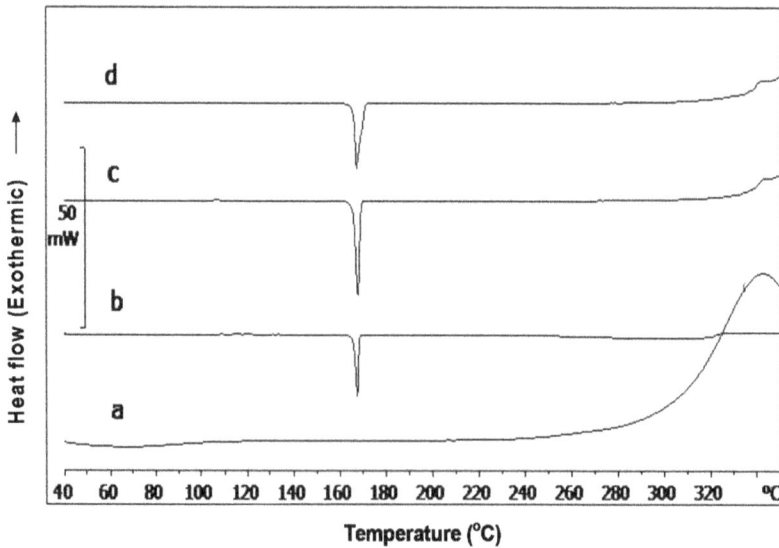

**Figure 4.** DSC thermograms of (**a**) chitin; (**b**) mannitol; (**c**) physical mixture of chitin-mannitol (2:8, w/w) and (**d**) co-processed chitin-mannitol (2:8 w/w) excipient (**Cop–CM**).

SEM was used to investigate particle surface morphology (Figure 5). When comparing the particle shape of mannitol (Figure 5a) with that of **Cop–CM** (Figure 5d), it is apparent that it has changed from rectangular rod granules to three-dimensional dense compacts for **Cop–CM**.

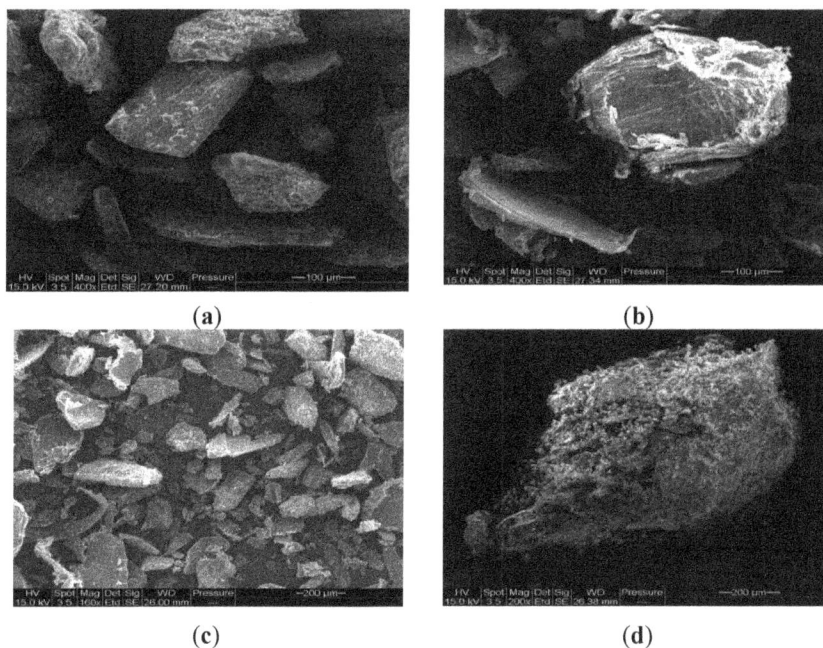

**Figure 5.** SEM images of (**a**) mannitol; (**b**) chitin; (**c**) physical mixture of chitin-mannitol (2:8, w/w); and (**d**) co-processed chitin-mannitol (2:8 w/w) excipient (**Cop–CM**).

## 2.3. Physical Properties of *Cop–CM Powder*

The physical properties of **Cop–CM** powders which passed through two different mesh size sieves (710 and 1000 μm) were evaluated. The two powders have a water content of about 1.5% w/w and a bulk density of 0.5–0.55 g/cm$^3$. The pH of a 5% (w/v) aqueous dispersion is in the range 6–8. The particle size distribution (D10, D50 and D90) of **Cop–CM** is given in Table 1.

Particle size and shape are critical parameters in powder characterization, particularly in DC formulations affecting powder performance, packing, consolidation, flowability and compaction. It is one of the prime considerations in selecting excipients to develop and optimize a pharmaceutical formulation. Ideally, DC excipients should exhibit narrow size distributions with moderate-to-coarse particle, having a mean particle size of 100–200 μm [36]. In ODT formulations, the control of particle size is essential for the water insoluble excipients to minimize the feeling of grittiness during tablet administration. The best results are obtained when using a smaller particle size for insoluble excipients. Another critical parameter for the DC excipient is the bulk density which can be used to describe the packing behavior of granules [36]. **Cop–CM** powder passed through a mesh size of 710 μm has a mean particle size of about 215 μm. A higher bulk density is advantageous in tabletting because of a reduction in the powder-fill volume of the die. **Cop–CM** powder sieved through a mesh size of 1000 μm has a bulk density of about 0.52 gm/mL and a tapped density of 0.59 gm/mL.

118

**Table 1.** The physical properties of co-processed chitin-mannitol (2:8 w/w) excipient (**Cop–CM**).

| Parameter | Value |
|---|---|
| Water content (w/w%) | 1.5 |
| pH | 6.0–8.0 |
| Bulk density (gm/mL) | 0.50–0.55 |
| Tapped density (gm/mL) | 0.55–0.65 |
| Particle size distribution: | |
| - Milling through 710 µm | D10: 5 µm; D50: 145 µm; D90: 496 µm |
| - Milling through 1000 µm | D10: 7 µm; D50: 170 µm; D90: 584 µm |
| Hausner Ratio | 1.13 |
| Carr Index | 11.86 |
| Angle of Repose | 32° |

On the other hand, Hausner Ratio ($H$) is an indirect index of ease of powder flow. It is calculated by using the formula [37]

$$H = \frac{TD}{BD} \tag{1}$$

where TD and BD are the tapped and bulk densities, respectively.

The simplest method of measurement of free flow of a powder is compressibility; an indication of the ease with which material can be induced to flow is given by Carr Index ($I$) which is calculated using the formula:

$$I = 100 \frac{(TD - BD)}{TD} \tag{2}$$

Carr Index of ≤10 indicates excellent flow, whereas $I$ values of 11–15 indicate good flow. Hausner Ratio of 1.0–1.11 indicates excellent flow whereas values of 1.12–1.18 indicate good flow (generally lower Carr Index and Hausner Ratio values represent better flow).

The change in density before and after tapping calculated as % compressibility (Carr Index) is an indicator of how fast granules can flow to their highest packing. The Carr Index calculated from the density data showed a value less than 12, and Hausner ratio of less than 1.13 further indicating the good flowability, which is an important factor for DC powders. Good flowability of powder is needed for content uniformity and less weight variation in the final tablets. According to US Pharmacopeia 31, General Chapter <1174>, an Angle of Repose of 25–30° indicates excellent flow, and 31–35° indicates good flow. The Hausner Ratio, Carr Index and Angle of Repose values for **Cop–CM** powder are shown in Table 1. From the data obtained, **Cop–CM** powder showed good flowability and compressibility.

*2.4. Moisture Uptake by Cop–CM*

The data in Figure 6 shows the water uptake by **Cop–CM** and commercial ODT bases (Phrmaburst C1, Isomalt 721, and Mannogem EZ) at 25 °C and different relative humidity. With up to 84% relative humidity for two weeks, all bases, except Pharmaburst C1, showed an insignificant increase in water uptake (Figure 6a). However, following equilibration for one day at 25 °C/45% relative humidity, Pharmaburst C1 lost the excess water absorbed (9%) to reach only 0.7% (Figure 6b). At high relative humidity (95%), the water uptake follows the order: **Cop–CM** (8%) < Mannogem EZ (14%) < Pharmaburst C1 (46%) < Isomalt galenIQ™ 721 (66%). Following equilibration for 1 day at 25 °C/45% relative humidity, all bases except Isomalt galenIQ™ 721 lost the excess water absorbed to give values less than 1% (Figure 6b). The relative humidity of Isomalt galenIQ™ 721 it is about 14% which is most probably due to partial dissolution of Isomalt at high relative humidity.

The difference in water uptake of different bases is due to the difference in their components and their morphology (e.g., crystalline *versus* amorphous). It seems that the RC of a large amount of mannitol (80% w/w) with chitin results in the coverage of the outer surface of chitin with mannitol; thus, **Cop–CM** powder is clearly non-hygroscopic due to the very minimal water uptake of mannitol.

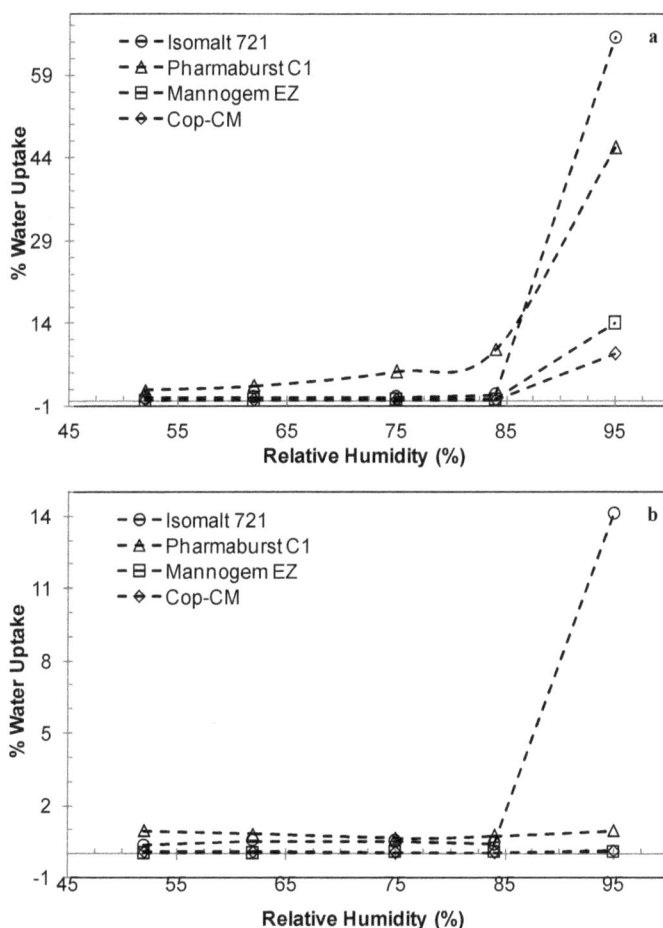

**Figure 6.** The water uptake by co-processed chitin–mannitol (2:8 w/w) excipient (**Cop–CM**) in comparison with some commercially available ODT bases after incubation at 25 °C and different relative humidity, (**a**) for two weeks; and (**b**) after equilibration at 25 °C/45% relative humidity for one further day.

## 2.5. Hygroscopicity of Tablets Prepared from **Cop–CM**

The water adsorption study was conducted for tablets prepared from **Cop–CM** at 75% relative humidity and room temperature. Results indicate that the tablets prepared from **Cop–CM** sorb very little, if any, water (less than 0.4% w/w). It is advantageous, in the pharmaceutical industry, to use non-hygroscopic ODT preparations, as this will reduce the cost of packaging which is usually used for moisture protection. Needless to say, wetting and ability to disintegrate must prevail.

## 2.6. Compression Profile of Tablet Prepared from **Cop–CM**

Data for the friability, disintegration and wetting times *versus* the corresponding crushing force for tablets prepared using **Cop–CM** powders which passed through either the 710 μm or 1000 μm sieves are shown in Figure 7. Generally, a reduction in particle size is associated with an increase in tablet mechanical strength. The increase in mechanical strength of the tablets is directly related to its physical properties (crushing force, disintegration time, friability, wetting time, *etc.*) and attributed to an increase in the surface area available for inter-particulate attraction [38]. However, when **Cop–CM** was used it was found that varying the particle size had no impact on the mechanical strength of the tablets. The mechanical strength of the tablets prepared from materials with a tendency to fragment, such as mannitol, dibasic calcium phosphate dihydrate and saccharose appear to be independent of particle size [39]. This could be the case for **Cop–CM** particles which contain an excess amount of mannitol (80% w/w) and undergo fragmentation [40] at the early stages of compression, thereby causing a minimal effect on tablet mechanical strength when varying the particle size.

The disintegration time of ODTs is generally less than one minute and the actual disintegration time that patients expect is less than 30 s. The general compendial method for performing disintegration tests for ODTs is not capable of detecting such a short disintegration time. The wetting time of the ODT is another important test, which gives an insight into the disintegration properties of the tablets. A lower wetting time indicates a quicker disintegration of the tablets [41]. With respect to tablet disintegration, **Cop–CM** showed a unique characteristic whereby tablet disintegration time was independent of particle size and tablet crushing force (Figure 7). Tablets produced from **Cop–CM** powders which passed through either the 710 μm or 1000 μm sieves, at an upper punch compression scale of 16–20 kN for each particle size, showed a superior disintegration time ranging from 11.5 to 59 s and from 14 to 64 s, respectively. This was achieved for tablet crushing force values ranging from 50 to 150 N. By increasing the crushing strength from 50 to 150 N, the wetting time of the tablet was increased from 9 to 35 s. This suggests that capillary action is the dominant mechanism for the disintegration of **Cop–CM** which is irrespective of the tablet crushing force [32]. In addition, the inter-particulate voids within the chitin particles in **Cop–CM**, as previously mentioned, remain intact and unchanged after using the RC procedure with mannitol and by varying the powder particle size. With respect to powder compressibility, chitin within **Cop–CM** mixture provides an effective means of obtaining hard tablets with low friability while persisting in its fast disintegration and wetting properties, as can be concluded from the data shown in Figure 7.

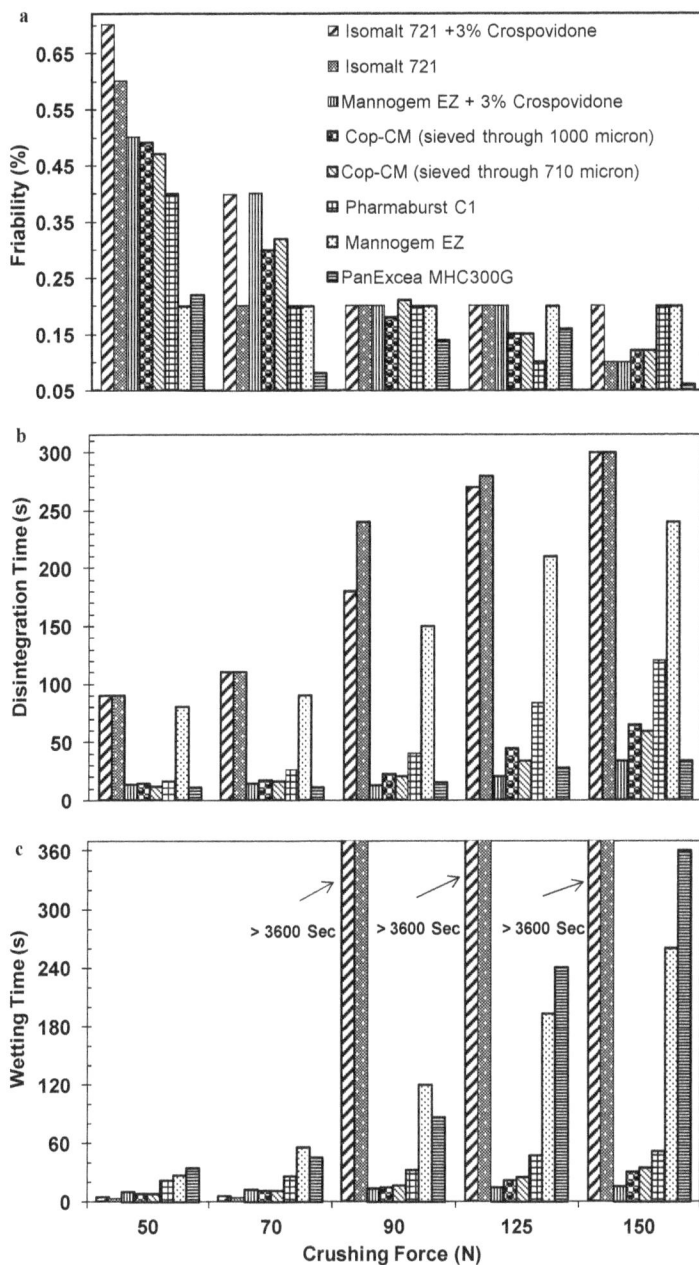

**Figure 7.** Plots of the crushing force (N) *versus* (**a**) friability; (**b**) disintegration time; and (**c**) wetting time for tablets prepared using co-processed chitin-mannitol (2:8 w/w) excipient (**Cop–CM**) which passed through either 710 μm or 1000 μm sieves in comparison with commercially available bases. The tablets were 10 mm in diameter and 250 mg in weight. All samples were lubricated with 1% (w/w) sodium stearyl fumarate.

Four commercially available ODT excipients were used for comparison purposes including, Isomalt galenIQ™ 721, Mannogem EZ, Pharmabust EZ and PanExcea MHC200G. The data in Table 2 shows the function and composition of these excipients. Crospovidone, a cross-linked polymer of N-vinyl-2-pyrrolidinone, is often used at concentrations up to 5.0% [11]. In this study, it was used as disintegrant in tablet preparations at 3% w/w level in both Isomalt galenIQ™ 721 and Mannogem EZ powders. Both PanExcea MC200G and Pharmaburst C1 already contain calcium silicate and crospovidone as disintegrant in their compositions, respectively.

**Table 2.** Function and composition of commercial oro-dispersible tablet excipients.

| Trade Name | Composition | Manufacturer | Advantages & Function |
|---|---|---|---|
| PanExcea MC200G | Mannitol (75%), calcium silicate (25%). Particle size: 50% (103 µm) | Avantor Performance Materials, Inc./Center Valley, PA, USA http://www.avantormaterials.com/ | High performance, rapid disintegration, direct compression excipient for oro-dissolving tablets formulation |
| Mannogem™ EZ | Spray dried direct compression mannitol Particle size: 60% (75–150 µm) | SPI Pharma™, Inc., New Castel, DE, USA http://www.spipharma.com | Assist in formulating difficult to use non-hygroscopic ODT containing fine drugs |
| Pharmaburst ™ C1 | Mannitol 84%, crospovidone 16%, silicon dioxide <1% | | High compactibility, high loading in small diameter tablets, smooth mouth feel, rapid disintegration |
| Isomalt galenIQ–721 | 1-O-D-glucopyranosyl-D-mannitol dehydrate and 6-O-D-glucopyranosyl-D-sorbitol (1:3) Particle size: 90% (360 µm), 50% (220 µm) | BENEO–Palatinit GmbH (Mannheim, Germany) http://www.beneo–palatinit.com/en/Pharma_Excipients /galenIQ/galenIQ_Grades/galenIQ721/ | Highly soluble agglomerated spherical isomalt for fast dissolving and very fast disintegrating direct compression tablet preparations |

In order to obtain a tablet crushing force in the range of 50–150 N, upper punch compression scales of 25.50–29.5 kN were applied to all excipients except for PanExcea in which case a scale range from 39 to 42 kN was applied. For all reference excipients used, increasing the crushing force from 50 to 150 N leads to a linear increase in the disintegration and wetting time of the tablets. The friability of the tablets was found to be within the acceptable limit [42] (less than 0.7% for Isomalt galenIQ™ 721 and 3% crospovidone) at the lower crushing force (50 N). Increasing tablet crushing force leads to decrease the friability (less than 0.2%). The reference excipients except for Mannogem EZ and Isomalt galenIQ™ 721 (with and without crospovidone) gave a disintegration time of less than 30 s at 50 N tablet crushing force. In addition, the wetting time for all reference excipients was less than 30 s at the same crushing force. The data in Figure 7 clearly shows that by increasing the tablet crushing force, the disintegration times and wetting times were increased accordingly. Only, Isomalt galenIQ™ 721 plus crospovidone and PanExcea MC200G tablets showed a short disintegration time (less than 33 s) at the highest crushing force (150 N), whereas for the other excipients a disintegration time range of 120–300 s were observed. At a tablet crushing force of 150 N, only pharmaburst C1 and Mannogem EZ plus crospovidone showed a short wetting time of less than 60 s (52 and 16 s, respectively).

For **Cop–CM**, it can be clearly observed that increasing the tablet crushing force up to 150 N does not affect both disintegration and wetting times. This property is extremely advantageous where hard tablets with very fast disintegration can be prepared using **Cop–CM** and simply packed in traditional packaging materials. This prevents the need of a special type of packaging to avoid the breakage of the tablets during removal from the package. A combination of Mannogem™ EZ and 3% crospovidone has showed similar behavior to **Cop–CM** at high tablets crushing forces. PanExcea MHC300G has preserved the very short disintegration time at 150 N tablet crushing force, while the tablet wetting time was increased. On the other hand, Pharmaburst C1 behaves in a different manner, whereby increasing the tablet crushing force to 150 N the disintegration time was relatively high (>2 min), while the tablet wetting time was not affected.

## 2.7. Powder Compressibility

The Kawakita equation (Equation (3)) is used to study powder compression using the degree of volume reduction, C. The basis for the Kawakita equation for powder compression is that particles subjected to a compressive load in a confined space are viewed as a system in equilibrium at all stages of compression, so that the product of the pressure term and the volume term is a constant [43]:

$$C = \frac{(V_o - V)}{V_0} = \frac{abP}{1 + bP} \tag{3}$$

where, $V_o$ is the initial volume and $V$ is the volume of powder column under an applied pressure, $P$. The constants $a$ and $b$ represent the minimum porosity before compression and plasticity of the material, respectively. The reciprocal of $b$ defines the pressure required to reduce the powder bed by 50% [44,45]. Equation (3) can be re-arranged in linear form as:

$$\frac{P}{C} = \frac{P}{a} + \frac{1}{ab} \tag{4}$$

The expression for particle rearrangement can be affected simultaneously by the two Kawakita parameters $a$ and $b$. The combination of these into a single value, *i.e.* the product of the Kawakita parameters ($ab$), may hence be used as an indicator of particle rearrangement during compression [46].

Figure 8 shows the Kawakita plots for mannitol, **Cop–CM** and chitin. The Kawakita constants $a$, $b$, $ab$ and $1/b$ were calculated from the intercept and slope of the plots (Table 3). The constant $a$, which represents the compressibility, is the highest for chitin ($a = 0.818$) and this is due to the large internal surface pores. The compressibility of **Cop–CM** is higher than mannitol alone ($a = 0.661$ and 0.576, respectively) and this is ascribed to the addition of the chitin to mannitol. This result emphasizes the fact that although the mannitol constitutes 80% of **Cop–CM** content, using RC techniques in the preparation of **Cop–CM** keeps the large chitin surface pores unoccupied and active. This is because mannitol physically adheres at the outer chitin surfaces.

The increase in the $ab$ value for **Cop–CM** (0.0592), which is a measure of the extent of particle rearrangement, indicates that the addition of chitin has improved the degree of particle rearrangement and packing during tabletting. The $1/b$ parameter is an inverse measure of the amount of plastic deformation occurring during the compression process [31,47]. Generally, a low value of $1/b$ is a reflection of the soft nature of the material and that the material is readily deformed plastically under pressure [48]. Chitin is a highly porous material and forms intermolecular hydrogen bonds between adjacent plastic, deformed chitin particles. The presence of moisture within the porous structure of chitin enforces the formation of hydrogen bond bridges which increase the internal binding upon compaction. Therefore, the use of a smaller amount of chitin (20%) with mannitol within **Cop–CM** decreases plastic deformation during compression [31,49].

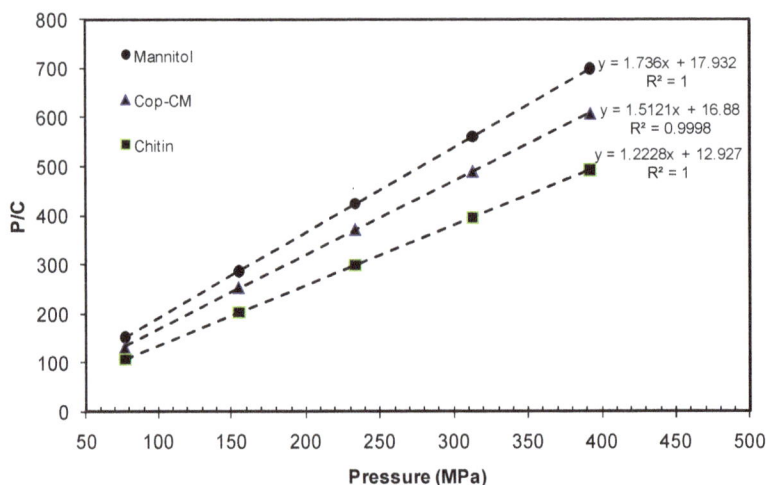

**Figure 8.** Kawakita plot for co-processed chitin-mannitol (2:8 w/w) excipient (**Cop–CM**). Tablets were 12 mm in diameter and 400 mg in weight.

**Table 3.** Kawakita parameters for mannitol, chitin and co-processed chitin-mannitol (2:8 w/w) excipient (**Cop–CM**).

| Material | Kawakita Parameters | | | | | |
|---|---|---|---|---|---|---|
| | Slope | Intercept | $a$ | $ab$ | $b$ | $1/b$ |
| Mannitol | 1.736 | 17.932 | 0.576 | 0.0558 | 0.0968 | 10.330 |
| Chitin | 1.223 | 12.927 | 0.818 | 0.0774 | 0.0946 | 10.570 |
| Cop–CM | 1.512 | 16.880 | 0.661 | 0.0592 | 0.0896 | 11.164 |

*2.8. Loading Capacity*

The loading capacity of **Cop–CM** excipient was studied by using metronidazole as a model drug for an incompressible material. Compressing metronidazole alone (100% as a reference) gives rise to tablets with low mechanical strength and long disintegration times. However, the effect of increasing the weight ratios of **Cop–CM**/metronidazole from 0/500 to 500/0 (wt/wt) on these properties were investigated. The results indicated that by increasing the quantity of **Cop–CM** in the matrix, compactability is improved and the disintegration time is decreased as shown Figure 9. As a result, **Cop–CM** is capable of accommodate poorly compressible drugs with high loading capacity without affecting the physical and mechanical properties.

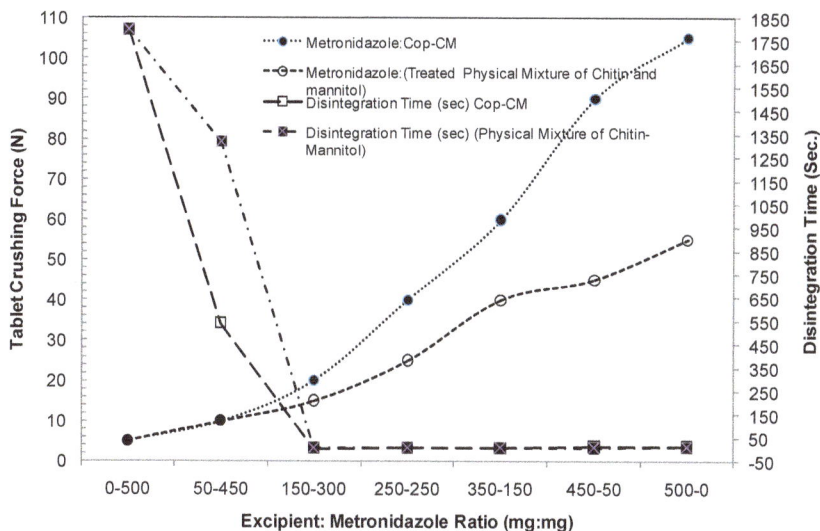

**Figure 9.** Relationship between tablet crushing force and disintegration time at different **Cop–CM**: metronidazole ratios using a physical mixture of chitin-mannitol (2:8, w/w) as a reference. Data are represented as the mean of $n = 10$. **Cop–CM** represents the co-processed chitin-mannitol (2:8 w/w) excipient.

## 2.9. Functionality

The functionality of **Cop–CM** as an excipient was investigated by examining different processing techniques including DC, RC and WG to prepare tablets. The three formulations containing **Cop–CM** and low strength drugs (montelukast and domperidone) were investigated. Different reported ODT formulations for these two drugs using almost DC technique are summarized in Table 4 [50–56]. In these formulations, several excipients were used to obtain fast disintegrating tablets. Mannitol and microcrystalline cellulose were used as diluents, in addition to deferent superdisintegrants such as croscarmellose sodium, crospovidone, sodium starch glycolate and starch. Combination of talc and magnesium stearate was used as a lubricant system [51,52,54,56]. Furthermore, co-processing of two disintegrants, e.g., crospovidone and sodium starch glycolate, using alcoholic solvent was proposed to obtain fast disintegrating tablets [51]. DC followed by sublimation at 60 °C was also proposed for ODT formulation [56]. In the present work, co-processed mixture of mannitol and chitin by RC (**Cop–CM**) is used as a multi-functional excipients (diluents and superdisintegrant), in addition to limited number of excipients (flavor, sweetening agent) and sodium stearyl fumarate as inert lubricant. Although a limited number of excipients were used with **Cop–CM** as ODT base to improve the taste and to prevent sticking of powder on punches and dies during tablet compression, the fast disintegration properties (≤30 s) was attained at relatively high tablet crushing force (crushing force: 60–80 N) values (Table 5). The tablets obtained from all the processing techniques showed high internal binding and friability <0.4% (Table 5). The results indicate that **Cop–CM** is compressible and preserves its functionality whether utilized in DC, RC or WG formulations. Hence, it can be used as a multifunctional base (binder, filler and disintegrant) in ODT formulations.

**Table 4.** Composition of various ODT formulations of montelukast sodium and domperidone.

| Montelukast Sodium | | | |
| --- | --- | --- | --- |
| **Singulair [50]** | **FDT [51]** | **ODT [52]** | **ODT [Present work]** |
| - Mannitol<br>- Microcrystalline cellulose<br>- Hydroxypropyl cellulose<br>- Croscarmellose sodium<br>- Aspartame<br>- Red ferric oxide<br>- Cherry flavor<br>- Magnesium stearate | - Mannitol<br>- Microcrystalline cellulose<br>- Crospovidone *<br>- Sodium starch glycolate *<br>- Sodium saccharin<br>- Mint flavor<br>- Talc<br>- Magnesium stearate | - Mannitol<br>- Microcrystalline cellulose<br>- Crospovidone or Croscarmellose sodium<br>- Aspartame<br>- Talc<br>- Magnesium stearate | - Mannitol $^+$<br>- Chitin $^+$<br>- Strawberry flavor<br>- Aspartame<br>- Sodium stearyl fumarate |

| Domperidone | | | |
| --- | --- | --- | --- |
| **Oroperidys [53]** | **FDT [54]** | **FDT [55]** | **FDT [56]** |
| - Mannitol<br>- Microcrystalline cellulose<br>- Maltodextrin<br>- Croscarmellose sodium<br>- Glucose<br>- Mint flavor<br>- Peppermint gasoline<br>- Anise oil<br>- Gasoline mint<br>- Levomentol<br>- Glycyrrhizate ammonium<br>- Gasoline cloves<br>- Acesulfame potassium<br>- Arabic gum<br>- Sulphur dioxide<br>- Magnesium stearate | - Mannitol<br>- Microcrystalline cellulose<br>- Sodium starch glycolate<br>- Lactose<br>- Talc<br>- Magnesium stearate | - Mannitol<br>- Microcrystalline cellulose<br>- Sodium starch glycolate<br>- Lactose<br>- Crospovidone<br>- Aspartame<br>- Citric acid<br>- Sodium bicarbonate<br>- Maize starch<br>- Starch 1500<br>- Colloidal anhydrous silica<br>- Lemon flavor<br>- Green lake color<br>- Menthol<br>- Magnesium stearate | - Mannitol<br>- Microcrystalline cellulose<br>- Camphor<br>- Ispaghula husk<br>- Povidone K30<br>- Crospovidone<br>- Guar gum<br>- Aspartame<br>- Colloidal anhydrous silica<br>- Orange flavor<br>- Talc<br>- Magnesium stearate |

* Co-processed together by alcoholic granulation, $^+$ Co-processed together by roll compaction, FDT: fast disintegrating tablet, ODT: oro-dispersible tablet.

**Table 5.** Composition and physical properties of montelukast and domperidone oro-dispersible tablets.

| Material | Composition (% w/w) | | | | | |
|---|---|---|---|---|---|---|
| | Montelukast | | | Domperidone | | |
| Drug | 01.77 | | | 03.40 | | |
| **Cop–CM** | 94.73 | | | 93.10 | | |
| Strawberry powder flavor | 02.00 | | | 02.00 | | |
| Aspartame | 00.50 | | | 00.50 | | |
| Sodium stearyl fumarate | 01.00 | | | 01.00 | | |
| **Tablet Physical Properties** | Tablet preparation process | | | | | |
| | DC | RC | WG | DC | RC | WG |
| Crushing force (N) | | 70–80 | | | 60–70 | |
| Friability (%) | 0.25 | 0.32 | 0.30 | 0.18 | 0.29 | 0.37 |
| Disintegration time(s) | 20 | 30 | 20 | 26 | 20 | 28 |

DC, RC and WG represent direct compression, roll compaction and wet granulation, respectively.
Cop–CM represents the co-processed chitin-mannitol (2:8 w/w) mixture.

## 2.10. Stability Studies

The stability of montelukast and domperidone tablets prepared by RC procedures in Section 2.9 (functionality) was investigated. Tablets were packed in aluminum/aluminum packs and incubated at 25 °C and 40 °C/75% relative humidity for different periods of time and then tested by HPLC methods. The HPLC method was initially tested for system suitability (*i.e.*, peak symmetry, repeatability, and resolution) and for validation parameters (*i.e.*, specificity, stability in solution, linearity and limit of quantitation (LOQ)) according to USP [57] and ICH guidelines [58]. The HPLC results showed a good separation between the drugs and their related impurities. Also, the methods were found to be suitable for stability studies, *i.e.*, the resolution, tailing factors and injection repeatability are within the acceptable criteria. In addition, analysis of samples obtained from stress testing studies in solutions (0.1 N NaOH, 0.1 N HCl, and 0.3% $H_2O_2$) indicated that the HPLC methods are stability indicating. The methods were linear over the range of ±50% of the target concentrations with $r^2$ of > 0.99. The LOQ values are within 0.08–0.4 and 0.05–0.14 (w/w %) for montelukast and domperidone tablets, respectively.

**Table 6.** Stability data for montelukast and domperidone oro-dispersible tablets.

| Product | Compound/Limit | Percentage (w/w) | | | |
|---|---|---|---|---|---|
| | | 25 °C/65%RH | | 40 °C/75% RH | |
| | | Initial | 24 Months | 3 Months | 6 Months |
| Montelukast | Drug/90%–110% | 99.4 | 104.8 | 102.8 | 98.2 |
| | Drug S–oxide/≤2.0% | 0.9 | 1.1 | 3.4 | 3.6 |
| | Drug *cis*–isomer/≤0.5% | 0.1 | 0.5 | 0.1 | 0.1 |
| | Any other ≤ 0.4% | 0.0 | 0.2 | 0.1 | 0.1 |
| | Total impurities ≤ 3.0% | 1.0 | 2.0 | 3.6 | 3.8 |
| Domperidone | Drug/95%–105% | 100.1 | – | 100.7 | 101.4 |
| | Any other/≤0.25% | 0.06 | – | 0.04 | 0.04 |
| | Total impurities/≤0.5% | 0.2 | – | 0.1 | 0.1 |

As shown in the data in Table 6, no significant decrease in the potency of montelukast and domperidone tablets occurred upon storage at 40 °C/75% RH for six months. Montelukast is liable to oxidation by heat [59] forming montelukast S-oxide; however, under shelf–life conditions (25 °C/65% RH) the degradation content of this product is within the limit (2.0%). Domperidone tablets display excellent stability when the fraction of impurities does not exceed 0.1% after 6 months incubation at 40 °C/75% RH. Both products showed fast disintegration (<30 s) and drug release (>90%) before and after incubation at 40 °C/75% RH indicating the absence of formulation ageing (Table 6).

## 3. Experimental Section

### 3.1. Materials

A-Chitin of average molecular weight 1000 KD, degree of acetylation of about 0.96 and a mean particle size of 90 μm (Zhejiang Jiande Biochemical, Jiande, China) and D-mannitol (Pearlitol), crystalline grade, with a mean particle size of 160 μm (Roquette, Lestrem, France) were used, Purified water of BP grade, Mannogem EZ and Pharmaburst C1 (SPI, Septemes-Les Vallons, France), Isomalt galenIQ™ 721 (BENEO–Palatinit GmbH, Mannheim, Germany), PanExcea MHC200G (Avantor Performance Materials, Inc./Center Valley, PA, USA), sodium stearyl fumarate (JRS, Patterson, NY, USA) and Crospovidone (Polyplasdone XL) with an average particle size of 110–140 (ISP, Wayne, NJ, USA) were also used. All active pharmaceutical ingredients employed *i.e.*, montelukast sodium (Mylan Lab., Hyderabad, India), domperidone (Xinshiji pharma, Fuzhou, Fujian, China) and metronidazole (Hubei Max Pharma, Wuhan, Hubei, China) were of pharmaceutical grade. All other excipients and reagents used were of pharmaceutical or analytical grades, respectively.

### 3.2. Methods

#### 3.2.1. Preparation of co-Processed Mannitol-Chitin Excipient

Three co–processed mixtures (each 1 kg) of chitin and mannitol of different ratios (1:9, 2:8 and 3:7 w/w) were prepared using different processing techniques, *i.e.*, direct mixing, RC and WG.

*Direct mixing:* The three mixtures were separately passed through a 1000 μm mesh sieve (Fritsch, Idar-Oberstein, Germany) and then mixed for 5 min at 10 rpm using a 1 L cubic blender equipped with a motor drive machine (Erweka, Heusenstamm, Germany).

*Roll compaction:* The three mixtures prepared by direct mixing were compacted using a roll compactor equipped with DPS type rolls (TFC–labo, Vector Corporation, Marion, IA, USA), set at about 5 MPa roll pressure, 4 rounds/minutes roll speed and 20 rounds/minutes screw control speed. The compacted powders were collected and passed through either the 710 μm or 1000 μm sieves using a milling machine equipped with a motor drive machine. Finally the granules were mixed for 5 min at 10 rpm using a 1-L cubic blender equipped with a motor drive machine.

*Wet granulation:* 350, 450 and 550 mL of 14.5% (w/v) of aqueous mannitol solutions were used as granulating agents to prepare the chitin-mannitol mixtures (1:9, 2:8 and 3:7 w/w ratio, respectively). The sieved chitin and the remaining quantity of mannitol were placed in granulation pans (Erweka,

Heusenstamm, Germany) and granulated with the mannitol solution using a mixing speed of 150 rpm. The wet masses were passed through a 9.5 mm sieve. Drying was performed at 60 °C using a drying oven (UT6200, Heraeous, Hanau, Germany). The granules were passed through the 1000 µm sieve and mixed using the same procedures as used for the RC preparation.

3.2.2. Characterization of Co-Processed Chitin-Mannitol (**Cop–CM**)

*Fourier transform infrared spectroscopy:* FT-IR measurements were undertaken using an FT-IR instrument (Paragon 1000, Perkin Elmer, Llantrisant, UK) by means of thin pellets containing 1 mg of each sample dispersed in 100 mg of KBr. The spectra were recorded at room temperature as an average of 30 scans, in the 400–4000 cm$^{-1}$ range with a spectral resolution of 1 cm$^{-1}$. In order to minimize the effects of traces of $CO_2$ and water vapour from the atmosphere of the sample compartment, the spectrometer was purged with nitrogen.

*X-ray powder diffractometry:* The XRPD patterns were measured using an X-ray diffractometer (PW1729, Philips, Amsterdam, The Netherlands). The radiation was generated using a *CoKα* source and filtered through Ni filters; a wavelength of 1.79025 Å at 40 mA and 35 kV was used. The instrument was operated over the 2θ range of 5–60°. The range and the chart speed were set at 2 × 103 cycles/s and 10 mm/2θ, respectively.

*Differential scanning calorimetry (DSC):* Samples (~5 mg) were hermetically sealed in aluminum pans and scanned over a range temperature of 0–300°C at a rate of 5 °C/min (DSC 25, Mettler Toledo, Greifensee, Germany). The instrument was calibrated using indium and the calorimetric data were analyzed using STAR software (version 9).

*Scanning electron microscopy:* The morphology of the samples were determined using a scanning electron microscope (Quanta 200 3D, FEI, Eindhoven, Netherland) operated at an accelerating voltage of 1200 V. The sample (0.5 mg) was mounted onto a 5 × 5 mm silicon wafer affixed via graphite tape to an aluminum stub. The powder was then sputter-coated for 105 s at a beam current of 20 mA/dm$^3$ with a 100 Å layer of gold/palladium alloy.

*Angle of Repose:* Angle of Repose (*q*) was determined using the funnel method [37]. The sample blends were poured through a funnel that could be raised vertically until a maximum cone height (*h*) was obtained. Radius of the heap (*r*) was measured and then *q* was calculated using the formula:

$$q = \tan^{-1}(\frac{h}{r}) \tag{5}$$

*Particle size:* The particle size distributions for all samples were measured by using a Malvern Mastersizer 2000 instrument (Malvern Instruments Ltd., Worcestershire, UK). Approximately 5 mL of powder was used for each measurement. The air pressure was set at 2.0 bar, and the feed rate was set at 50%. The particle size distributions D10, D50 and D90 were recorded. Each sample was measured three times.

*Bulk density (BD) and tapped density (TD):* Approximately 100 mL of powder was gently poured into a tarred graduated cylinder and the initial volume and weight of the material recorded. The graduated cylinder is placed on a tap density tester (SVM, Tapped volumeter, Erweka, Heusenstamm, Germany) and the final volume is recorded after 200 taps. *BD* and *TD* are calculated by dividing the initial and final volume of powder by the weight of powder, respectively [37].

*Water content:* The water content of the powders was measured using a Karl Fischer Titrator (DL38, Mettler Toledo, Greifensee, Switzerland).

*pH measurement:* The pH was measured using a a pH-meter (3030, Jenway, Staffordshire, UK).

*Hygroscopicity:* Samples (2.5 g) were stored in desiccators containing water saturated salt solutions at room temperature (20 °C) for 10 and 14 days. The media compositions were set according to the Handbook of Chemistry and Physics [60] to obtain relative humidity's (RHs) of 52%, 62%, 75%, 84% and 95% using $Ca(NO_3).4H_2O$, $NH_4NO_3$, $NaCl$, $KCl$ and $Na_2HPO_4.12H_2O$, respectively. The samples were withdrawn after a fixed time period and kept at 20 °C for 1 and 24 h before weighing and calculating the fractional gain in mass compared to the original mass under the different RH conditions.

3.2.3. Physical and Chemical Properties of Tablets Prepared from **Cop–CM**

*Crushing force, disintegration and friability:* The crushing force (6D, Schelenuiger, Thun, Switzerland), disintegration (2T31, Erweka, Heusenstamm, Germany) and friability (Erweka, Heusenstamm, Germany) tests were performed following the general tests in the BP [42].

*Influence of particle size on tablet properties:* Samples of **Cop–CM** powders were passed through either 710 μm or 1000 μm sieves and individually mixed with 1.0% (w/w) of sodium stearyl fumarate as a lubricant and then compressed using a single punch tabletting machine (SF3, Chadmach Machinery, Ahmedabad, India) at different crushing force values of 30, 50, 70, 90, 110, 130 and 150 N, using a 10 mm circular punch to produce tablets of 250 mg weight. The disintegration time and friability were measured at each tablet crushing force point. Some of the commercially available ODT bases (Pharmaburst C1, Isomalt galenIQ™ 721, Mannogem EZ and PanExcea MHC 200G) in addition to Mannogem EZ and 3% crospovidone, Isomalt galenIQ™ 721 and 3% crospovidone powders were lubricated using 1% w/w sodium stearyl fumarate and used as reference materials.

*Moisture uptake studies:* Moisture uptake studies were conducted in order to assess the physical stability of the ODTs composed of **Cop–CM** base. Twenty tablets were kept in a desiccator over calcium chloride at 37 °C for 24 h. The tablets were then weighed and exposed to 75% relative humidity, at room temperature for 14 days. The required humidity was achieved by the use of saturated sodium chloride solution at the bottom of the desiccators for 72 h. Tablets were weighed and the fractional increase in mass was recorded [60].

*Wetting time:* A piece of tissue paper (8 cm in diameter), folded twice was placed in a Petri dish (8.5 cm in diameter) containing 6 mL of water. One tablet was carefully placed on the surface of the tissue paper and allowed to wet completely [60]. The time required for the water to reach the upper surface of the tablet was recorded as the wetting time.

*Loading capacity:* A study was undertaken to measure the impact of the drug load on the performance of **Cop–CM** as tablet excipient. Tablets were prepared by DC using a SF3 single punch tablet press machine equipped with D-type tooling. The seven experiments were performed using **Cop–CM** and metronidazole, containing, 0%, 10%, 30%, 50%, 70%, 90% and 100% (for comparison) of metronidazole lubricated with 0.3% sodium stearyl fumarate. The prepared tablets were circular in shape with a diameter of 12 mm and a mass of 500 mg. Tablets from each experiment were evaluated for crushing force and disintegration time.

*Functionality*: To investigate the functionality of **Cop–CM**, two drug models as small strength tablets were studied including montelukast sodium and domperidone. The tablets for the two drugs were prepared by DC, RC as well as WG methods. The montelukast and domperidone tablets contained 1.77% and 3.4% of drug and 94.7% and 93.1% of **Cop–CM**, respectively. In addition, both drugs formulations contained strawberry powder (2.0%), aspartame (0.5%) and sodium stearyl fumarate (1.0%). For the DC experiments, montelukast and all excipients, except sodium stearyl fumarate, were first mixed for 2 min and then sodium stearyl fumarate was added and further mixed for another 2 min.

For the RC procedure, montelukast (1.77% w/w), **Cop–CM** (25% w/w, intra–granular) and sodium stearyl fumarate (0.6% w/w) were compacted by employing a DP roll type compaction using 10 MPa roll pressure, 3 rounds/minutes roll speed and 43 rounds/minutes screw control speed and then passed through a 1000 μm sieve. The remaining amount of **Cop–CM** was added and mixed for 2 min followed by the addition of sodium stearyl fumarate (0.4% w/w). The powder was then further mixed for 2 min.

For the WG procedure, montelukast (1.77% w/w) and **Cop–CM** (35% w/w, intra-granular) were granulated with 50% (w/v) ethanol in water, dried at 60 °C, and then sieved using the 1000 μm sieve. The remaining amount of **Cop–CM** was added and mixed for 2 min; sodium stearyl fumarate (1%) was then added and mixed for a further 2 min. The same procedures were repeated for domperidone. The prepared mixtures for each drug were compressed at 300 mg tablet weight, for which 10 mm shallow concave punches and dies were used. Dissolution tests (DT–80; Erweka, Heusenstamm, Germany) for montelukast and domperidone were performed according to the USP [61], FDA [62] and BP [63] published dissolution methods. The released fraction of montelukast and domperidone were determined spectrophotometrically (Du-650i, Beckman Coulter, Brea, CA, USA) by measuring the first derivative absorbance modes at 290 nm for montelukast and absorbance mode at 280 nm for domperidone.

*Compressibility:* Mannitol, chitin and **Cop–CM** powder samples were compressed using a universal testing machine (RKM 50, PR–F system, ABS Instruments, Tamilnadu, Germany) equipped with 12 mm round, flat face upper and lower punches as well as dies; punch speed was fixed at 10 mm/min. Different compression forces from 80 to 390 MPa were applied. Three tablets were prepared to ensure reproducibility. Compression was carried out at 400 mg tablet weight. The compression behavior of the samples was evaluated using Kawakita analysis [43–46].

*Stability studies:* Montelukast and domperidone tablets prepared by DC were packed in aluminum/aluminum strips and stored at 25 °C/60% RH and 40 °C/75% RH for 24 and 6 months, respectively. At different interval times, tablets were withdrawn and tested for dissolution and content of drug and its related substances by stability indicating and validated HPLC methods [57,59,64]. The HPLC instrument was equipped with a P1000 pump and a UV1000 detector (TSP, Alexandria, VA, USA). For montelukast tablets, a mixture of acetate buffer (0.385% ammonium acetate in water adjusted with acetic acid to pH 3.5) and methanol (15:85, v/v) was used as the mobile phase and an octadecylsilyl silica column as the stationary phase (250 × 4 mm, 10 μm). UV detection at 254 nm, a flow rate of 1 mL/min, and 20 μL injection volumes of the test solutions (0.2 mg montelukast /mL of 70% ethanol) were used. While for domperidone tablets, methanol and 0.5% ammonium acetate in water were used as the mobile phases A and B, respectively. A linear gradient elution with a flow rate of 1.5 mL/min was programmed as follows: time 0 min: 30, 70, time 10 min: 100, 0, and time 12 min: 100, 0 for mobile phase A and B, respectively. A based-deactivated, end capped L7 column was used as the stationary phase (Hypersil C8 BDS, 100 × 4.6 mm, 3 μm). UV detection at 280 nm and a 10 μL injection volume of the test solutions (5 mg domperidone/mL of 0.1 M·HCl in 50% ethanol) were employed. The HPLC method was initially tested for system suitability (*i.e.*, peak symmetry, repeatability, and resolution) and for validation parameters (*i.e.*, specificity, recovery, stability in solution, linearity, and limit of quantitation (LOQ)) according to USP guidelines [57].

## 4. Conclusions

Co-processing of crystalline mannitol with α-chitin by RC offers an excellent multifunctional base for ODT formulations. The novel excipient displayed fast disintegration and wetting properties over a wide range of tablet crushing force values in comparison with commercially available ODT bases. Regardless of the preparation method (DC, WG or DG), the functionality of the novel excipient was preserved. Moreover, the excipient can accommodate a high amount of drug without affecting its functionality. Utilization of the novel excipient in ODT containing active pharmaceutical ingredients offers very fast disintegration and wetting rates, excellent chemical stability and binding properties. Consequently, the need to use expensive packaging materials for ODT will be eliminated as tablets will no long be prone to breaking during patient use.

## Author Contributions

Adnan A. Badwan, Babur Z. Chowdhry and Stephen A. Leharne conceived and designed the experiments; Nidal Daraghmeh performed the experiments; Nidal Daraghmeh analyzed the data; Adnan A. Badwan contributed reagents/materials/analysis tools; Nidal Daraghmeh and Mahmoud M.H. Al Omari wrote the paper.

## Conflicts of Interest

The authors declare no conflict of interest.

## References

1. Jivraj, M.; Martini, L.G.; Thomson, C.M. An overview of the different excipients useful for the direct compression of tablets. *Pharm. Sci. Tech. Today* **2000**, *3*, 58–63.
2. Bhattacharyya, L.; Shuber, S.; Sheehan, S.; William, R. Excipients: background/Introduction. In *Excipient Development for Pharmaceutical, Biotechnology, and Drug Delivery Systems*; Katdare, A., Chaubal, M.V., Eds.; Informa Healthcare Inc.: New York, NY, USA, 2006; pp. 1–3.
3. Jonwal, N.; Mane, P.; Mokati, S.; Meena, A. Preparation and *in vitro* evaluation of mouth dissolving tablets of domperidone. *Int. J. Pharm. Pharm. Sci.* **2010**, *3*, 975–1491.

4.  U.S. Department of Health and Human Services, Food and Drug Administration, Centre for Drug Evaluation and Research (CDER). Guidance for industry: Orally disintegrating tablets, 2007. Available online: http://www.fda.gov/downloads/Drugs/GuidanceComplianceRegulatoryInformation/ Guidances/ucm070578.pdf (accessed on 2 February 2015).

5.  Orodispersible tablets. In *European Pharmacopeia*, 8th ed.; Council of Europe: Strasbourge, France, 2014; Volume 1, p. 811.

6.  Polyplasdone® crospovidone: Superdisintegrants for orally disintegrating and chewable tablets. Available online: http://www.anshulindia.com/pdfs/Polyplasdone%20for%20odt%20Lit.pdf (accessed on 3 February 2015).

7.  Deshpande, K.B.; Ganesh, N.S. Formulation and evaluation of orodispersible tablets of propranolol hydrochloride. *Int. J. Res. Pharm. Biomed. Sci.* **2011**, *2*, 529–534.

8.  Bandari, S.; Mittapalli, R.K.; Gannu, R.; Rao, Y.M. Orodispersible tablets: An overview. *Asian J. Pharm.* **2008**, *2*, 2–11.

9.  Pfister, W.R.; Ghosh, T.K. Orally disintegrating tablets, products, technologies, and development issues. Pharmaceutical Technology. Available online: http://www.pharmtech.com/node/ 238195?rel=canonical (accessed on 3 February 2015).

10. Schiermeier, S.; Schmidt, P.C. Fast dispersible ibuprofen tablets. *Eur. J. Pharm. Sci.* **2002**, *15*, 295–305.

11. Raymond, C.R.; Paul, J.S.; Siân, C.O. *Handbook of Pharmaceutical Excipients*, 5th ed.; Pharmaceutical Press: Greyslake, IL, USA; American Pharmacists Association: Washington, DC, USA, 2006.

12. Mannogem® Mannitol. Available online: http://www.spipharma.com/product.php? id=15&prodtype=p (accessed on 3 February 2015).

13. Dolson, L. Low Carb Diets: What are sugar alcohols? Comparisons and blood sugar impact. Available online: http://lowcarbdiets.about.com/od/whattoeat/a/sugaralcohols.htm (accessed on 3 February 2015).

14. Ghosh, T.; Ghosh, A.; Prasad, D. A review on new generation orodispersible tablets and its future prospective. *Int. J. Pharm. Pharm. Sci.* **2011**, *3*, 1–7.

15. Erik, L.; Philippe, L.; Jose, L. Pulverulent Mannitol and Process for Preparing it. U.S. Patent 6743447, 1 June 2004.

16. Debord, B.; Lefebvre, C.; Guyothermann, A.M.; Hubert, J.; Bouche, R.; Guyot, J.C. Study of different crystalline forms of mannitol: Comparative behavior under compression. *Drug Dev. Ind. Pharm.* **1987**, *13*, 1533–1546.

17. Patil, J.; Vishwajith, V.; Gopal, V. Formulation development and evaluation of chewable tablets containing non-sedating antihistamine. *J. Pharm. Sci. Innov.* **2012**, *1*, 112–117.

18. Muzzarelli, R.A.; Tubertini, O. Chitin and chitosan as chromatographic supports and adsorbents for collection of metal ions from organic and aqueous solutions and sea-water. *Talanta* **1969**, *16*, 1571–1577.

19. Datta, P.K.; Basu, P.S.; Datta, T.K. Isolation and characterization of *Vicia faba* lectin affinity purified on chitin column. *Prep. Biochem.* **1984**, *14*, 373–387.

20. Songkroah, C.; Nakbanpote, W.; Thiravetyan, P. Recovery of silver-thiosulphate complexes with chitin. *Proc. Biochem.* **2004**, *39*, 1553–1559.

21. Krajewska, B. Application of chitin- and chitosan-based materials for enzyme immobilizations: A review. *Enzyme Microb. Tech.* **2004**, *35*, 126–139.

22. Yusof, N.L.; Wee, A.; Lim, L.Y.; Khor, E. Flexible chitin films as potential wound-dressing materials: wound model studies. *J. Biomed. Mater. Res. A* **2003**, *66*, 224–232.

23. Rathke, T.D.; Hudson, S.M. Review of chitin and chitosan as fiber and film formers. *J. Macromol. Sci. C* **1994**, *34*, 375–437.

24. Pierson, Y.; Chen, X.; Bobbink, F.D.; Zhang, J.; Yan, N. Acid-catalyzed chitin liquefaction in ethylene glycol. *ACS Sustain. Chem. Eng.* **2014**, *2*, 2081–2089.

25. Chen, X.; Chew, S.L.; Kerton, F.M.; Yan, N. Direct conversion of chitin into a *N*-containing furan derivative. *Green Chem.* **2014**, *16*, 2204–2212.

26. Bobbink, F.D.; Zhang, J.; Pierson, Y.; Chen, X.; Yan, N. Conversion of chitin derived *N*-acetyl-D-glucosamine (NAG) into polyols over transition metal catalysts and hydrogen in water. *Green Chem.* **2015**, *17*, 1024–1031.

27. Daraghmeh, N.H.; Chowdhry, B.Z.; Leharne, S.A.; Al Omari, M.M.; Badwan, A.A. Chitin. In *Profiles of Drug Substances, Excipients and Related Methodology*; Brittain, H., Ed.; Elsevier Inc.: New York, NY, USA, 2011; Volume 36, pp. 35–102.

28. Muzzarelli, R.A.A. *Chitin*; Pergamon Press: Oxford, UK, 1977.

29. Gupta, P.; Nachaegari, S.K.; Bansal, A.K. Improved Excipient Functionality by Co-Processing. In *Excipient Development for Pharmaceutical, Biotechnology, and Drug Delivery Systems*; Katdare, A., Chaubal, M.V., Eds.; Informa Healthcare Inc.: New York, NY, USA, 2006; pp. 109–124.

30. Rashid, I.; Daraghmeh, N.; Al-Remawai, M.; Leharne, S.A.; Chowdhry, B.Z.; Badwan, A. Characterization of chitin-metal silicates as binding superdisintegrants. *J. Pharm. Sci.* **2009**, *98*, 4887–4901.

31. Rashid, I.; Al-Remawi, M.; Eftaiha, A.; Badwan, A. Chitin–silicon dioxide coprecipitate as a novel superdisintegrant. *J. Pharm. Sci.* **2008**, *97*, 4955–4969.

32. Daraghmeh, N.; Rashid, I.; Al Omari, M.M.H.; Leharne, S.A.; Chowdhry, B.Z.; Badwan, A. Preparation and characterization of a novel co-processed excipient of chitin and crystalline mannitol. *AAPS Pharm. Sci. Tech.* **2010**, *11*, 1558–1571.

33. Kablan, T; Clément, Y. Bi, Y.; Françoise, K.A.; Mathias, O.K. Determination and modelling of moisture sorption isotherms of chitosan and chitin. *Acta Chim. Slov.* **2008**, *55*, 677–682.

34. Silva, S.S.; Duarte, A.R.C.; Carvalho, A.P.; Mano, J.F.; Reis, R.L. Green processing of porous chitin structures for biomedical applications combining ionic liquids and supercritical fluid technology. *Acta Biomater.* **2011**, *7*, 1166–1172.

35. Kharade, S.; Bhutkar, M.A. Novel superdisintegrants interpolymeric chitosan-alginate complex and chitin in the formulation of orodispersible tablets. *Int. J. Pharm. Res. Dev.* **2013**, *5*, 87–94.

36. Glenn, T.C.; Bruno, C.H. A Comparison of Physical and Mechanical Properties of Common Tableting Diluents. In *Excipient Development for Pharmaceutical, Biotechnology, and Drug Delivery Systems*; Katdare A., Chaubal M.V., Eds.; Informa Healthcare Inc.: New York, NY, USA, 2006; pp. 127–151.

37. Khinchi, M.P.; Gupta, M.K.; Bhandari, A.; Sharma, N.; Agarwal, D. Design and development of orally disintegrating tablets of famotidine prepared by direct compression method using different superdisintegrants. *J. App. Pharm. Sci.* **2011**, *1*, 50–58.

38. Nyström, C.; Alderborn, G.; Duberg, M.; Karehill, P.G. Bonding surface area and bonding mechanism-two important factors for the understanding of powder compactibility. *Drug Dev. Ind. Pharm.* **1993**, *19*, 2143–2196.

39. Alderborn, G.; Börjesson, E.; Glazer, M.; Nyström, C. Studies on direct compression of tablets. XIX: The effect of particle size and shape on the mechanical strength of sodium bicarbonate tablets. *Acta Pharm. Suec.* **1988**, *25*, 31–40.

40. Juppo, A.M. Change in porosity parameters of lactose, glucose and mannitol granules caused by low compression force. *Int. J. Pharm.* **1996**, *130*, 149–157.

41. Bhowmik, D.; Chiranjib, B.; Krishnakanth, P.; Chandira, R.M. Fast dissolving tablet: An overview. *J. Chem. Pharm. Res.* **2009**, *1*, 163–177.

42. Disintegration, Friability of Uncoated Tablets, Resistance to Crushing of Tablets. In *British Pharmacopeia*; The Stationary Office: London, UK, 2014; Volume V, pp. A333–A378, A493, A495.

43. Kawakita, K.; Lüdde, K.H. Some considerations on powder compression equations. *Powder Technol.* 1071, *4*, 61–68.

44. Shivanand, P.; Sprockel, O.L. Compaction behaviour of cellulose polymers. *Powder Technol.* **1992**, *69*, 177–184.

45. Lin, C.; Cham, T. Compression behaviour and tensile strength of heat-treated polyethylene glycols. *Int. J. Pharm.* **1995**, *118*, 169–179.

46. Nordström, J.; Klevan, I.; Alderborn, G. A particle rearrangement index based on the Kawakita powder compression equation. *J. Pharm. Sci.* **2008**, *98*, 1053–1063.

47. Adetunji, O.A.; Odeniyi, M.A.; Itiola, O.A. Compression, mechanical and release properties of chloroquine phosphate tablets containing corn and trifoliate yam starches as binders. *Trop. J. Pharm. Res.* **2006**, *5*, 589–596.

48. Martins, E.; Christiana, I.; Olobayo, K. Effect of grewia gum on the mechanical properties of paracetamol tablet formulations. *African J. Pharm. Pharmacol.* **2008**, *2*, 1–6.

49. Zhang, Y.; Law, Y.; Chakrabarti, S. Physical properties and compact analysis of commonly used direct compression binders. *AAPS Pharm. Sci. Tech.* **2005**, *4*, Article 62.

50. U.S. Food and Drug Administration. Singulair® (montelukast sodium) Tablets, Chewable Tablets, and Oral Granules. Available online: http://www.accessdata.fda.gov (accessed on 29 January 2015).

51. Mahesh, E.; Kiran Kumar, G.B.; Ahmed, M.G.; Kiran Kumar, P. Formulation and evaluation of montelukast sodium fast dissolving tablets. *Asian J. Biomed. Pharm. Sci.* **2012**, *2*, 75–82.

52. Chhajed, M.; Tiwari, D.; Malve, A.; Godhwani, T.; Chhajed, A.; Shrivastava, A.K. Formulation development and evaluation of montelukast sodium orodispersible tablets: A new trend in asthma treatmentInt. *J. Pharm. Res. Sci.* **2012**, *1*, 127–139.

53. Oroperidys 10 mg cp Orodispers, Vidal Homepage. Available online: http://www.vidal.fr/Medicament/oroperidys-75053.htm (accessed on 29 January 2015).

54. Parmar, R.B.; Baria, A.H.; Tank, H.M.; Faldu, S.D. Formulation and evaluation of domperidone fast dissolving tablets. *Int. J. Pharm. Tech. Res.* **2009**, *1*, 483–487.

55. Islam, A.; Haider, S.S.; Reza, M.S. Formulation and evaluation of orodispersible tablet of domperidone. *Dhaka Univ. J. Pharm. Sci.* **2011**, *10*, 117–122.

56. Sutradhar, K.B.; Akhter, D.T.; Uddin, R. Formulation and evaluation of taste masked oral dispersible tablets of domperidone using sublimation method. *Int. J. Pharm. Pharm. Sci.* **2012**, *4*, 727–732.

57. Validation of Compendia Procedures <1225>. In *United States Pharmacopeia and National Formulary (USP37-NF32)*; US Pharmacopoeia Convention: Rockville, MD, USA, 2014; Volume I, pp. 1157–1162.

58. Validation of Analytical Procedures: Text and Methodology, European Medicines Agency. Available online: http://www.ema.europa.eu/docs/en_GB/document_library/Scientific_guideline/2009/09/WC500002662.pdf (accessed on 3 February 2015).

59. Al Omari, M.M.; Zoubi, R.M.; Hasan, E.I.; Khader, T.Z.; Badwan, A.A. Effect of light and heat on the stability of montelukast in solution and in its solid state. *J. Pharm. Biomed. Anal.* **2007**, *45*, 465–471.

60. Weast, R.C. *Handbook of Chemistry and Physics*, 55th ed.; CRC Press: Boca Raton, FL, USA, 1974–1975; p. E-46.

61. Dissolution <711>. In *United States Pharmacopeia and National Formulary (USP37-NF32)*; US Pharmacopoeia Convention: Rockville, MD, USA, 2014; Volume 1, pp. 344–351.

62. *Dissolution Method*; U.S. Food and Drug Administration: Rockville, MD, USA. Available online: http://www.accessdata.fda.gov/scripts/cder/dissolution/dsp_SearchResults_Dissolutions.cfm?PrintAll=1 (accessed on 3 February 2015).

63. Domperidone Tablets. In *British Pharmacopeia*; The Stationary Office: London, UK, 2014; Volume III, p. 469.

64. Badwan, A.A. The Jordanian Pharmaceutical Manufacturing Co. (JPM), Amman, Jordan. Unpublished work, 2014.

# Design of Chitosan-Grafted Carbon Nanotubes: Evaluation of How the –OH Functional Group Affects Cs$^+$ Adsorption

Shubin Yang, Dadong Shao, Xiangke Wang, Guangshun Hou, Masaaki Nagatsu, Xiaoli Tan, Xuemei Ren and Jitao Yu

**Abstract:** In order to explore the effect of –OH functional groups in Cs$^+$ adsorption, we herein used the low temperature plasma-induced grafting method to graft chitosan onto carbon nanotubes (denoted as CTS-g-CNTs), as raw-CNTs have few functional groups and chitosan has a large number of –OH functional groups. The synthesized CTS-g-CNT composites were characterized using different techniques. The effect of –OH functional groups in the Cs$^+$ adsorption process was evaluated by comparison of the adsorption properties of raw-CNTs with and without grafting chitosan. The variation of environmental conditions such as pH and contact time was investigated. A comparison of contaminated seawater and simulated groundwater was also evaluated. The results indicated that: (1) the adsorption of Cs$^+$ ions was strongly dependent on pH and the competitive cations; (2) for CNT-based material, the –OH functional groups have a positive effect on Cs$^+$ removal; (3) simulated contaminated groundwater can be used to model contaminated seawater to evaluate the adsorption property of CNTs-based material. These results showed direct observational evidence on the effect of –OH functional groups for Cs$^+$ adsorption. Our findings are important in providing future directions to design and to choose effective material to remedy the removal of radioactive cesium from contaminated groundwater and seawater, crucial for public health and the human social environment.

Reprinted from *Mar. Drugs*. Cite as: Yang, S.; Shao, D.; Wang, X.; Hou, G.; Nagatsu, M.; Tan, X.; Ren, X.; Yu, J. Anticancer and Cancer Preventive Properties of Marine Polysaccharides: Some Results and Prospects. *Mar. Drugs* **2015**, *13*, 3116-3131.

## 1. Introduction

Radioactive cesium is of serious social and environment concern as it readily dissolves in water, it has a high fission yield (6.09%), and a long half-life (T$_{1/2}$ = 30.17 years) [1,2]. The major source of radioactive cesium is from the leaks of nuclear reactors, such as the nuclear disaster that occurred at Fukushima Daiichi in 2011 [3–5]. It is important to highlight that radioactive cesium can make its way into the food chain when present in wastewater, and do great harm to human health as well as to the living creatures in the aquatic environment [2,6,7]. Therefore, when accidentally released to the ground and sea, it is crucial for both the natural and the human social environment to find an effective material for removal of radioactive cesium from contaminated groundwater and seawater.

Over the past 50 years, various effective materials for capturing Cs$^+$ ions have been developed. Datta *et al.* [1] designed a novel vanadosilicate with hexadeca-coordinated Cs$^+$ ions as highly effective for Cs$^+$ removal. Torad *et al.* [8] showed a large Cs$^+$ adsorption capability of nano-structured Prussian blue particles. However, there are few reports about the effect of functional groups on Cs$^+$ adsorption. In addition, the effects of functional groups and structure determine the direction for design and for choosing material for the uptake of radioactive cesium ions. Dwivedi *et al.* [9] considered that the high affinity of resorcinol-formaldehyde resin for $Cs^+$ ions was attributed to the presence of the –OH group. In addition, the pH-dependence of $Cs^+$ adsorption was usually attributed to the competition exchange of hydrogen in the –OH groups. However, to the best of our knowledge, direct observational evidence on the effect of the –OH functional group in $Cs^+$ adsorption is still not available.

Carbon nanotubes (CNTs) and CNT-based materials gained widespread attention owing to their good chemical stability, relatively large specific area, and large average pore diameter [10–12]. Their size, shape, and physicochemical properties make them principal rivals for exploiting the growth of a potentially revolutionary material for diverse applications [13–15]. Conventional methods such as X-ray photoelectron spectroscopy (XPS), and X-ray powder diffraction (XRD) have been explicated to detect the structure and functional groups of CNTs. They reveal that regardless of the graphene structure, possession of few functional groups is the essential trait of pristine CNTs. Therefore, a significant amount of research activity into surface modification of CNTs was carried out to create functional groups on the nanotubes to explore their potential applications.

Conventional chemistry modification involving acid treatment and ultrasound may introduce wall damage of CNTs and cleave them into shorter pieces which is not especially environmentally friendly [16,17]. Low-temperature pressure plasma-induced grafting technique is an efficient method to graft functional groups onto CNT surfaces in the field of surface modifications and green eco-friendly chemistry [18]. Chitosan is one of the most abundant nontoxic biopolymers in nature with abundant hydroxyl groups. Diverse methods were applied to modify material by grafting chitosan to change its physical or chemical properties [2,19,20].

With these in mind, we herein designed novel chitosan grafted carbon nanotubes (CTS-g-CNTs) as $Cs^+$ remover. The composite was synthesized by a radio frequency Ar-plasma-induced grafting method. The variance of environmental conditions such as pH, ionic strength, and adsorbent content was taken into account. We determined the effect of the hydroxyl group on the $Cs^+$ adsorption process by comparison of the adsorption properties of CNTs with and without grafting chitosan. A comparison of contaminated seawater and simulated groundwater was also evaluated.

## 2. Results and Discussion

### 2.1. Material Characterization

The morphology and size of the raw-CNTs and CTS-g-CNTs were characterized by SEM and TEM. The CNTs (Figure 1A) have very smooth surfaces and the nanotubes are entangled, with a diameter of about 30 nm. From Figure 1B we can clearly observe the graphene sheet structure of raw-CNTs with an inner diameter of about 8.48 nm. However, the effective hydrated radius of cesium ions is only 0.33 nm, much smaller than the inner diameter of raw-CNTs [21–23]. Therefore, the cesium ions could easily diffuse into the inner part (pore) of the nanotubes, indicating that the pore filling is also one of the possible main mechanisms for the capture of $Cs^+$ ions by CNT-based material. A large number of previous studies have emphasized the importance of physical adsorption in the adsorption mechanism of heavy metal ions [12,24,25]. For instance, Omura *et al.* [25] designed a size-controlled nanospace of hexacyanoferrate applied in trapping Cs$^+$ ions. In Figure 1C, a more extensive three-dimensional network of the surface morphology between raw-CNTs and CTS-g-CNTs is observed. The CTS-g-CNTs depict large nanostructures of about 0.5–0.8 μm in diameter coated on the surface of CNTs. The obvious differences in the SEM images indicate that the CTS-g-CNTs composites have been synthesized successfully.

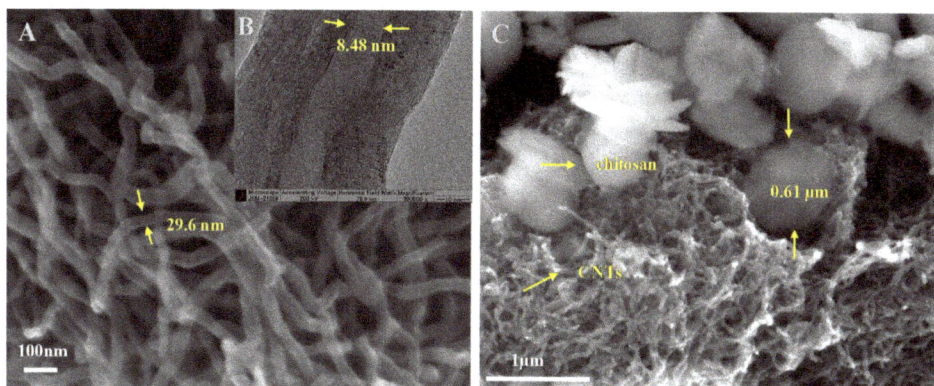

**Figure 1.** SEM (**A**) and TEM (**B**) images of raw-CNTs; and SEM image of CTS-g-CNTs (**C**).

The surface properties of the samples were analyzed by XPS, which was used to ensure the elemental composition at the surface. The grafted chitosan was evidenced by the following XPS analysis. In our system, nitrogen only exists in chitosan; therefore, the nitrogen content can be an indication of the extent of surface coverage by chitosan [26]. Figure 2A illustrates the N 1s spectrum of CTS-g-CNTs, a nitrogen peak at 400.5 eV was observed, which was attributed to the amino groups of chitosan. Besides, obvious differences of the O 1s spectrum (Figure 2B) between raw-CNTs and CTS-g-CNTs were also observed. After chitosan coating, the O 1s (533 eV) peak intensity of CTS-g-CNTs significantly increased with regard to that of CNTs, which was attributed to the hydroxyl groups of chitosan.

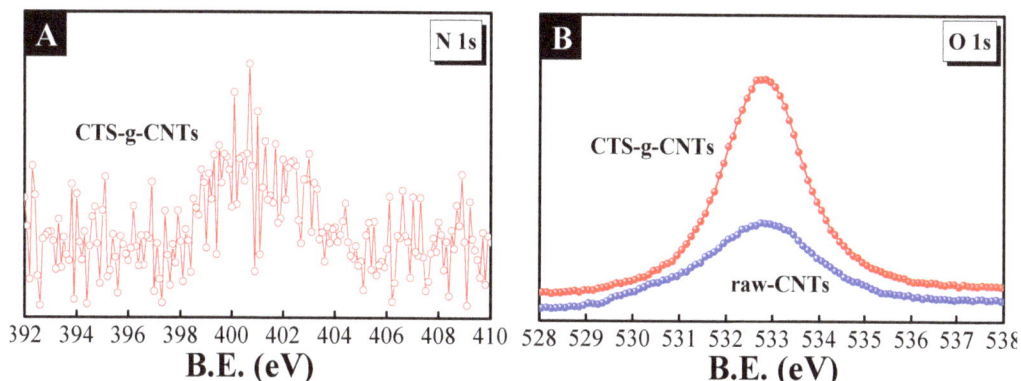

**Figure 2.** X-ray photoelectron spectroscopy (XPS) spectra of N 1s (**A**) and O 1s (**B**).

In addition, the C 1s XPS spectra of raw-CNTs, plasma treated CNTs (denoted as: CNTs-treated) and CTS-g-CNTs are shown in Figure 3. The more detailed analysis of the XPS C 1s spectra is shown in Table 1. All of the C 1s XPS spectra have three characteristic peaks: C=C (284.4 eV), C–C (285.4 eV) and C–O (286.2 eV) peak. As can be seen from the quantitative analysis in Table 1, after plasma treated, the peak fraction of C=C decreases, whereas the peak fraction of C–C increases. Ar plasma can activate the C=C bonds of the CNTs surface to increase the reactivity of CNTs during the pre-treatment as previously reported [27–29]. These activated C=C bonds can interact with chitosan, resulting in a decrease in the peak fraction of C=C, whereas there is an increase in the fractions of C–C and C–O. These XPS analyses are valid indication of the effective connection of chitosan onto the CNTs structure. The CTS-g-CNT composites were synthesized successfully which was consistent with the results of SEM analysis.

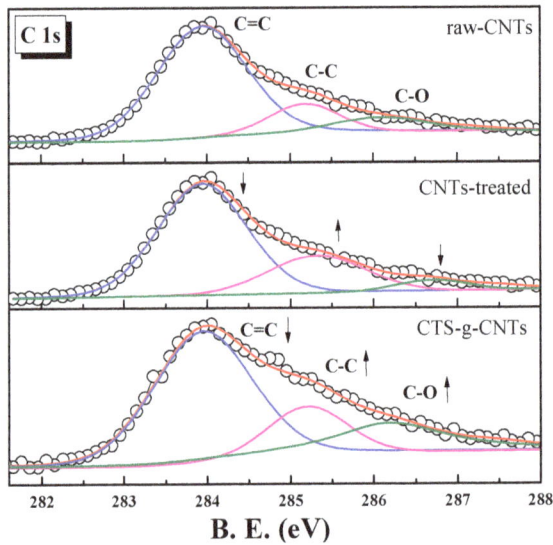

**Figure 3.** XPS spectra of C 1s.

X-ray diffraction (XRD) can provide useful information on the structural properties of CNT-based materials [17,30,31]. Figure 4A shows the XRD patterns of CNTs, CNTs-treated, CTS-g-CNTs and chitosan. For CNTs, a strong diffraction peak at $2\theta = 26.0°$ was observed, corresponding to the (002) planes of graphite. The peaks of the raw-CNT and CNTs-treated material are very intense and pointed, indicating a nanotube with excellent crystallinity. In addition, the XRD patterns of CNTs-treated and CNTs are very similar, meaning that there is only minor alteration in the structure of CNTs after Ar plasma treatment. The plasma treatment only activated the surface of CNTs without damaging the original orientation of CNTs alignment, as previously reported [27,32]. For CTS-g-CNTs, the peak at $2\theta = 26.2°$ is related to the characteristic of raw-CNTs. The dominant peak at $2\theta = 26.2°$ is still intense and sharp, indicating the CTS-g-CNTs composite shows a good crystallinity. Thus, the nanotube framework still shows strong influence on the properties of CTS-g-CNT composite. After loading with chitosan, many new miscellaneous and low intensity peaks appeared indicating lower crystallinity of the CTS-g-CNTs phase due to embedded chitosan. Namely, the CTS-g-CNTs composite had been synthesized. It was also observed that chitosan led to a small positive shift of the (002) plane of graphite, indicating that the distance between planes is reduced instead of increased. From Bragg's Law [33,34], we can see that the chitosan addition does not have a significant impact on the mean distance between graphitic walls. The broad peak in the XRD pattern of chitosan indicates the amorphous state of chitosan. The narrow and weak peak at $2\theta = 20.8°$ in the XRD pattern of CTS-g-CNTs corresponds to the characteristics of chitosan. From the XRD studies it is observed that grafted chitosan affects both the intensity and peak position of the CNTs phase. Combined with these phenomena, it was proposed that they were related to a phase change in the structure of CNTs, in which chitosan had connected to the CNTs.

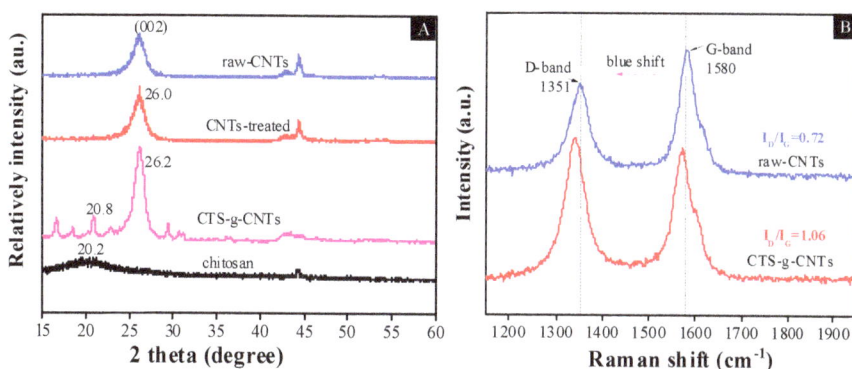

**Figure 4.** X-ray diffraction (XRD) patterns (**A**); and Raman spectra (**B**) of raw-CNTs and CNT-based materials.

**Table 1.** Curve fitting results of X-ray photoelectron spectroscopy (XPS) C 1s spectra.

|  | C=C (%) | C–C (%) | C–O (%) |
| --- | --- | --- | --- |
| raw-CNTs | 74.2 | 15.5 | 10.3 |
| CNTs-treated | 67.5 | 23.7 | 8.8 |
| CTS-g-CNTs | 60 | 17.8 | 22.2 |

Raman spectroscopy provides valuable information about the disorder in these materials. The Raman spectra of raw-CNTs and CTS-g-CNT composite are shown in Figure 4B. It is obvious that the spectrum of CNTs shows two characteristic bands at 1351 cm$^{-1}$ (D-band) for the presence of defects (sp$^3$ carbons, foreign atoms, *etc.*) of nanotubes and at 1580 cm$^{-1}$ (G-band) for the tangential modes of CNTs. However, after chitosan had grafted, a blue shift of the characteristic peaks was observed. The slight shifts of the D-band and G-band could be related to some molecule embedding, which has been reported earlier [15,35]. The intensity relation between the two bands ($I_G/I_D$) is the most widely used tool to evaluate the grafting of carbon nanotubes [17,36]. According to the Raman data, the CTS-g-CNTs composite shows a higher $I_G/I_D$ ratio due to the defects created along the nanotube surface during the plasma-induced grafting process.

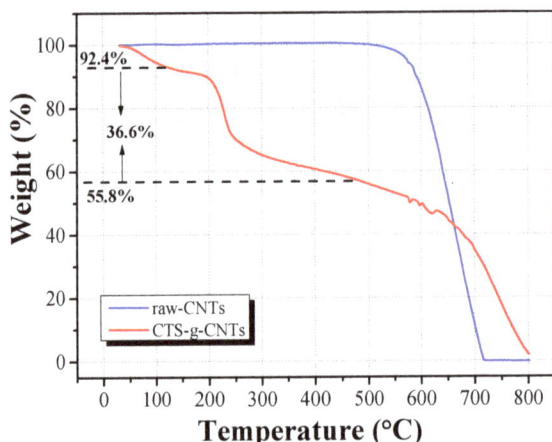

**Figure 5.** Thermogravimetric analysis (TGA) curves of raw-CNTs and CTS-g-CNT composite.

The weight percentage of grafted chitosan in CTS-g-CNTs composite can be estimated by thermogravimetric analysis (TGA). Figure 5 shows the TGA curves of CNTs and CTS-g-CNTs under 25% Ar/75% air atmosphere from 35 to 800 °C. For the TGA curve of CNTs, the weight loss of CNTs is negligible before 500 °C. For CTS-g-CNTs, there are three clearly separated weight loss stages in the range of 35–130 °C, 130–500 °C and 500–800 °C, which are mainly attributed to the combustion of the absorbed water, grafted chitosan, and CNTs, respectively. Assuming that the grafted chitosan was completely decomposed, the content of grafted chitosan was about 36.6% in the CTS-g-CNT composites.

*2.2. Adsorption Experiment*

It has become an important point for researchers and enterprises to know how environmental conditions such as pH, contact time, sorbent content, *etc.*, influence $Cs^+$ sorption capacity. Figure 6A shows how the pH influences $Cs^+$ adsorption in contaminated simulated groundwater using 0.6 g/L adsorbents. It is noted that the removal percentage of $Cs^+$ ions depends on pH value. We considered that there are two main reasons for the effect of pH value. The first is the surface properties of materials involving the surface charge of material and the protonation state of functional groups on the materials. At high pH, the material should possess a negative charge and more deprotonated functional groups, resulting in more $Cs^+$ ions being adsorbed through electrostatic interaction. The second one is the fierce competition between hydronium ions ($H_3O^+$, 0.28 nm) and hydrated cesium ions (0.33 nm) [37,38]. At high pH, it is expected that low concentration of $H_3O^+$ will compete for the adsorption sites with hydrated cesium ions. As can be seen from the effect of pH in Figure 6A, the difference of the $Cs^+$ removal percentage onto CNTs or CNT-treated material is negligible (<2.0%). Therefore, the plasma treatment cannot improve the adsorption capacity of CNTs in the removal of $Cs^+$ ions. By comparison with raw-CNTs, the adsorption capacity of CTS-g-CNTs is much higher by 11%–24%. We should note that the adsorption of $Cs^+$ ions on CTS-g-CNTs at pH >6.5 increases more quickly than that of $Cs^+$ on raw-CNTs. This is due to the increased –OH functional groups which are closely related to the grafted chitosan. With the increase of pH, more –OH functional groups could react with $Cs^+$ ions, leading to a rapid increase of the adsorption percentage. Therefore, for CNT-based material, –OH functional groups have a positive effect on $Cs^+$ removal.

The effect of contact time in the removal of $Cs^+$ from contaminated simulated groundwater by 0.6 g/L CTS-g-CNTs at pH = 7 was detected (Figure 6B). It was noted that the adsorption of $Cs^+$ reached equilibrium in about 10 h. Therefore, the shaking time (contact time) of 24 hours is sufficient to reach full equilibrium state. The adsorption of $Cs^+$ by 0.6 g/L CTS-g-CNTs at pH = 7 as a function of sorbent content is shown in Figure 6C. It is expected that the removal of $Cs^+$ ions increases with increasing solid content; the more solid content the more active efficient sites for $Cs^+$ ions.

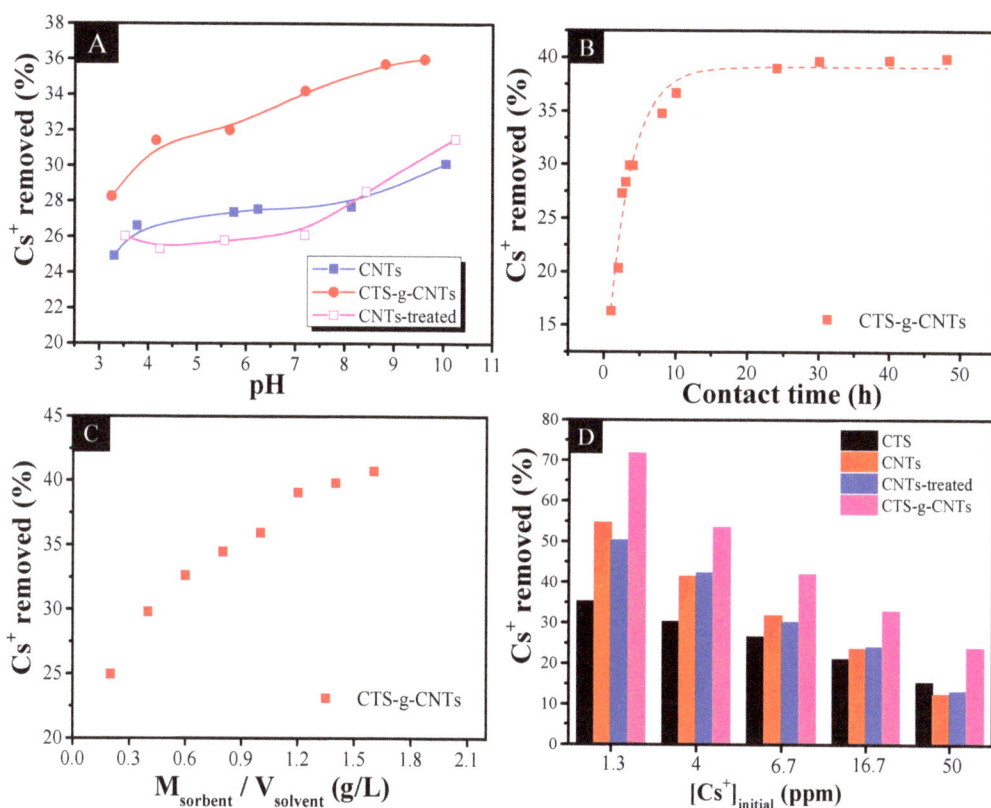

**Figure 6.** Effects of initial pH (**A**); contact time (**B**); sorbent content (**C**) and initial $Cs^+$ concentration for $Cs^+$ adsorption in contaminated simulated groundwater by CNTs-based materials with $m_{sorbent}/V_{solvent}$ = 0.6 g/L, $[Cs^+]_{initial}$ = 10.0 mg/L.

The comparison of the degree of $Cs^+$ removal for CTS, CNTs, CNTs-treated and CTS-g-CNTs sorbents at 1.3 ppm $\leq Cs^+ \leq$ 50 ppm, $m_{sorbent}/V_{solvent}$ = 0.6 g/L, and pH = 7 is shown in Figure 6D. The removal efficiency of the different sorbents was in the order of CTS < CNTs $\approx$ CNTs-treated < CTS-g-CNTs. Obviously, there is almost no difference between CNTs and CNT-treated while a clear increase was shown in CTS-g-CNT. We consider that there are two reasons for the enhanced efficiency of CTS-g-CNT. Dwivedi *et al.* [9] reported the high affinity of resorcinol-formaldehyde resin for $Cs^+$ ions to be attributed to the presence of the –OH group. In addition, chitosan is a nontoxic biopolymer with abundant hydroxyl groups. Therefore, we consider that the improved efficiency of CTS-g-CNTs is largely due to the increased –OH functional groups which are closely related to the grafted chitosan. The low removal efficiency of CTS is related to the peculiar structure of chitosan which appears lamellar when mixed with CNTs, while it is amorphous when considered alone in XRD patterns.

In addition, chitosan is a nontoxic biopolymer with abundant hydroxyl groups. Therefore, we consider that the improved efficiency of CTS-g-CNTs is largely due to the increased –OH functional groups which are closely related to the grafted chitosan.

An additional important characteristic of $Cs^+$ sorption is competitive cation dependence (Figure 7). Many researches have shown that ion exchange is an important principle in $Cs^+$ adsorption process. We can see that the adsorption of $Cs^+$ by CTS-g-CNTs in Figure 7 is strongly dependent on the competitive cations. In the presence of different competitive cations, the removal percentage of $Cs^+$ ions decreased in the order of $Li^+$ (48.5%) > $Na^+$ (32.8%) > $K^+$ (12.9%). This is closely related to the hydrated radii of cesium and the competitive cations. The hydrated radii of cations [23,39–41] decreased in the order of $Li^+$ (0.38 nm) > $Na^+$ (0.36 nm) > $K^+$ (0.33 nm) ≈ $Cs^+$ (0.33 nm), therefore, $K^+$ ions are the most important inhibitors of $Cs^+$ adsorption.

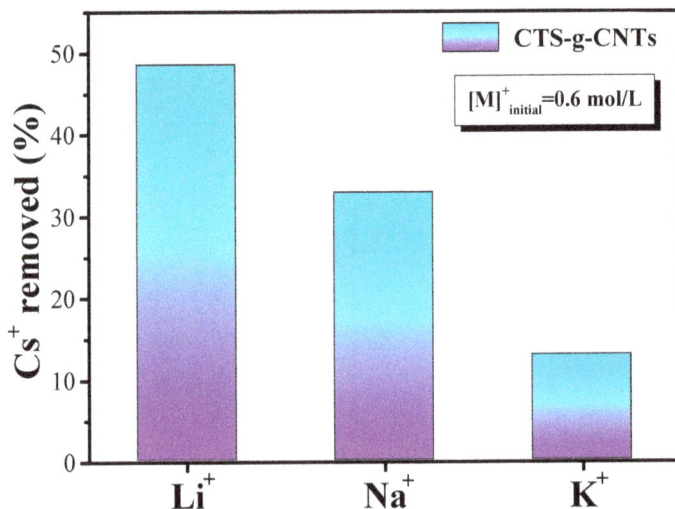

**Figure 7.** Comparison of the removal percentage of $Cs^+$ ions obtained using CTS-g-CNTs in presence of competitive cations with $m_{sorbent}/V_{solvent}$ = 0.6 g/L and $[Cs^+]_{initial}$ = 10.0 mg/L.

In addition, the distribution coefficient ($K_d$) of $Cs^+$ in the presence of competitive cations and for various materials collected from the recent references is listed in Table 2. It can be seen that the $K_d$ value substantially decreased in the same order of $Li^+$ > $Na^+$ > $K^+$. In addition, the $K_d$ value expresses the chemical binding affinity of $Cs^+$ ion to the sorbents, which is helpful for us in understanding the relative efficiency of the materials. It is obvious that the CTS-g-CNTs composite shows a bigger distribution coefficient than the other sorbents, indicating the CTS-g-CNTs composite shows a higher adsorption capacity (Table 2). Therefore, the CTS-g-CNTs composite could be a good candidate for the remediation of radioactive cesium nuclear waste water.

**Table 2.** Comparison of $K_d$ values obtained using different materials in the presence of competitive cations.

| Materials | Competitive Cations | $K_d$ (mL/g) | References |
|---|---|---|---|
| CTS-g-CNTs | 0.1 M Li$^+$ | 152.8 | This work |
| | 0.1 M Na$^+$ | 118.6 | |
| | 0.1 M K$^+$ | 94.7 | |
| CA | 3.5 mM Na$^+$ | 69.8 | [42] |
| | 2.1 mM K$^+$ | 66.5 | |
| IA | 3.5 mM Na$^+$ | 43.2 | [42] |
| | 2.1 mM K$^+$ | 26.6 | |
| PB-coated MNP | 0.1 M Na$^+$ | 56.4 | [43] |
| | 0.1 M Mg$^{2+}$ | 112.5 | |
| | 0.1 M K$^+$ | 14.3 | |

Two comparisons of Cs$^+$ adsorption isotherms are shown in Figure 8. We used the Langmuir [37,44] and Freundlich [45] isotherm models, both of which are the most widely used ones among the abundant isotherm models, to fit the experimental data in order to understand the adsorption mechanism. The Langmuir (1) and Freundlich (2) equations are expressed as follow:

$$Q_e = \frac{Q_{max} K_L C_e}{1 + K_L C_e}$$ (1)

$$Q_e = K_F C_e^{1/n}$$ (2)

where $Q_e$ is the equilibrated cesium ion concentration, $Q_{max}$ (mg/g) is the maximum sorption capacity, $K_L$ (L/mg) is the Langmuir adsorption constant and $1/n$ is the Freundlich adsorption constant.

The related parameters of the two models are listed in Table 3. From the correlation coefficient ($R^2$), the Langmuir model fits the experimental data better than the Freundlich model. The first comparison (Figure 8A) is between the raw-CNTs and CTS-g-CNTs for Cs$^+$ adsorption capacity, as it is very useful to understand the effect of –OH functional groups. The maximum adsorption capacity ($Q_{max}$) of Cs$^+$ on CTS-g-CNTs is 0.340 mmol/g, and much higher than that of Cs$^+$ on raw-CNTs (0.224 mmol/g). Therefore, after having added many –OH functional groups, which are derived from the grafted chitosan, the adsorption capacity of CNTs is enhanced by about 52%. In a word, the effect of –OH functional groups in our system is positive, which is consistent with results showed in Figure 6A. The second comparison (Figure 8B) is between the contaminated seawater and simulated groundwater for Cs$^+$ adsorption capacity by CTS-g-CNTs. The purposes of this comparison were to detect the stability of CTS-g-CNTs in seawater and to evaluate the simulated groundwater. The adsorption isotherm in contaminated seawater is similar to that in contaminated simulated groundwater, indicating that the CTS-g-CNTs could remain stable in seawater. In addition, the $Q_{max}$

for $Cs^+$ ions by CTS-g-CNTs in contaminated simulated groundwater (0.340 mmol/g) is a bit larger than that of $Cs^+$ ions in contaminated seawater (0.272 mmol/g), which is attributed to the higher concentration of competitive cations in seawater. Therefore, to a certain extent, we can consider that the simulated groundwater can be used to model the seawater in our system.

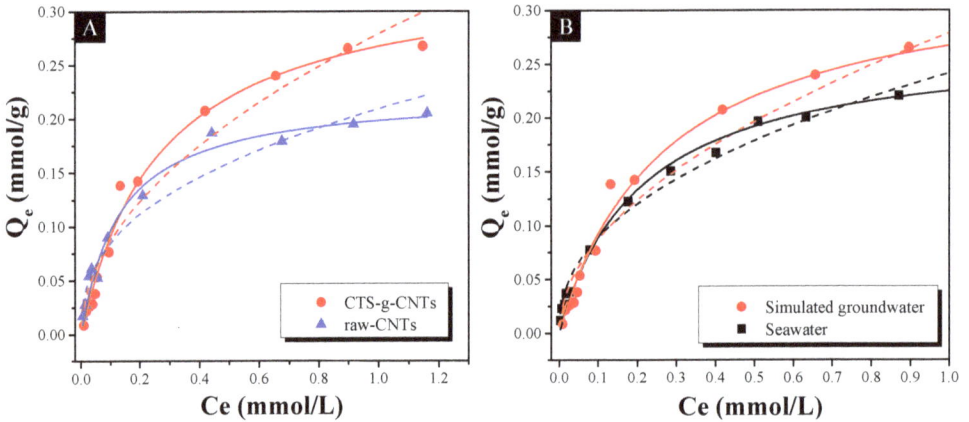

**Figure 8.** Adsorption isotherms of $Cs^+$ on CTS-g-CNTs and raw-CNTs in simulated groundwater (**A**) and adsorption isotherms of $Cs^+$ on CTS-g-CNTs in contaminated stimulated groundwater and seawater (**B**) with pH = 7.0 and $m_{sorbent}/V_{solvent}$ = 0.6 g/L. Symbols denote experimental data, solid lines represent model fitting of the Langmuir equation, and dash lines represent the model fitting of the Freundlich equation.

**Table 3.** Sorption constants for Langmuir and Freundlich isotherm models.

| System | Sorbent | Langmuir | | | Freundlich | | |
|---|---|---|---|---|---|---|---|
| | | $Q_{max}$ (mmol/g) | $K_L$ (L/mmol) | $R^2$ | $n$ | $K_F$ (mmol/g) | $R^2$ |
| Simulated | raw-CNTs | 0.224 | 7.62 | 0.976 | 2.55 | 0.209 | 0.951 |
| groundwater | CTS-g-CNTs | 0.340 | 3.67 | 0.988 | 1.97 | 0.279 | 0.944 |
| Seawater | CTS-g-CNTs | 0.272 | 4.79 | 0.987 | 2.30 | 0.242 | 0.986 |

# 3. Experimental Section

## 3.1. Materials

The CNTs used in this work are multi-walled CNTs, and were prepared by chemical vapor deposition as previously reported [27,36]. Chitosan 100, cesium chloride, sodium hydroxide, and other reagents were purchased from Wako Pure Chemical Industries, Ltd. (Osaka, Japan). All chemicals used were analytical grade and the solutions were prepared with Milli-Q water. The seawater ($Cl^-$: 19,400 ppm, $Na^+$: 10,800 ppm, $Mg^{2+}$: 1270 ppm, $Ca^{2+}$: 412 ppm, $K^+$: 392 ppm, pH = 7.6) used in this study was taken from the Pacific Ocean near Hamamatsu city, which is in the eastern coast of Japan. The simulated groundwater was prepared by $Na^+$: 230 ppm, $Mg^{2+}$: 240 ppm, $Li^+$: 70 ppm, $K^+$: 390 ppm, pH = 5.0.

## 3.2. Synthesis of CTS-g-CNTs

The CTS-g-CNT composites were synthesized by the plasma-induced grafting method involving surface activation by radio frequency Ar plasma and chitosan grafting procedures. An amount of 0.1 g of raw-CNTs was firstly pre-treated by Ar plasma at a pressure of 50 Pa. The treatment time was for 10 min and the plasma power was 80 W. Then 150 mL 1.0% w/v of chitosan solution prepared in 1% v/v acetic acid was immediately injected into the plasma treated CNTs. The mixture was heated to 80 °C and the temperature maintained with fast stirring for 24 h. The CTS-g-CNT composites were collected by centrifuging, washed, dried, and analyzed by SEM (JSM-7001F, JEOL, Tokyo, Japan), XRD equipped with Cu Kα radiation ($\lambda = 0.154$ nm), LabRam HR Raman spectrometry, XPS (ESCA-3400, Shimadzu, Kyoto, Japan) with Mg Kα X-ray source and TGA (DTG-60A, Shimadzu, Kyoto, Japan) under 25% Ar/75% air atmosphere with a heating rate of 10 °C/min from 35 to 800 °C.

The schematic view of the inductively-coupled radio frequency plasma device is described in Figure 9. The schematic of the formation of CTS-g-CNTs and the schematic illustration of the research approach are shown in Figure 10.

## 3.3. Cesium Adsorption Experiment

An amount of 6 mg of CTS-g-CNT composites was added to the simulated groundwater or seawater, then a dilute CsCl solution with different amounts of $Cs^+$ was added into the above mixture solution to control the solution volume of 6 mL, and the concentration of $Cs^+$ ranging from 1.0 to 42 ppm. The desired pH was adjusted by adding small volumes of HCl or NaOH (0.01 or 0.1 mol/L). The suspension was then shaken at ambient conditions. The shaking time was fixed at 24 h to ensure that the adsorption could achieve full equilibrium. Finally, the solid and liquid phases were separated by centrifuging at 14,000 rpm for 30 min, and the concentration of $Cs^+$ in solution was determined by atomic absorption spectroscopy.

The distribution coefficient ($K_d$, mL/g) and the percentage of $Cs^+$ removed by the adsorbents were calculated according to the following equations:

$$K_d = \frac{(C_o - C_t)V}{132.9W} \tag{3}$$

$$Cs^+ \ removed(\%) = \frac{(C_o - C_t)}{C_o} \times 100\% \tag{4}$$

where $C_o$ is the initial concentration of $Cs^+$ (mg/L), $C_t$ represents the concentration of $Cs^+$ at time $t$, $V$ represents the total volume of the solution (L), $W$ is the mass of adsorbent (g) and 132.9 is the standard atomic weight of cesium.

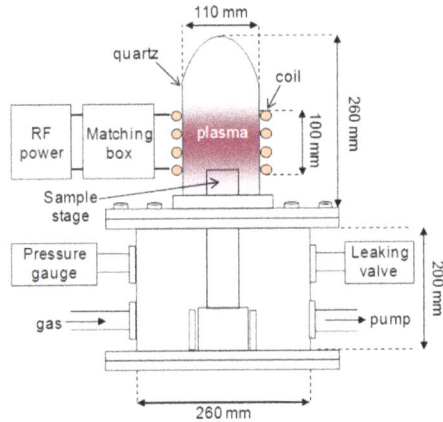

**Figure 9.** Schematic view of the experimental setup for inductively coupled radio frequency plasma.

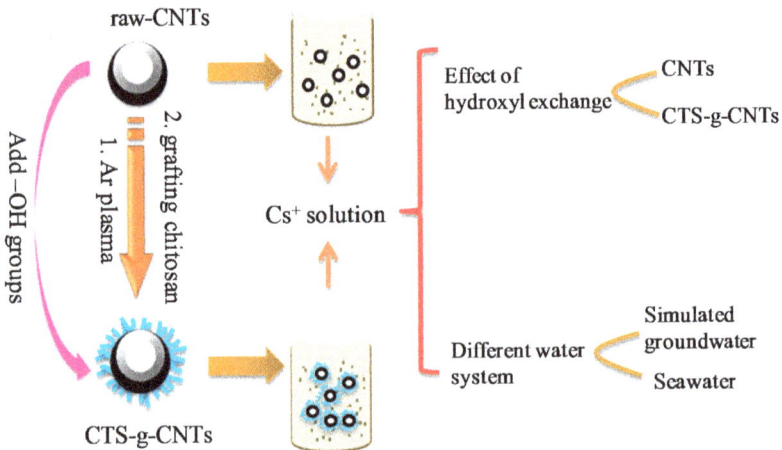

**Figure 10.** Schematic illustration of the designed research approach.

## 4. Conclusions

To summarize, we synthesized CTS-g-CNT composites by the plasma-induced grafting method to explore the effect of the –OH functional groups in $Cs^+$ adsorption. The variation of environmental conditions such as pH, contact time, *etc.* were taken into account. A comparison of contaminated seawater and simulated groundwater was also performed. The adsorption of $Cs^+$ ions was strongly dependent on pH and the competitive cations. By examining the materials and the two aqueous solution systems, one can see that: (1) modification with many –OH functional groups can increase the adsorption capacity for $Cs^+$ ions to a certain extent; (2) we can use the simulated groundwater to model the contaminated seawater to evaluate the adsorption property of CNTs-based material. These results showed the direct observational evidence on the effect of the –OH functional group for $Cs^+$

adsorption. Our findings are important to provide future directions to design and choose effective materials to remedy the removal of radioactive cesium from contaminated groundwater and seawater, which is crucial for both the natural environment and the human social environment.

## Acknowledgments

This work was supported by the National Natural Science Foundation of China (21225730, 91326202, 21377132, 21307135), the Jiangsu Provincial Key Laboratory of Radiation Medicine and Protection and the Priority Academic Program Development of Jiangsu Higher Education Institutions. We also thank Yanxia Yang to revise the grammar and language of this paper.

## Author Contributions

Cesium adsorption experiment: Shubin Yang and Guangshun Hou; Synthesis of CNTs and CTS-g-CNTs: Dadong Shao; Theoretical guidance: Xiangke Wang and Masaaki Nagatsu; Material characterization: Xiaoli Tan; Analysis of characterization results: Xuemei Ren; Analysis of experimental data: Jitao Yu.

## Conflicts of Interest

The authors declare no conflict of interest.

## References

1. Datta, S.J.; Moon, W.K.; Choi, D.Y.; Hwang, I.C.; Yoon, K.B. A novel vanadosilicate with hexadeca-coordinated $Cs^+$ ions as a highly effective $Cs^+$ remover. *Angew. Chem. Int. Ed.* **2014**, *53*, 7203–7208.
2. Yang, S.; Han, C.; Wang, X.; Nagatsu, M. Characteristics of cesium ion sorption from aqueous solution on bentonite- and carbon nanotube-based composites. *J. Hazard. Mater.* **2014**, *274*, 46–52.
3. Sato, K.; Fujimoto, K.; Dai, W.; Hunger, M. Molecular mechanism of heavily adhesive Cs: Why radioactive Cs is not decontaminated from soil. *J. Phys. Chem. C* **2013**, *117*, 14075–14080.
4. Tanaka, K.; Sakaguchi, A.; Kanai, Y.; Tsuruta, H.; Shinohara, A.; Takahashi, Y. Heterogeneous distribution of radiocesium in aerosols, soil and particulate matters emitted by the Fukushima Daiichi Nuclear Power Plant accident: Retention of micro-scale heterogeneity during the migration of radiocesium from the air into ground and river systems. *J. Radioanal. Nucl. Chem.* **2013**, *295*, 1927–1937.
5. Mizuno, T.; Kubo, H. Overview of active cesium contamination of freshwater fish in Fukushima and eastern Japan. *Sci. Rep.* **2013**, *3*, 1–4.
6. Yang, D.; Sarina, S.; Zhu, H.; Liu, H.; Zheng, Z.; Xie, M.; Smith, S.V.; Komarneni, S. Capture of radioactive cesium and iodide ions from water by using titanate nanofibers and nanotubes. *Angew. Chem. Int. Ed.* **2011**, *50*, 10594–10598.

7. Celestian, A.J.; Kubicki, J.D.; Hanson, J.; Clearfield, A.; Parise, J.B. The mechanism responsible for extraordinary Cs ion selectivity in crystalline silicotitanate. *J. Am. Chem. Soc.* **2008**, *130*, 11689–11694.

8. Torad, N.L.; Hu, M.; Imura, M.; Naito, M.; Yamauchi, Y. Large Cs adsorption capability of nanostructured Prussian Blue particles with high accessible surface areas. *J. Mater. Chem.* **2012**, *22*, 18261–18267.

9. Dwivedi, C.; Kumar, A.; Ajish, J.K.; Singh, K.K.; Kumar, M.; Wattal, P.K.; Bajaj, P.N. Resorcinol-formaldehyde coated XAD resin beads for removal of cesium ions from radioactive waste: Synthesis, sorption and kinetic studies. *RSC Adv.* **2012**, *2*, 5557–5564.

10. Long, R.Q.; Yang, R.T. Carbon nanotubes as superior sorbent for dioxin removal. *J. Am. Chem. Soc.* **2001**, *123*, 2058–2059.

11. Premkumar, T.; Mezzenga, R.; Geckeler, K.E. Carbon nanotubes in the liquid phase: Addressing the issue of dispersion. *Small* **2012**, *8*, 1299–1313.

12. Ren, X.M.; Chen, C.L.; Nagatsu, M.; Wang, X.K. Carbon nanotubes as adsorbents in environmental pollution management: A review. *Chem. Eng. J.* **2011**, *170*, 395–410.

13. Belloni, F.; Kütahyali, C.; Rondinella, V.V.; Carbol, P.; Wiss, T.; Mangione, A. Can carbon nanotubes play a role in the field of nuclear waste management? *Environ. Sci. Technol.* **2009**, *43*, 1250–1255.

14. Yavari, R.; Huang, Y.D.; Ahmadi, S.J. Adsorption of cesium(I) from aqueous solution using oxidized multiwall carbon nanotubes. *J. Radioanal. Nucl. Chem.* **2011**, *287*, 393–401.

15. Kaper, H.; Nicolle, J.; Cambedouzou, J.; Grandjean, A. Multi-method analysis of functionalized single-walled carbon nanotubes for cesium liquid–solid extraction. *Mater. Chem. Phys.* **2014**, *147*, 147–154.

16. Yu, X.Y.; Luo, T.; Zhang, Y.X.; Jia, Y.; Zhu, B.J.; Fu, X.C.; Liu, J.H.; Huang, X.J. Adsorption of lead(II) on $O_2$-plasma-oxidized multiwalled carbon nanotubes: Thermodynamics, kinetics, and desorption. *ACS Appl. Mater. Interfaces* **2011**, *3*, 2585–2593.

17. Yang, S.B.; Shao, D.D.; Wang, X.K.; Nagatsu, M. Localized *in situ* polymerization on carbon nanotube surfaces for stabilized carbon nanotube dispersions and application for cobalt(II) removal. *RSC Adv.* **2014**, *4*, 4856–4863.

18. Chen, C.L.; Ogino, A.; Wang, X.K.; Nagatsu, M. Plasma treatment of multiwall carbon nanotubes for dispersion improvement in water. *Appl. Phys. Lett.* **2010**, *96*, doi:10.1063/1.3377007.

19. Shao, D.D.; Hu, J.; Wang, X.K. Plasma induced grafting multiwalled carbon nanotube with chitosan and its application for removal of $UO_2^{2+}$, $Cu^{2+}$, and $Pb^{2+}$ from aqueous solutions. *Plasma Process. Polym.* **2010**, *7*, 977–985.

20. Swayampakula, K.; Boddu, V.M.; Nadavala, S.K.; Abburi, K. Competitive adsorption of Cu(II), Co(II) and Ni(II) from their binary and tertiary aqueous solutions using chitosan-coated perlite beads as biosorbent. *J. Hazard. Mater.* **2009**, *170*, 680–689.

21. Nightingale, E.R. Phenomenological theory of ion solvation effective radii of hydrated ions. *J. Phys. Chem.* **1959**, *63*, 1381–1387.

22. Heyrovska, R. Dependences of molar volumes in solids, partial molal and hydrated ionic volumes of alkali halides on covalent and ionic radii and the golden ratio. *Chem. Phys. Lett.* **2007**, *436*, 287–293.

23. Tansel, B.; Sager, J.; Rector, T.; Garland, J.; Strayer, R.F.; Levine, L.; Roberts, M.; Hummerick, M.; Bauer, J. Significance of hydrated radius and hydration shells on ionic permeability during nanofiltration in dead end and cross flow modes. *Sep. Purif. Technol.* **2006**, *51*, 40–47.

24. Lu, H.; Zhang, W.; Yang, Y.; Huang, X.; Wang, S.; Qiu, R. Relative distribution of $Pb^{2+}$ sorption mechanisms by sludge-derived biochar. *Water Res.* **2012**, *46*, 854–862.

25. Omura, A.; Moritomo, Y. $Cs^+$ trapping in size-controlled nanospaces of hexacyanoferrates. *Appl. Phys. Express* **2012**, *5*, 057101.

26. Yang, M.H.; Jong, S.B.; Lu, C.Y.; Lin, Y.F.; Chiang, P.W.; Tyan, Y.C.; Chung, T.W. Assessing the responses of cellular proteins induced by hyaluronic acid-modified surfaces utilizing a mass spectrometry-based profiling system: Over-Expression of CD36, CD44, CDK9, and PP2A. *Analyst* **2012**, *137*, 4921–4933.

27. Chen, C.L.; Liang, B.; Ogino, A.; Wang, X.K.; Nagatsu, M. Oxygen functionalization of multiwall carbon nanotubes by microwave-excited surface-wave plasma treatment. *J. Phys. Chem. C* **2009**, *113*, 7659–7665.

28. Saraswati, T.E.; Ogino, A.; Nagatsu, M. Plasma-activated immobilization of biomolecules onto graphite-encapsulated magnetic nanoparticles. *Carbon* **2012**, *50*, 1253–1261.

29. Shao, D.D.; Ren, X.M.; Hu, J.; Chen, Y.X.; Wang, X.K. Preconcentration of $Pb^{2+}$ from aqueous solution using poly(acrylamide) and poly(*N,N*-dimethylacrylamide) grafted multiwalled carbon nanotubes. *Colloids Surf. A* **2010**, *360*, 74–84.

30. Cao, A.; Xu, C.; Liang, J.; Wu, D.; Wei, B. X-ray diffraction characterization on the alignment degree of carbon nanotubes. *Chem. Phys. Lett.* **2001**, *344*, 13–17.

31. Yusa, H.; Watanuki, T. X-ray diffraction of multiwalled carbon nanotube under high pressure: Structural durability on static compression. *Carbon* **2005**, *43*, 519–523.

32. Chen, C.L.; Liang, B.; Lu, D.; Ogino, A.; Wang, X.K.; Nagatsu, M. Amino group introduction onto multiwall carbon nanotubes by $NH_3/Ar$ plasma treatment. *Carbon* **2010**, *48*, 939–948.

33. Lee, A.F.; Baddeley, C.J.; Hardacre, C.; Ormerod, R.M.; Lambert, R.M.; Schmid, G.; West, H. Structural and catalytic properties of novel Au/Pd bimetallic colloid particles: EXAFS, XRD, and acetylene coupling. *J. Phys. Chem.* **1995**, *99*, 6096–6102.

34. Guo, J.; Chen, S.; Liu, L.; Li, B.; Yang, P.; Zhang, L.; Feng, Y. Adsorption of dye from wastewater using chitosan-CTAB modified bentonites. *J. Colloid Interface Sci.* **2012**, *382*, 61–66.

35. Burghard, M. Electronic and vibrational properties of chemically modified single-wall carbon nanotubes. *Surf. Sci. Rep.* **2005**, *58*, 1–109.

36. Yang, S.B.; Hu, J.; Chen, C.L.; Shao, D.D.; Wang, X.K. Mutual effects of Pb(II) and humic acid adsorption on multiwalled carbon nanotubes/polyacrylamide composites from aqueous solutions. *Environ. Sci. Technol.* **2011**, *45*, 3621–3627.

37. Volkov, A.G.; Paula, S.; Deamer, D.W. Two mechanisms of permeation of small neutral molecules and hydrated ions across phospholipid bilayers. *Bioelectrochem. Bioenerg.* **1997**, *42*, 153–160.

38. Zhou, J.; Lu, X.; Wang, Y.; Shi, J. Molecular dynamics study on ionic hydration. *Fluid Phase Equilib.* **2002**, *194–197*, 257–270.

39. Volkov, A.G. Liquid-liquid interfaces. In *Theory and Methods*; Deamer, D.W., Ed.; CRC Press: Boca Raton, NY, USA, 1996.

40. Gourary, B.S.; Adrian, F.J. Wave functions for electron-excess color centers in alkali halide crystals. In *Solid State Physics*; Frederick, S., David, T., Eds.; Academic Press: Waltham, MA, USA, 1960; pp. 127–247.

41. O'M, B.J. Review: Ionic hydration in chemistry and biophysics, by B.E. Conway, Elsevier Publishing Company, 1981. *J. Solut. Chem.* **1982**, *11*, 221–222.

42. Awual, M.R.; Suzuki, S.; Taguchi, T.; Shiwaku, H.; Okamoto, Y.; Yaita, T. Radioactive cesium removal from nuclear wastewater by novel inorganic and conjugate adsorbents. *Chem. Eng. J.* **2014**, *242*, 127–135.

43. Thammawong, C.; Opaprakasit, P.; Tangboriboonrat, P.; Sreearunothai, P. Prussian blue-coated magnetic nanoparticles for removal of cesium from contaminated environment. *J. Nanopart. Res.* **2013**, *15*, 1–10.

44. Markham, E.C.; Benton, A.F. The adsorption of gas mixtures by silica. *J. Am. Chem. Soc.* **1931**, *53*, 497–507.

45. Digiano, F.A.; Baldauf, G.; Frick, B.; Sontheimer, H. A simplified competitive equilibrium adsorption model. *Chem. Eng. Sci.* **1978**, *33*, 1667–1673.

# Chapter II:
# Medicinal Biology

# Emerging Biomedical Applications of Nano-Chitins and Nano-Chitosans Obtained via Advanced Eco-Friendly Technologies from Marine Resources

Riccardo A. A. Muzzarelli, Mohamad El Mehtedi and Monica Mattioli-Belmonte

**Abstract:** The present review article is intended to direct attention to the technological advances made in the 2010–2014 quinquennium for the isolation and manufacture of nanofibrillar chitin and chitosan. Otherwise called nanocrystals or whiskers, n-chitin and n-chitosan are obtained either by mechanical chitin disassembly and fibrillation optionally assisted by sonication, or by e-spinning of solutions of polysaccharides often accompanied by poly(ethylene oxide) or poly(caprolactone). The biomedical areas where n-chitin may find applications include hemostasis and wound healing, regeneration of tissues such as joints and bones, cell culture, antimicrobial agents, and dermal protection. The biomedical applications of n-chitosan include epithelial tissue regeneration, bone and dental tissue regeneration, as well as protection against bacteria, fungi and viruses. It has been found that the nano size enhances the performances of chitins and chitosans in all cases considered, with no exceptions. Biotechnological approaches will boost the applications of the said safe, eco-friendly and benign nanomaterials not only in these fields, but also for biosensors and in targeted drug delivery areas.

Reprinted from *Mar. Drugs*. Cite as: Muzzarelli, R.A.A.; El Mehtedi, M.; Mattioli-Belmonte, M. Emerging Biomedical Applications of Nano-Chitins and Nano-Chitosans Obtained via Advanced Eco-Friendly Technologies from Marine Resources. *Mar. Drugs* **2014**, *12*, 5468-5502.

## 1. Introduction and Scope

Discovered over two centuries ago, chitin plays today protagonist roles in innovative research. A number of current research works are inspired by the natural chitin structure: the occurrence of chitin in living organisms since the Cambrian life explosion is explained by the recognition of its very good performance and versatility in perception, protection, aggression, feeding, reproduction and fertilization, locomotion and flight [1–7].

Chitin nanofibers are mainly prepared from crustacean and diatomaceous chitin powders according to newly adopted approaches and protocols. In particular, recent articles deal with the following advances: (I) n-chitin isolated after hydrolysis in diluted HCl; (II) n-chitin isolated mechanically in the presence of minor amounts of acetic acid; (III) n-chitosan obtained from partially deacetylated chitin; (IV) mechanical fibrillation; (V) fibrillation with the aid of sonication; (VI) manufacture of chitin nanofibers by e-spinning; (VII) preparation and spinning of chitin solutions in ionic liquids; (VIII) manufacture of aerogels. These advances are of such importance that they overshadow the technology developed during the previous years, as it will be apparent below.

In his review, Araki [8] introduced recent results on electrostatic and steric stabilizations of nanofibrils, together with brief and basic descriptions of their stabilization mechanisms. Chitin nanofibers were isolated from the cell walls of five types of mushrooms by the removal of glucans, minerals, and proteins, followed by a simple grinding treatment under acidic conditions. The width of the nanofibers depended on the type of mushrooms and varied in the range 20–28 nm; the crystalline structure was maintained and glucans remained on the nanofiber surface [9]. By similar means, chitin nanofibers ($\Phi$ 10–20 nm) were isolated from prawn shells under mild conditions [10].

Once isolated, chitin nanofibers can be derivatized to modify their surfaces permanently: for example they are fully acetylated with acetic anhydride in warm anhydrous pyridine. The acetylation can be controlled by changing the reaction time; it proceeds heterogeneously from the surface to the core [11]. As an example of elaborated application, covalent coupling of chitin nanofibrils with magnetic nanoparticles in aqueous media was proposed for DNA extraction [12].

The e-spun composite nanofibers are of great significance owing to their large surface area to volume ratio, besides porosity, stability, and permeability. The functionality and applicability of these nanostructures were further improved by incorporating secondary phases that include magnetic metal oxides, carbon nanotubes, precious metals, and hydroxyapatite. Nanofibrous materials compatible with the extracellular matrix and capable to promote the adhesion of cells are being developed as engineered scaffolds for the skin, heart, cornea, nerves, bone, blood vessels, and other tissues. The review article by Sahay *et al.* [13] discusses the applicability of these composite fibers in energy, filters, biotechnology, sensors, packaging materials, and indicates technological issues, research challenges, and emerging trends. The reader is referred to fundamental works [14–27] for complementary information.

### 1.1. β-Chitin: The Simplest 2D Hydrogen Bonded Polymorph

β-Chitin is found in association with proteins in squid pens: the dry pen contains 31% chitin whose viscosity average MW is over 2 MDa, and the crystallinity index is 75%. The degree of acetylation was found to be 0.96 [28]. The content of inorganic compounds is very low. The crystal structure of β-chitin [29–33] lacks hydrogen bonds along the b axis (Figure 1), and therefore it is more susceptible than α-chitin to intra-crystalline swelling, acid hydrolysis even at low acid concentrations, and loss of scarcely crystalline fractions. In the squid gladius, the chitin molecules are known to form nano-crystallites of monoclinic lattice symmetry wrapped in a protein layer, resulting in β-chitin nanofibrils [34]. Three β-chitin structures (anhydrous, dihydrate, and mono-ethylenediamine) were recently determined by synchrotron X-ray and neutron fiber diffraction [35]. The optimal deproteination and demineralisation conditions were defined by Youn *et al.* [36].

**Figure 1.** Projections of the structure of β-chitin: no linkage exists along the b axis. The polymer can be easily fibrillated by acting on this point of weakness. Courtesy of Riccardo A. A. Muzzarelli.

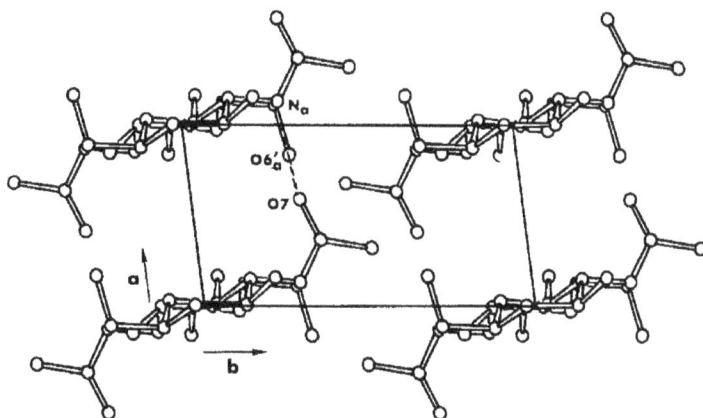

*1.2. α-Chitin: The 3D Hydrogen Bonded Polymorph*

α-Chitin is the most abundant polymorph; it occurs in fungal and yeast cell walls, and in the arthropod cuticle in general: the biological composite materials forming the exoskeleton of the lobster *Homarus americanus* and the crab *Cancer pagurus* have shown that all parts of the exoskeleton were optimized to fulfill different functions according to different eco-physiological strains sustained by the animals [37–45]. The hard chitinous tissues found in some invertebrate marine organisms are paradigms for robust, lightweight materials. Examples of the superior performances of chitin nanofibrils *in vivo* are the oral grasping spines of Chaetognaths, *Sagitta* in particular, [46,47], and the filaments of the seaweed *Phaeocystis* [48,49]. Polyplacophorans, or chitons, are an important group of molluscan invertebrates deemed to have retained many features of the molluscan body plan. They feed on microbes detached from the rocks by the scraping action of the radula, a ribbon-like organ endowed with rows of mineralized teeth. The radular teeth of *Cryptochiton stelleri* are three-fold harder than human enamel [50–54].

In the crystal structures of α- and β-chitins, the chains are organized in sheets and held in place by a number of intra-sheet hydrogen bonds, including the rather strong C–O...NH hydrogen bonds, that maintain the chains at a distance of about 0.47 nm along the a axis of the unit cell. In the α-chitin there are also some inter-sheet hydrogen bonds along the b axis of the unit cell, involving the hydroxymethyl groups of adjacent chains: as already noted, this feature is not found in the structure of β-chitin [55–57].

*1.3. Scope of the Present Review*

The scope of this review article is to draw attention to the sudden upsurge of research activity on n-chitin production, development, and biomedical applications. Creative and inspired works dated 2010–2014 are considered here as priority. While n-chitin bearing materials have enhanced mechanical characteristics, it should be underlined that these properties are of outmost importance for biomedical uses of all kinds: for example they permit minimization of the load bearing stress of prosthetic materials, they offer easy handling of surgical aids, and favor cell growth and differentiation.

## 2. Advanced Approaches to the Preparation of Chitin Nanofibrils

### 2.1. Nanochitin Isolation under Mild Oxidative Conditions

In the frame of an early project intended for the preparation of hyaluronan surrogates, chitins were regiospecifically oxidized at C-6 with NaOCl in the presence of the stable nitroxyl radical 2,2,6,6-tetramethyl-1-piperidinyloxy (Tempo®, Aldrich, Milan, Italy) and NaBr at 25 °C in water. The obtained anionic oxychitins are fully soluble (pH 3–12); they exert metal chelation, polyelectrolyte complexation with biopolymers such as chitosan, and generate microspheres and beads; they precipitate a variety of proteins, including papain, lysozyme and other hydrolases. Remarkably, 6-oxychitin was assayed for the regeneration of bone [58].

Tempo®-oxidized chitin nanocrystals were used to cast films that were fully characterized. They were labeled with a fluorescent imidazoisoquinolinone dye, and simultaneously conjugated with carbohydrate ligands, resulting in dually functionalized nanocrystals. The biorecognition properties of the nanocrystals were probed with lectins and bacteria, resulting in selective interactions with their corresponding cognate carbohydrate-binding proteins. These works represent a new approach to multifunctional nanomaterials based on naturally occurring polymers [59–61].

A significant factor that affects transparency of the dispersions, weight ratio of water-insoluble fractions, shape, length, and width of the chitin nanocrystals obtained, is the carboxylate content in the Tempo® oxidized chitins or the amount of NaClO added in the oxidation of α-chitin. The chitin nanocrystals typically had fiber widths smaller than 15 nm, and average widths of 8 nm. The carboxylate groups generated by Tempo®-mediated oxidation solely at C6 of the α-chitin at the fibril surface, promote the individualization of the fibrils by mild mechanical treatment. In fact, the preparation of chitin nanofibrils from squid β-chitin by Tempo®-mediated oxidation, only requires mild mechanical agitation in water at pH 3–4.8 [62,63].

This was a real breakthrough: since then, the preparation of chitin nanofibrils has been definitely simplified in terms of expenditures, duration, yield, eco-compatibility, and laboratory safety. For instance, the hydrochloric acid concentration was reduced from 3 M to 5 mM; the temperature from 102 °C down to room temperature. Most importantly, in recent works acetic acid has replaced HCl.

### 2.2. Nanochitin Disassembly and Fibrillation by Mechanical and Hydraulic Means

Mechanical treatment under mild acidic conditions is the key to fibrillating dry chitin. The method by Dutta et al. includes a chitin powder dispersion in water at 1% followed by addition of acetic acid to adjust the pH to 3 [64]. The slurry is then passed through a high pressure water-jet system equipped with a ball-collision chamber for mechanical disintegration and nano-fibrillation. The resulting n-chitin, further dispersed in water (0.1%), yields films with uniform surface and thickness of ca. 25 μm when dried at 40 °C.

Grinders and high speed blenders are also useful for the mechanical conversion of chitin to nanofibers. At pH 3–4, the cationization of amino groups on the fiber surface assists nanofibrillation by exerting an electrostatic repulsive force, in the same way as the carboxyl group generated by Tempo®. Even though the degree of deacetylation might be as low as 0.04, the protonation of the amino groups generates repulsion forces that overcome the hydrogen bonds between the nanofibers. The fibrillated chitin samples exhibited uniform structure endowed with high aspect ratio, the fibril width being 10–20 nm. By a grinding treatment, chitin nanofibers were isolated from never-dried crustacean shells after removing inorganics and proteins: equivalent results were obtained. Furthermore, it was confirmed that nanofibers could be conveniently extracted from the natural chitin + protein + inorganic composites of crab shells: on the other hand the acetyl group was not hydrolyzed and the crystalline structure survived intact [65].

α-Chitin powder (<100 μm, acetylation 0.90) was treated to reach a degree of acetylation of 0.70–0.74 by using 33% NaOH in the presence of NaBH₄ at 90 °C for 2–4 h, with a yield of 85%–90% [66]. The crystallinity index and the crystal size of the α-chitin did not change, showing that deacetylation took place on the crystallite surface. (When 50% NaOH at 90 °C is used, deacetylation occurs instead within the whole mass of the crystallites, thus leading to a decrease of the crystallinity index). Therefore, the said conditions are mandatory for limited and regioselective deacetylation of the crystallite surfaces because, of course, the said treatment with 33% NaOH avoids the generation of highly deacetylated chitosans that disappointingly would dissolve as soon as they are immersed into acidic aqueous media.

The convenient features of the newly developed α-chitin nanofibrils are: (1) commercially available α-chitins can be used as starting materials; (2) nanofibrils are obtained in high yields (85%–90%); (3) the rod-like morphology of the nanofibrils supports the high yields; (4) the α-chitin nanofibril dispersions has high UV-vis transmittance hence high transparency, indicating individualization of α-chitin fibrils; (5) lower costs are involved: no disposal of the brown HCl solution, no handling of enormous quantities of acidic wash water, no cumbersome filtration; (6) the procedure is safer compared with the traditional one and simpler than with Tempo®, hence, considering the higher yields, potential applications can be expanded to numerous fields; (7) β-chitins are transformed into α-chitins during treatment with aqueous NaOH, as justified on thermodynamic grounds [67].

*2.3. Emerging Novel Approaches*

Recent investigations still based on the previous hydrolytic approach claimed the isolation of long α-chitin nanofibrils from *Homarus americanus* carapace, suitable for the preparation of nanostructured membranes [68]. Close inspection of the reported data, however, points out the omission of key data from the preparation protocol, such as temperature values and production yields, accompanied by debatable choices such as deproteination protracted for 14 days but leading in any case to partial removal of proteins, depigmentation with the aid of 96% ethanol (instead of more appropriately ethylacetate). Of course unrealistic research planning does not permit economical feasibility studies. Instead, a more pragmatic approach is that followed by Wijesena *et al.* along the lines set forth by the Ifuku group and other researchers [69]: in practice duly cleaned and powdered crab (*Portunus pelagicus*) shells were treated with 2.5 M HCl for 2 days at room temperature under stirring to remove CaCO₃. After washing, the sample was treated with 1 M NaOH for 2 days at room temperature to remove proteins completely. The pigments were bleached with 3% $H_2O_2$ at pH $10.5 \pm 0.5$ (Na acetate) for 20 min at 80 °C. The sample dispersed in water (1%, pH 3–4 upon subsequent addition of acetic acid) was sonicated for 2 h to yield a stable bluish dispersion of n-chitin.

The work just mentioned, as well as some others, resulted in the preparation of n-chitosan, besides n-chitin: in fact, Watthanaphanit *et al.* have prepared n-chitosan via deacetylation with NaOH and borohydride, with consequent lowering of the molecular weight to 59 kDa, and the degree of deacetylation to 0.50 [70]; the 1.13% suspension was of colloidal nature. Under milder conditions, Fan *et al.* carrie out the deacetylation of a finely milled chitin powder [66], that yielded viscous birefringent dispersions of n-chitosan at pH values 3–4 [66,71]. Chitin nanofibrils were instead easily produced via gelation of a commercial chitin powder by soaking it at room temperature in the ionic liquid 1-allyl-3-methylimidazoliumbromide, followed by heating at 100 °C. Subsequent sonication gave a chitin dispersion from which chitin nanofibrils were regenerated [72]. When PVA was added, the SEM images of the composite (weight ratio of chitin to PVA 1.0:0.3) provided evidence that the nanofibrillar morphology was preserved. This technique for the preparation of chitin nanofibrils has great advantages compared to the early methods because special equipment and chemical modifications are not necessary.

## 2.4. Self-Assembled Nanofibrils

Despite the desirable nano-dimensional attributes of chitin nanofibrils, abundant surface polar groups cause them to self-assemble upon drying, losing their unique individual nano-domain features. Wet-grinding and high-pressure homogenization were combined to fibrillate chitosan (Φ 50 nm, length *ca.* 1 micron): the obtained nanofiber assembled into a high strength liquid crystal film by self-organization. The thus fabricated transparent liquid crystal film had high tensile strength (*ca.* 100 MPa) and Young's modulus (*ca.* 2.2 GPa) owing to its ordered, layered structure. The chitosan nanofibrous film presented the characteristic cholesteric texture of a liquid crystal (Figure 2) after self-organization from colloidal suspension [73].

From homogeneous LiCl + dimethylacetamide solutions, chitin nanofibrils precipitated upon the addition of water (10–25 times the original volume). Nanofibers prepared in this fashion generally had a larger diameter (Φ $10.2 \pm 2.9$ nm) than those prepared from HFIP. However, both types of nanofibers had similar lengths. The resulting nanofibers were made of highly crystalline α-chitin [74]. The crystallization of α-chitin was favored with respect to β-chitin because of the higher number of hydrogen bonds and higher thermodynamic stability of α-chitin [67].

**Figure 2.** SEM (**a**); TEM (**b**) micrographs of chitosan nanofibrils; and polarized optical microscopy micrographs of chitosan liquid crystal film (**c,d**). Reprinted with permission. Copyright © 2011 Elsevier [73].

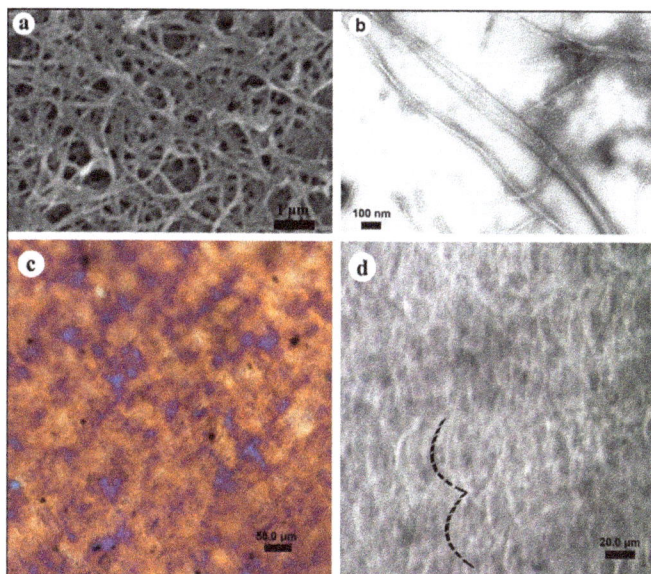

To mimic the association of chitin with proteins *in vivo*, silk was added to solutions of squid pen β-chitin in HFIP, which were dried to yield homogeneous films made of ultrafine (~3 nm) chitin nanofibrils embedded in a silk fibroin matrix [75]. The chitin nanofiber content of the biocomposite was easily tunable by varying the chitin/silk ratio in solution. This desirable feature afforded a simple strategy to fine-tune the biocomposite properties. Transparent chitin-silk films co-assembled from solution were easily manipulated with soft-lithography skill to manufacture optical devices such as diffraction gratings (Figure 3) [76,77].

On the chitin micropatterned supports, cells with a spindle-like morphology aligned their cytoskeleton along the major axis of the pattern features (contact guidance, Figure 4a,b). In contrast, the cells grown on the control chitin supports had no preferred orientation (Figure 4c). After 5 days of cell culture a larger proportion of the cells aligned within the 0–10° preferred angle (Figure 4d,e) as opposed to control (Figure 4f). This proof-of-concept data showed the potential of self-assembled chitin nanofibers to create robust and flexible micropatterned materials intended for tissue engineering, that in any case need to be easily retrievable, to be mechanically robust to provide substantial support for the generation of new tissues, and to maintain proper handling characteristics [78]. The versatility of chitosan-based nanofibers with controllable size and directional alignment as well as highly ordered and customized patterns was also demonstrated by Fuh *et al.* who used PEO-chitosan nanofibers [79]. Analogous investigations were carried out on the manufacture of chitin nanofiber templates for artificial neural networks: chitin nanofiber surfaces were deacetylated to form chitosan nanofibers ($\Phi$ 4 nm and 12 nm) that were coupled with poly-D-lysine. In fact, the 4 nm chitosan nanofibers with poly-D-lysine supported 37.9% neuron viability compared to only 13.5% on traditional poly-D-lysine surfaces after 7-day culture [80].

**Figure 3.** Microcontact printing of chitin nanofibers onto glass supports. Topographic AFM images of chitin nanofiber patterns printed from 0.05% (w/v) ink. The PDMS stamp is replicated from a holographic diffraction grating with 1200 grooves/mm. Scale bars: (**a**) 4 μm and (**b**) 400 nm. Reprinted with permission. Copyright © 2011 Elsevier [76].

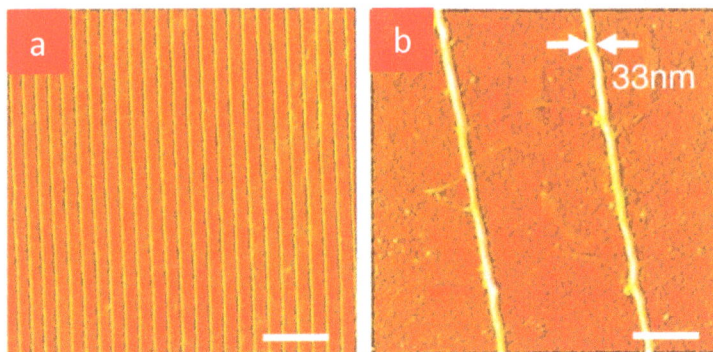

**Figure 4.** Fluorescence images of the actin cytoskeleton of the cells on: (**a**) G1; (**b**) G2 support; and (**c**) control sample after five days of culture. Scale bars 50 μm. The white arrow shows the longitudinal direction of the patterns; (**d**–**f**) Distribution of alignment angles of cell nuclei on the patterned samples and control. Note: G1 is a pattern with 3.2 μm spacing (smaller than the average cell diameter) and G2 with 11.2 μm spacing (slightly larger than the average cell diameter). Reprinted with permission. Copyright © 2013 Elsevier [78].

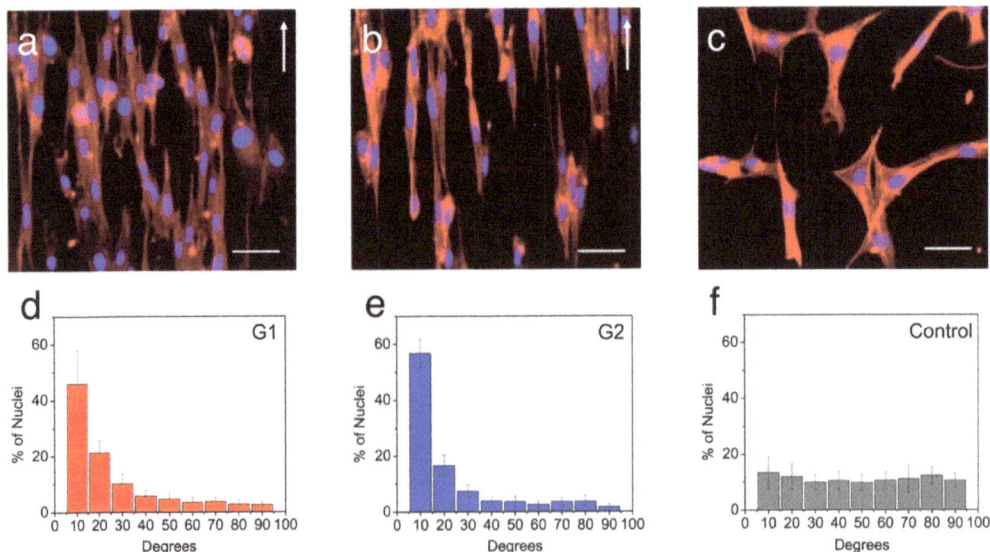

A facile freeze-drying approach to assemble chitin nanofibers ($\Phi$ 20 nm) into a variety of structures whose size and morphology are tunable by adjusting freezing temperature and heat transfer characteristics was adopted by Wu J *et al.* [81]. Notwithstanding the fact that the described self-assembly has proven to be viable, it would be better to use solvents exempt from toxicity and volatility. One approach is based on ionic liquids considered as green solvents capable to replace organic compounds [82], whilst the second approach is based on urea in alkaline solution [83–86]. In addition, self-assembled chitin nanofibers are important for the study of randomly oriented nanofiber networks.

## 2.5. Chitin Foams and Transparent Films Obtained by Sonication

A transparent nanofibril suspension is readily obtained by sonicating purified squid pen powder in water. The $\beta$-chitin nanofibrils were 3–10 nm in width and several microns in length, with acetylation degree of 0.84, *i.e.*, 10% lower than controls. The suspension could be transformed into stable 3-D hydrogel by simply heating at 180 °C for 1–4 h in an autoclave. Experimental evidence was provided that hydrophobic interaction between fibrils has a role in self-assembling into hydrogels. The physical properties of the hydrogels could be easily modulated. The suspension of 1% (w/v) fibrils (4 h, 180 °C) generated a hydrogel with 99.3% water content, fibrils with 87% crystallinity and mechanical strength of 0.7 N breaking force. The chitin hydrogels, molded into desired shapes and prepared without chemical crosslinkers, could be of interest for wound dressing and tissue engineering [87].

Likewise, $\alpha$-chitin nanofibers were fabricated with dried shrimp shells via a simple high-intensity ultrasonic treatment (60 KHz, 300 W, pH = 7). The diameter of the obtained chitin nanofibers could be controlled within 20–200 nm by simply adjusting the sonication time. This high-intensity sonication treatment separates nanofibers from natural matrices after the purified chitin is dispersed in water. The pulsed sonication disassembled chitin into high-aspect-ratio nanofibrils with a uniform width (19.4 nm after 30 min) (Figure 5). The $\alpha$-chitin crystalline structure and molecular structure were preserved; interestingly, ultrasonication slightly increased the degree of crystallinity. Furthermore, highly transparent chitin films (transmittance 90.2% at 600 nm) and flexible ultralight chitin foams were prepared from chitin nanofiber hydrogels.

Optically transparent nanocomposites using chitin nanofibers with acrylic resin were prepared to examine the fibrillation process of dry chitin, and the nanofiber homogeneity. Since dried chitin was fully fibrillated, the optical losses of these composites were less than 2% even after the drying process [88,89]. The nanofibrils were small enough to preserve the transparency of the neat polymethylmethacrylate resin; furthermore the extremely low thermal expansion of nano-chitin films improved the thermal stability of PMMA [90,91] even in the presence of glycerol [92]. Nano-chitin transparent films are thermally stable up to 200 °C for a long period of time [93].

Transparent and highly viscous liquids were obtained by sonication of the partially deacetylated chitins in water at pH 3–4. Transmission electron microscopy revealed that the liquids consisted mainly of independent nanofibrils with average width and length 6–7 nm and 100–200 nm, respectively. In fact, some $\alpha$-chitin nano-fibrils of >500 nm in length were present. Because the acetylation values 0.70–0.74 correspond to 1.34–1.56 mmol/g amino group content, positive charges form on the α-chitin fibril surfaces in high density by protonation in water at pH 3–4 [66].

The ultrasonication used for physical fibrillation, could disassemble the micro-fibres into nanofibrils in water via cavitation. The shockwaves, generated by the implosion of the cavity, break the relatively weak chitin interfibrillar hydrogen bonding and the Van der Waals forces to gradually yield nanofibrils [94]. The method of degradation of chitosan by hydrodynamic cavitation, has some advantages such as a high degradation rate, low energy consumption, equipment which is easy to obtain, the ability to handle large quantities of sample, and no pollution risk to the environment [95].

**Figure 5.** SEM micrographs of (**a**) dry shell; (**b**) after 5 min sonication; and (**c**) after 30 min sonication; (**d–f**) are the distributions of the fiber diameters respectively, and insets are EDS spectra. Reprinted with permission. Copyright © 2013 Elsevier [94].

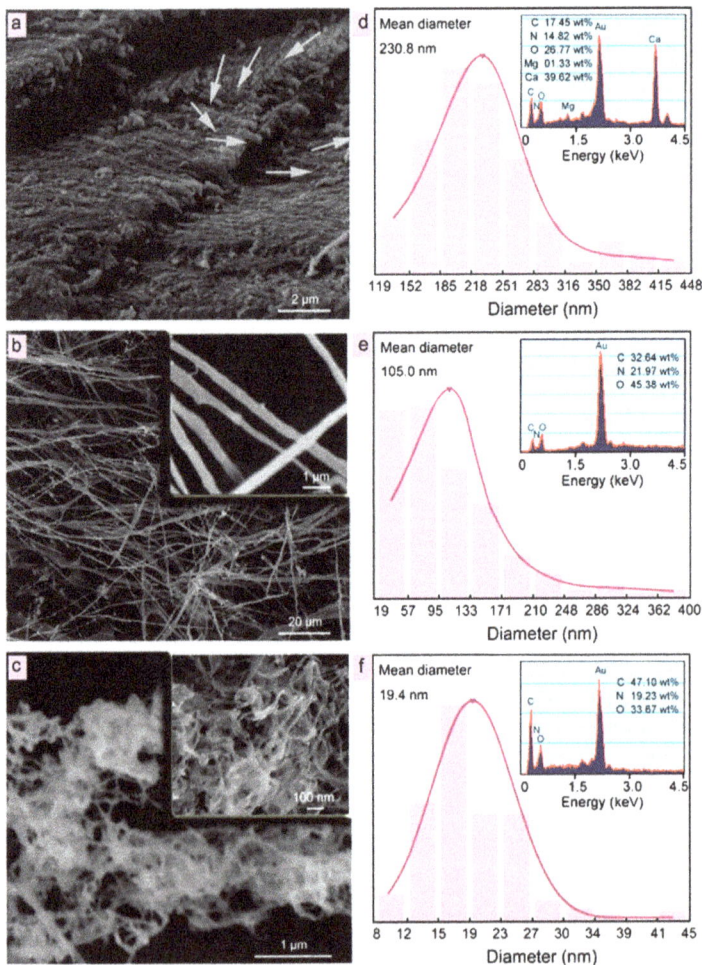

## 3. Manufacture of Chitin Nanofibers via Electrospinning

Recent reviews on spinning methods and e-spun fibers testify the increasing interest in this technology, notwithstanding the high costs of the solvents and the challenges faced in scaling-up [96–100]. It should be underlined that the term nanofibers refers to fibers with diameters in the nano range and undefined length, whilst the terms nanofibrils, nanocrystals and whiskers refer to highly crystalline objects having both diameter and length in the nano range, unless otherwise specified.

### 3.1. Electrospinning of Chitin

Besides the already mentioned *N,N*-dimethylacetamide + LiCl, other solvents such as hexafluoroacetone, hexafluoro-2-propanol, methanol and ethanol saturated with calcium chloride dissolve chitin which can then undergo e-spinning when accompanied by some other polymer; moreover, chitin nanofibrils can be incorporated into certain e-spinnable compounds.

For example, in the work of Junkasem *et al.* fiber mats of e-spun poly(vinyl alcohol) (PVA) were made containing α-chitin nanofibrils prepared from shrimp shells. The as-prepared chitin nanofibrils exhibited lengths in the range 231–969 nm and widths in the range 12–65 nm. The incorporation of chitin nanofibrils within the as-spun fiber mats increased the Young's modulus by 4–8 times over that of the neat as-spun PVA fiber mat. The maximum tensile strength $5.7 \pm 0.6$ MPa was obtained when the chitin to PVA ratio was ca. 5.1%. Similarly, composite nanofibers based on PVA and nanocrystals of α-chitin (Φ *ca.* 31 nm, length *ca.* 549 nm) have been prepared (Φ 175–218 nm). The addition itself and the increase of the amount of the nanofibrils caused the crystallinity of PVA within the nanocomposite materials to decrease and the glass transition to increase [101,102]. We can best appreciate these results if we recall that certain early patents on chitin surgical sutures obtained by wet spinning chitin in dimethylacetamide + LiCl could not be exploited solely because the fibers scarcely had knot resistance [103,104].

To manufacture biodegradable scaffolds, chitin + poly(glycolic acid) nanofibers e-spun in hexafluoro-2-propanol (Φ *ca.* 140 nm) were investigated: the nanofibrous mats with PGA to chitin ratio 1:3 (and with bovine serum albumin coating) were the best in terms of cell attachment and spreading for normal human fibroblasts [105]. *In vitro*, the blend fibers degraded faster than pure PGA fibers at pH 7.2. Shalumon *et al.* developed e-spun carboxymethyl chitin + PVA blends that were exposed to glutaraldehyde vapors to make them water insoluble, *i.e.*, suitable for tissue engineering applications [106].

It is important to underline that the surface area of n-chitin e-spun mats is definitely smaller than the surface area of n-chitin aerogels obtained from hydrogels submitted to low-power ultrasonication, and dried by using supercritical $CO_2$ (surface area 58–261 $m^2/g$). Chitin was also fabricated into nanoporous aerogels by using aqueous NaOH + urea chaotropic solution as solvent (surface area up to 366 $m^2/g$) [107,108].

## 3.2. Electrospinning of Chitosan

Review articles dealing with this specific topic are available [109–112]. Nanofibrous mats were produced by e-spinning of chitosan + poly(ethylene oxide) (PEO) solution. In the presence of poly(hexamethylene biguanide), thinner fibers ($\Phi$ 60–240 nm) were obtained [113]. Chitosan and alginate were e-spun together with the aid of a dual jet system: PEO was applied to increase the viscosity of polymer solutions, and to yield nanofibers with appropriate morphology [114].

Novel biodegradable sutures were manufactured via coaxial e-spinning. Poly(lactic acid), a hydrophobic polyester, has good biocompatibility and mechanical properties, therefore, e-spun poly(lactic acid) nanofibers with uniaxial alignment were coated with chitosan and applied as tissue sutures: *in vivo* they exhibited better histocompatibility than silk, optimum mechanical resistance in clinical trials, and promoted cell growth. It is important to underline that they exhibited tensile and knot strengths similar to those of a commercial suture [115]. Some works have been devoted to the manufacture of PLA + chitosan composites, among which the one by Li YJ *et al.* who used Na lauryl sulfate to promote the distribution of chitosan in the periphery of the nanofibers; these materials supported growth and attachment of mouse fibroblasts [116].

It should also be considered that the preparation of nanostructured scaffolds is based on the chemical and morphological transformation of chitin nanofibrils into highly deacetylated n-chitosan. Upon deacetylation the chitin nanofibrils yield a colloidal chitosan solution, whose viscosity increase suggests that the n-chitosan network behaves as a polymer bulk in the solution. Facile chemical modifications of the chitosan nanoscaffold with lactose or maltose leads to white fluffy mesoporous chitosans whose characteristic properties (surface area, pore size, zeta potential) are quite suitable for tissue engineering [117].

It is also true that the preformed nanofibrillar mats of n-chitin can be deacetylated: in this case n-chitin becomes n-chitosan, but the texture remains practically the same as shown in Figure 6 [118], and amply confirmed by Pereira *et al.* [119].

Further utilization of chitosan nanofibrous mats e-spun from chitosan solutions in trifluoroacetic acid with or without chloromethane as the modifying co-solvent was found to be limited by the loss of the fibrous structure when the mats were in contact with neutral or weak basic aqueous solutions due to complete dissolution of the mats [120]; the effect of the degree of deacetylation was also studied [121]. Much improvement in the neutralization method was achieved with a saturated $Na_2CO_3$ solution. Torres-Giner *et al.* also developed porous e-spun chitosan nanofibers by using chloromethane [122].

The second solvent system demonstrated to effectively produce nanofibers was 30% acetic acid: thin nanofibers ($\Phi$ 40 nm) were produced together with large beads, but at 90% concentration the fiber's diameter increased to 130 nm without bead formation. Thus uniform mats of 130 nm fibers were obtained by e-spinning aqueous 90% acetic acid containing 7% chitosan in a 4 kV/cm electric field. These studies showed that the acetic acid concentration in water strongly influenced the surface tension of chitosan solutions [123]. Net charge density of the chitosan solution linearly increased with acetic acid concentration in water resulting in more charged ions available for charge repulsion.

A fibrous scaffold comprising chitosan and PCL was e-spun from mixture of formic acid and acetone [124]. The PCL e-spun mats exhibited hydrophilicity when the n-chitin content was >25 wt% [125].

**Figure 6.** Electrospun mats of nano-chitin (left) are transformed into mats of nano-chitosan (right) by chemical deacetylation up to 0.85, without significant dimensional change (no shrinkage). Reprinted with permission. Copyright © 2004 Elsevier [118].

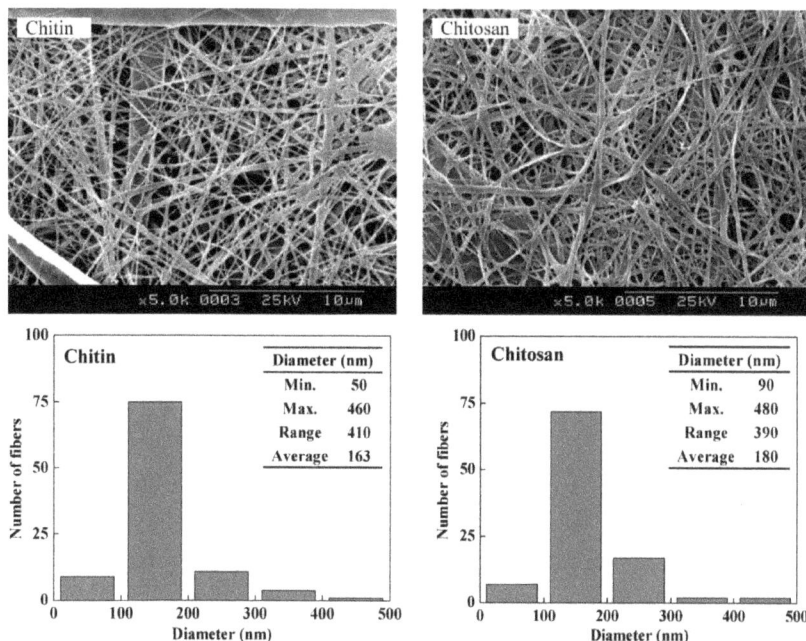

Rosic *et al.* demonstrated that interfacial, rather than bulk, rheological parameters can be used to predict the results of the e-spinning process [99]. By using the interfacial parameters (viscosity, $G'$, $G''$) of samples with homologous compositions, solutions of chitosan and PEO with differences in polymer ratio that form smooth nanofibers, can be identified. The bulk parameters are determined by polymer concentration and directly affect jet initiation, while the interfacial parameters determine the continuation of the jet and fiber formation.

Microfluidic-based pure chitosan microfibers (*ca.* 1 m long, $\Phi$ 70–150 μm) were fabricated without any chemical additive, and hepatoma HepG2 cells were seeded onto them. The functionality of the hepatic cells cultured on chitosan microfibers, analyzed by measuring albumin secretion and urea synthesis, was satisfactory; the microfiber chip could be useful for liver regeneration [126,127].

*3.3. Electrospinning of DBC-Chitin*

Dibutyryl chitin (DBC), a lipophilic chitin diester, is fully soluble in various organic solvents, thus it has been processed into fibers via conventional dry spinning from acetone, and wet spinning from dimethylformamide. Fine DBC fibers ($\Phi$ 300 nm) have been e-spun from ethanol and then regenerated with alkali for the preparation of nonwoven wound dressings. Although the preparation of DBC was initially made with the aid of perchloric acid, the adoption of less dangerous acids has simplified the preparation and made possible the scaling-up of the production. The most favorable characteristics of DBC are: hemocompatibility, lack of thrombogenicity, full biocompatibility toward human fibroblasts and keratinocytes, as well as documented technical feasibility of medication items such as plasters and dressings [128–132]. The effect of e-spun non-woven mats of dibutyryl chitin + poly(lactic acid) blends and other formulations were assayed for the purpose of wound healing [133–135].

## 4. Biomedical Applications of Nano-Chitins

Major biomedical applications of chitin and chitosan nanofibers have been recognized as emerging in the areas of tissue engineering, wound dressing, cosmetic and skin health, stem cell technology, anti-cancer treatments, drug delivery, anti-inflammatory aids, antimicrobial agents, biosensors, and reduction of obesity [136,137]. Nano-sized materials of interest for pharmaceutical uses have been reviewed as well as polysaccharide nanocarriers for therapeutic applications [138,139]. The state of the art and perspectives of the hemostatic polymers have been reviewed [140].

### 4.1. Hemostasis and Wound Healing

Chitin nanofibrils Talymed® manufactured from marine diatoms by Marine Polymer Tech., MA, USA, have an average length of *ca.* 80 μm. Gamma irradiation resulted in length shortening down to 4–7 μm, width of 100–150 nm, and thickness of 40–60 nm. Treatment of cutaneous wounds with the said FDA approved n-chitin (mainly used for hemostasis) resulted in more rapid wound closure in diabetic animal models, owing to increased expression of several cytokines, growth factors, and innate immune activation, besides activating angiogenesis, cell proliferation and re-epithelialization, as known long since [141].

Standard care for venous leg ulcers has remained unchanged over several decades despite high rates of initial treatment failure and ulcer recurrence. Kelechi *et al.* evaluated the efficacy, safety, and tolerability of Talymed® among patients with leg ulcers [142]. In a randomized, multi-center study, 86.4% of patients experienced complete wound healing when receiving multilayer compression plus Talymed® *vs.* 45% receiving multilayer compression alone. The pilot study suggested that n-chitin is well tolerated and effective. Results reported by Fischer *et al.* provide evidence that n-chitin nanofibers activate platelets and accelerate the clotting of blood, and on how best to achieve surface hemostasis when patients are coagulopathic because of shock or treatment with antiplatelet drugs [143].

n-Chitin promoted the expression of α- and β-defensins in endothelial cells and β-defensins in keratinocytes. Lindner *et al.* assessed the antimicrobial efficacy of n-chitin [144]: *S. aureus* infected wounds were either treated with n-chitin or left untreated for three and five days. Animals treated with n-chitin showed significant reduction in Gram positive staining by day 5 post wounding as compared with untreated wounds. Given that defensins are part of the innate immune system, activation of these pathways precludes the generation of resistant organisms and also allows for the antibiotic-independent clearance of bacterial infection. Thus they concluded that n-chitin enhances wound healing while concomitantly limiting wound infection. Antimicrobial n-carriers such as n-emulsions, n-liposomes, n-particles and n-fibers were reviewed by Blanco-Padilla *et al.* [145].

The reasons for the exceptional performances reside in the chemical nature and tertiary/quaternary structure of the chitin/chitosan whose surface is recognized by the platelets: via the staining of the activation marker P-selectin, it was possible to reveal the sudden activation of the platelets whose pseudopodia make a robust contact immediately upon activation [146]. The influence of altered platelet function by treatment with the ADP inhibitor Clopidogrel® (Sanofi, Paris, France) on wound healing and the ability of n-chitin to repair wounds in diabetic mice treated with Clopidogrel® were studied by Scherer *et al.* [147]. With the growing number of patients being treated with antiplatelet drugs, chitin nanofiber mats may be useful more generally for enhancing wound healing and restoring homeostasis.

Vacuum-assisted closure has become the preferred mode to treat many complex wounds, but could be further improved by methods that minimize bleeding and facilitate wound epithelialization. Membranes consisting entirely of chitin nanofibers were applied to dorsal excisional wounds of db/db mice followed by application of a vacuum device. Results included significant expression of PDGF, TGF-β, EGF, superior granulation tissue formation rich in collagen-I as well as epithelialization and wound contraction. Thus the application of membranes containing n-chitin, prior to the application of the polyurethane foam interface of vacuum devices, leads to most satisfactory healing and represents an advantage that reduces the risk of bleeding [148].

*4.2. Joints and Bones*

The early stages of degenerative disc disease primarily affect the disc nucleus pulposus. The product used by Gorapalli *et al.* was a relatively high MW n-chitosan [149]. The nanofibers were then manufactured as thin membranes by simple filtration and drying. Membranes were suspended in 40% NaOH at 80 °C for 3 h for deacetylation. Gel 1 consisted of 33.3 mg/mL of a sulphated n-chitosan having approximately 60%–70% of the sugar residues sulphated and 70% deacetylated (~500 kDa), plus 30 mg/mL of n-chitosan (pH 8.3). Gel 2 consisted of 10 mg/mL of irradiated (LMW) n-chitin and 30 mg/mL of n-chitosan (pH 6.8). These shortened nanofibers were 5–7 μm in length instead of 80 μm of the original nanofibers. Gel formulations were developed so as to be injectable into the nucleus pulposus of the intervertebral disc. The sulphated, deacetylated n-chitin hydrogel demonstrated most evident biological effects on cell viability, metabolic activity, and proteoglycan expression. RT-PCR and immunohistochemical data corroborated the expression of characteristic disc markers, aggrecan and collagen type II in cultured cells. The sulphated n-chitosan hydrogel possesses convincing characteristics, although results cannot yet be extrapolated to *in vivo* situations [149].

Muise-Helmericks *et al.* drilled circular holes (Φ 2.0 mm) in the femurs of rabbits and implanted n-chitin [150]. All the 15 n-chitin test sites were found to have new bone tissue present. Hematoxylin and eosin histology of the n-chitin-treated sites showed the presence of osteoblasts, osteocytes, and trabeculae of new bone at the end of the 28-day study period. The n-chitin mats activated the regeneration of new bone tissue in a rabbit model after 28 days of implantation, whereas the control bone did not. It is known that large bone defects do not heal unless treated with suitably modified chitosans, the plain chitosan itself being inactive [151–153]. A totally original approach was adopted in a bio-inspired work by Malho *et al.* who used a genetically modified protein to functionalize superficially the chitin nanofibers with a mineralization domain [154]. The said protein has two distinct groups, the first one (for binding chitin) the chitin-binding domain of bacterial chitinases, and the second one (for binding minerals) a fragment of aspein, a shell-specific protein from the oyster *Pinctada fucata* [155]. The charge density enabled the combination of $CaCO_3$ crystals with the chitin, thus providing a composite material endowed with enhanced mechanical and biochemical properties, probably suitable for bone surgery.

### 4.3. Ulcers and Traumatic Wounds

Azuma *et al.* found that n-chitin alleviates the clinical symptoms and suppresses the onset of ulcerative colitis in an animal model [156], in agreement with Ifuku *et al.* [10]; furthermore, n-chitin suppressed myeloperoxidase activation in the colon and decreased serum interleukin-6 concentration. In contrast, the application of chitin powder did not produce any anti-inflammatory action. Actually, 5-aminosalicylate is the only drug available, not exempt from side-effects [157–159]. Further work showed that α-chitin nanofibrils decreased positive areas of NF-kB staining in the colon tissue (7.2 in the chitin nanofibrils group *vs.* 10.7%/fields in the control). Chitin nanofibrils also decreased serum monocyte chemotactic protein-1 concentration in ulcerative colitis (24.1 in the chitin nanofibrils group *vs.* 53.5 pg/mL in the control). Moreover, the nanofibrils depressed the positive areas of Masson's trichrome staining in colon tissue (6.8 in the chitin nanofibrils group *vs.* 10.1%/fields in the control) [160].

Chitin nanofibrils suspended in water were incorporated into chitosan glycolate upon simple addition of the proper amount of chitosan powder and glycolic acid crystals. No aggregation or precipitation of chitin nanofibrils was observed in the course of several months. The wound dressing included a flexible support made of non-woven dibutyryl chitin (0.8 g), chitosan glycolate solution 1.0% (8 g), containing chitin nanofibrils (2 g/L), and chlorhexidine at physiological pH. The preparations were freeze-dried and sterilized. Ulcers and wounds in 75 patients were treated for 60 days. In the treatment of torpid and slowly healing lesions or ulcers, the association of the chitin + chitosan gel with a foam-like dressing induced physiological repair. A remarkable advantage was that the glycolic acid solutions are capable to preserve chitosan from microbial spoilage. Moreover, the nanofibrillar chitin + chitosan glycolate composites exert control over certain biochemical and physiological processes, besides hemostasis: while chitosan provides moderate antimicrobial activity, cell stimulation and filmogenicity, chitin nanofibrils slowly release *N*-acetylglucosamine, and recognize growth factors [161]. In fact, the introduction of chitin nanofibrils (0.1%–0.3%) in a chitosan solution influences the orientation of the chitosan macromolecules and leads to an increase in the strength and Young modulus of the chitosan + n-chitin composite fibers. The orientation of the chitosan macromolecules on the surface of the chitin nanofibrils was confirmed by the molecular dynamics simulation of systems containing one chitosan molecule on the chitin nanocrystallite surface [24,162].

Rod-like chitin nanofibrils were used to reinforce chitosan films, and composite membranes were prepared by casting/evaporation. The films with 3% chitin content had a tensile strength 2.8 times higher than that of plain chitosan film. Sterilized transparent film disks (Φ 7 cm) were placed on the inoculated media: after 24 h at 37 °C the composite film effectively inhibited all of the three strains tested, namely *S. aureus*, *E. coli* and *Corinebacterium michiganense*, thus providing preliminary indications on its suitability as an antibacterial film [163,164]. Genipin, as a crosslinker of the chitosan film assures the endurance of the composite in the culture environment for a prolonged period of time [165]. Chitosan films reinforced with chitin nanofibrils in admixture with tannic acid were conveniently crosslinked via amide formation by simply keeping them at 105 °C for 90 min [166].

Therefore, the presence of chitin nanocrystals into chitin fibers ($\Phi$ 223–966 nm) had a positive impact on the mechanical properties of e-spun mats further crosslinked with genipin. Those with a tensile strength of 64.9 MPa, modulus of 10.2 GPa and surface area 35 $m^2/g$ were considered for wound dressing. The water vapor transmission rate of the mats was between 1290 and 1548 $g\,m^{-2}day^{-1}$, and was in the range suitable for injured skin or wounds. The e-spun fiber mats showed compatibility with adipose derived stem cells [167].

According to Tchemtchoua *et al.* the best concentrations for e-spinning were 7.9% medical-grade chitosan and 1% PEG (900 kDa) in 6.5% acetic acid. The chitosan nanofiber mats produced by e-spinning were compared with evaporated films and xerogels. The nanofibrillar structure strongly improved cell adhesion and proliferation *in vitro*. When implanted in mice, the nanofibrillar scaffold was colonized by mesenchymal cells and blood vessels. When used as a dressing, covering full thickness skin wounds in mice, chitosan nanofibres induced a faster regeneration of both epidermis and dermis. They shortened the healing time of skin wounds by stimulating migration, invasion, and proliferation of the relevant cutaneous resident cells [168].

### 4.4. Dermal Protection

Stable PCL + chitin nanofibrous mats were manufactured from blended solutions of PCL and chitin dissolved in the co-solvent hexafluoro-2-propanol and trifluoroacetic acid [169]. The PCL-chitin nanofibrils ($\Phi$ 340 nm) showed decreased water contact angles as the proportion of chitin increased. Instead, the tensile properties of mats containing 30%–50% wt/wt chitin were enhanced compared with PCL mats. The viability of human dermal fibroblasts in culture for up to seven days was higher on composite than on PCL nanofibrous mats, with viability directly correlated with chitin concentration. Therefore PCL-chitin nanofibrous mats are useful as implantable substrates to modulate the viability of human dermal fibroblasts [169].

Ito *et al.* suggested that the application of n-chitin to skin, protects the epithelial cells, owing to its capacity to prevent moisture evaporation [170]. Moreover, the n-chitin (pH 6) group scored higher on histological data after the first 8 h of application, indicating that n-chitin is a very effective dermal protector in the long term even in comparison with GlcNAc. Thus n-chitin protects and hydrates the skin while not being allergenic.

### 5. Biomedical Applications of n-Chitosan

From the standpoint of this review article, a major difference between n-chitin and n-chitosan resides in the capacity of the latter to form polyelectrolyte complexes owing to its high cationicity. Polyelectrolyte complexation is an effective strategy for enhancing the mechanical properties of nanofibrous scaffolds. For the improvement of the mechanical and biochemical properties of chitosan intended for pharmaceutical and biomedical applications, blending with other polymers is important, since the native ECM is a complex of polysaccharides and proteins with nanofibrous porous structure. Moreover, crosslinking is often adopted, in particular with the use of genipin, a commercially available plant pigment ten thousand fold less cytotoxic than glutaraldehyde; moreover n-chitosan promptly undergoes other reactions such as reductive amination of aldehydes and ketones [171].

A number of drugs and other significant compounds can be added to the chitosan solutions for incorporation in the nanofibers in the case of e-spinning. For example, *Garcinia mangostana* extracts were incorporated into chitosan + EDTA + PVA solution and e-spun. The fibrous mats exhibited antioxidant and antibacterial activity and accelerated the wound healing process [172]. Polyethylene terephthalate fibrous mats e-spun in the presence of honey were proposed as potential wound dressings owing to their improved characteristics besides their suitable structural properties [173].

*5.1. Epithelial Tissue Regeneration*

Polyelectrolyte complexation enhances the mechanical properties of the nanofibrous scaffolds [174]. With the aid of the e-spun chitosan + gelatin model, it was measured that the storage modulus of a nanofiber mat is at least one thousand-fold higher than that of plain chitosan or gelatin membranes. Further, the annealing process promotes the conjugation of the oppositely charged polymers and thus the tensile modulus becomes 1.9-fold more elevated. When the molar ratio of the anhydroglucosamine units in chitosan to carboxyl units in gelatin was 1:1, the complex nanofiber mats displayed the highest mechanical strength. The characteristic properties of chitosan-gelatin edible films were reported by Jridi *et al.* and Tsai *et al.* [175,176].

Collagen has been widely used for tissue-engineering, in consideration of its biological origin, and ubiquitous presence in living organisms. Chitosan forms polyelectrolyte complexes with collagen: for example, chitosan + collagen composites were prepared by dissolving collagen in HFP, and chitosan in HFP + TFA [177,178]. The samples were e-spun at room temperature, and crosslinked with glutaraldehyde vapor. The authors examined the expression of ICAM-1 and VCAM-1, for which the chitosan + collagen scaffold can act as a stimulus. ICAM-1 and VCAM-1, adhesive proteins of the immunoglobulin superfamily, occur on the endothelial cell membrane and regulate the adhesion process of the leucocytes to these cells: they were used as primers for RT-PCR. Results showed that the chitosan + collagen nanofibrous scaffold enhanced the attachment, spreading, and proliferation of porcine iliac artery endothelial cells. The endothelial cells grown on the e-spun chitosan + collagen scaffolds maintained the capacity to regulate the cell cycle via the p53 mRNA expression and hence to function as tumor suppressors. E-spun chitosan mats coated with collagen were proposed for skin engineering [179] and curcumin-loaded mats were studied for wound healing [180]. Du *et al.* mimicked the natural blood vessel microenvironment by using heparinization and immobilization of vascular endothelial growth factor in the chitosan + PCL. As a consequence, the anti-thrombogenic properties of these scaffolds were enhanced [181].

Catalase, a redox enzyme, is generally recognized as an efficient agent for protecting cells against hydrogen peroxide. The immobilization of catalase was accomplished by depositing the PEC made of cationic chitosan and anionic catalase on e-spun cellulose nanofibrous mats via e-spinning and layer-by-layer deposition. The immobilized catalase protected cells against cytotoxic effects produced by $H_2O_2$ as demonstrated by TEM and SEM [182].

Another protein of interest is fibroin: the silk fibroin + chitosan composite nanofibers ($\Phi$ 185.5–484.6 nm) were easily e-spun in mixtures of hexafluoro-2-propanol and trifluoroethanol. Because the fibers as such are promptly water-soluble, they were then crosslinked with glutaraldehyde. The fibroin helps e-spin chitosan and contributes to the biocompatibility. The mats were found to promote the attachment and proliferation of murine fibroblasts [183].

**Figure 7.** Appearance of (left) n-cellulose, (middle) n-chitin, (right) n-cellulose + n-chitin + sericin. The latter contains glutaraldehyde. Reprinted with permission. Copyright © 2014 Elsevier [184].

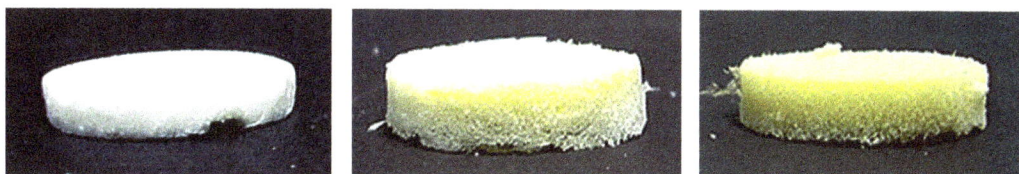

Composites of n-cellulose, n-chitin, and sericin were developed by Ang-atikarnkul *et al.* [184]: n-cellulose was used because of its nanofibrillar structure with high aspect ratio. n-Chitin was chosen as addtional component owing to its ability to promote the repair of wounds. The n-cellulose + n-chitin + sericin scaffolds with different compositions were prepared by freeze-drying and then treated with glutaraldehyde vapor (Figure 7). The release of the sericin from the nanocomposites was assessed in terms of blend composition, presence of lysozyme, and NaCl concentration. Sericin, a glue-like protein found in silk cocoons, was found to have good moisturizing and antioxidant capacity.

The water-soluble *N*-carboxyethyl chitosan was synthesized straightforwardly via a Michael addition reaction of chitosan with acrylic acid. Because of unsatisfactory e-spinning of aqueous mixtures of *N*-carboxyethyl chitosan and silk fibroin, PVA was selected as a polymeric additive to produce e-spun nanofibrous mats owing to its good fiber-forming, biocompatibility, and chemical resistance properties. Indirect *in vitro* cytotoxicity assessment of e-spun nanofiber mats with mouse fibroblasts indicated good biocompatibility. These composites might be assayed for wound dressing [185]. Fibroin-chitosan scaffolds with aligned nanofibrous structures were fabricated by Dunne *et al.* to guide vasculature in tissue engineering and repair [186]. The use of nanofibers for cardiovascular tissue engineering was discussed by Oh & Lee [187].

It is also interesting to note that n-chitosan can accompany other polysaccharides. For example, e-spun chitosan nanofibers were deposited onto cellulose treated with atmospheric plasma to generate a composite bandage with higher adhesion, better handling properties, enhanced bioactivity, and suitability for moisture management [188].

Repeated freeze/thaw cycles induced packing and phase separation of the hydrogels made of hemicelluloses, chitin nanofibrils and PVA (average length *ca.* 200 nm, width 40 nm). Large pores led to remarkable swelling, whereas the formation of a compact structure resulted in good mechanical strength and thermal stability. The chitin nanofibrils were embedded homogeneously in the PVA + hemicellulose matrix and limited the packing process, leading to the improvement of compressive strength and crystallinity of the hydrogels [189,190]. Analogous work was done on n-chitin incorporated into carboxymethylcellulose films [191].

Cytocompatible composite films were prepared by adding chitin nanofibrils to a cellulose solution in NaOH + urea. HeLa and T293 cells seeded onto the surface of the said films showed absence of toxicity to both cell types, and cell adhesion and proliferation were enhanced by chitin nanofibrils [192]. Experimental observations were reported in the case of ulvan + chitosan + PEG nanofibrous mats obtained with a strongly acidic polysaccharide from the plant *Ulva rigida*. The nanofibrous structure of these constructs, mimicking the fibrous part of the extracellular matrix, favored the excellent attachment of the osteoblasts [193].

*5.2. Bone and Dental Tissue Regeneration*

Tan *et al.* demonstrated that chitosan increases collagen-I and osteopontin expression, promotes osteoblast proliferation and osteogenesis in mesenchymal stem cells, and reduces osteoclastogenesis [194]. Norowski *et al.* prepared e-spun chitosan mats crosslinked with minor amounts of genipin, and showed that the obtained mats were cytocompatible and supported fibroblast cell proliferation for nine days; they did not activate monocytes to produce nitric oxide *in vitro* in the absence of lipopolysaccharide [195]. As a consequence of high surface area, decreased crystallinity degree (−14%), and decreased molecular weight of chitosan (−75%), the ultimate suture pullout strength was significantly lower (−51%) than that of commercially available collagen membranes. However, when genipin was used to crosslink nanofibrous chitosan made to incorporate hydroxyapatite nanoparticles, the Young's modulus value of the composite was $142 \pm 13$ MPa, which is similar to that of the natural periosteum. Pure chitosan and hydroxyapatite-chitosan composites supported adhesion, proliferation and osteogenic differentiation of murine 7F2 osteoblast-like cells. Likewise, cells cultured on hydroxyapatite + chitosan had the highest rate of osteonectin mRNA expression over two weeks, indicating enhanced osteoinduction exerted by the composite. The role of composite scaffolds containing chitosan on periosteal cell behavior (*i.e.*, on bone tissue regeneration) was strengthened in the work by Gentile *et al.* [196]. Therefore, Frohberg *et al.* proposed that these scaffolds might be useful for repair of maxillofacial defects and injuries (Figure 8) [197]. In fact, films crosslinked with genipin significantly promoted adhesion, proliferation, and differentiation of pre-osteoblasts.

Resin-based sealants containing chitosan nanofibers were developed by Mahapoka *et al.* and reviewed by Li XM *et al.* [198,199]. Chitosan whiskers were incorporated into dimethacrylate monomer at various ratios by weight. The dimethacrylate-based sealant containing chitosan nanofibers had a greater antimicrobial activity than control sealant and they were comparable with commercial sealants. The inclusion of the whiskers did not reduce the curing depth, and the reduction in hardness was minimal. In conclusion, resin-based sealants containing chitosan nanofibers are effective antimicrobial pit and fissure sealants with enhanced performances as dental restorative materials.

**Figure 8.** Electrospun chitosan microfibers (**A**); and the fibrous mat (**B**). Scale bar for (**A**) is 200 μm, and for (**B**) is 1 cm. Reprinted with permission. Copyright © 2012 Elsevier [196].

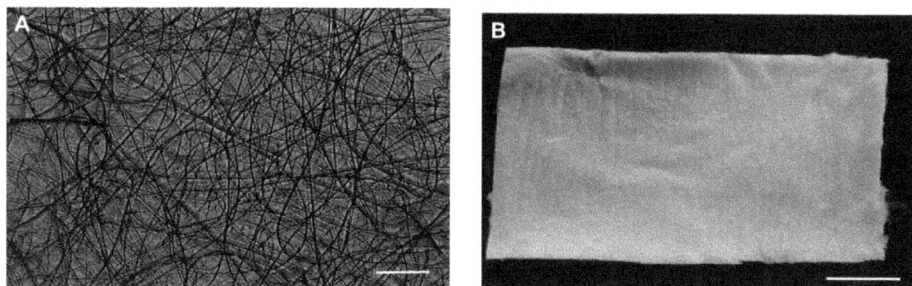

## 5.3. Bacteria, Fungi, and Viruses

By using Na hypochlorite, Dutta *et al.* substituted the hydrogen atom in the N-H group of chitin with a chlorine atom, to generate the N-Cl bond on the n-chitin surface, while maintaining the characteristic n-chitin morphology [200]. Although plain chitosan can be *N*-chlorinated [201], there is interest in preferring n-chitin because the latter is stably dispersed in water, and has large surface area, excellent mechanical properties, and prompt filmogenicity, as points of superiority compared with plain chitosan. The antimicrobial properties of *N*-chlorine stem from the direct transfer of the oxidative chlorine from the n-chitin films to the most susceptible parts of the microbes, thus effectively dismantling or inhibiting their enzymatic or metabolic processes.

Thus, n-chitin in *N*-halamine form kills microorganisms without the release of free chlorine. Upon depletion, the chloramine function is rechargeable with another NaClO treatment. Table 1 shows some data of bacteriological interest. Moreover, the films exerted 100% and 80% inhibition of fungal spore germination against *Alternaria alternata* and *Penicillium digitatum*, respectively [200]. *N*-(2-Hydroxy-3-trimethylammonium)propyl chitosan and *N*-benzyl-*N*,*N*-dimethyl chitosan were prepared in the form of e-spun mats. Both *S. aureus* and *E. coli* did not survive after 4 h contact with each of them [202].

**Table 1.** Percentage reduction of *E. coli* and *S. aureus* by chlorinated nano-chitin films [200].

| Contact Time, Min | *Escherichia coli*, % | *Staphylococcus aureus*, % |
|---|---|---|
| 5 | 86.4 | 46.7 |
| 10 | 99.9 | 87.8 |
| 30 | 100.0 | 100.0 |
| 60 | 100.0 | 100.0 |

Bacterial concentrations were 108–109 CFU/mL. The chlorinated n-chitin film contained 2.69% of active chlorine. The non chlorinated chitosan did not affect the bacteria. Cellulose membranes were used as negative control.

As for viruses, the *N*-(2-hydroxy-3-trimethylammonium)propyl chitosan was e-spun into nanofibers with PVA, to yield a mat with a large surface area that is a major requirement for effective adsorption. The nanofibers were crosslinked with glutaraldehyde to impart stability in aqueous media, thus the swelling of the fibers after 6 h in water was limited to 30%. Tests for their capacity to remove the non-enveloped porcine parvovirus and the enveloped Sindbis virus yielded values that came close to or exceeded the EPA regulation values for virus removal processes [203].

## 6. Conclusions and Perspectives

The above study of the current literature indicates that the nano size enhances the performances of chitins and chitosans, with no exceptions, ranging from human tissue regeneration to microbicidal activity; the most impressive data being those indicating that n-chitin alleviates the clinical symptoms and suppresses the onset of ulcerative colitis in an animal model.

The chitin nanofibrils are today isolated by quite simple mechanical means, that do not present scaling-up problems. It should be remarked however that for n-chitin itself and especially for n-chitosan, the bottleneck seems to reside in the deacetylation of the raw chitin. In particular the deacetylation is always carried out with the aid of boiling NaOH, which can be a dangerous and expensive operation.

A totally different panorama is offered by e-spinning. Although e-spun materials have been available for a long time, and the technique has been claimed to be versatile, their structure is either fluffy or offers too small pores, so that cellular infiltration is precluded. Moreover, e-spinning is based exclusively on ejection from a needle at extremely low speed, and scaling-up is quite a problem. New approaches such as force-spinning might be developed as described by Lozano *et al.* but it seems that there is still a long way to go to take e-spun materials to the clinical use [204]. On the other hand, e-spinning is a powerful stimulus for doing basic research on nano materials.

Turning to realistic perspectives, it would seem that biotechnological approaches are available immediately to modify certain situations that delay the exploitation of the chitin resources. For the sake of clarity let us consider some examples. (**a**) The study of the enzymatic deacetylation of n-chitin has not been undertaken so far, notwithstanding the fact that engineered deacetylases are available today [205]. No information exists on the behavior of deacetylases on n-chitin; (**b**) *Serratia marcescens* B742 mutants were prepared to improve the deproteination of shrimp shell powders, in fact 91.4% was achieved after three days of fermentation [206]; (**c**) Yeast spores can be deprived of their outermost dityrosine layer by genetic engineering, thus exposing their chitosan layer which becomes available for collection of metals, enzymes, sterols, and for use in medication [207]; (**d**) Certain agroindustrial discards (corn steep liquor and molasses) can be converted into chitosan by *Rhizopus arrhizus* and *Cunninghamella elegans* [208]; (**e**) The fisheries themselves have much to gain by using n-chitin and n-chitosan for the improved preservation of crustaceans [209]; (**f**) The treatment of fresh by-products from the canning factories should be revised in the light of existing advanced technologies [210].

The production of medical-grade chitosan took many years of effort in coordinating the activities of the fisheries with those of industries and research laboratories for quality assessment and certification. The currently marketed medical-grade chitosan derives from purified chitins that are also suitable for the isolation of n-chitin: for n-chitin, therefore, the development stage might be shorter, but it demands the same endeavor.

## Acknowledgments

The authors are grateful to Marilena Falcone, Central Library, Polytechnic University, Ancona, Italy, for assistance in handling the bibliographic information, and to Maria Weckx for help with the preparation of the manuscript. This work stemmed from a spontaneous initiative of the authors, and was not financially supported.

## Conflict of Interest

The authors declare no conflict of interest.

## References

1. Muzzarelli, R.A.A. Chitin nanostructures in living organisms. *Chitin Formation and Diagenesis*; Springer: Dordrecht, The Netherlands, 2011; Volume 34, pp. 1–34.
2. Muzzarelli, R.A.A. Nanochitins and nanochitosans, paving the way to eco-friendly and energy-saving exploitation of marine resources. *Polym. Sci. Compr. Ref.* **2012**, *10*, 153–164.
3. Muzzarelli, R.A.A.; Boudrant, J.; Meyer, D.; Manno, N.; DeMarchis, M.; Paoletti, M.G. A tribute to Henri Braconnot, precursor of the carbohydrate polymers science, on the chitin bicentennial. *Carbohydr. Polym.* **2012**, *87*, 995–1012.
4. Muzzarelli, R.A.A.; Muzzarelli, C. *Chitin and Chitosan: Opportunities and Challenges*; Dutta, P.K., Ed.; SSM International: Contai, India, 2005; pp. 129–146.
5. Muzzarelli, R.A.A. Biomedical exploitation of chitin and chitosan via mechano-chemical disassembly, electrospinning, dissolution in imidazolium ionic liquids, and supercritical drying. *Mar. Drugs* **2011**, *9*, 1510–1533.
6. Muzzarelli, R.A.A. New techniques for optimization of surface area and porosity in nanochitins and nanochitosans. In *Advances in Polymer Science: Chitosan for Biomaterials*; Jayakumar, R., Prabaharan, A., Muzzarelli, R.A.A., Eds.; Springer-Verlag: Berlin, Germany, 2011; Volume 2, pp. 167–186.
7. Muzzarelli, R.A.A. *Chitin*; Pergamon: Oxford, UK, 1977.
8. Araki, J. Electrostatic or steric? Preparations and characterizations of well-dispersed systems containing rod-like nanowhiskers of crystalline polysaccharides. *Soft Matter* **2013**, *9*, 4125–4141.
9. Ifuku, S.; Nomura, R.; Morimoto, M.; Saimoto, H. Preparation of chitin nanofibers from mushrooms. *Materials* **2011**, *4*, 1417–1425.
10. Ifuku, S.; Nogi, M.; Abe, K.; Yoshioka, M.; Morimoto, M.; Saimoto, H.; Yano, H. Simple preparation of chitin nanofibers with a width of 10–20 nm from prawn shell under neutral conditions. *Carbohydr. Polym.* **2011**, *84*, 762–764.
11. Ifuku, S.; Saimoto, H. Chitin nanofibers: Preparations, modifications, and applications. *Nanoscale* **2012**, *4*, 3308–3318.
12. Chatrabhuti, S.; Chirachanchai, S. Single step coupling for multi-responsive water-based chitin/chitosan magnetic nanoparticles. *Carbohydr. Polym.* **2013**, *97*, 441–450.

13. Sahay, R.; Kumar, P.S.; Sridhar, R.; Sundaramurthy, J.; Venugopal, J.; Mhaisalkar, S.G.; Ramakrishna, S. Electrospun composite nanofibers and their multifaceted applications. *J. Mater. Chem.* **2012**, *22*, 12953–12971.

14. Neville, A.C. *Biology of Fibrous Composites: Development beyond the Cell Membrane*; Cambridge University Press: New York, NY, USA, 1993.

15. Muzzarelli, R.A.A.; Jeuniaux, C.; Gooday, G.W. *Chitin in Nature and Technology*; Plenum: New York, NY, USA, 1986.

16. Stankiewicz, B.A.; van Bergen, P. *Nitrogen-Containing Macromolecules in the Bio- and Geosphere*; ACS-707; American Chemical Society: Washington, DC, USA, 1998.

17. Jollès, P.; Muzzarelli, R.A.A. *Chitin and Chitinases*; Birkhauser: Basel, Switzerland, 1999.

18. Kurita, K. Chitin and chitosan: Functional biopolymers from marine crustaceans. *Mar. Biotechnol.* **2006**, *8*, 203–226.

19. Ravi Kumar, M.N.V.; Muzzarelli, R.A.A.; Muzzarelli, C.; Sashiwa. H.; Domb, A.J. Chitosan chemistry and pharmaceutical perspectives. *Chem. Rev.* **2004**, *104*, 6017–6084.

20. Keong, L.C.; Halim, A.S. *In vitro* models in biocompatibility assessment for biomedical-grade chitosan derivatives in wound management (Review). *Int. J. Mol. Sci.* **2009**, *10*, 1300–1313.

21. Desbrieres, J.; Babak, V.G. Interfacial properties of amphiphilic systems on the basis of natural polymers-chitin derivatives. *Russ. J. Gen. Chem.* **2008**, *78*, 2230–2238.

22. Muzzarelli, R.A.A. Chitins and chitosans as immunoadjuvants and non-allergenic drug carriers. *Mar. Drugs* **2010**, *8*, 292–312.

23. Grunenfelder, L.K.; Herrera, S.; Kisailus, D. Crustacean-derived biomimetic components and nanostructured composites. *Small* **2014**, *10*, 3207–3232.

24. Yan, W.X.; Shen, L.B.; Ji, Y.L.; Yang, Q.; Shen, X.Y. Chitin nanocrystal reinforced wet-spun chitosan fibers. *J. Appl. Polym. Sci.* **2014**, *131*, doi:10.1002/app.40852.

25. Sashiwa, H.; Aiba, S.I. Chemically modified chitin and chitosan as biomaterials. *Prog. Polym. Sci.* **2004**, *29*, 887–908.

26. Gomez d'Ayala, G.; Malinconico, M.; Laurienzo, P. Marine derived polysaccharides for biomedical applications: Chemical modification approaches. *Molecules* **2008**, *13*, 2069–2106.

27. Mincea, M.; Negrulescu, A.; Ostafe, V. Preparation, modification, and applications of chitin nanowhiskers: A review. *Rev. Adv. Mater. Sci.* **2012**, *30*, 225–242.

28. Cortizo, M.S.; Berghoff, C.F.; Alessandrini, J.L. Characterization of chitin from *Illex argentinus* squid pen. *Carbohydr. Polym.* **2008**, *74*, 10–15.

29. Yui, T.; Taki, N.; Sugiyama, J.; Hayashi, S. Exhaustive crystal structure search and crystal modeling of beta-chitin. *Int. J. Biol. Macromol.* **2007**, *40*, 336–344.

30. Lavall, R.L.; Assis, O.B.G.; Campana, S.P. Beta-Chitin from the pens of *Loligo* sp.: Extraction and characterization. *Bioresour. Technol.* **2007**, *98*, 2465–2472.

31. Chandumpai, A.; Singhpibulporn, N.; Faroongsarng, D.; Sornprasit, P. Preparation and physico-chemical characterization of chitin and chitosan from the pens of the squid species, *Loligo lessoniana* and *Loligo formosana*. *Carbohydr. Polym.* **2004**, *58*, 467–474.

32. Nishiyama, Y.; Noishiki, Y.; Wada, M. X-ray Structure of Anhydrous beta-Chitin at 1 angstrom Resolution. *Macromolecules* **2011**, *44*, 950–957.

33. Sawada, D.; Nishiyama, Y.; Langan, P.; Forsyth, V.T.; Kimura, S.; Wada, M. Water in crystalline fibers of dihydrate beta-chitin results in unexpected absence of intramolecular hydrogen bonding. *PLoS One* **2012**, *7*, e39376.

34. Yang, F.C.; Peters, R.D.; Dies, H.; Rheinstadter, M.C. Hierarchical, self-similar structure in native squid pen. *Soft Matter* **2014**, *10*, 5541–5549.

35. Sawada, D.; Ogawa, Y.; Kimura, S.; Nishiyama, Y.; Langan, P.; Wada, M. Solid-solvent molecular interactions observed in crystal structures of beta-chitin complexes. *Cellulose* **2014**, *21*, 1007–1014.

36. Youn, D.K.; No, H.K.; Prinyawiwatkul, W. Preparation and characteristics of squid pen beta-chitin prepared under optimal deproteination and demineralisation condition. *Int. J. Food Sci. Technol.* **2013**, *48*, 571–577.

37. Fabritius, H.; Sachs, C.; Raabe, D.; Nikolov, S.; Friak, M.; Neugebauer, J. Chitin in the exoskeletons of arthropoda: From ancient design to novel materials science. In *Chitin Formation and Diagenesis: 34*; Springer: Dordrecht, The Netherland, 2011; pp. 35–60.

38. Fabritius, H.O.; Karsten, E.S.; Balasundaram, K.; Hild, S.; Huemer, K.; Raabe, D. Correlation of structure, composition and local mechanical properties in the dorsal carapace of the edible crab *Cancer pagurus*. *Zeitschrift Fur Kristallographie* **2012**, *227*, 766–776.

39. Raabe, D.; Al-Sawalmih, A.; Romano, P.; Sachs, C.; Brokmeier, H.G.; Yi, S.B.; Servos, G.; Hartwig, H.G. Structure and crystallographic texture of arthropod bio-composites. *Icotom 14: Texture Materi.* **2005**, *495–497*, 1665–1674.

40. Raabe, D..; Romano, P.; Sachs, C. The crustacean exoskeleton as an example of a structurally and mechanically graded biological nanocomposite material. *Acta Mater.* **2005**, *53*, 4281–4292.

41. Raabe, D.; Romano, P.; Sachs, C.; Al-Sawalmih, A.; Brokmeier, H.G.; Yi, S.B.; Servos, G.; Hartwig, H.G. Discovery of a honeycomb structure in the twisted plywood patterns of fibrous biological nanocomposite tissue. *J. Cryst. Growth* **2005**, *283*, 1–7.

42. Raabe, D.; Romano, P.; Sachs, C.; Fabritius, H.; Al-Sawalmih, A.; Yi, S.B.; Servos, G.; Hartwig H.G. Microstructure and crystallographic texture of the chitin-protein network in the biological composite material of the exoskeleton of the lobster *Homarus americanus*. *Mater. Sci. Eng.* **2006**, *421*, 143–153.

43. Raabe, D.; Al-Sawalmih, A.; Yi, S.B.; Fabritius, H. Preferred crystallographic texture of alpha-chitin as a microscopic and macroscopic design principle of the exoskeleton of the lobster *Homarus americanus*. *Acta Biomater.* **2007**, *3*, 882–895.

44. Nikolov, S.; Fabritius, H.; Petrov, M.; Friak, M.; Lymperakis, L.; Sachs, C.; Raabe, D.; Neugebauer, J. Robustness and optimal use of design principles of arthropod exoskeletons studied by ab initio-based multiscale simulations. *J. Mech. Behav. Biomed. Mater.* **2011**, *4*, 129–145.

45. Raue, L.; Klein, H.; Raabe, D. The exoskeleton of the american lobster: From texture to anisotropic properties. *Texture Anisotropy Polycrystals III* **2010**, *160*, 287–294.

46. Saito, Y.; Okano, T.; Chanzy, H.; Sugiyama, J. Structural study of alpha-chitin from the grasping spines of the arrow worm *Sagitta* spp. *J. Struct. Biol.* **1995**, *114*, 218–228.

47. Bone, Q.; Ryan, K.; Pulsford, A.L. The structure and the composition of the teeth and grasping spines of Chaetognaths. *J. Mar. Biol. Assoc. UK* **1983**, *63*, 929–939.

48. Chretiennot-Dinet, M.J.; Giraud-Guille, M.M.; Vaulot, D.; Putaux, J.L.; Saito, Y.; Chanzy, H. The chitinous nature of filaments ejected by *Phaeocystis* (Prymnesiophyceae). *J. Phycol.* **1997**, *33*, 666–672.

49. Rousseau, V.; Lantoine, F.; Rodriguez, F.; LeGall, F.; Chretiennot-Dinet, M.J.; Lancelot, C. Characterization of *Phaeocystis globosa* (Prymnesiophyceae), the blooming species in the Southern North Sea. *J. Sea Res.* **2013**, *76*, 105–113.

50. Barbosa, S.S.; Kelaher, B.P.; Byrne, M. Patterns of abundance, growth and size of the tropical intertidal chiton *Acanthopleura gemmate*. *Molluscan Res.* **2010**, *30*, 48–52.

51. Kelly, R.P.; Eernisse, D.J. Reconstructing a radiation: The chiton genus Mopalia in the north Pacific. *Invertebr. Syst.* **2008**, *22*, 17–28.

52. Evans, L.A.; Macey, D.J.; Webb, J. Characterization and structural organization of the organic matrix of the radula teeth of the chiton *Acanthopleura hirtosa*. *Philos. Trans. R. Soc. Lond. B* **1990**, *329*, 87–96.

53. Shaw, J.A.; Macey, D.J.; Brooker, L.R. Radula synthesis by three species of iron mineralizing molluscs: Production rate and elemental demand. *J. Mar. Biol. Assoc. UK* **2008**, *88*, 597–601.

54. Wang, Q.Q.; Nemoto, M.; Li, D.S.; Weaver, J.C.; Weden, B.; Stegemeier, J.; Bozhilov, K.N.; Wood, L.R.; Milliron, G.W.; Kim, C.S.; *et al.* Phase transformations and structural developments in the radular teeth of *Cryptochiton stelleri*. *Adv. Funct. Mater.* **2013**, *23*, 2908–2917.

55. Minke, R.; Blackwell, J. The structure of alpha chitin. *J. Mol. Biol.* **1978**, *120*, 167–181.

56. Noishiki, Y.; Nishiyama, Y.; Wada, M.; Okada, S.; Kuga, S. Inclusion complex of beta-chitin and aliphatic amines. *Biomacromolecules* **2003**, *4*, 944–949.

57. Miserez, A.; Li, Y.L.; Waite, J.H.; Zok, F. Jumbo squid beaks: Inspiration for design of robust organic composites. *Acta Biomater.* **2007**, *3*, 139–149.

58. Muzzarelli, R.A.A.; Muzzarelli, C.; Cosani, A.; Terbojevich, M. 6-Oxychitins, novel hyaluronan-like regiospecifically carboxylated chitins. *Carbohydr. Polym.* **1999**, *39*, 361–367.

59. Lai, C.; Zhang, S.J.; Chen, X.C.; Sheng, L.Y. Nanocomposite films based on TEMPO-mediated oxidized bacterial cellulose and chitosan. *Cellulose* **2014**, *21*, 2757–2772.

60. Fan, Y.M.; Fukuzumi, H.; Saito, T.; Isogai, A. Comparative characterization of aqueous dispersions and cast films of different chitin nanowhiskers/nanofibers. *Int. J. Biol. Macromol.* **2012**, *50*, 69–76.

61. Zhou, J.; Butchosa, N.; Jayawardena, H.S.N.; Zhou, Q.; Yan, M.D.; Ramstrom, O. Glycan-functionalized fluorescent chitin nanocrystals for biorecognition applications. *Bioconjug. Chem.* **2014**, *25*, 640–643.

62. Fan, Y.M.; Saito, T.; Isogai, A. Preparation of chitin nanofibers from squid pen beta-chitin by simple mechanical treatment under acid conditions. *Biomacromolecules* **2008**, *9*, 1919–1923.

63. Fan, Y.M.; Saito, T.; Isogai, A. Chitin nanocrystals prepared by TEMPO-mediated oxidation of alpha-chitin. *Biomacromolecules* **2008**, *9*, 192–198.

64. Dutta, A.K.; Yamada, K.; Izawa, H.; Morimoto, M.; Saimoto, H.; Ifuku, S. Preparation of chitin nanofibers from dry chitin powder by star burst system: Dependence on number of passes. *J. Chitin Chitosan Sci.* **2013**, *1*, 59–64.

65. Ifuku, S.; Nogi, M.; Abe, K.; Yoshioka, M.; Morimoto, M.; Saimoto, H.; Yano, H. Preparation of chitin nanofibers with a uniform width as alpha-chitin from crab shells. *Biomacromolecules* **2009**, *10*, 1584–1588.

66. Fan, Y.M.; Saito, T.; Isogai, A. Individual chitin nano-whiskers prepared from partially deacetylated alpha-chitin by fibril surface cationization. *Carbohydr. Polym.* **2010**, *79*, 1046–1051.

67. Abe, K.; Ifuku, S.; Kawata, M.; Yano, H. Preparation of tough hydrogels based on beta-chitin nanofibers via NaOH treatment. *Cellulose* **2014**, *21*, 535–540.

68. Mushi, N.E.; Butchosa, N.; Salajkova, M.; Zhoua, Q.; Berglund, L.A. Nanostructured membranes based on native chitin nanofibers prepared by mild process. *Carbohydr. Polym.* **2014**, *112*, 255–263.

69. Wijesena, R.; Tissera, N.; Kannankgara, Y.; Lin, Y.; Amaratunga, G.; de Silva, N. A method for top down preparation of chitosan nanoparticles and nanofibers. *Carbohydr. Polym.* **2014**, in press.

70. Watthanaphanit, A.; Supaphol, P.; Tamura, H.; Tokura, S.; Rujiravanit, R. Wet-spun alginate/chitosan whiskers nanocomposite fibers: Preparation, characterization and release characteristic of the whiskers. *Carbohydr. Polym.* **2010**, *79*, 738–746.

71. Ifuku, S.; Ikuta, A.; Egusa, M.; Kaminaka, H.; Izawa, H.; Morimoto, M.; Saimoto, H. Preparation of high-strength transparent chitosan film reinforced with surface-deacetylated chitin nanofibers. *Carbohydr. Polym.* **2013**, *98*, 1198–1202.

72. Kadokawa, J.; Takegawa, A.; Mine, S.; Prasad, K. Preparation of chitin nanowhiskers using an ionic liquid and their composite materials with poly(vinyl alcohol). *Carbohydr. Polym.* **2011**, *84*, 1408–1412.

73. Liu, D.G.; Wu, Q.L.; Chang, P.R.; Gao, G.Z. Self-assembled liquid crystal film from mechanically defibrillated chitosan nanofibers. *Carbohydr. Polym.* **2011**, *84*, 686–689.

74. Saito, Y.; Putaux, J.L.; Okano, T.; Gaill, F.; Chanzy, H. Structural aspects of the swelling of beta chitin in HCl and its conversion into alpha chitin. *Macromolecules* **1997**, *30*, 3867–3873.

75. Jin, J.; Hassanzadeh, P.; Perotto, G.; Sun, W.; Brenckle, M.A.; Kaplan, D.; Omenetto, F.G.; Rolandi, M. A biomimetic composite from solution self-assembly of chitin nanofibers in a silk fibroin matrix. *Adv. Mater.* **2013**, *25*, 4482–4487.

76. Zhong, C.; Kapetanovic, A.; Deng, Y.X.; Rolandi, M. A chitin nanofiber ink for airbrushing, replica molding, and microcontact printing of self-assembled macro-, micro-, and nanostructures. *Adv. Mater.* **2011**, *23*, 4776–4781.

77. Rolandi, M.; Rolandi, R. Self-assembled chitin nanofibers and applications. *Adv. Colloid Interface Sci.* **2014**, *207*, 216–222.

78. Hassanzadeh, P.; Kharaziha, M.; Nikkhah, M.; Shin, S.R.; Jin, J.; He, S.; Sun, W.; Zhong, C.; Dokmeci, M.R.; Khademhosseini, A.; *et al*. Chitin nanofiber micropatterned flexible substrates for tissue engineering. *J. Mater. Chem. B* **2013**, *1*, 4217–4224.

182

79. Fuh, Y.K.; Chen, S.Z.; Jang, J.S.C. Direct-write, well-aligned chitosan-poly(ethylene oxide) nanofibers deposited via near-field electrospinning. *J. Macromol. Sci. A* **2012**, *49*, 845–850.

80. Cooper, A.; Zhong, C.; Kinoshita, Y.; Morrison, R.S.; Rolandi, M.; Zhang, M.Q. Self-assembled chitin nanofiber templates for artificial neural networks. *J. Mater. Chem.* **2012**, *22*, 3105–3109.

81. Wu, J.; Meredith, J.C. Assembly of chitin nanofibers into porous biomimetic structures via freeze drying. *Acs Macro Lett.* **2014**, *3*, 185–190.

82. Wu, Y.; Sasaki, T.; Irie, S.; Sakurai, K. A novel biomass-ionic liquid platform for the utilization of native chitin. *Polymer* **2008**, *49*, 2321–2327.

83. Hu, X.W.; Du, Y.M.; Tang, Y.F.; Wang, Q.; Feng, T.; Yang, J.H.; Kennedy, J.F. Solubility and property of chitin in NaOH/urea aqueous solution. *Carbohydr. Polym.* **2007**, *70*, 451–458.

84. Hu, X.W.; Tang, Y.F.; Wang, Q.; Li, Y.; Yang, J.H.; Du, Y.M.; Kennedy, J.F. Rheological behaviour of chitin in NaOH/urea aqueous solution. *Carbohydr. Polym.* **2011**, *83*, 1128–1133.

85. Huang, Y.; Zhong, Z.B.; Duan, B.; Zhang, L.N.; Yang, Z.X.; Wang, Y.F.; Ye, Q.F. Novel fibers fabricated directly from chitin solution and their application as wound dressing. *J. Mater. Chem. B* **2014**, *2*, 3427–3432.

86. Li, G.X.; Du, Y.M.; Tao, Y.Z.; Liu, Y.T.; Li, S.; Hu, X.W.; Yang, J. Dilute solution properties of four natural chitin in NaOH/urea aqueous system. *Carbohydr. Polym.* **2010**, *80*, 970–976.

87. Nata, I.F.; Wang, S.S.S.; Wu, T.M.; Lee, C.K. β-Chitin nanofibrils for self-sustaining hydrogels preparation via hydrothermal treatment. *Carbohydr. Polym.* **2012**, *90*, 1509–1514.

88. Ifuku, S.; Morooka, S.; Morimoto, M.; Saimoto, H. Acetylation of chitin nanofibers and their transparent nanocomposite films. *Biomacromolecules* **2010**, *11*, 1326–1330.

89. Ifuku, S.; Iwasaki, M.; Morimoto, M.; Saimoto, H. Graft polymerization of acrylic acid onto chitin nanofiber to improve dispersibility in basic water. *Carbohydr. Polym.* **2012**, *90*, 623–627.

90. Chen, C.C.; Li, D.G.; Deng, Q.Y.; Zheng, B.T. Optically transparent biocomposites: Polymethylmethacrylate reinforced with high-performance chitin nanofibers. *Bioresources* **2012**, *7*, 5960–5971.

91. Chen, C.C.; Li, D.G.; Hu, Q.Q.; Wang, R. Properties of polymethyl methacrylate-based nanocomposites: Reinforced with ultra-long chitin nanofiber extracted from crab shells. *Mater. Des.* **2014**, *56*, 1049–1056.

92. Ifuku, S.; Ikuta, A.; Izawa, H.; Morimoto, M.; Saimoto, H. Control of mechanical properties of chitin nanofiber film using glycerol without losing its characteristics. *Carbohydr. Polym.* **2014**, *101*, 714–717.

93. Shams, M.I.; Yano, H. Simplified fabrication of optically transparent composites reinforced with nanostructured chitin. *J. Polym. Environ.* **2013**, *21*, 937–943.

94. Lu, Y.; Sun, Q.F.; She, X.L.; Xia, Y.Z.; Liu, Y.X.; Li, J.; Yang, D.J. Fabrication and characterisation of α-chitin nanofibers and highly transparent chitin films by pulsed ultrasonication. *Carbohydr. Polym.* **2013**, *98*, 1497–1504.

95. Huang, Y.C.; Wu, Y.; Huang, W.C.; Yang, F.; Ren, X.E. Degradation of chitosan by hydrodynamic cavitation. *Polymer. Degrad. Stab.* **2013**, *98*, 37–43.

96. Gao, Y.; Truong, Y.B.; Zhu, Y.G.; Kyratzis, I.L. Electrospun antibacterial nanofibers: Production, activity, and *in vivo* applications. *J. Appl. Polym. Sci.* **2014**, *131*, doi:10.1002/app.40797.

97. Goh, Y.F.; Shakir, I.; Hussain, R. Electrospun fibers for tissue engineering, drug delivery and wound dressing. *J. Mater. Sci.* **2013**, *48*, 3027–3054.

98. Jayakumar, R.; Prabaharan, M.; Nair, S.V.; Tamura, H. Novel chitin and chitosan nanofibers in biomedical applications. *Biotechnol. Adv.* **2010**, *28*, 142–150.

99. Rosic, R.; Pelipenko, J.; Kocbek, P.; Baumgartner, S.; Bester-Rogac, M.; Kristl, J. The role of rheology of polymer solutions in formation by electrospinning. *Eur. Polym. J.* **2012**, *48*, 1374–1384.

100. Wang, X.F.; Ding, B.; Sun, G.; Wang, M.R.; Yu, J.Y. Electro-spinning/netting: A strategy for the fabrication of three-dimensional polymer nano-fiber/nets. *Prog. Mater. Sci.* **2013**, *58*, 1173–1243.

101. Junkasem, J.; Rujiravanit, R.; Supaphol, P. Fabrication of alpha-chitin whisker-reinforced poly(vinyl alcohol) nanocomposite nanofibres by electrospinning. *Nanotechnology* **2006**, *17*, 4519–4528.

102. Junkasem, J.; Rujiravanit, R.; Grady, B.P.; Supaphol, P. X-ray diffraction and dynamic mechanical analyses of alpha-chitin whisker-reinforced poly(vinyl alcohol) nanocomposite nanofibers. *Polym. Int.* **2010**, *59*, 85–91.

103. Austin, P.R. Chitin solvents and solubility parameters. In *Chitin, Chitosan, and Related Enzymes*; Zikakis, J.P., Ed.; Academic: Orlando, FL, USA, 1984; pp. 57–75.

104. Austin, P.R.; Brine, C.J.; Castle, J.E.; Zikakis, J.P. Chitin: New facets of research. *Science* **1981**, *212*, 749–753.

105. Park, K.E.; Kang, H.K.; Lee, S.J.; Min, B.M.; Park, W.H. Biomimetic nanofibrous scaffolds: Preparation and characterization of PGA/chitin blend nanofibers. *Biomacromolecules* **2006**, *7*, 635–643.

106. Shalumon, K.T.; Binulal, N.S.; Selvamurugan, N.; Nair, S.V.; Menon, D.; Furuike, T.; Tamura, H.; Jayakumar, R. Electrospinning of carboxymethyl chitin/poly(vinyl alcohol) nanofibrous scaffolds for tissue engineering applications. *Carbohydr. Polym.* **2009**, *77*, 863–869.

107. Heath, L.; Zhu, L.F.; Thielemans, W. Chitin nanowhisker aerogels. *Chemsuschem* **2013**, *6*, 537–544.

108. Ding, B.B.; Cai, J.; Huang, J.C.; Zhang, L.N.; Chen, Y.; Shi, X.W.; Du, Y.M.; Kuga, S. Facile preparation of robust and biocompatible chitin aerogels. *J. Mater. Chem.* **2012**, *22*, 5801–5809.

109. Elsabee, M.Z.; Naguib, H.F.; Morsi, R.E. Chitosan based nanofibers, a review. *Mater. Sci. Eng. C-Mater. Biol. Appl.* **2012**, *32*, 1711–1726.

110. Mucha, M.; Balcerzak, J.; Michalak, I.; Tylman, M. Biopolymeric matrices based on chitosan for medical applications. *E-Polymers* **2011**, *11*, 21–28.

111. Nirmala, R.; Il, B.W.; Navamathavan, R.; El-Newehy, M.H.; Kim, H.Y. Preparation and characterizations of anisotropic chitosan nanofibers via electrospinning. *Macromol. Res.* **2011**, *19*, 345–350.

112. Ohkawa, K.; Cha, D.I.; Kim, H.; Nishida, A.; Yamamoto, H. Electrospinning of chitosan. *Macromol. Rapid Commun.* **2004**, *25*, 1600–1605.

113. Dilamian, M.; Montazer, M.; Masoumi, J. Antimicrobial electrospun membranes of chitosan/poly(ethylene oxide) incorporating poly(hexamethylene biguanide) hydrochloride *Carbohydr. Polym.* **2013**, *94*, 364–371.

114. Hu, W.W.; Yu, H.N. Co-electrospinning of chitosan/alginate fibers by dual-jet system for modulating material surfaces. *Carbohydr. Polym.* **2013**, *95*, 716–727.

115. Hu, W.; Huang, Z.M. Biocompatibility of braided poly(L-lactic acid) nanofiber wires applied as tissue sutures. *Polym. Int.* **2010**, *59*, 92–99.

116. Li, Y.J.; Chen, F.; Nie, J.; Yang, D.Z. Electrospun poly(lactic acid)/chitosan core-shell structure nanofibers from homogeneous solution. *Carbohydr. Polym.* **2012**, *90*, 1445–1451.

117. Mathew, A.P.; Laborie, M.P.G.; Oksman, K. Cross-linked chitosan/chitin crystal nanocomposites with improved permeation selectivity and pH stability. *Biomacromolecules* **2009**, *10*, 1627–1632.

118. Min, B.M.; Lee, S.W.; Lim, J.N.; You, Y.; Lee, T.S.; Kang, P.H.; Park, W.H. Chitin and chitosan nanofibers: Electrospinning of chitin and deacetylation of chitin nanofibers. *Polymer* **2004**, *45*, 7137–7142.

119. Pereira, A.G.B.; Muniz, E.C.; Hsieh, Y.L. Chitosan-sheath and chitin-core nanowhiskers. *Carbohydr. Polym.* **2014**, *107*, 158–166.

120. Sangsanoh, P.; Supaphol, P. Stability improvement of electrospun chitosan nanofibrous membranes in neutral or weak basic aqueous solutions. *Biomacromolecules* **2006**, *7*, 2710–2714.

121. Nam, Y.S.; Park, W.H.; Ihm, D.; Hudson, S.M. Effect of the degree of deacetylation on the thermal decomposition of chitin and chitosan nanofibers. *Carbohydr. Polym.* **2010**, *80*, 291–295.

122. Torres-Giner, S.; Ocio, M.J.; Lagaron, J.M. Development of active antimicrobial fiber based chitosan polysaccharide nanostructures using electrospinning. *Eng. Life Sci.* **2008**, *8*, 303–314.

123. Geng, X.Y.; Kwon, O.H.; Jang, J.H. Electrospinning of chitosan dissolved in concentrated acetic acid solution. *Biomaterials* **2005**, *26*, 5427–5432.

124. Shalumon, K.T.; Anulekha, K.H.; Girish, C.M.; Prasanth, R.; Nair, S.V.; Jayakumar, R. Single step electrospinning of chitosan/poly(caprolactone) nanofibers using formic acid/acetone solvent mixture. *Carbohydr. Polym.* **2010**, *80*, 413–419.

125. Ji, Y.L.; Liang, K.; Shen, X.Y.; Bowlin, G.L. Electrospinning and characterization of chitin nanofibril/polycaprolactone nanocomposite fiber mats. *Carbohydr. Polym.* **2013**, *101*, 68–74.

126. Bhattarai, N.; Edmondson, D.; Veiseh, O.; Matsen, F.A.; Zhang, M. Electrospun chitosan-based nanofibers and their cellular compatibility. *Biomaterials* **2005**, *26*, 6176–6184.

127. Lee, K.H.; Shin, S.J.; Kim, C.B.; Kim, J.K.; Cho, Y.W.; Chung, B.G.; Lee, S.H. Microfluidic synthesis of pure chitosan microfibers for bio-artificial liver chip. *Lab Chip* **2010**, *10*, 1328–1334.

128. Casettari, L.; Cespi, M.; Castagnino, E. Evaluation of dibutyrylchitin as new excipient for sustained drug release. *Drug Dev. Ind. Pharm.* **2012**, *38*, 979–984.

129. Castagnino, E.; Ottaviani, M.F.; Cangiotti, M.; Morelli, M.; Casettari, L.; Muzzarelli, R.A.A. Radical scavenging activity of 5-methylpyrrolidinone chitosan and dibutyryl chitin. *Carbohydr. Polym.* **2008**, *74*, 640–647.

130. Jeon, I.H.; Mok, J.Y.; Park, K.H.; Hwang, H.M.; Song, M.S.; Lee, D.; Lee, M.H.; Lee, W.Y.; Chai, K.Y.; Jang, S.I.; *et al.* Inhibitory effect of dibutyryl chitin ester on nitric oxide and prostaglandin E-2 production in LPS-stimulated RAW 264.7 cells. *Arch. Pharm. Res.* **2012**, *35*, 1287–1292.

131. Muzzarelli, C.; Francescangeli, O.; Tosi, G.; Muzzarelli, R.A.A. Susceptibility of dibutyryl chitin and regenerated chitin fibres to deacylation and depolymerization by lipases. *Carbohydr. Polym.* **2004**, *56*, 137–145.

132. Muzzarelli, R.A.A.; Guerrieri, M.; Goteri, G.; Muzzarelli, C.; Armeni, T.; Ghiselli, R.; Cornelissen, M. The biocompatibility of dibutyryl chitin, in the context of wound dressings. *Biomaterials* **2005**, *26*, 5844–5854.

133. Bogun, M.; Krucinska, I.; Kommisarczyk, A.; Mikolajczyk, T.; Blazewicz, M.; Stodolak-Zych, E.; Menaszek, E.; Scislowska-Czarnecka, A. Fibrous polymeric composites based on alginate fibres and fibres made of poly-epsilon-caprolactone and dibutyryl chitin for use in regenerative medicine. *Molecules* **2013**, *18*, 3118–3136.

134. Jang, S.I.; Mok, J.Y.; Jeon, I.H.; Park, K.H.; Thuy, T.T.N.; Park, J.S.; Hwang, H.M.; Song, M.S.; Lee, D.; Chai, K.Y.; *et al.* Effect of electrospun non-woven mats of dibutyryl chitin/poly(lactic acid) blends on wound healing in hairless mice. *Molecules* **2012**, *17*, 2992–3007.

135. Schoukens, G. Bioactive dressings to promote wound healing. *Adv. Text. Wound Care* **2009**, *85*, 114–152.

136. Azuma, K.; Ifuku, S.; Osaki, T.; Okamoto, Y.; Minami, S. Preparation and biomedical applications of chitin and chitosan nanofibers. *J. Biomed. Nanotechnol.* **2014**, *10*, 2891–2920.

137. Ding, F.Y.; Deng, H.B.; Du, Y.M.; Shi, X.W.; Wang, Q. Emerging chitin and chitosan nanofibrous materials for biomedical applications. *Nanoscale* **2014**, *6*, 9477–9493.

138. Jin, S.B.; Li, S.L.; Wang, C.X.; Liu, J.; Yang, X.L.; Wang, P.C.; Zhang, X.; Liang, X.J. Biosafe nanoscale pharmaceutical adjuvant materials. *J. Biomed. Nanotechnol.* **2014**, *10*, 2393–2419.

139. Singh, D.; Han, S.S.; Shin, E.J. Polysaccharides as nanocarriers for therapeutic applications. *J. Biomed. Nanotechnol.* **2014**, *10*, 2149–2172.

140. DiLena, F. Hemostatic polymers: The concept, state of the art and perspectives. *J. Mater. Chem. B* **2014**, *2*, 3567–3577.

141. Muzzarelli, R.A.A. Biochemical significance of exogenous chitins and chitosans in animals and patients. *Carbohydr. Polym.* **1993**, *20*, 7–16.

142. Kelechi, T.J.; Mueller, M.; Hankin, C.S.; Bronstone, A.; Samies, J.; Bonham, P.A. A randomized, investigator-blinded, controlled pilot study to evaluate the safety and efficacy of a poly-*N*-acetyl glucosamine-derived membrane material in patients with venous leg ulcers. *J. Am. Acad. Dermatol.* **2012**, *66*, E209–E215.

143. Fischer, T.H.; Hays, W.E.; Valeri, C.R. Poly-*N*-acetyl glucosamine fibers accelerate hemostasis in patients treated with antiplatelet drugs. *J. Trauma-Inj. Infect. Crit. Care* **2011**, *71*, S176–S182.

144. Lindner, H.B.; Zhang, A.G.; Eldridge, J.; Demcheva, M.; Tsichilis, P.; Seth, A.; Vournakis, J.; Muise-Helmericks, R.C. Anti-bacterial effects of poly-*N*-acetyl-glucosamine nanofibers in cutaneous wound healing: Requirement for Akt1. *PLoS One* **2011**, *6*, 556–569.

145. Blanco-Padilla, A.; Soto, K.M.; Iturriaga, M.H.; Mendoza, S. Food antimicrobials nanocarriers. *Sci. World J.* **2014**, *2014*, 837215; doi:10.1155/2014/837215.

146. Busilacchi, A.; Gigante, A.; Mattioli-Belmonte, M.; Muzzarelli, R.A.A. Chitosan stabilizes platelet growth factors and modulates stem cell differentiation toward tissue regeneration. *Carbohydr. Polym.* **2013**, *98*, 665–676.

147. Scherer, S.S.; Pietramaggiori, G.; Matthews, J.C.; Gennaoui, A.; Demcheva, M.; Fischer, T.H.; Valeri, C.R.; Orgill, D.P. Poly-*N*-acetyl glucosamine fibers induce angiogenesis in ADP inhibitor-treated diabetic mice. *J. Trauma-Inj. Infect. Crit. Care* **2011**, *71*, S183–S186.

148. Erba, P.; Adini, A.; Demcheva, M.; Valeri, C.R.; Orgill, D.P. Poly-*N*-acetyl glucosamine fibers are synergistic with vacuum-assisted closure in augmenting the healing response of diabetic mice. *J. Trauma-Inj. Infect. Crit. Care* **2011**, *71*, S187–S193.

149. Gorapalli, D.; Seth, A.; Vournakis, J.; Whyne, C.; Akens, M.; Zhang, A.G.; Demcheva, M.; Qamirani, E.; Yee, A. Evaluation of a novel poly *N*-acetyl glucosamine (pGlcNAc) hydrogel for treatment of the degenerating intervertebral disc. *Life Sci.* **2012**, *91*, 1328–1335.

150. Muise-Helmericks, R.C.; Demcheva, M.; Vournakis, J.N.; Seth, A. Poly-*N*-acetyl glucosamine fibers activate bone regeneration in a rabbit femur injury model. *J. Trauma-Inj. Infect. Crit. Care* **2011**, *71*, S194–S196.

151. Muzzarelli, R.A.A. Chitins and chitosans for the repair of wounded skin, nerve, cartilage and bone. *Carbohydr. Polym.* **2009**, *76*, 167–182.

152. Muzzarelli, R.A.A.; Mattioli-Belmonte, M.; Tietz, C.; Brunelli, M.A.; Fini, M.; Giardino, R.; Ilari, P.; Biagini, G. Stimulatory effect on bone formation exerted by a modified chitosan. *Biomaterials* **1994**, *15*, 1075–1081.

153. Mattioli-Belmonte, M.; Nicoli-Aldini, N.; DeBenedittis, A.; Sgarbi, G.; Amati, S.; Fini, M.; Biagini, G.; Muzzarelli, R.A.A. Morphological study of bone regeneration in the presence of 6-oxychitin. *Carbohydr. Polym.* **1999**, *40*, 23–27.

154. Malho, J.M.; Heinonen, H.; Kontro, I.; Mushi, N.E.; Serimaa, R.; Hentze, H.P.; Linder, M.B.; Szilvay, G.R. Formation of ceramophilic chitin and biohybrid materials enabled by a genetically engineered bifunctional protein. *Chem. Commun.* **2014**, *50*, 7348–7351.

155. Nakayama, S.; Suzuki, M.; Endo, H.; Iimura, K.; Kinoshita, S.; Watabe, S.; Kogure, T.; Nagasawa, H. Identification and characterization of a matrix protein in the periostracum of the pearl oyster, Pinctada fucata. *FEBS Open Biol.* **2013**, *3*, 421–427.

156. Azuma, K.; Osaki, T.; Wakuda, T.; Ifuku, S.; Saimoto, H.; Tsuka, T.; Imagawa, T.; Okamoto, Y.; Minami, S. Beneficial and preventive effect of chitin nanofibrils in a dextran sulfate sodium-induced acute ulcerative colitis model. *Carbohydr. Polym.* **2012**, *87*, 1399–1403.

157. Baker, D.E.; Kane, S. The short and long-term safety of 5-aminosalicylate products in the treatment of ulcerative colitis. *Rev. Gastroenterol. Disord.* **2004**, *4*, 86–91.

158. Kane, S.; Bjorkman, D.J. The efficacy of oral 5-ASA in the treatment of active ulcerative colitis: A systematic review. *Rev. Gastroenterol. Disord.* **2013**, *3*, 210–218.

159. Lowry, P.W.; Franklin, C.L.; Weaver, A.L.; Szumlanski, C.L.; Mays, D.C.; Loftus, E.V.; Tremaine, W.J.; Lipsky, J.J.; Weinshilboum, R.M.; Sandborn, W.J.; *et al.* Leucopenia resulting from a drug interaction between azathioprine or 6-mercaptopurine and mesalamine, sulphasalazine or balsalazide. *Gut* **2001**, *49*, 656–664.

160. Azuma, K.; Osaki, T.; Ifuku, S.; Saimoto, H.; Tsuka, T.; Imagawa, T.; Okamoto, Y.; Minami, S. α-Chitin nanofibrils improve inflammatory and fibrosis responses in inflammatory bowel disease mice model. *Carbohydr. Polym.* **2012**, *90*, 197–200.

161. Muzzarelli, R.A.A.; Morganti, P.; Morganti, G.; Palombo, P.; Palombo, M.; Biagini, G.; Belmonte, M.M.; Giantomassi, F.; Orlandi, F.; Muzzarelli, C.; *et al.* Chitin nanofibrils/chitosan glycolate composites as wound medicaments. *Carbohydr. Polym.* **2007**, *70*, 274–284.

162. Yudin, V.E.; Dobrovolskaya, I.P.; Neelov, I.M.; Dresvyanina, E.N.; Popryadukhin, P.V.; Ivan'kova, E.M.; Elokhovskii, V.Y.; Kasatkin, I.A.; Okrugin, B.M.; Morganti, P.; *et al.* Wet spinning of fibers made of chitosan and chitin nanofibrils. *Carbohydr. Polym.* **2014**, *108*, 176–182.

163. Ma, B.M.; Qin, A.W.; Li, X.; Zhao, X.Z.; He, C.J. Bioinspired design and chitin whisker reinforced chitosan membrane. *Mater. Lett.* **2014**, *120*, 82–85.

164. Ma, B.M.; Qin, A.W.; Li, X.; Zhao, X.Z.; He, C.J. Structure and properties of chitin whisker reinforced chitosan membranes. *Int. J. Biol. Macromol.* **2014**, *64*, 341–346.

165. Colosi, C.; Costantini, M.; Latini, R.; Ciccarelli, S.; Stampella, A.; Barbetta, A.; Massimi, M.; Devirgiliis, L.C.; Dentini, M. Rapid prototyping of chitosan-coated alginate scaffolds through the use of a 3D fiber deposition technique. *J. Mater. Chem.* **2014**, *2*, 6779–6791.

166. Rubentheren, V.; Ward, T.A.; Chee, C.Y.; Tang, C.K. Processing and analysis of chitosan nanocomposites reinforced with chitin whiskers and tannic acid as a crosslinker. *Carbohydr. Polym.* **2015**, *115*, 379–387.

167. Naseri, N.; Algan, C.; Jacobs, V.; John, M.; Oksman, K.; Mathew, A.P. Electrospun chitosan-based nanocomposite mats reinforced with chitin nanocrystals for wound dressing. *Carbohydr. Polym.* **2014**, *109*, 7–15.

168. Tchemtchoua, V.T.; Atanasova, G.; Aqil, A.; Filee, P.; Garbacki, N.; Vanhooteghem, O.; Deroanne, C.; Noel, A.; Jerome, C.; Nusgens, B.; *et al.* Development of a chitosan nanofibrillar scaffold for skin repair and regeneration. *Biomacromolecules* **2011**, *12*, 3194–3204.

169. Kim, M.S.; Park, S.J.; Gu, B.K.; Kim, C.H. Polycaprolactone-chitin nanofibrous mats as potential scaffolds for tissue engineering. *J. Nanomater.* **2012**, *2012*, doi:10.1155/2012/635212.

170. Ito, I.; Osaki, T.; Ifuku, S.; Saimoto, H.; Takamori, Y.; Kurozumi, S.; Imagawa, T.; Azuma, K.; Tsuka, T.; Okamoto, Y.; *et al.* Evaluation of the effects of chitin nanofibrils on skin function using skin models. *Carbohydr. Polym.* **2014**, *101*, 464–470.

171. Muzzarelli, R.A.A. Genipin-chitosan hydrogels as biomedical and pharmaceutical aids. *Carbohydr. Polym.* **2009**, *77*, 1–9.

172. Charernsriwilaiwat, N.; Rojanarata, T.; Ngawhirunpat, T.; Sukma, M.; Opanasopit, P. Electrospun chitosan-based nanofiber mats loaded with *Garcinia mangostana* extracts. *Int. J. Pharm.* **2013**, *452*, 333–343.

173. Arslan, A.; Simsek, M.; Aldemir, S.D.; Kazaroglu, N.M.; Gumusderelioglu, M. Honey-based PET or PET/chitosan fibrous wound dressings: Effect of honey on electrospinning process. *J. Biomater. Sci.-Polym. Ed.* **2014**, *25*, 999–1012.

174. Xu, J.; Cai, N.; Xu, W.X.; Xue, Y.A.; Wang, Z.L.; Dai, Q.; Yu, F.Q. Mechanical enhancement of nanofibrous scaffolds through polyelectrolyte complexation. *Nanotechnology* **2013**, *24*, 025701; doi:10.1088/0957-4484/24/2/025701.

175. Jridi, M.; Hajji, S.; Ben Ayed, H.; Lassoued, I.; Mbarek, A.; Kammoun, M.; Souissi, N.; Nasri, M. Physical, structural, antioxidant and antimicrobial properties of gelatin-chitosan composite edible films. *Int. J. Biol. Macromol.* **2014**, *67*, 373–379.

176. Tsai, R.Y.; Hung, S.C.; Lai, J.Y.; Wang, D.M.; Hsieh, H.J. Electrospun chitosan-gelatin-polyvinyl alcohol hybrid nanofibrous mats: Production and characterization. *J. Taiwan Inst. Chem. Eng.* **2014**, *45*, 1975–1981.

177. Chen, Z.G.; Wang, P.W.; Wei, B.; Mo, X.M.; Cui, F.Z. Electrospun collagen-chitosan nanofiber: A biomimetic extracellular matrix for endothelial cell and smooth muscle cell. *Acta Biomater.* **2010**, *6*, 372–382.

178. Wang, P.W.; Liu, J.L.; Zhang, T. *In vitro* biocompatibility of electrospun chitosan/collagen scaffold. *J. Nanomater.* **2013**, doi:10.1155/2013/958172.

179. Sarkar, S.D.; Farrugia, B.L.; Dargaville, T.R.; Dhara, S. Chitosan-collagen scaffolds with nano/microfibrous architecture for skin tissue engineering. *J. Biomed. Mater. Res. A* **2013**, *101*, 3482–3492.

180. Dhurai, B.; Nachimuthu, S.; Maheswaran; Kumar, G.; Babu, R. Electrospinning of chitosan nanofibres loaded with curcumin for wound healing. *J. Polym. Mater.* **2013**, *30*, 471–483.

181. Du, F.Y.; Wang, H.; Zhao, W.; Li, D.; Kong, D.L.; Yang, J.; Zhang, Y.Y. Gradient nanofibrous chitosan/poly epsilon-caprolactone scaffolds as extracellular microenvironments for vascular tissue engineering. *Biomaterials* **2012**, *33*, 762–770.

182. Huang, R.; Deng, H.B.; Cai, T.J.; Zhan, Y.F.; Wang, X.K.; Chen, X.X.; Ji, A.L.; Li, X.Y. Layer-by-layer immobilized catalase on electrospun nanofibrous mats protects against oxidative stress induced by hydrogen peroxide. *J. Biomed. Nanotechnol.* **2014**, *10*, 1346–1358.

183. Cai, Z.X.; Mo, X.M.; Zhang, K.H.; Fan, L.P.; Yin, A.L.; He, C.L.; Wang, H.S. Fabrication of chitosan + silk fibroin composite nanofibers for wound-dressing applications. *Int. J. Mol. Sci.* **2010**, *11*, 3529–3539.

184. Ang-atikarnkul, P.; Watthanaphanit, A.; Rujiravanit, R. Fabrication of cellulose nanofiber/chitin whisker/silk sericin bionanocomposite sponges and characterizations of their physical and biological properties. *Compos. Sci. Technol.* **2014**, *96*, 88–96.

185. Zhou, Y.S.; Yang, H.J.; Liu, X.; Mao, J.; Gu, S.J.; Xu, W.L. Electrospinning of carboxyethyl chitosan/poly(vinyl alcohol)/silk fibroin nanoparticles for wound dressings. *Int. J. Biol. Macromol.* **2013**, *53*, 88–92.

186. Dunne, L.W.; Iyyanki, T.; Hubenak, J.; Mathur, A.B. Characterization of dielectrophoresis-aligned nanofibrous silk fibroin-chitosan scaffold and its interactions with endothelial cells for tissue engineering applications. *Acta Biomater.* **2014**, *10*, 3630–3640.

187. Oh, B.; Lee, C.H. Nanofiber for cardiovascular tissue engineering. *Expert Opin. Drug Deliv.* **2013**, *10*, 1565–1582.

188. Nawalakhe, R.; Shi, Q.; Vitchuli, N.; Noar, J.; Caldwell, J.M.; Breidt, F.; Bourham, M.A.; Zhang, X.; McCord, M.G. Novel atmospheric plasma enhanced chitosan nanofiber/gauze composite wound dressings. *J. Appl. Polym. Sci.* **2013**, *129*, 916–923.

189. Guan, Y.; Bian, J.; Peng, F.; Zhang, X.M.; Sun, R.C. High strength of hemicelluloses based hydrogels by freeze/thaw technique. *Carbohydr. Polym.* **2014**, *101*, 272–280.

190. Guan, Y.; Zhang, B.; Bian, J.; Peng, F.; Sun, R.C. Nanoreinforced hemicellulose-based hydrogels prepared by freeze-thaw treatment. *Cellulose* **2014**, *21*, 1709–1721.

191. Hatanaka, D.; Yamamoto, K.; Kadokawa, J. Preparation of chitin nanofiber-reinforced carboxymethyl cellulose films. *Int. J. Biol. Macromol.* **2014**, *69*, 35–38.

192. Huang, Y.; Zhang, L.N.; Yang, J.; Zhang, X.Z.; Xu, M. Structure and properties of cellulose films reinforced by chitin whiskers. *Macromol. Mater. Eng.* **2013**, *298*, 303–310.

193. Toskas, G.; Heinemann, S.; Heinemann, C.; Cherif, C.; Hund, R.D.; Roussis, V.; Hanke, T. Ulvan and ulvan/chitosan polyelectrolyte nanofibrous membranes as a potential substrate material for the cultivation of osteoblasts. *Carbohydr. Polym.* **2012**, *89*, 997–1002.

194. Tan, M.L.; Shao, P.; Friedhuber, A.M.; van Moorst, M.; Elahy, M; Indumathy, S.; Dunstan, D.E.; Wei, Y.Z.; Dass, C.R. The potential role of free chitosan in bone trauma and bone cancer management. *Biomaterials* **2014**, *35*, 7828–7838.

195. Norowski, P.A.; Mishra, S.; Adatrow, P.C.; Haggard, W.O.; Bumgardner, J.D. Suture pullout strength and *in vitro* fibroblast and RAW 264.7 monocyte biocompatibility of genipin crosslinked nanofibrous chitosan mats for guided tissue regeneration. *J. Biomed. Mater. Res. A* **2012**, *100*, 2890–2896.

196. Gentile, P.; Mattioli-Belmonte, M.; Chiono, V.; Ferretti, C.; Baino, F.; Tondo-Turo, C.; Vitale-Brovarone, C.; Pashkuleva, I.; Reis, R.L.; Ciardelli, G.; *et al.* Bioreactive glass/polymer composite scaffold mimiking bone tissue. *J. Biomed. Mater. Res. A* **2012**, *100*, 2654–2667.

197. Frohbergh, M.E.; Katsman, A.; Botta, G.R.; Lazarovici, P.; Schauer, C.L.; Wegst, U.G.K.; Lelkes, P.I. Electrospun hydroxyapatite-containing chitosan nanofibers crosslinked with genipin for bone tissue engineering. *Biomaterials* **2012**, *33*, 9167–9178.

198. Mahapoka, E.; Arirachakaran, P.; Watthanaphanit, A.; Rujiravanit, R.; Poolthong, S. Chitosan whiskers from shrimp shells incorporated into dimethacrylate-based dental resin sealant. *Dent. Mater. J.* **2012**, *31*, 273–279.

199. Li, X.M.; Liu, W.; Sun, L.W.; Aifantis, K.E.; Yu, B.; Fan, Y.B.; Feng, Q.L.; Cui, F.Z.; Watari, F. Resin composites reinforced by nanoscaled fibers or tubes for dental regeneration. *BioMed Res. Int.* **2014**, *2014*, 542958; doi:10.1155/2014/542958.

200. Dutta, A.K.; Egusa, M.; Kaminaka, H.; Izawa, H.; Morimoto, M.; Saimoto, H.; Ifuku, S. Facile preparation of surface *N*-halamine chitin nanofiber to endow antibacterial and antifungal activities. *Carbohydr. Polym.* **2014**, *115*, 342–347.

201. Shin, H.K.; Park, M.; Chung, Y.S.; Kim, H.Y.; Jin, F.L.; Park, S.J. Antimicrobial characteristics of *N*-halaminated chitosan salt/cotton knit composites. *J. Ind. Eng. Chem.* **2014**, *20*, 1476–1480.

202. Kangwansupamonkon, W.; Tiewtrakoonwat, W.; Supaphol, P.; Kiatkamjornwong, S. Surface modification of electrospun chitosan nanofibrous mats for antibacterial activity. *J. Appl. Polym. Sci.* **2014**, *131*, doi:10.1002/app.40981.

203. Mi, X.; Vijayaragavan, K.S.; Heldt, C.L. Virus adsorption of water-stable quaternized chitosan nanofibers. *Carbohydr. Res.* **2014**, *387*, 24–29.

204. Xu, F.; Weng, B.; Gilkerson, R.; Materon, L.A.; Lozano, K. Development of tannic acid/chitosan/pullulan composite nanofibers from aqueous solution for potential applications as wound dressing. *Carbohydr. Polym.* **2015**, *115*, 16–24.

205. Zhao, Y.; Park, R.D.; Muzzarelli, R.A.A. Chitin deacetylases: Properties and applications. *Mar. Drugs* **2010**, *8*, 24–46.

206. Zhang, H.C.; Fang, J.Y.; Deng, Y.; Zhao, Y.Y. Optimized production of *Serratia marcescens* B742 mutants for preparing chitin from shrimp shells powders. *Int. J. Biol. Macromol.* **2014**, *69*, 319–328.

207. Zhang, H.N.; Tachikawa, H.; Gao, X.D.; Nakanishi, H. Applied usage of yeast spores as chitosan beads. *Appl. Environ. Microbiol.* **2014**, *80*, 5098–5105.

208. Berger, L.R.R.; Stamford, T.C.M.; Stamford-Arnaud, T.M.; de Alcantara, S.R.C.; da Silva, A.C.; da Silva, A.M.; do Nascimento, A.E.; de Campos-Takaki, G.M. Green conversion of agroindustrial wastes into chitin and chitosan by *Rhizopus arrhizus* and *Cunninghamella elegans* strains. *Int. J. Mol. Sci.* **2014**, *15*, 9082–9102.

209. Chantarasataporn, P.; Yoksan, R.; Visessanguan, W.; Chirachanchai, S. Water-based nano-sized chitin and chitosan as seafood additive through a case study of Pacific white shrimp (*Litopenaeus vannamei*). *Food Hydrocoll.* **2013**, *32*, 341–348.

210. Xu, Y.M.; Bajaj, M.; Schneider, R.; Grage, S.L.; Ulrich, A.S.; Winter, J.; Gallert, C. Transformation of the matrix structure of shrimp shells during bacterial deproteination and demineralization. *Microb. Cell Factories* **2013**, *12*, doi:10.1186/1475-2859-12-90.

# Delivery of Berberine Using Chitosan/Fucoidan-Taurine Conjugate Nanoparticles for Treatment of Defective Intestinal Epithelial Tight Junction Barrier

Shao-Jung Wu, Trong-Ming Don, Cheng-Wei Lin and Fwu-Long Mi

**Abstract:** Bacterial-derived lipopolysaccharides (LPS) can cause defective intestinal barrier function and play an important role in the development of inflammatory bowel disease. In this study, a nanocarrier based on chitosan and fucoidan was developed for oral delivery of berberine (Ber). A sulfonated fucoidan, fucoidan-taurine (FD-Tau) conjugate, was synthesized and characterized by Fourier transform infrared (FTIR) spectroscopy. The FD-Tau conjugate was self-assembled with berberine and chitosan (CS) to form Ber-loaded CS/FD-Tau complex nanoparticles with high drug loading efficiency. Berberine release from the nanoparticles had fast release in simulated intestinal fluid (SIF, pH 7.4), while the release was slow in simulated gastric fluid (SGF, pH 2.0). The effect of the berberine-loaded nanoparticles in protecting intestinal tight-junction barrier function against nitric oxide and inflammatory cytokines released from LPS-stimulated macrophage was evaluated by determining the transepithelial electrical resistance (TEER) and paracellular permeability of a model macromolecule fluorescein isothiocyanate-dextran (FITC-dextran) in a Caco-2 cells/RAW264.7 cells co-culture system. Inhibition of redistribution of tight junction ZO-1 protein by the nanoparticles was visualized using confocal laser scanning microscopy (CLSM). The results suggest that the nanoparticles may be useful for local delivery of berberine to ameliorate LPS-induced intestinal epithelia tight junction disruption, and that the released berberine can restore barrier function in inflammatory and injured intestinal epithelial.

Reprinted from *Mar. Drugs*. Cite as: Wu, S.-J.; Don, T.-M.; Lin, C.-W.; Mi, F.-L. Delivery of Berberine Using Chitosan/Fucoidan-Taurine Conjugate Nanoparticles for Treatment of Defective Intestinal Epithelial Tight Junction Barrier. *Mar. Drugs* **2014**, *12*, 5677-5697.

## 1. Introduction

Intestinal epithelial tight junctions provide the barrier function in preventing the invasion of bacterial endotoxin and subsequent contact with the immune system. Bacterial-derived lipopolysaccharides (LPS) can cause defective intestinal barrier function which increases the risk of development of inflammatory bowel disease [1]. Berberine (Ber) is an isoquinoline alkaloid in the *Berberis* species which has many antimicrobial activities against fungal, bacterial and viral infections [2]. Berberine also exhibited potential anti-inflammatory activity both *in vitro* and *in vivo* [3]. Several studies reported that berberine promoted tightness of the intestinal epithelial tight junction (TJ) barrier and ameliorated TJ barrier impairment by suppressing the production of proinflammatory cytokines [4–8]. However, its application in oral administration is limited mainly due to the low local concentration, short residence time, and poor absorption in the intestinal tract [9]. To overcome these problems, the development of a drug delivery system with both mucoadhesive and pH-sensitive properties is required to increase the local berberin concentration by reducing the dissolution rate of berberin in gastric juice and also by prolonging the residence time of berberin in intestinal mucus. Nanocarriers have been used to localize berberine to the gastric epithelium for the treatment of *H. pylori* infection [10,11].

Chitosan (CS), a linear polysaccharide obtained by partial deacetylation of chitin, has been widely used in the biomedical field and drug delivery applications [12–14]. The naturally occurring polymer has many favorable characteristics, including mucoadhesive and pH-sensitive properties [15,16]. Chitosan-based nanoparticles have gained increasing attention for their efficient oral delivery of proteins and drugs [17,18]. Fucoidan (FD) is extracted from marine brown seaweed that has a backbone composed of sulfated esters of fucose and glucuronic acid or other monosaccharides [19]. Fucoidan can exert a wide variety of pharmacological activities, such as anti-inflammatory, anti-angiogenic, antitumor, and antithrombotic activities [20,21]. Suppression of inflammatory cytokine production in the Caco-2/RAW264.7 co-culture model by fucoidan was reported [22]. Moreover, recent studies have found that fucoidan enhanced epithelial barrier function via up-regulating the expression of the tight junction protein Claudin-1 [23].

Chitosan-based nanoparticles have been investigated in recent years for developing oral drug delivery carriers. However, the studies focused on preparing nanoparticles composed of a chitosan shell, thus the nanoparticles had the ablity to open the intestinal epithelial tight junctions. The nanoparticles were usually prepared by adding polyanions into excess amounts of chitosan solution to obtain nanoparticles covered with positively charged chitosan. In recent years, increased attention has been focused on the development of chitosan/fucoidan (CS/FD) complex nanoparticles for drug delivery [24–30]. Our previous study developed a chitosan/fucoidan (FD) nanoparticle with chitosan dominant at an outer layer. The highly positively charged nanoparticles could open the tight junction for the transport of anti-angiogenic sulfated polysaccharides across Caco-2 cell monolayers. However, the aim of this work was to develop a berberine-loaded chitosan/FD-Tau nanoparticles for treatment of the defective intestinal TJ barrier induced by bacterial endotoxin. Because berberine could attenuate pro-inflammatory cytokine-induced tight junction disruption, it should be targeted to the intestinal epithelial Caco-2 cells, but not the sublayer macrophage cells. Thus, the nanoparticles were not designed to open the tight junction for transepithelial transport of berberine.

To achieve the goal, FD was first conjugated with taurine (Tau) to obtain a fucoidan-taurine (FD-Tau) conjugate. Taurine can inhibit lipopolysaccharide-induced release of inflammatory factors to attenuate dysfunction in epithelial cells [31]. Moreover, the sulfonate group of taurine is a very strong acid which can increase the negative-charge density on fucoidan. Subsequently, a reverse of the CS/FD-Tau mixing process was developed to prepare negatively charged nanoparticles by adding CS solution into an excess amount of FD-Tau solution. This method was able to produce a FD-Tau-shelled nanoparticle because the excessive FD-Tau could be precipitated on the surface of the nanoparticles through the spontaneous formation of polyelectrolyte complex with chitosan. The nanoparticles shelled with FD-Tau are of benefit to the intestinal TJ barrier because fucoidan and taurine have been reported to attenuate dysfunction in epithelial cells. Furthermore, fucoidan can help the nanoparticles to target intestinal epithelial cells due to the fucose receptor on the epithelial cells. The prepared Ber-loaded CS/FD-Tau nanoparticles were then used for the treatment of defective intestinal epithelial TJ barrier caused by bacterial endotoxin. These nanoparticles were suitable to deliver berberine to epithelial Caco-2 cells without inducing the impairment of the intestinal barrier function. Berberine release from the nanoparticles could attenuate the intestinal epithelial impairment resulting from the inflammatory cytokine which was produced by endotoxin-activated macrophage. However, berberine could be delivered to the Caco-2 cell, thus the pro-inflammatory cytokines-mediated NF-κB signaling pathway in the cell could be inhibited and the epithelial TJ junction could be protected.

Moreover, the pH-sensitivity property and berberine release behavior of the Ber-loaded CS/FD-Tau nanoparticles were investigated in simulated gastric fluid (SGF) and intestinal fluid (SIF). The effect of the nanoparticles on LPS-induced TJ barrier dysfunction was investigated by measuring transepithelial electrical resistance (TEER) and paracellular flux of fluorescein isothiocyanate-dextran (FITC-dextran) in an intestinal epithelial Caco-2 cells/macrophage RAW264.7 cells co-culture system. Redistribution of ZO-1 TJ proteins was observed using confocal laser scanning microscopy (CLSM).

## 2. Results and Discussion

### 2.1. Characterization of FD-Tau Conjugate

A schematic diagram of the preparation of Ber-loaded CS/FD-Tau nanoparticles and construction of the Caco-2/RAW 264.7 cells co-culture system for estimating the protective effect of nanoparticles against LPS-caused barrier dysfunction is shown in Figure 1. Figure 2A shows the schematic diagram of the fucoidan-taurine (FD-Tau) conjugation reaction. FD-Tau conjugate was synthesized through activation of carboxyl groups by EDC in MES buffer followed by the formation of amide bonds between the activated carboxyl groups of fucoidan and the amino groups of taurine. As shown in Figure 2B, the FTIR spectrum of fucoidan (FD) shows the absorption band due to asymmetric and symmetric stretching vibration bands of O=S=O (1246 cm$^{-1}$) and C–O–S stretch (833 cm$^{-1}$), indicating the presence of a sulfate ester linkage. The carbonyl stretch C=O of a carboxylic acid appears at 1632 cm$^{-1}$ and 1733 cm$^{-1}$, indicating the presence of glucuronic acid in fucoidan. The FD-Tau conjugate demonstrated the asymmetric and symmetric stretching vibration bands of O=S=O at around 1203 cm$^{-1}$ due to the sulfonate groups on taurine, while a lower intensity shoulder near 1557 cm$^{-1}$ is due to the formation of amide bonds after conjugation. These results indicated that taurine has been successfully coupled to fucoidan. TNBS assay of the fucoidan/taurine reaction mixture showed 71.3% of unreacted primary amine of taurine. Accordingly, the taurine substitution ratio of the FD-Tau conjugate was estimated to be 223 μg taurine/mg FD-Tau conjugate.

### 2.2. Characterization of Berberine-Loaded Nanoparticles

Fucoidan is a polysaccharide extracted from marine brown seaweed which contains negatively charged sulfate and carboxyl groups. The electrostatic interactions between fucoidan and oppositely charged chitosan lead to the formation of stable colloidal nanoparticles. However, the nanoparticles were found to disintegrate in simulated gastric fluid (SGF, pH 2.0) rapidly because fucoidan contains carboxyl groups which are less acidic (pKa near 3.0). In this study, a FD-Tau conjugate was pre-synthesized to reduce the carboxyl groups and increase the more acidic sulfonate groups (pKa 1.5). Berberine is an isoquinoline alkaloid possessing a strong positive charge on its quaternary ammonium group. The FD-Tau conjugate was able to assemble with berberine to form stable Ber/FD-Tau nanoparticles. The particle size of Ber/FD-Tau nanoparticles could be varied over a wide range by adjusting the weight ratio of berberine to FD-Tau. As shown in Table 1, the average particle size increased from $111.7 \pm 2.7$ to $156.3 \pm 5.5$ nm by decreasing the Ber/FD-Tau weight ratio from 2/1 to 2/4. The zeta potentials were negative and also decreased with the decrease of the Ber/FD-Tau weight ratio, demonstrating that FD-Tau was increasingly exposed on the surfaces of the nanoparticles. The large polydispersity (PDI) of the Ber/FD-Tau nanoparticle systems indicated a wide range of particle size distribution. Moreover, berberine-loading efficiency was low (Table 1), suggesting that berberine was poorly retained in the nanoparticles because berberine and FD-Tau could not produce well-organized nanoparticles.

**Figure 1.** Schematic diagram of the preparation of berberine (Ber)-loaded chitosan (CS)/fucoidan-taurine (FD-Tau) nanoparticles and construction of the human colon carcinoma cell line (Caco-2 cells)/murine macrophage cell line (RAW 264.7 cells) co-culture system for estimating the protective effect of nanoparticles against lipopolysaccharides (LPS)-caused barrier dysfunction.

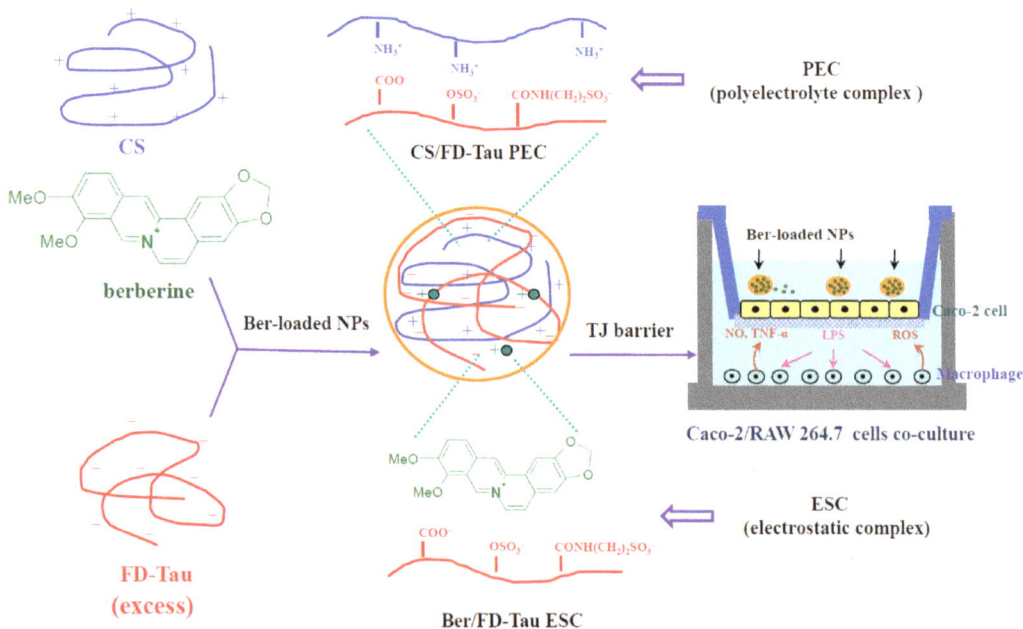

**Figure 2. (A)** Schematic diagram of the fucoidan-taurine (FD-Tau) conjugation reaction; **(B)** Fourier transform infrared (FTIR) spectra of fucoidan, taurine, and fucoidan-taurine (FD-Tau) conjugate.

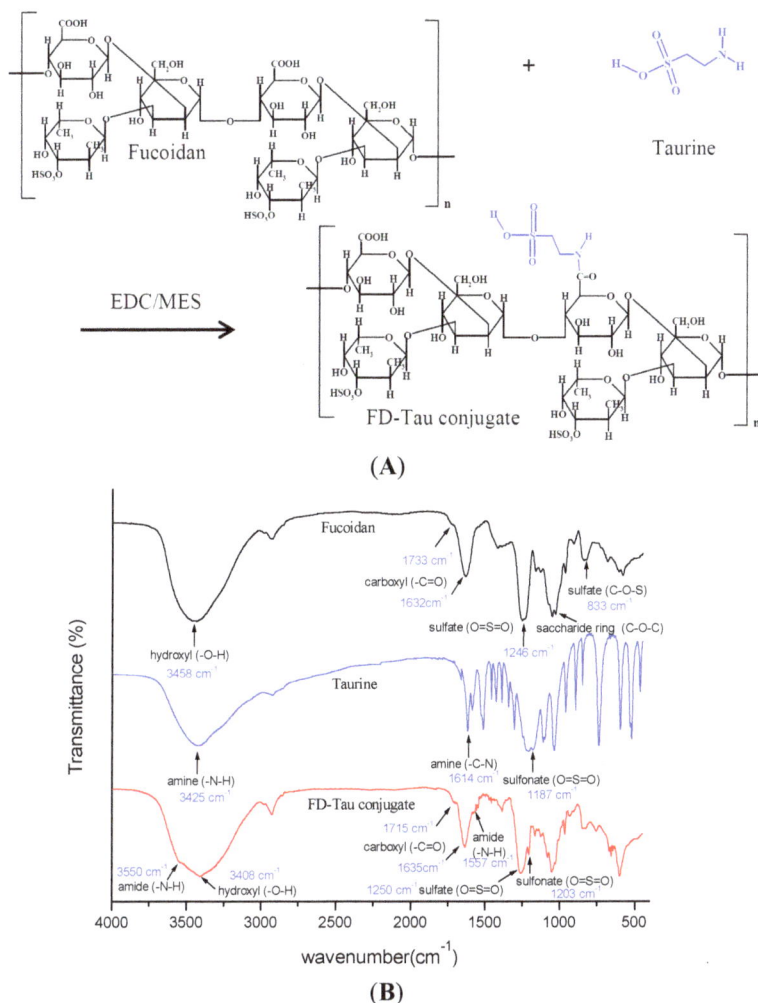

**(A)**

**(B)**

**Table 1.** Average particle size, particle size distribution (polydispersity, PDI), zeta potential, berberine-loading content of Ber/FD-Tau nanoparticles prepared from berberine (Ber) (1.0 mg/mL, 1 mL) and fucoidan-taurine (FD-Tau) (0.5, 1.0, 1.5, 2.0 mg/mL, 1 mL) aqueous solution.

| FD-Tau (mg/mL) | Ber/FD-Tau Weight Ratio | Average Size (nm) | Zeta Potential (mV) | Drug Loading (%) | PDI |
|---|---|---|---|---|---|
| 0.5 | 2/1 | 111.7 ± 2.7 | −14.7 ± 1.4 | 10.3 ± 0.4 | 0.41 ± 0.01 |
| 1.0 | 2/2 | 120.9 ± 4.1 | −20.4 ± 0.7 | 13.1 ± 0.5 | 0.39 ± 0.02 |
| 1.5 | 2/3 | 147.4 ± 4.8 | −27.1 ± 0.9 | 9.7 ± 0.8 | 0.47 ± 0.01 |
| 2.0 | 2/4 | 156.3 ± 5.5 | −31.4 ± 1.8 | 12.8 ± 0.3 | 0.46 ± 0.02 |

To enhance the berberine-loading efficiency of the nanoparticle system, chitosan was employed to form a polyelectrolyte complex with FD-Tau to obtain Ber-loaded CS/FD-Tau nanoparticles. We found that stable nanoparticles could only be prepared if both concentrations of berberine and FD-Tau were no more than 1.0 mg/mL. Therefore, the concentrations of berberine and FD-Tau were kept at 1.0 mg/mL in order to form a polyelectrolyte complex with chitosan. As shown in Table 2, the zeta potentials of the CS/FD-Tau nanoparticles were almost negative, suggesting that the reversed mixing process used in this study was able to produce FD-Tau-shelled nanoparticles because the excessive FD-Tau could be precipitated on the surface of the nanoparticles. The average particle size of Ber-loaded CS/FD-Tau nanoparticles increased noticeably when the chitosan amount was increased. In the presence of positively charged berberine, low-positively charged nanoparticles could be produced, depending on the chitosan/berberine/FD-Tau weight ratios (Table 2). Figure 3A shows the TEM micrographs of Ber/FD-Tau and Ber-loaded CS/FD-Tau nanoparticles. The Ber/FD-Tau nanoparticles are irregular in shape while the Ber-loaded CS/FD-Tau nanoparticles are spherical. Figure 3B shows the FTIR spectra of berberine, FD-Tau, chitosan and the Ber-loaded nanoparticles. The charcteristic bands of berberine at 1602 cm$^{-1}$ (quaternary iminium ion, -C=N-) and 1505 cm$^{-1}$ (C=C stretching vibration in the aromatic ring) are observed from the spectrum of the Ber-loaded nanoparticles. The characteristic peak of chitosan at 1589 cm$^{-1}$ (the amino group, -NH$_2$) and the absorption peak of fucoidan at 1632 cm$^{-1}$ (carboxylic ion, -COO$^-$) respectively shift to 1602 and 1630 cm$^{-1}$, accompanied by alteration in intensity of band signals. These results suggest that berberine was successfully incorporated in the nanoparticles through the formation of polyelectrolyte complex between fucoidan and chitosan.

**Table 2.** Average particle size, particle size distribution (polydispersity, PDI), zeta potential, berberine-loading content of Ber-loaded CS/FD-Tau nanoparticles (NPs) prepared from the mixed solutions (1 mL) of CS/Ber with different weight ratios and FD-Tau aqueous solution (1.0 mg/mL, 2 mL).

| CS/Ber (mg/mg) | CS/Ber/FD-Tau Weight Ratio | Average Particle Size (nm) | PDI | Zeta Potential (mV) | Ber-Loading Content (%) |
|---|---|---|---|---|---|
| | | CS/FD-Tau NPs | | | |
| 0.5/0.0 | 1/0/4 | 225.6 ± 3.4 | 0.32 ± 0.02 | −38.2 ± 1.4 | – |
| 1.0/0.0 | 2/0/4 | 208.1 ± 5.5 | 0.35 ± 0.02 | −35.7 ± 2.1 | – |
| 1.5/0.0 | 3/0/4 | 204.5 ± 4.2 | 0.29 ± 0.02 | −11.7 ± 1.7 | – |
| 2.0/0.0 | 4/0/4 | 179.7 ± 3.9 | 0.33 ± 0.02 | +17.1 ± 1.6 | – |
| | | Ber-loaded CS/FD-Tau NPs | | | |
| 0.5/1.0 | 1/2/4 | 145.9 ± 2.7 | 0.27 ± 0.01 | −13.1 ± 0.8 | 32.3 ± 0.4 |
| 1.0/1.0 | 2/2/4 | 187.4 ± 6.2 | 0.21 ± 0.01 | +7.6 ± 0.5 | 50.1 ± 2.5 |
| 1.5/1.0 | 3/2/4 | 359.4 ± 4.7 | 0.39 ± 0.02 | +15.6 ± 0.6 | 62.7 ± 3.4 |
| 2.0/1.0 | 4/2/4 * | – | – | – | – |

*: Aggregation and precipitation of nanoparticles were found at CS/Ber/FD-Tau weight ratio of 4/2/4.

**Figure 3. (A)** Transmission electron microscopy (TEM) micrographs of Ber/FD-Tau (**a**) and Ber-loaded CS/FD-Tau (**b**) nanoparticles; (**B**) FTIR spectra of FD-Tau conjugate, chitosan, berberine, and Ber-loaded nanoparticles.

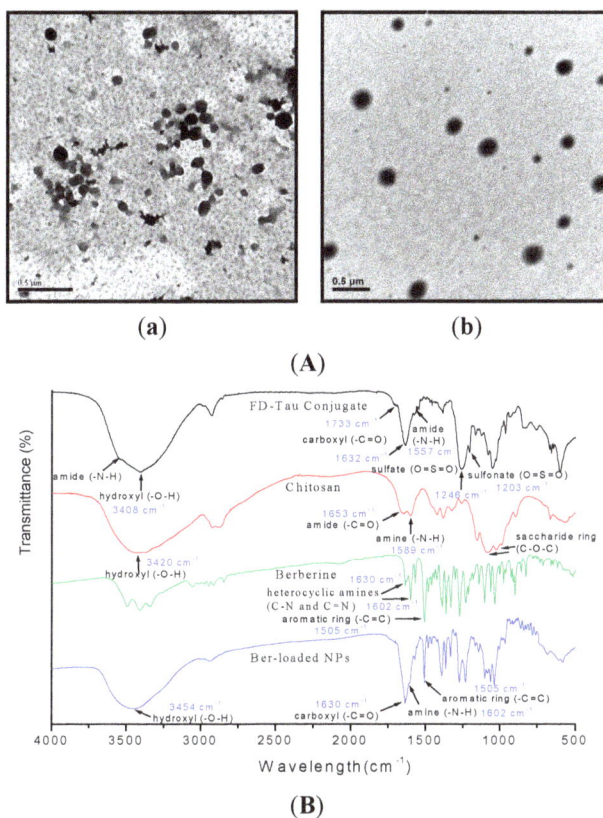

*2.3. Berberine Release*

The loading efficiency and PDI of the Ber-loaded CS/FD-Tau nanoparticles prepared at a CS/Ber/FD-Tau weight ratio = 2/2/4 were 50.1% ± 2.5% and 0.21 ± 0.01, respectively (Table 2). Therefore, the nanoaprticles with optimal drug loading and size distribution were chosen for drug release and cell culture. The sustained release profile of berberine from nanoparticles was investigated in the dissolution mediums of SGF (pH 2.0) and SIF (pH 7.4). Factors affecting the berberine release rate were the hydrophilicity and stability of various nanoparticle systems and the pH of the release medium. Fucoidan is a polysaccharide composed of sulfated esters of fucose and glucuronic acid. The pKa values of sulfate esters in sulfated fucose are around 1.5 while the pKa value of the carboxylate group in glucuronic acid is about 3.0. At pH 2.0, strong acid protonated the carboxylate ions (-COO$^-$) in fucoidan, the polyelectrolyte complex of chitosan and fucoidan thus could be rapidly broken down [28]. After chemical modification, the carboxylate group decreased in amount but the sulfonate group increased due to the conjugation of taurine with the glucuronic acid residue of fucoidan. Accordingly, more negative charge was retained on the FD-Tau conjugate in

SGF than on the original fucoidan. The burst release was not obvious because the positively charged berberine could form a strong electrostatic interaction with FD-Tau during the preparation of the nanoparticles. As shown in Figure 4, after 12 h of dissolution test at pH 2.0, there was only 31.2% berberine released from the Ber-loaded nanoparticles. Under these conditions, the protonaed chitosan (pKa value of the primary amine is around 6.5) and negatively charged FD-Tau conjugate can form stable and well-organized nanoparticles, thus providing a slow and continuous release of berberine. On the other hand, at neutral pH (pH 7.4), chitosan was deprotonated and berberine was rapidly released from the disintegrating nanoparticles [10]. It is worth noting that, at pH 7.4, the electrostatic attractions between chitosan and FD-Tau conjugate became weaker than those at pH 2.0 because chitosan was deprotonated. The nanoparticles released 85.7% of loaded berberine within 12 h (Figure 4). The result suggests that the CS/Tau-FD nanoparticles can release berberine in response to the change in pH value of the simulated gastrointestinal fluids. The intestinal pH (near neutrality) facilitates the release of berberine, indicating that the nanoparticles may be a potential intestinal delivery carrier for berberine.

**Figure 4.** Cumulative release of berberine from nanoparticles at pH 2.0 (simulated gastric fluid, SGF) and pH 7.4 (simulated intestinal fluid, SIF).

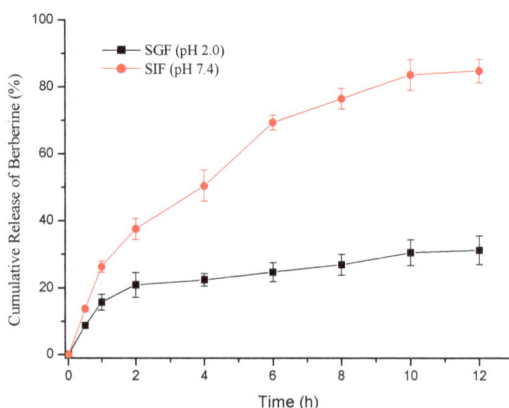

*2.4. Cytotoxicity of Berberine and Nanoparticles*

The berberine-free nanoparticles did not exhibit significant cytotoxicity. Cell viability of Caco-2 cells was higher than 90% by treating the cells with 250 µg/mL nanoparticles (Figure 5A). Figure 5 shows the dose-dependent cytotoxicity of Ber-loaded nanoparticles on Caco-2 cells. It was reported that cell viability of A549 cells incubated with CS/FD nanoparticles at a concentration below 3 mg/mL was higher than 80% [29]. Both berberine and Ber-loaded nanoparticles induced low cytotoxicity in the concentration range of 5–40 µg/mL as measured by the MTT assay (Figure 5B). Therefore, the nanoparticle samples were used at a Ber equivalent concentration of 30 µg/mL for the following studies.

**Figure 5.** Dose-dependent cytotoxicity of berberine-free nanoparticles (**A**) and berberine-loaded nanoparticles (**B**) on Caco-2 cells.

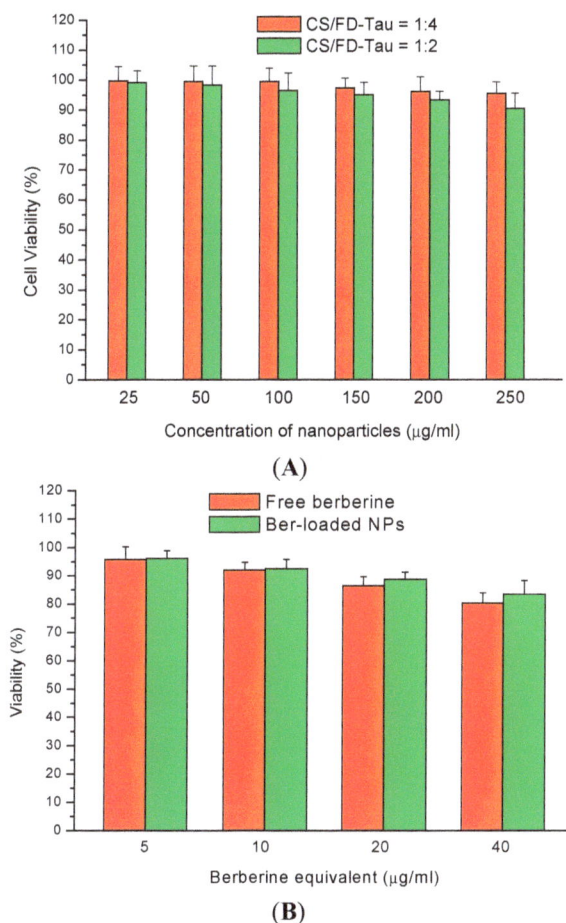

(**A**)

(**B**)

## 2.5. Inhibition of NO and TNF-α Production

Bacterial-derived lipopolysaccharides (LPS) can cause impaired barrier function, leading to a leak-flux diarrhea by enhancing uptake of antigen across the intestinal epithelium tight junction (TJ). Most types of intestinal inflammation are associated with disorder of the intestinal epithelial TJ barrier function. LPS regulates proinflammatory cytokine which is produced by macrophage and can cause intestinal epithelial barrier dysfunction. The protective effect of Ber-loaded nanoparticles on epithelial barrier function of Caco-2 cell monolayer co-cultured with LPS-treated RAW 264.7 cells was evaluated by TEER and FITC-dextran permeability.

**Figure 6.** (**A**) Nitric oxide (NO) and (**B**) TNF-α production in RAW264.7 cells stimulated by 100 ng/mL of LPS in presence of berberine-free nanoparticles (NPs) and berberine-loaded nanoparticles (Ber-loaded NPs) by adding 30 μg/mL berberine equivalent of the nanoparticles to the apical and basolateral sides respectively (*n* = 5). ** *p* < 0.01 compared with the control; ## *p* < 0.01 compared with the LPS-treated group.

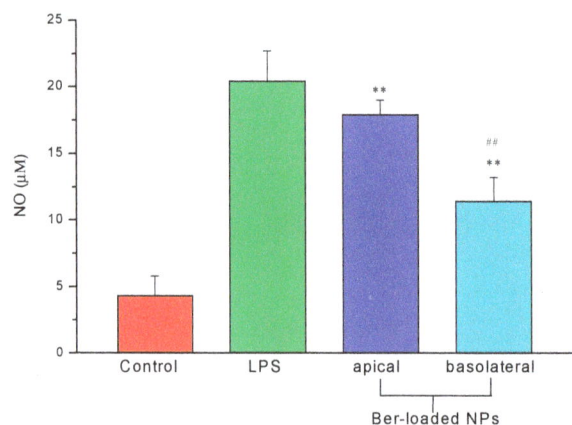

(**A**)

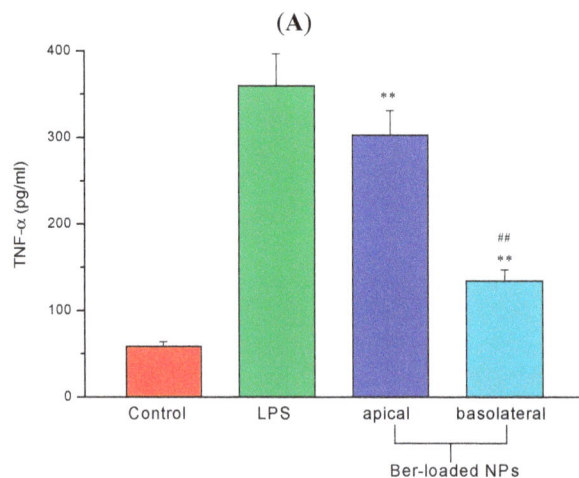

(**B**)

 To identify the protective effect of the Ber-loaded nanoparticles on the tight junction which was disrupted by inflammation, macrophages were incubated with the nanoparticles alone or in the presence of LPS. LPS is known to secrete inflammatory cytokines like TNF-α which are involved in immune responses and induces epithelial destruction [32]. LPS-stimulated nitric oxide (NO) production in macrophage can be easily determined and used as an index of inflammation. As shown in Figure 6, without LPS, the presence of Ber-free nanoparticles (control) produced only low amounts of NO and TNF-α protein. Yet, the presence of PLS alone induced a large amount of them. As evidenced from Figure 6A, further addition of Ber-loaded nanoparticles to the basolateral side considerably inhibited NO production in LPS-activated macrophages. The reduction in NO production indicated that iNOS protein expression, a key factor in oxidant-induced disruption of intestinal Caco-2 monolayer barrier, was inhibited by the Ber-loaded nanoparticles. Moreover, the expression of TNF-α protein by LPS-activated macrophages was markedly inhibited by the Ber-loaded nanoparticles (Figure 6B). This agrees with the report from Jeong *et al.*, that berberine could inhibit LPS-induced expression of proinflammatory genes in peritoneal macrophages and RAW 264.7 cells [33]. Besides, chitosan-based nanoparticles have been widely studied as drug carriers in mucosal and targeting drug delivery [34,35].

However, the addition of Ber-loaded nanoparticle to the apical side did not significantly reduce NO and TNF-α production by RAW 264.7 cells. The results suggest that the nanoparticles cannot effectively permeate through the TJ barrier to inhibit the inflammatory response in macrophage. The nanoparticles must be localized to macrophage and subsequently release berberine to inhibit the production of NO and pro-inflammatory cytokines by macrophage.

*2.6. Intestinal TJ Permeability*

As shown in Figure 7A, Ber-free nanoparticles or Ber-loaded nanoparticles alone did not result in reduction in TEER. The zeta potentials of the nanoparticles were −35.7 ± 2.1 and 7.6 ± 0.5 mV, respectively (Table 2). Berberine and fucoidan have been shown to improve intestinal barrier function and reduce intestinal epithelial permeability [6,23]. On the other hand, when the LPS (100 ng/mL) was applied to the basolateral compartment, it caused a significant decrease in TEER after 48 h incubation with the co-culture system of intestinal epithelial Caco-2 cells/macrophage RAW264.7 cells. However, the decrease in TEER induced by LPS-activated macrophage could be retarded by berberine treatment. To determine whether the Ber-loaded nanoparticles could reduce inflammation-induced TJ disruption, polarized Caco-2 monolayer was exposed to the nanoparticles after LPS treatment; and the TEER was monitored for 72 h. We found that the released berberine could effectively inhibit the LPS-induced disruption of TJ. For comparison, by adding Ber-free nanoparticles after LPS treatment, the decreasing trend of the TEER value was relatively close to that of the negative control group (LPS treatment). This indicated that the nanoparticles did not exhibit a significant protective effect on epithelial cell injury. Moreover, it was found that TEER values of Caco-2 monolayer exposed to the Ber-loaded nanoparticles 2 h before LPS treatment remained at a high level. These results suggested that the preventive effect of nanoparticles on LPS-induced destruction of the intestinal epithelial barrier was dependent on the incorporated berberine.

LPS play an essential role in inducing inflammatory response in macrophages and the subsequent TJ disassembly in intestinal epithelia accompanied by an increase in paracellular permeability. The effect of LPS-induced intestinal epithelial barrier dysfunction was determined by measuring the paracellular flux of FITC-dextran. The permeability of TJ increased after stimulating the cell monolayer with LPS. As shown in Figure 7B, LPS caused a significant increase in the permeability coefficient (Papp) of FITC-dextran. The increase in FITC-dextran flux from the apical to the basal side corresponded to the increase in the Caco-2 TJ permeability as indicated by the increased TEER. However, as the Caco-2 intestinal monolayer was co-treated with the LPS and Ber-loaded nanoparticles, the permeability of FITC-dextran through the Caco-2 cells was significantly reduced. The Ber-loaded nanoparticles thus lessened the increase of paracellular flux induced by LPS. These results indicated that Ber-loaded nanoparticles can be used to reduce the effects of LPS-induced impairment of epithelial barrier function.

**Figure 7.** Epithelial barrier function determined by measurements of transepithelial electrical resistance (TEER) (**A**) and Fluorescein isothiocyanate (FITC) labeled dextrans (FITC-dextran) permeability (**B**). Caco-2 cell monolayers were co-cultured with RAW264.7 stimulated by 100 ng/mL of LPS in the presence of berberine (Ber), and berberine-free (NPs) and loaded nanoparticles (Ber-loaded NPs, 30 µg/mL berberine equivalent) ($n = 5$). ** $p < 0.01$ compared with the control; ## $p < 0.01$ compared with the LPS-treated group.

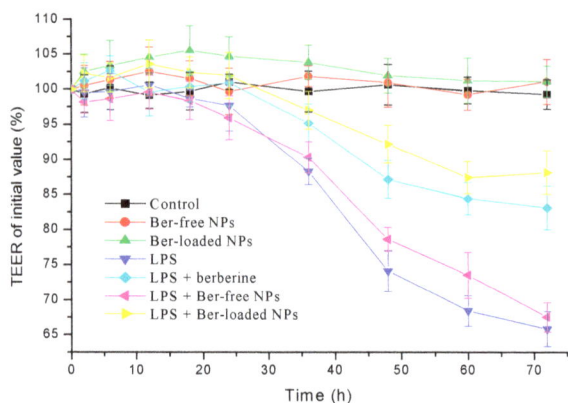

(**A**)

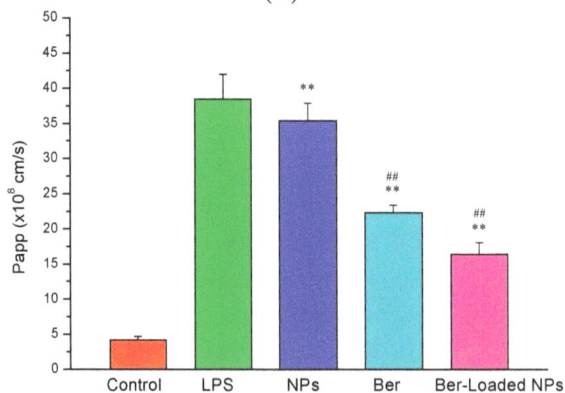

(**B**)

Although the above mentioned results suggested that the Ber-loaded nanoparticle cannot effectively permeate through TJ barrier to inhibit the production of NO and pro-inflammatory cytokines by macrophage (Figure 6A,B), the effect of the nanoparticles on attenuating inflammation-induced tight junction dysfunction was significant (Figure 7A,B). Berberine is a traditional Chinese medicine used for the treatment of gastroenteritis and infective diarrhea. Berberine could be delivered to the Caco-2 cell, but not to the sublayer macrophage, thus the pro-inflammatory cytokines mediating NF-κB signaling pathway in the cell could be inhibited to protect the TJ junction. In this study, the decrease in TEER and increase in paracellular permeability induced by LPS were moderated by Ber-loaded nanoparticles. Berberine has a considerable effect in decreasing intestinal epithelial permeability without affecting TJ proteins. Li *et al.*, (2010) reported that berberine can inhibit pro-inflammatory cytokines such as TNF-α and IFN-γ induced intestinal epithelial tight junction damage [8]. Another study showed that increased intestinal permeability and tight junction disruption induced by LPS in mice could be efficaciously suppressed by berberine [6]. Those results revealed that berberine plays an important role in ameliorating intestinal epithelial TJ damage. On the other hand, fucoidan demonstrated superior immunomodulatory activity of suppressing TNF-α production in macrophage. Fucoidan also improves intestinal epithelial barrier function by reducing IL-8 gene expression and upregulating the expression of claudin-1 in Caco-2 cells [36,37]. Moreover, taurine is a potent compound against intestinal inflammation by repressing TNF-α induced Caco-2 cell damage [38]. Incorporation of berberine with the FD-Tau conjugate into the nanoparticle system was thus able to increasingly protect the intestinal epithelial barrier function under LPS-induced inflammation by macrophage, compared with berberine alone in solution (Figure 7A,B). Moreover, the Ber-loaded nanoparticles anchored with the mucoadhesive polymer, chitosan, might prolong the residence time of the nanoparticles on the intestinal mucous layer and subsequently localize the released berberine to the intestinal epithelial cells in an inflammatory bowel disease.

*2.7. Immunostaining of ZO-1 Protein*

LPS is known to induce intestinal barrier dysfunction and disruption of epithelial tight junction due to the production of pro-inflammatory cytokines such as TNF-α. The effect of TNF-α on the epithelial barrier function is associated with the redistribution of TJ proteins in polarized Caco-2 cell. Zonula occludens-1 (ZO-1) is a tight junction protein that links transmembrane proteins of the TJ to the actin cytoskeleton. As shown in Figure 8A, in the control group (without TNF-α), the stained Caco-2 cell visualized by CLSM exhibited a normally smooth ZO-1 distribution. Exposure of Caco-2 cells to TNF-α led to slight disruption of the TJ structure in polarized Caco-2 monolayers. The disrupted ZO-1 proteins were not recovered after the removal of TNF-α, suggesting that the TJ was irreversibly disrupted by LPS. Treatment of the cells by the Ber-loaded nanoparticles prevented the TJ protein from disruption by TNF-α. The ZO-1 proteins remained intact after directly treating Caco-2 cells with TNF-α in the presence of the nanoparticles (Figure 8A). Several studies have demonstrated that berberine or fucoidan could directly induce changes in TJ protein expression, consequently improving intestinal epithelial barrier functions.

ROS is known to induce disruption of intestinal epithelial barrier function [39,40]. CLSM was carried out to investigate the oxidative stress induced by LPS in RAW 264.7 cells and the ROS scavenging activity of the nanoparticles in the LPS-treated cells. The fluorescent images of intracellular ROS levels in RAW 264.7 cells after 24 h of incubation with LPS are shown in Figure 8B. The green fluorescence was from ROS-sensitive fluorescence dye (DCFDA) whereas the blue fluorescence was from DAPI dye. The merged image of the fluorescence from DCFDA and DAPI dyes showed that the blue fluorescence in nuclei was surrounded by green fluorescence.

Visualization of the green fluorescent signal in the cells indicated the production of intracellular oxidative stress by LPS. Pretreatment of the cells with 30 µg/mL berberine equivalent of nanoparticles quenched the green fluorescence of the ROS-sensitive dye in RAW 264.7 cells (Figure 8B). The nanoparticles therefore seemed to be a promising carrier to deliver berberine to scavenge the intracellular ROS in macrophage.

Figure 8. (A) Confocal laser scanning microscopy (CLSM) visualization of protective effect of berberine in TNF-α induced epithelial barrier disruption. ZO-1 protein of Caco-2 cells treated without (a) or with (b) berberine-loaded nanoparticles (Ber-loaded NPs) in the absence of TNF-α for 72 h; (B) CLSM visualization of intracellular ROS levels in RAW 264.7 cells treated without (a) or with (b) berberine-loaded nanoparticles in the absence of LPS for 72 h.

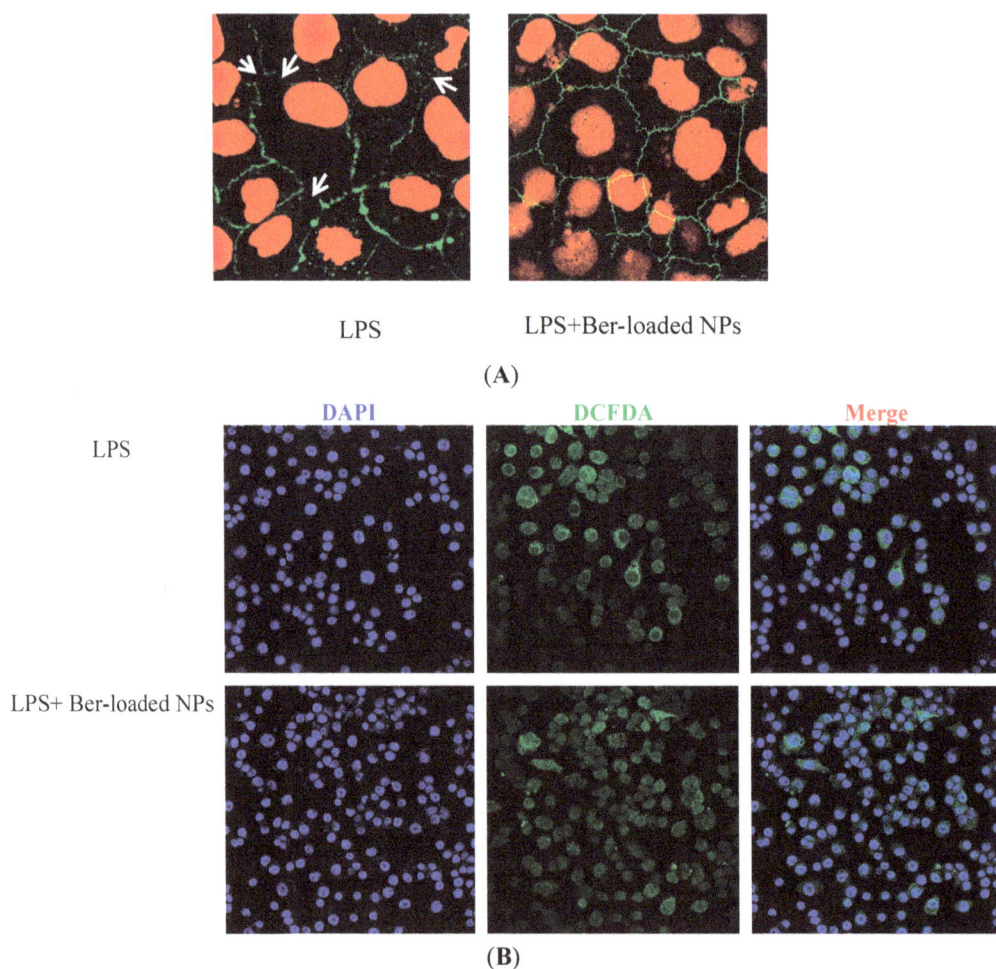

LPS          LPS+Ber-loaded NPs

(A)

(B)

## 3. Experimental Section

### 3.1. Materials

Lipopolysaccharides (LPS) from *Salmonella enterica* serotype typhimurium (L6143), Taurine, 1-ethyl-3-(3-(dimethylamino)propyl)carbodiimide hydrochloride (EDC), berberine, Dulbecco's modified Eagle medium (DMEM), 2-(*N*-Morpholino)ethanesulfonic acid sodium salt (MES), Griess reagent, berberine, fluorescein isothiocyanate–dextran (FITC-dextran, 4000 kD), 2′,7′-Dichlorofluorescin diacetate (DCFDA), and MTT reagent were purchased from Sigma-Aldrich (St Louis, MO, USA).

### 3.2. Synthesis and Characterization of Fucoidan-Taurine (FD-Tau) Conjugates

FD-Tau conjugates were synthesized following a modified procedure described by Yu *et al.* [41]. Briefly, the carboxyl group on the glucuronic acid residues of fucoidan (MW 80 kDa, NOVA Pharma & Liposome Biotech Co., Ltd, Kaohsiung, Taiwan) was activated by EDC in MES buffer (25 mM, pH 5.0) and the activated fucoidan solution was added with an adequate amount of taurine (weight ratio of fucoidan/taurine/EDC = 1:1:1.5), and the resulting mixture was allowed to react for 48 h. Both reactions were quenched by adding hydroxylamine, and adjusting the pH of the reaction medium to 8.0. The obtained FD-Tau polymer conjugates were dialyzed against water and then lyophilized. The purified products were analyzed by FTIR spectrometer (Perkin-Elmer Spectrum RX1, Waltham, MA, USA). The taurine substitution ratio of the FD-Tau conjugate was estimated by reacting free taurine with 2,4,6-trinitrobenzenesulfonic acid (TNBS) and subsequently measuring the absorbance at 420 nm.

### 3.3. Preparation of Berberine-Loaded CS/FD-Tau Nanoparticles

Berberine and FD-Tau solutions were prepared by respectively dissolving adequate amounts of berberine and FD-Tau in DI water. Berberine/FD-Tau nanoparticles were then prepared by adding the berberine solution (1.0 mg/mL, 1 mL) into the FD-Tau solution (0.5, 1.0, 1.5, 2.0 mg/mL, 1 mL) at various weight ratios (as shown in Table 1). Berberine-loaded CS/FD-Tau nanoparticles were prepared by dissolving chitosan (MW 60 kDa, deacetylation degree 85%, Koyo Chemical Co. Ltd. Hyogo, Japan) and berberine (1.0 mg/mL) together in DI water at different chitosan-to-berberine weight ratios (as shown in Table 2). Subsequently, the berberine/chitosan solution (chitosan/berberine weight ratio = 0.5 mg/1.0 mg, 1.0 mg/1.0 mg, 1.5 mg/1.0 mg, and 2.0 mg/1.0 mg, 1 mL) was added to the aqueous FD-Tau solution (1.0 mg/mL, 2 mL) to obtain self-assembled nanoparticles. A Malvern Zetasizer (3000HS, Worcestershire, UK) was used to measure the particle size and zeta potential of the nanoparticle suspensions. Transmission electron microscopy (TEM, Hitachi H-600, Tokyo, Japan) was used observe the morphology of nanoparticles after drying the suspension on a copper grid (300 mesh) coated with carbon film.

206

*3.4. In Vitro Release Study*

The nanoparticles were ultracentrifugated to remove free berberine molecules; and the loading efficiency (LE) was determined by measuring the concentration of free berberine in the supernatant using high performance liquid chromatography (HPLC) coupled with an ultraviolet (UV) absorption detector operated at 360 nm. Quantification of berberine was performed using a reverse-phase C18 column (150 mm × 4.6 mm, 5 µm), with a mobile phase of acetonitrile—0.04 M $H_3PO_4$ (42:58 vol.%)—and a flow rate of 1.0 mL/min. Berberine release from the nanoparticles was investigated in SGF (0.01 N HCl, pH 2.0) and SIF (PBS, pH 7.4) at 37 °C under agitation. Samples were collected at several pre-determined times. After centrifugation, the supernatants were used for berberine assay. The fraction of drug release was calculated based on the initial amount of berberine incorporated in the nanoparticles. The release study was repeated four times for each time point to obtain the average and standard deviation (SD).

*3.5. MTT Assay for Cell Viability*

The Caco-2 cell (BCRC 60182, Hsinchu, Taiwan) was maintained in DMEM medium containing 10% fetal bovine serum (FBS), 1% penicillin (100 U/mL)-streptomycin (100 µg/mL), and 4mM glutamine. Caco-2 cells were cultured in 96-well plates at a density of $2 \times 10^4$ cells per well. Subsequent to adherence, berberine (5, 10, 20 and 40 µg/mL), Ber-loaded nanoparticles (the same berberine equivalents), Ber-free nanoparticles (25, 50, 100, 150, 200 and 250 µg/mL) were added to the cells and incubated for 24 h. After 48 h incubation at 37 °C, the medium was aspirated and the cells were washed with PBS. The colorimetric determination of cell viability was performed by adding 20 µL MTT solution (5 mg/mL) to each well. After 4 h of incubation, the culture medium was removed carefully. The supernatant was aspirated, and 100 µL dimethyl sulfoxide (DMSO) was added to dissolve the formazan crystal. The optical intensity of color (absorbance) was measured on a Perkin Elmer EnSpire 2300 multimode plate reader (PerkinElmer, Inc., Waltham, MA, USA) at 570 nm. Cytotoxicity was expressed as the relative viability (% control).

*3.6. Caco-2/Macrophage Co-Culture System*

Caco-2 cells were seeded at $4 \times 10^5$ cells/well and monolayers were grown in Costar Transwell 6 wells/plates (Corning Costar Corp., NY, USA) with a 3 µm pore size filter insert. The electrical resistances of the filter-grown monolayers were measured using a Millicell®-Electrical Resistance System (Millipore Corporation, Billerica, MA, USA). Monolayers were maintained for 14–20 days in an atmosphere of 95% air and 5% $CO_2$ at 37 °C until the transepithelial electrical resistance (TEER) reached a value in the range of 900–1000 Ω $cm^2$. RAW264.7 cells were seeded into the bottom plate at a density of $7.5 \times 10^5$ cells/well and the insert with polarized Caco-2 monolayer was added into the Transwell plate preloaded with RAW264.7 cells (BCRC 60001, Hsinchu, Taiwan). The anti-inflammatory effect of Ber-loaded nanoparticles was examined by addition of 100 ng/mL LPS to the basolateral side subsequent to adding 30 µg/mL berberine equivalent of the nanoparticles to the apical side. For comparison, 30 µg/mL berberine equivalent of the nanoparticles was directly added to the basolateral side (RAW264.7 cells). Nitric oxide and TNF-α productions were determined by culture supernatant collected from the basolateral side after 24 h.

## 3.7. Colorimetric Nitric Oxide Assay

Griess reagent (0.1% $N$-(1-naphthyl)-ethylenediamine dihydrochloride and 1% sulfanilamide) was used to measure LPS-induced nitric oxide levels (NO) in RAW 264.7 macophage. At the end of incubation, 50 μL of Griess solution was added to the same volume of the supernatant for 10 min. The absorbance of the final product was measured at a wavelength of 540 nm using a Perkin Elmer EnSpire 2300 multimode plate reader to determine the nitrite concentration with a calibration curve constructed using a standard solution of NaNO$_2$.

## 3.8. Enzyme-Linked Immunosorbent Assay (ELISA) for TNF-α

Subsequent to LPS treatment, the TNF-α concentration in culture supernatant was determined by a sandwich enzyme-linked immunosorbent assay (ELISA). Thermo Scientific 96-well immunoplate was coated with anti-mouse TNF-α monoclonal antibody (R & D Systems) and blocked using 4% bovine serum albumin (BSA) in PBS. After the addition of 100 μL diluted sample to the wells, an anti-mouse TNF-α polyclonal antibody (R & D Systems, Minneapolis, MN, USA) was added to the ELISA plate. The plate was developed by horseradish peroxidase for 2 h and the color development was terminated with the addition of a 1 N H$_2$SO$_4$ solution. The absorbance was read at 450 nm using a Perkin Elmer EnSpire 2300 multimode plate reader (PerkinElmer, Inc., Waltham, MA, USA).

## 3.9. Measurement of TEER and Paracellular Permeability

$S.$ $typhimurium$ LPS (100 ng/mL, L6143, Sigma Chemical Co., St. Louis, MO, USA) was added to the basolateral side (cultured with RAW264.7 cells) of Transwell plate to induce the inflammatory response. The effect of the Ber-loaded nanoparticles on attenuating LPS-induced tight junction disruption was evaluated by adding 30 μg/mL berberine equivalent of the nanoparticles to the apical side (insert with Caco-2 cells monolayer). For comparison, the system in which the cells were not treated by LPS was used as a control. Moreover, the cells were pre-treated with 30 μg/mL berberine equivalent of the nanoparticles for 2 h, followed by adding LPS to RAW264.7 cells to induce tight junction damage in Caco-2 monolayer. Changes in TEER were measured using the above mentioned method.

The transepithelial permeability was quantified by measuring the paracellular flux of fluorescein isothiocyanate (FITC) labeled dextrans (FITC-dextran). Transport of FITC-dextran (500 μg/mL in the apical compartment) across Caco-2 cell monolayer was quantitatively analyzed by measuring fluorescence intensity in the receiver compartment (basolateral side) at different time periods. The intensity of fluorescence emission (FL intensity) was determined by a Perkin Elmer EnSpire 2300 multimode plate reader, with excitation and emission wavelengths set to 488 and 519 nm, respectively. The amount of transported FITC-dextran was calculated using the calibration curve of FITC-dextran. The apparent permeability coefficient (Papp) was determined as follows:

$$\text{Papp (cm/s)} = (\Delta Q/\Delta t)/(A \times C_0)$$

where $\Delta Q/\Delta t$ ($\mu$g/s) is the cumulative amount transported, $A$ is the diffusion area (4.67 cm$^2$), and $C_0$ is the initial FITC-dextran concentration in the donor side ($\mu$g/mL).

### 3.10. CLSM Visualization of Immunostained TJ Protein

Cells grown on glass cover slips in a 6-well plate were directly incubated with the pro-inflammatory cytokines, TNF-$\alpha$ (10 ng/mL), in the presence or absence of the Ber-loaded nanoparticles (30 $\mu$g berberine equivalent/mL). After removal of culture medium, cells were fixed with 3.7% paraformaldehyde. Subsequently, cells were permeabilized with 0.1% Triton X-100 at room temperature for 10 min. The cells were incubated with rabbit anti-ZO-1 monoclonal antibody (Zymed Laboraties, Inc., San Francisco, CA, USA) and subsequently stained by a Cy-3 conjugated goat anti-rabbit IgG (Jackson ImmunoResearch Laboratories, West Grove, PA, USA). Dislocation of ZO-1 protein in Caco-2 cells was examined under a confocal laser scanning microscopy (CLSM, Leica TCS SP2, Bensheim, Germany). To determine reactive oxygen species (ROS) induced by LPS (100 ng/mL) in RAW264.7 cells, the culture medium was removed and the cells were washed with PBS. Subsequently, the cells were incubated in the dark with DCFDA (20 $\mu$M) which could passively diffuse across the cell membrane. The diacetate of nonfluorescent DCFDA was cleaved by intracellular esterase and then reacted with intracellular ROS to produce fluorescence. Fluorescence images of ROS generated in RAW264.7 cells were visualized using CLSM.

### 3.11. Statistical Analysis

All measurements were replicated three times and data were expressed as the mean ± standard deviation. Statistical analysis was performed by one-way analysis of variance and the determination of confidence intervals at $p < 0.05$ using SAS version 9.1 (SAS Institute, Cary, NC, USA).

## 4. Conclusions

In this work, Ber-loaded CS/FD-Tau nanoparticles were developed and acted as an epithelial protective material to prevent redistribution of TJ protein caused by bacterial endotoxin (LPS). The pH-responsive nanoparticles were stable at pH 2.0 but became unstable as the pH increased to 7.4. The release rate of berberine from the nanoparticle was slow in SGF but fast in SIF. Measurements of TEER and paracellular flux of FITC-dextran in Caco-2 intestinal monolayers showed that the Ber-loaded nanoparticles were able to diminish the LPS-induced increment in intestinal epithelial TJ permeability. CLSM confirmed that the Ber-loaded nanoparticles prevented redistribution of ZO-1 proteins mediated by TNF-$\alpha$ induced TJ disruption. These findings suggested that the Ber-loaded nanoparticle is a potential carrier for site-specific delivery of berberine to the intestine for the inhibition of impaired intestinal barrier function. The nanoparticles might serve as an appropriate therapy for the treatment of disease associated with intestinal epithelial TJ dysfunction.

## Acknowledgments

This work was supported by a grant from Taipei Medical University (TMU101-AE1-B39), Taiwan.

## Author Contributions

Fwu Long Mi conceived and designed the experiments, and wrote the manuscript. Shao Jung Wu, Trong Ming Don, and Cheng-Wei Lin contributed to performing experimental works and proofreading the manuscript.

## Conflicts of Interest

The authors declare no conflict of interest.

## References

1. Guo, S.; Al-Sadi, R.; Said, H.M.; Ma, T.Y. Lipopolysaccharide causes an increase in intestinal tight junction permeability *in vitro* and *in vivo* by inducing enterocyte membrane expression and localization of TLR-4 and CD14. *Am. J. Pathol.* **2013**, *182*, 375–387.
2. Amin, A.H.; Subbaiah, T.V.; Abbasi, K.M. Berberine sulfate: Antimicrobial activity, bioassay, and mode of action. *Can. J. Microbiol.* **1969**, *15*, 1067–1076.
3. Kuo, C.L.; Chi, C.W.; Liu, T.Y. The anti-inflammatory potential of berberine *in vitro* and *in vivo*. *Cancer Lett.* **2004**, *203*, 127–137.
4. Li, G.X.; Wang, X.M.; Jiang, T.; Gong, J.F.; Niu, L.Y.; Li, N. Berberine prevents damage to the intestinal mucosal barrier during early phase of sepsis in rat through mechanisms independent of the NOD-like receptors signaling pathway. *Eur. J. Pharmacol.* **2014**, *730*, 1–7.
5. Cao, M.; Wang, P.; Sun, C.; He, W.; Wang, F. Amelioration of IFN-gamma and TNF-alpha-induced intestinal epithelial barrier dysfunction by berberine via suppression of MLCK-MLC phosphorylation signaling pathway. *PLoS One* **2013**, *8*, e61944.
6. Gu, L.; Li, N.; Gong, J.; Li, Q.; Zhu, W.; Li, J. Berberine ameliorates intestinal epithelial tight-junction damage and down-regulates myosin light chain kinase pathways in a mouse model of endotoxinemia. *J. Infect. Dis.* **2011**, *203*, 1602–1612.
7. Amasheh, M.; Fromm, A.; Krug, S.M.; Amasheh, S.; Andres, S.; Zeitz, M.; Fromm, M.; Schulzke, J.D. TNFα-induced and berberine-antagonized tight junction barrier impairment via tyrosine kinase, Akt and NFκB signaling. *J. Cell Sci.* **2010**, *123*, 4145–4155.
8. Li, N.; Gu, L.; Qu, L.; Gong, J.; Li, Q.; Zhu, W.; Li, J. Berberine attenuates pro-inflammatory cytokine-induced tight junction disruption in an *in vitro* model of intestinal epithelial cells. *Eur. J. Pharmacol. Sci.* **2010**, *40*, 1–8.
9. Tan, X.S.; Ma, J.Y.; Feng, R.; Ma, C.; Chen, W.J.; Sun, Y.P.; Fu, J.; Huang, M.; He, C.Y.; Shou, J.W.; *et al.* Tissue distribution of berberine and its metabolites after oral administration in rats. *PLoS One* **2013**, *8*, e77969.

10. Chang, C.H.; Huang, W.Y.; Lai, C.H.; Hsu, Y.M.; Yao, Y.H.; Chen, T.Y.; Wu, J.Y.; Peng, S.F.; Lin, Y.H. Development of novel nanoparticles shelled with heparin for berberine delivery to treat Helicobacter pylori. *Acta. Biomater.* **2011**, *7*, 593–603.

11. Lin, Y.H.; Lin, J.H.; Chou, S.C.; Chang, S.J.; Chung, C.C.; Chen, Y.S.; Chang, C.H. Berberine-loaded targeted nanoparticles as specific *Helicobacter pylori* eradication therapy: *In vitro* and *in vivo* study. *Nanomedicine* **2014**, *1*, 1–15.

12. Muzzarelli, R.A. Chitins and chitosans as immunoadjuvants and non-allergenic drug carriers. *Mar. Drugs* **2010**, *8*, 292–312.

13. Sashiwa, H.; Aiba, S.I. Chemically modified chitin and chitosan as biomaterials. *Prog. Polym. Sci.* **2004**, *29*, 887–908.

14. Harris, R.; Lecumberri, E.; Heras, A. Chitosan-genipin microspheres for the controlled release of drugs: Clarithromycin, tramadol and heparin. *Mar. Drugs* **2010**, *8*, 1750–1762.

15. Eftaiha, A.F.; Qinna, N.; Rashid, I.S.; Al Remawi, M.M.; Al Shami, M.R.; Arafat, T.A.; Badwan, A.A. Bioadhesive controlled metronidazole release matrix based on chitosan and xanthan gum. *Mar. Drugs* **2010**, *8*, 1716–1730.

16. Kavianinia, I.; Plieger, P.G.; Kandile, N.G.; Harding, D.R.K. *In vitro* evaluation of spray-dried chitosan microspheres crosslinked with pyromellitic dianhydride for oral colon-specific delivery of protein drugs. *J. Appl. Polym. Sci.* **2014**, *131*, doi:10.1002/app.40514.

17. Korkiatithaweechai, S.; Umsarika, P.; Praphairaksit, N.; Muangsin, N. Controlled release of diclofenac from matrix polymer of chitosan and oxidized konjac glucomannan. *Mar. Drugs* **2011**, *9*, 1649–1663.

18. Chen, M.C.; Mi, F.L.; Liao, Z.X.; Hsiao, C.W.; Sonaje, K.; Chung, M.F.; Hsu, L.W.; Sung, H.W. Recent advances in chitosan-based nanoparticles for oral delivery of macromolecules. *Adv. Drug. Deliv. Rev.* **2013**, *65*, 865–879.

19. Ale, M.T.; Mikkelsen, J.D.; Meyer, A.S. Important determinants for fucoidan bioactivity: A critical review of structure-function relations and extraction methods for fucose-containing sulfated polysaccharides from brown seaweeds. *Mar. Drugs* **2011**, *9*, 2106–2130.

20. Li, B.; Lu, F.; Wei, X.; Zhao, R. Fucoidan: Structure and bioactivity. *Molecules* **2008**, *13*, 1671–1695.

21. Fitton, J.H. Therapies from fucoidan; multifunctional marine polymers. *Mar. Drugs* **2011**, *9*, 1731–1760.

22. Tanoue, T.; Nishitani, Y.; Kanazawa, K.; Hashimoto, T.; Mizuno, M. *In vitro* model to estimate gut inflammation using co-cultured Caco-2 and RAW264.7 cells. *Biochem. Biophys. Res. Commun.* **2008**, *374*, 565–569.

23. Iraha, A.; Chinen, H.; Hokama, A.; Yonashiro, T.; Kinjo, T.; Kishimoto, K.; Nakamoto, M.; Hirata, T.; Kinjo, N.; Higa, F.; *et al.* Fucoidan enhances intestinal barrier function by upregulating the expression of claudin-1. *World J. Gastroenterol.* **2013**, *19*, 5500–5507.

24. Hamman, J.H. Chitosan based polyelectrolyte complexes as potential carrier materials in drug delivery systems. *Mar. Drugs* **2010**, *8*, 1305–1322.

25. Murakami, K.; Aoki, H.; Nakamura, S.; Nakamura, S.; Takikawa, M.; Hanzawa, M.; Kishimoto, S.; Hattori, H.; Tanaka, Y.; Kiyosawa, T.; *et al.* Hydrogel blends of chitin/chitosan, fucoidan and alginate as healing-impaired wound dressings. *Biomaterials* **2010**, *31*, 83–90.

26. Venkatesan, J.; Bhatnagar, I.; Kim, S.K. Chitosan-alginate biocomposite containing fucoidan for bone tissue engineering. *Mar. Drugs* **2014**, *12*, 300–316.

27. Huang, Y.C.; Liu, T.J. Mobilization of mesenchymal stem cells by stromal cell-derived factor-1 released from chitosan/tripolyphosphate/fucoidan nanoparticles. *Acta Biomater.* **2012**, *8*, 1048–1056.

28. Yu, S.H.; Tang, D.W.; Hsieh, H.Y.; Wu, W.S.; Lin, B.X.; Chuang, E.Y.; Sung, H.W.; Mi, F.L. Nanoparticle-induced tight-junction opening for the transport of an anti-angiogenic sulfated polysaccharide across Caco-2 cell monolayers. *Acta Biomater.* **2013**, *9*, 7449–7459.

29. Huang, Y.C.; Li, R.Y. Preparation and characterization of antioxidant nanoparticles composed of chitosan and fucoidan for antibiotics delivery. *Mar. Drugs* **2014**, *12*, 4379–4398.

30. Da Silva, L.C.; Garcia, T.; Mori, M.; Sandri, G.; Bonferoni, M.C.; Finotelli, P.V.; Cinelli, L.P.; Caramella, C.; Cabral, L.M. Preparation and characterization of polysaccharide-based nanoparticles with anticoagulant activity. *Int. J. Nanomedicine* **2012**, *7*, 2975–2986.

31. Miao, J.; Fa, Y.; Gu, B.; Zhu, W.; Zou, S. Taurine attenuates lipopolysaccharide-induced dysfunction in mouse mammary epithelial cells. *Cytokine* **2012**, *59*, 35–40.

32. Lee, D.U.; Kang, Y.J.; Park, M.K.; Lee, Y.S.; Seo, H.G.; Kim, T.S.; Kim, C.H.; Chang, K.C. Effects of 13-alkyl-substituted berberine alkaloids on the expression of COX-II, TNF-alpha, iNOS, and IL-12 production in LPS-stimulated macrophages. *Life Sci.* **2003**, *73*, 1401–1412.

33. Jeong, H.W.; Hsu, K.C.; Lee, J.W.; Ham, M.; Huh, J.Y.; Shin, H.J.; Kim, W.S.; Kim, J.B. Berberine suppresses proinflammatory responses through AMPK activation in macrophages. *Am. J. Physiol. Endocrinol. Metab.* **2009**, *296*, E955–E964.

34. Cheng, M.; Gao, X.; Wang, Y.; Chen, H.; He, B.; Xu, H.; Li, Y.; Han, J.; Zhang, Z. Synthesis of glycyrrhetinic acid-modified chitosan 5-fluorouracil nanoparticles and its inhibition of liver cancer characteristics *in vitro* and *in vivo*. *Mar. Drugs* **2013**, *11*, 3517–3536.

35. Van der Lubben, I.M.; Verhoef, J.C.; Borchard, G.; Junginger, H.E. Chitosan and its derivatives in mucosal drug and vaccine delivery. *Eur. J. Pharm. Sci.* **2001**, *14*, 201–207.

36. Do, H.; Pyo, S.; Sohn, E.H. Suppression of iNOS expression by fucoidan is mediated by regulation of p38 MAPK, JAK/STAT, AP-1 and IRF-1, and depends on up-regulation of scavenger receptor B1 expression in TNF-alpha- and IFN-gamma-stimulated C6 glioma cells. *J. Nutr. Biochem.* **2010**, *21*, 671–679.

37. Mizuno, M.; Nishitani, Y.; Hashimoto, T.; Kanazawa, K. Different suppressive effects of fucoidan and lentinan on IL-8 mRNA expression in in vitro gut inflammation. *Biosci. Biotechnol. Biochem.* **2009**, *73*, 2324–2325.

38. Mochizuki, T.; Satsu, H.; Nakano, T.; Shimizu, M. Regulation of the human taurine transporter by TNF-alpha and an anti-inflammatory function of taurine in human intestinal Caco-2 cells. *BioFactors* **2004**, *21*, 141–144.

39. Cuzzocrea, S.; Mazzon, E.; de Sarro, A.; Caputi, A.P. Role of free radicals and poly(ADP-ribose) synthetase in intestinal tight junction permeability. *Mol. Med.* **2000**, *6*, 766–778.

40. Rao, R.K.; Baker, R.D.; Baker, S.S.; Gupta, A.; Holycross, M. Oxidant-induced disruption of intestinal epithelial barrier function: Role of protein tyrosine phosphorylation. *Am. J. Physiol.* **1997**, *273*, G812–G823.

41. Yu, S.H.; Mi, F.L.; Pang, J.C.; Jiang, S.C.; Kuo, T.H.; Wu, S.J.; Shyu, S.S. Preparation and characterization of radical and pH-responsive chitosan–gallic acid conjugate drug carriers. *Carbohydr. Polym.* **2011**, *84*, 794–802.

# Mucoadhesive Microparticles for Gastroretentive Delivery: Preparation, Biodistribution and Targeting Evaluation

Jing-Yi Hou, Li-Na Gao, Fan-Yun Meng and Yuan-Lu Cui

**Abstract:** The aim of this research was to prepare and characterize alginate-chitosan mucoadhesive microparticles containing puerarin. The microparticles were prepared by an emulsification-internal gelatin method using a combination of chitosan and $Ca^{2+}$ as cationic components and alginate as anions. Surface morphology, particle size, drug loading, encapsulation efficiency and swelling ratio, *in vitro* drug released, *in vitro* evaluation of mucoadhesiveness and Fluorescence imaging of the gastrointestinal tract were determined. After optimization of the formulation, the encapsulation efficiency was dramatically increased from 70.3% to 99.2%, and a highly swelling ratio was achieved with a change in particle size from $50.3 \pm 11.2$ μm to $124.7 \pm 25.6$ μm. In ethanol induced gastric ulcers, administration of puerarin mucoadhesive microparticles at doses of 150 mg/kg, 300 mg/kg, 450 mg/kg and 600 mg/kg body weight prior to ethanol ingestion significantly protected the stomach ulceration. Consequently, significant changes were observed in inflammatory cytokines, such as prostaglandin $E_2$ ($PGE_2$), tumor necrosis factor (TNF-α), interleukin 6 (IL-6), and interleukin1β (IL-1β), in stomach tissues compared with the ethanol control group. In conclusion, core-shell type pH-sensitive mucoadhesive microparticles loaded with puerarin could enhance puerarin bioavailability and have the potential to alleviate ethanol-mediated gastric ulcers.

Reprinted from *Mar. Drugs*. Cite as: Hou, J.-Y.; Gao, L.-N.; Meng, F.-Y.; Cui, Y.-L. Mucoadhesive Microparticles for Gastroretentive Delivery: Preparation, Biodistribution and Targeting Evaluation. *Mar. Drugs* **2014**, *12*, 5764-5787.

## 1. Introduction

Gastric ulcers, primarily defined as damage in the gastric mucosa that penetrates through the muscularis mucosa into the submucosa [1], is a common disease, affecting an estimated 10% of the population. The basic physiopathology of gastric ulcers results from an imbalance between the defensive (mucus secretion, mucus-bicarbonate barrier, blood flow, cellular regeneration and endogenous protective agents) and aggressive (pepsin secretion, hydrochloric acid, stress and alcohol consumption) functions of the gastric system [2]. Barry Marshall and Robin Warren, who explained the relationship between the bacterium *Helicobacter pylori* and gastric ulcers, won the Nobel Prize in Medicine or Physiology in 2005 [3,4].

Various formulations for oral drug delivery in the treatment of gastric ulcers, such as tablets, capsules and float tablets, have been challenged given their incomplete eradication of *H. pylori*. One reason for the incomplete eradication of *H. pylori* is likely due to the short residence time of drugs in the stomach; thus, effective treatment concentrations cannot be achieved in the gastric mucous layer or epithelial cell surfaces where *H. pylori* exists [5,6]. Another reason might be due to poor stability of drugs or formulations in gastric acid or poor permeability of the drugs across the mucus layer [5,7]. Thus, many researchers have developed several new formulations, such as nanoparticles, mucoadhesive tablets, pH-sensitive excipient composition mucoadhesive microspheres, *etc.*, to increase the time that the drugs reside in the gastrointestinal tract to enhance *H. pylori* eradication [8–11]. Among these formulations, mucoadhesive microparticles have obtained considerable attention due to their ability to contact with the absorbing mucosa, thereby prolonging the drug's residence time at or above the site of drug absorption and resulting in an increased concentration gradient that favors drug absorption and localization in specified regions to enhance the drug's bioavailability [12–14].

Over recent decades, a considerable amount of attention has been paid to the utilization of natural polymers for the development of various drug delivery systems owing to their availability, non-toxic properties, cost effectiveness, biodegradability and biocompatibility [15]. Among these polymers, sodium alginate has been investigated widely given its unique characteristic of forming hydrogel beads in the presence of various metal ions, such as $Ca^{2+}$, $Ba^{2+}$, $Zn^{2+}$, $Al^{3+}$, *etc.*, due to an ionic interaction between the carboxylic acid groups located on the polymer backbone and these cations [16,17]. Various drugs have been successfully incorporated in ionotropically cross-linked alginate hydrogels and release profiles depending on their physicochemical properties and method of preparation [18–20]. However, the drug release properties of ionotropically cross-linked alginate hydrogels have some disadvantages when used as drug carriers. First, the drug could leak during gel formation due to the long immersion time, which decreased the encapsulation efficiency. Moreover, the burst release of the drug from pure cross-linked alginate microparticles/beads is severe due to the rapid breakdown of beads during the *in vitro* release process [21,22].

Chitosan, a natural polysaccharide [23] derived from chitin by alkaline deacetylation, is one of the most abundant natural polymers on earth and serves as a structural polysaccharide for many phyla of lower plants and animals. Given its suitable biodegradability; biocompatibility; immunological, antibacterial, and wound-healing properties; and its good mechanical and film-forming properties, [24] chitosan has been widely applied in biomedical fields as a hemostat, [25] scaffolds for tissue engineering [26], wound dressing [27], controlled drug [28], and gene [29], delivery vehicle. At the same time, chitosan has been used to reinforce alginate microspheres [30] base on the electrostatic interaction between carboxylate alginate groups and ammonium chitosan groups. The chitosan-alginate complex degrades slowly in phosphate buffer, and this behavior results in suppression of the initial release of drugs occurring for uncoated microspheres [31]. Chitosan is a mucoadhesive polymer with permeation enhancing properties [32]; it facilitates the opening of epithelial tight junctions [4], which prevent sialic acid from eroding mucosa. This may attributed to the electrostatic attraction between its positively charged D-glucose-amine residues and the negatively charged sialic acid residues of mucin. In addition, hydrophobic interactions might contribute to its mucoadhesive properties [33]. As chitosan precipitates at pH values above 6.5, it loses its mucoadhesive and permeability properties. Collectively, these effects reduce the drug's release in the intestinal tract, thereby making it suitable for gastroretentive delivery. Based on the need for a gastroretentive delivery system as well as the physical and chemical characteristics of chitosan and sodium alginate, we designed a novel core-shell type pH-sensitive mucoadhesive microparticles delivery system. The mucoadhesive microparticles are prepared using a two-stage method, wherein Ca-Alginate (Ca-Alg) gel beads loading puerarin are recovered as a core and subsequently coated with chitosan as the shell (Figure 1), and these techniques are amenable to industrial production.

**Figure 1.** Depiction of a core-shell microparticle containing a drug-loaded Ca-alginate microsphere as the core and chitosan as the outer shell.

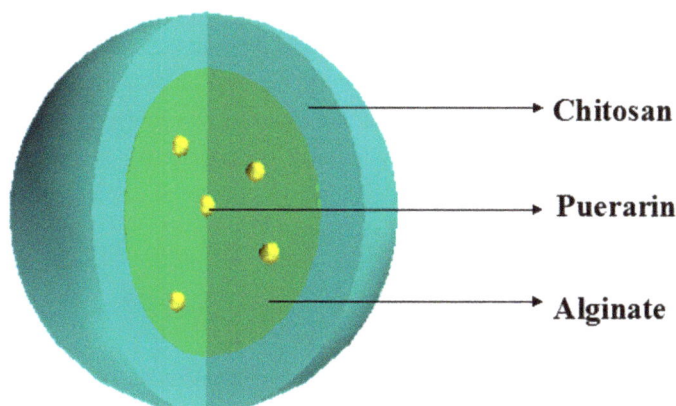

Puerarin (4′,7-dihdroxy-8-β-glucosylisoflavone), a major isoflavone found in a number of plants and herbs, has been used as a functional food and medicine for a long time. Its comprehensive biological actions have been well-documented by numerous studies, indicating its protective effects in gynecological diseases, diabetic nephropathy, cognitive capability, osteoporosis and cardiovascular diseases [34]. Many researchers have reported that puerarin has a variety of activities, including anti-inflammatory [35], anti-apoptosis [36] and anti-oxidative activities. In addition, puerarin has been administered to treat alcohol-related problems, acting as an anti-intoxication agent [37,38]. It also has exhibited preventive effects on immunological injury [3] and liver damage [39]. Increasing evidence suggests that puerarin can protect gastric mucosa from stress-induced injury [40].

In the present study, we developed a novel core-shell type pH-sensitive mucoadhesive microparticle. Sodium alginate acts as the drug-loaded core beads, and chitosan serves as the coating shell. The complex not only targets puerarin into the gastric mucosa but maintains sustained release. Additionally, we explored the gastric protection and mechanisms of mucoadhesive microparticles loaded with puerarin.

## 2. Experimental Section

### 2.1. Materials and Animals

Puerarin (purity > 99%; molecular structure presented in Figure 2) was obtained from Xi'an Qing Yue Biotechnology Co., Ltd. (Xi'an, Shanxi, China). Sodium alginate, chitosan (with 95% deacetylation and a molecular weight of 650,000) and fluorescein isothiocyanate (FITC) were obtained from Sangon Biotech, Co., Ltd. (Shanghai, China). The omeprazole was purchased from the Youcare Pharmaceutical Group Co., Ltd. (Beijing, China). The rebamipide was obtained from the Otsuka Pharmaceutical Co., Ltd. (Hangzhou, Zhejiang, China). Liquid paraffin was supplied by Beifang Tianyi Chemical Reagent Co. (Tianjin, China). Span-80 and Tween-80 were purchased from Sigma-Aldrich Co. (St. Louis, MO, USA). Micronized $CaCO_3$ (40 nm) was provided by Wangyong Technology, Ltd. (Beijing, China). Methanol for HPLC analysis was obtained from Merck Co. (Darmstadt, Germany). Deionized water was obtained from a Milli-Q water purification system (Merck Millipore, Bedford, MA, USA).The simulated gastric fluid (SGF, pH 1.2) composed of 7 mL 36.5% HCl, 2g NaCl and 1000 mL deionized water and the simulated intestinal fluid (SIF, pH 6.8) composed of 6.8g $K_2HPO_4$, 1.2g NaOH and 1000 mL distilled water were prepared as described in Chinese Pharmacopoeia 2010. All other solvents and reagents were analytical grade and used without further modification. The Prostaglandin $E_2$ Express EIA Monoclonal Kit was obtained from R&D (Ann Arbor, MI, USA). The IL-6 Mouse ELISA Kit, IL-1β Mouse ELISA Kit and TNF-α Mouse ELISA Kit were obtained from eBioscience (San Diego, CA, USA).

Male Sprague Dawley rats weighing 180–200 g and C57 black mice (6 weeks old, weighing 18–22 g) were obtained from the Vital River Laboratory Animal Technology Co., Ltd. (Beijing, China). The animals were housed under standard conditions of temperature (24 ± 1 °C), relative humidity (55% ± 10%), and 12 h/12 h light/dark cycle and fed standard pellet and water *ad libitum*. Animals were housed for 5 days under these conditions to adapt to the experimental environment. Animals described as fasted were deprived of food for 24 h but had free access to water. All protocols used in this study were in accordance with NIH Guide for the Care and Use of Laboratory Animals and approved by the Ethics Committee of Tianjin University of Traditional Chinese Medicine (TCM-2009-037-E15).

**Figure 2.** Chemical structure of puerarin.

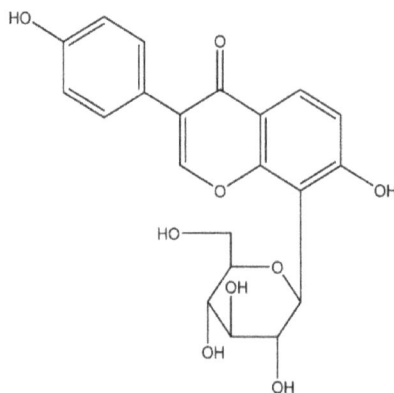

*2.2. Preparation of Mucoadhesive Microparticles*

A modified emulsification-internal gelatin method was employed to prepare Ca-Alg gel beads as described previously [41]. Briefly, 0.20 g of calcium carbonate was added to 20 mL of 1.0% (w/v) sodium alginate solution containing 0.50 g puerarin and placed in an ultrasonic bath for 10 min. The suspension was dispersed into 100 mL of light mineral oil containing 1.0% (v/v) Span 80 and 1.0% (v/v) acetic acid at a stirring speed of 500× *g* at 37 °C for 15 min. The Puerarin-Ca-Alg gel beads were rinsed with 200 mL of 1% (v/v) Tween 80 in aqueous solution and then with 100 mL of deionized water thrice to remove any traces of oil from the Puerarin-Ca-Alg gel bead surface. Puerarin microparticles were prepared by immersing 0.5 mL of Puerarin-Ca-Alg gel beads into a chitosan acetic acid solution (1%, v/v) for 20 min at room temperature. During the coating process, Puerarin-Ca-Alg gel beads were gently shaken to ensure a uniform reaction. Afterwards, Puerarin microparticles were frozen and lyophilized in a Savant ModulyoD freeze-drier (Thermo, Holbrook, NK, USA). The properties of the microparticles are listed in Table 1 (formulations A0-A5). Three batches of microparticles were prepared for further study.

**Table 1.** The mean size of different composition microparticles prepared by emulsification-internal gelatin method.

| Formulation | Composition (as(w/w) Ratio) | | Coagulation Fluid (%(w/v)) | Mean Size (μm) (±S.D.) |
| --- | --- | --- | --- | --- |
| | Alginate | Puerarin | Chitosan | |
| A1 | 1 | 0.5 | 0 | 50.3 ± 11.2 |
| A2 | 1 | 0.5 | 0.4 | 69.3 ± 17.6 |
| A3 | 1 | 0.5 | 0.7 | 86.3 ± 20.5 |
| A4 | 1 | 0.5 | 1 | 112.3 ± 7.8 |
| A5 | 1 | 0.5 | 1.3 | 124.7 ± 25.6 |

*2.3. Characterization of the Microparticles*

2.3.1. Morphological Examination

The morphology of the microparticles was observed via optical microscopy (Nikon FA-35, Tokyo, Japan) and scanning electron microscopy (SEM, Hitachi SU70, Tokyo, Japan). For optical microscopy, the microparticles were directly observed under magnification. Prior to SEM examination, lyophilized microparticles were mounted on mental stubs using double-sided tape and coated with a 150 Å layer of gold under vacuum.

2.3.2. Particle Size Measurement

The particle size of the microparticles was measured using a stage micrometer scale. Dry microparticles (3 mg) were suspended in distilled water and ultrasonicated for 10 s. A drop of suspension was placed on a clean glass slide, and the microparticles were counted under optical microscopy. A minimum of 200 microparticles was counted per batch.

2.3.3. Differential Scanning Calorimetry (DSC) Analysis

DSC was recorded on a Perkin-Elmer DSC7 (Perkin-Elmer, Norwalk, CT, USA). The samples of sodium alginate (A); chitosan (B); puerarin (C); blank microparticles (D) and puerarin microparticles (E) were freeze-dried. Lyophilized samples (5–8 mg) were heated from 30 to 350 °C in crimped standard aluminum hermetic pans at a heating rate of 10 °C per min with a constant purging of nitrogen at 100 mL per min. The system was calibrated with indium (melting point of 156.86 °C).

2.3.4. Fourier Transform Infrared Spectroscopy (FT-IR)

The FT-IR transmission spectra were recorded on a Bio-Rad FTS 3000 spectrophotometer (Bio-Rad, Richmond, CA, USA) in the wave number range 4000–400 cm$^{-1}$ using KBr pellets. The samples of sodium alginate (A); chitosan (B); puerarin (C); blank microparticles (D) and puerarin microparticles (E) were freeze-dried, and a total of 2% (w/w) of samples were mixed with potassium bromide. The mixtures were ground into fine powders, and disks were compressed for scanning. Each sample was assessed in triplicate at a minimum.

*2.4. Determination of Drug Loading, Encapsulation Efficiency and Swelling Ratio*

Drug loading and encapsulation efficiency were measured after extracting drug from the prepared puerarin microparticles. Briefly, 100 mg of drug-loaded microparticles were added to 10 mL of methanol and sonicated for 30 min to ensure the complete extraction of puerarin. Each test group was performed in triplicate. After equilibrium was attained, the samples were filtered through 0.22-μm pore size syringe filters and assayed by HPLC. Determination was performed on a Waters 2695 system (Waters, New York, NY, USA) equipped with a 2487 dual λ absorbance detector. 5 μL of samples were injected onto a Thermo Hypersil ODS-2 Column (250 mm × 4.6 mm, 5 μm) at 25 °C. All samples were detected with a mobile phase of a mixture of methanol-water (75:25, v/v) at a flow rate of 1.0 mL/min. Chromatograms were monitored at 250 nm. The drug loading (%) and encapsulation efficiency (%) were calculated using the following equations, respectively:

$$drug\ loading(\%) = \frac{weight\ of\ drug\ in\ sample}{weight\ of\ sample} \times 100 \tag{1}$$

$$Encapsulation\ efficiency(\%) = \frac{weight\ of\ drug\ in\ sample}{theoretical\ drug\ loading} \tag{2}$$

The swelling properties of puerarin microparticles were assessed in the SGF (pH 1.2). Puerarin microparticles (0.10 g) were placed in the baskets of intelligent dissolution apparatus (ZRS-8G, Tianjin University Wireless factory, Tianjin, China) containing 200 mL of SGF (pH 1.2) and stirred at 37 ± 0.5 °C at 50 rpm. The swelled beads were removed at predetermined time intervals and weighed after drying the surface with tissue paper. The swelling ratio was determined using following formula:

$$Swelling\ ration = \frac{Weight\ of\ beads\ after\ swelling - Dry\ weight\ of\ beads}{Dry\ weight\ of\ beads} \times 100 \tag{3}$$

*2.5. Drug Release Study in Vitro*

*In vitro* release experiments were performed using the USP 30 NO. 2 dissolution test apparatus fixed with six rotating paddles (ZRS-8G, Tianjin University Wireless Factory, Tianjin, China). The release media are SGF (pH 1.2) and SIF (pH 6.8) (500 mL, 37.5 ± 0.5 °C), and the rotation speed was 50 ± 1 rpm. The dried microparticles (500 mg) were placed into each cup, and 5 mL of solution was withdrawn from the release medium at regular intervals, and the same amount of the fresh buffer solution was added to maintain a constant volume. The collected solution (2 mL) was filtered through a membrane with a pore size of 0.22 μm. Each test group was performed in triplicate. The concentration of puerarin was assayed using the above mentioned HPLC method, and then the cumulative percentage of puerarin released was obtained. The dissolution results were the average of three measurements.

## 2.6. Evaluation of Mucoadhesiveness in Vitro

The puerarin microparticles were tested for mucoadhesiveness according to the method designed by Rao and Buri [42]. Briefly, the stomachs obtained from male Sprague-Dawley rats (180–200 g) subjected to fasting 24 h were opened along the great curvature and rinsed in SGF (pH 1.2). In addition, the small intestines (jejunum) obtained from the same rats were cut longitudinally and rinsed in physiological saline. The experiment to evaluate the adhesive properties began within 2 h after dissection. Stomach tissue was cut into $2 \times 1$ cm pieces, and jejunum tissue (4 cm in length) was prepared. Two-hundred microspheres of each were scattered uniformly on the surface of the stomach mucosa. Then, the mucosa with the microparticles was placed in a chamber maintained at 93% relative humidity and room temperature. After 20 min, the tissues were removed and fixed on a polyethylene support at a 45° angle. The stomach and intestine tissues were rinsed with SGF (pH 1.2) and SIF (pH 6.8) for 5 min at a rate of 22 mL/min. The microparticles remaining at the surface of the gastric mucosa were counted, and the percentage of the remaining microparticles was calculated and statistically analyzed.

## 2.7. Fluorescence Imaging of the Gastrointestinal Tract

To observe the behavior of microparticles *in vivo* more precisely, chitosan was labeled with FITC via chemical reaction at the isothiocyanate group of FITC and the primary amino group of chitosan [43]. In brief, FITC-labeled chitosan was synthesized by adding 10 mL of methanol followed by 5 mL of FITC in methanol (2.0 mg/mL) to 10 mL of chitosan (1% in 0.1 M CH$_3$COOH) in the dark at ambient temperature. After 5 h, the labeled polymer was precipitated in 0.2 M NaOH. The precipitate was pelleted at $35,000 \times g$ (15 min) and washed with methanol: water (70:30, v/v). The washing and pelletization were repeated until no fluorescence was detected in the supernatant (Perkin-Elmer LS-5B Luminescence spectrometer, Beaconsfield, England, $\lambda_{exc}$ = 490 nm, $\lambda_{emi}$ = 520 nm). Finally, the labeled chitosan was frozen and lyophilized.

C57 black mice were fasted overnight with free access to water before the experiments. A certain amount of FITC-labeled chitosan (FITC-CS)-coated microparticles was administered into fifteen male C57 black mice. At certain times (0, 2, 4, 6, and 8 h), the mice were sacrificed. Then, the stomach, duodenum, jejunum and colon were excised and observed using the Kodak In-vivo Imaging System FX Pro (Kodak, Rochester, NY, USA).

*2.8. Gastro-Protective Studies in Rats*

2.8.1. Ethanol-Induced Gastric Injury in Rats

The rats were deprived of food but had *ad libitum* access to tap water for overnight before ulcer induction. Gastric mucosal damage was induced in conscious rats by gavage of 5.0 mL/kg of absolute ethanol. Puerarin microparticles were suspended in normal saline. Animals were randomized into eight groups ($n$ = 6): control, ethanol, omeprazole (20 mg/kg) + ethanol, rebamipide (100 mg/kg) + ethanol, puerarin microparticles (150 mg/kg) + ethanol, puerarin microparticles (300 mg/kg) + ethanol, puerarin microparticles (450 mg/kg) + ethanol, and puerarin microparticles (600 mg/kg) + ethanol. All of the rats in groups were pre-treated by gavages with puerarin microparticles and control drugs (omeprazole and rebamipide) 120 min prior to ethanol administration. Four hours later, the animals were sacrificed, and their stomachs were excised. Each stomach was cut along the greater curvature and rinsed thoroughly with normal saline; then, macroscopic determination of the gastric mucosal injury index was performed.

2.8.2. Determination of the Ulcer Index and Percent Inhibition

The ulcer index (UI) and percent inhibition were calculated in ethanol-induced rats. To determine the ulcer index, the stomach was examined for ulceration using a simple dissecting microscope. The stomach was examined under the microscope to observe erosions. The stomachs were scored using the following scale: 1, small round hemorrhagic erosion; 2, hemorrhagic erosions <1 mm; 3, hemorrhagic erosion 2–3 mm in size; and 4, hemorrhagic erosion >4 mm. The scores were multiplied by 2 when the width of the erosion was larger than 1 mm [44].The UI for each animal was calculated as the mean ulcer score ($mm^2$). The percentage of inhibition (I %) was calculated using the following formula:

$$I\% = \left( \frac{U\,A_{control} - U\,A_{treated}}{U\,A_{control}} \right) \times 100 \qquad (4)$$

2.8.3. Histopathology

A small fragment of the gastric wall from each animal was fixed in 10% buffered formalin solution followed by tissue dehydrated with alcohol and xylene. Then, each sample was embedded in paraffin wax and sectioned into 5-μm slides prior to staining. To evaluate mucus production, periodic acid Schiff Base (PAS) was used for initiative staining following the manufacturer's instructions (Periodic Acid-Schiff (PAS) Kit, Sigma-Aldrich Co., St. Louis, MO, USA). Then, some slides were also stained with hematoxylin and eosin (H & E).

2.8.4. Measurement of Cytokine, Production (TNF-α, 1L-1β, IL-6 and PGE2)

A 10% (v/w) gastric mucosa homogenate was prepared in PBS buffer (10 mM phosphate buffer, pH 7.4, 130 mM NaCl, and 4 mM KCl) and centrifuged at 12,000× $g$ for 10 min at 4 °C. The resultant supernatant was used to evaluate TNF-α, IL-6, 1L-1β and PGE2 levels in rat stomach tissues using corresponding ELISA kits according to the manufacturers' instructions. Total protein concentrations in the supernatants were determined using a Pierce BCA Protein Assay Kit (Rockford, IL, USA). Furthermore, the relative amounts of TNF-α, IL-6, 1L-1β and $PEG_2$ were determined as milligram of total protein in the gastric mucosa tissues.

## 2.9. Statistical Analysis

The results analysis for the *in vitro* acitvity of puerarin microparticles were expressed as means ± S.D. and the results of *in vivo* activity of puerarin micropartivles were expressed as means ± S.E. The statistical analysis was performed by analysis of variance (ANOVA) followed by Dunnett's test. The data were evaluated with SPSS 17.0 (SPSS Inc., Chicago, IL, USA). The criterion for statistical significance was $p < 0.01$ or $p < 0.05$.

## 3. Results and Discussion

### 3.1. Characterization of the Puerarin Microparticles

#### 3.1.1. Morphological Observations of Puerarin Microparticles

The morphological characterization of the puerarin microparticles was performed by optical microscopy and SEM (Figure 3). As shown in Figure 3B, microparticles prepared by this method appeared as well-rounded spheres with uniform size distribution under optical microscopy. This arrangement was attributed to the fact that the alginate gel beads were formed from the interaction between $Ca^{2+}$ and guluronic acid residues of alginate, and puerarin microparticles were obtained by chitosan solidification. Figure 3A indicates that after lyophilization, the puerarin microparticles exhibited very rough surfaces with characteristic large wrinkles. This phenomenon may be caused by the unique structure of the Ca-Alg gel, which contains 99%–99.5% water [45]. Interestingly, the coarse and wrinkled microparticle surface might improve its mucoadhesion *in vivo* [46].

#### 3.1.2. Particle Size

Previous reports suggested that the size of the beads increases with increasing concentrations of chitosan in the coagulation fluid [2]. In this study, the mean particle size of the microparticles (formulations A0–A5) increased from 50.3 to 124.7 μm as the concentration of chitosan increased in the coagulation fluid (Table 1). Furthermore, Figure 3C indicates a narrow particle size distribution of microspheres.

**Figure 3.** The morphological characterization of the puerarin microparticles. The SEM micrograph of puerarin microparticles (**A**); optical micrograph of puerarin microparticles (**B**); and particle size distribution of puerarin microparticles (**C**).

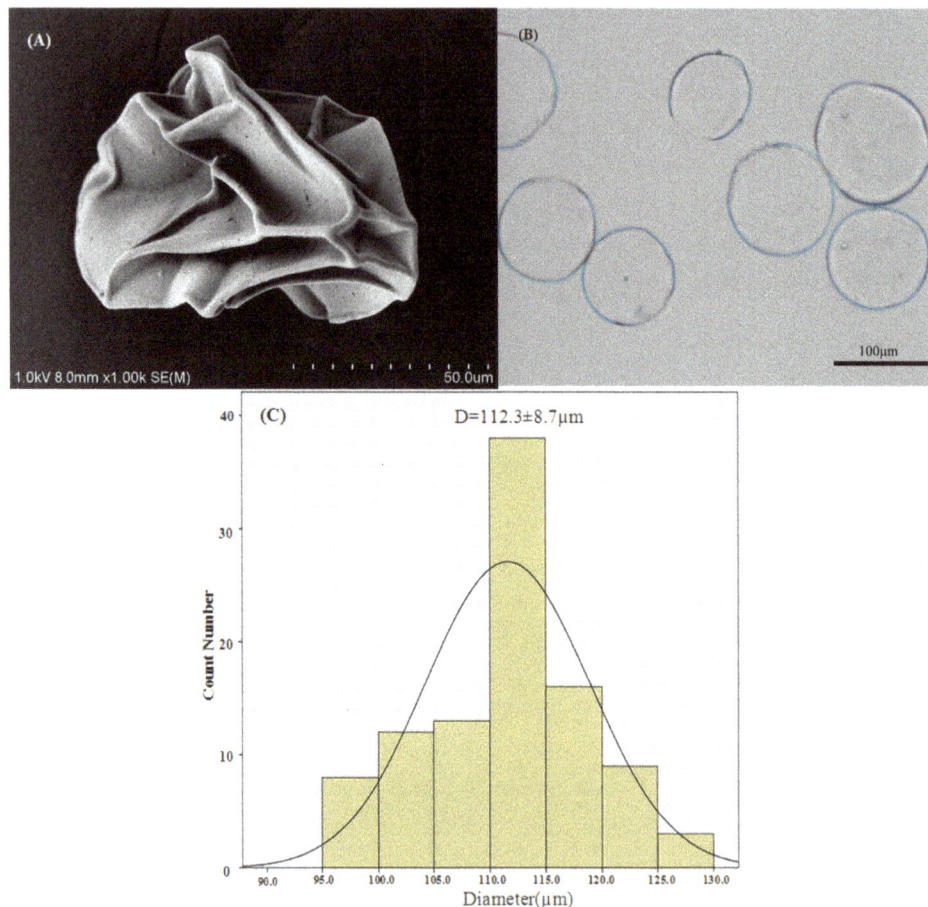

## 3.1.3. DSC analysis

The DSC characteristics of sodium alginate (A); chitosan (B); puerarin (C); blank microparticles (D) and puerarin microparticles (E) are presented. All of the curves were merged into one picture after standardizing the units and scales. In the calorimetric studies, the thermogram of sodium alginate is characterized by an exothermic peak at 246.1 °C due to polymer degradation and exhibits the temperature for sodium alginate degradation (Figure 4A). The DSC scans of chitosan demonstrate an exothermic baseline deviation at approximately 305 °C, which indicates the onset of chitosan degradation (Figure 4B). The puerarin powder exhibited a sharp but wide endothermic peak at 234.56 °C and 207.11 °C, indicating the melting points and that puerarin was in the polymorphs. However, Figure 4D indicates that the spectrum of puerarin microparticles exhibited neither a single nor a double characteristic exothermic peak of two polymers but rather a slightly broad band at a range of 222–277 °C, which indicates the interaction between chitosan and alginate in the blank microparticles. As shown in Figure 4E, the melting point of puerarin microparticles was slightly changed from 217.2 °C to 240.4 °C. The shapes of the peaks were also altered as the peak at 217.2 °C was reduced and the peak at 240.2 °C was stronger.

**Figure 4.** DSC thermograms of sodium alginate (**A**); chitosan (**B**); puerarin (**C**); blank microparticles (**D**) and puerarin microparticles (**E**).

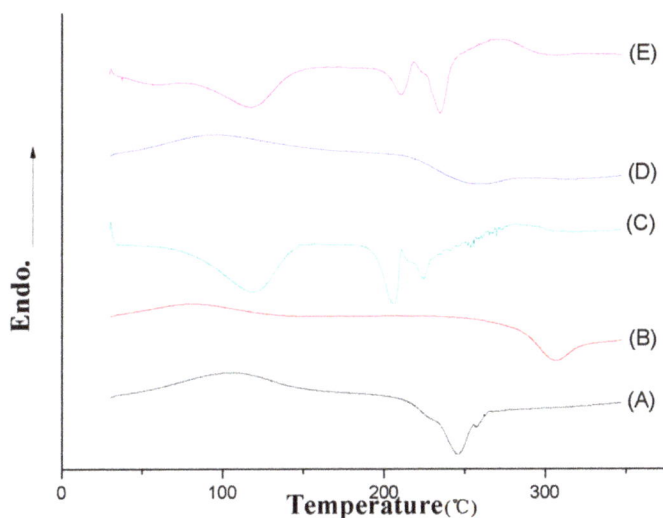

3.1.4. FT-IR Spectroscopy

FT-IR analysis allows for the observation of vibration modes for the specific groups of compounds analyzed [47]. Therefore, infrared spectra of sodium alginate (A); chitosan (B); puerarin (C); blank microparticles (D) and puerarin microparticles (E) are presented in Figure 5. In the sodium alginate IR spectrum (Figure 5A), we observed vibration mode in the band of 1596 to 1421 cm$^{-1}$, which can be attributed to carboxyl group (COO-). A wide absorption band around 1031 cm$^{-1}$ was observed due to the C-OH stretch. Moreover, the IR spectrum of chitosan (Figure 5B) exhibits peaks at 1662, 1590, and 1428 cm$^{-1}$, characterizing the amino groups (-NH$^{3+}$); a band around 1070 cm$^{-1}$ can be attributed to –CH-OH stretch. As shown in Figure 5C, there are three absorption peaks at 1630, 1588 and 1260 cm$^{-1}$, which correspond to the aldehyde group (C=O) stretching vibration, benzene skeleton vibration, and C-O absorption peak. By analyzing the IR spectra of the absorption spectrum of the blank microparticles (Figure 5D), differences were noted in the vibration modes of their peaks compared with the polymers alone. In detail, the appearance of the bands at 1631 cm$^{-1}$, 1447 cm$^{-1}$ and 2922 cm$^{-1}$ as well as the disappearance of the band at 1590 cm$^{-1}$ (the characteristic peak of the chitosan amino group) suggest the formation of a polyelectrolyte complex between sodium alginate and chitosan. As shown in Figure 5E, two wide absorption band around 1447 and 1060 cm$^{-1}$ are noted that are similar to the infrared spectrum of the blank microparticles, indicating a polyelectrolyte complex has been formed. In addition, two characteristic peaks of puerarin at 1630 and 1260 cm$^{-1}$

in the infrared spectra of puerarin microparticles are evident, which indicates that puerarin has been loaded into the microparticles.

Figure 5. The FT-IR spectra of different compounds of puerarin microparticles. FT-IR spectra of sodium alginate (A); chitosan (B); puerarin (C); blank microparticles (D) and puerarin microparticles (E).

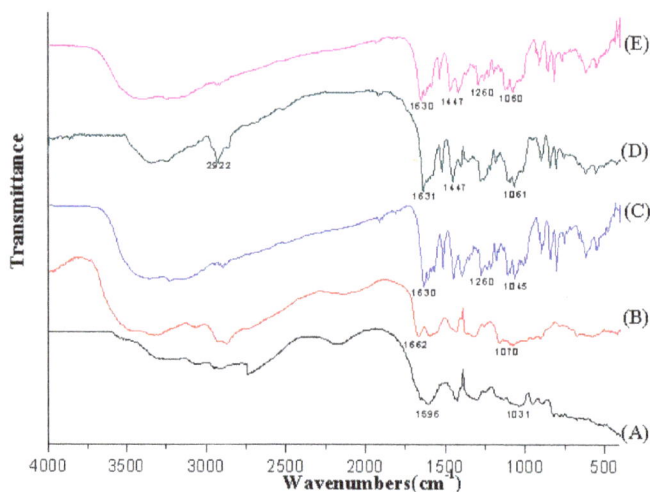

*3.2. Drug Loading, Encapsulation Efficiency and Swelling*

Variation in the concentrations of chitosan greatly impacts drug loading and encapsulation efficiency in chitosan-alginate beads. In the absence of chitosan, the drug loading of microparticles was very low (5.1%, Table 2, A1), which is potentially attributed to insufficient cross-linking and the fact that the structure of the gel network allows puerarin diffusion. The addition of 0.4%–1.0% of chitosan to the coagulation fluid (A2, A3, and A4) resulted in a large increase of the drug loading and encapsulation efficiency owing to increased firmness in the alginate-chitosan complex between the carboxylate groups in the alginate and the protonated amine groups in the chitosan. As a result, less puerarin was lost during gelation. In the presence of more chitosan, this process also occurs due to the increased number of alginate-chitosan ionic linkages. However, the drug loading may be relatively low than others, which may be attributed to the multilayer chitosan microparticles (A5).

Previous articles reported that the adhesive properties and cohesiveness of mucoadhesive polymers are generally affected by their swelling behavior [48]. Mucoadhesive microparticles take up water from the underlying mucosal tissue by absorbing, swelling, and capillary effects, leading to considerably stronger adhesion [49]. Alginate beads coated with chitosan exhibited increased swelling ability (132%–222%), with an optimal chitosan concentration of 1% (w/v) with 222% swelling ratio that was reduced to 179% with 0.7% (w/v) chitosan. The lower chitosan concentration may be insufficient to protect air bubbles inside the beads from the surrounding medium, resulting in shrinking. Higher (1.3% (w/v)) chitosan exhibited a swelling ratio comparable to 0.7% (w/v) chitosan owing to an increased concentration of coagulation fluid, which yielded larger, thicker beads. The thicker chitosan layer may cause solution uptake, leading to a higher bulk density than the external medium and shrinking [50]. Based on the drug loading, encapsulation efficiency and swelling ratio data, 1% chitosan was chosen as the optimal coagulation fluid.

**Table 2.** The entrapment and swelling ratio of different compositions microparticles prepared by emulsification-internal gelatin method.

| Formulation | Entrapment Efficiency (%) | Drug Loading (%) | Swelling Ratio (%) (±S.D.) |
|---|---|---|---|
| A1 | 70.3 | 5.1 | 69 ± 11 |
| A2 | 84.3 | 10.4 | 132 ± 18 |
| A3 | 90.8 | 15.9 | 179 ± 12 |
| A4 | 98.5 | 34.7 | 222 ± 2 |
| A5 | 99.2 | 23.2 | 175 ± 11 |

*3.3. In Vitro Drug Release Results*

The *in vitro* drug release studies were performed for puerarin mucoadhesive microparticles composite beads in SGF (pH 1.2) and SIF (pH 6.8) (500 mL, 37.5 ± 0.5 °C) for 12 h, respectively. As shown in Figure 6, the puerarin release profile from microparticles in SGF exhibited different behaviors compare with that in SIF. The time taken to release stable in SGF and SIF was 7 ± 0.2, 5 ± 0.3 h, respectively. After 12 h, the cumulative release of the puerarin microparticles was 93.50% in SGF, considerably higher than that in SIF (52.18%). The increased release of puerarin from microparticles might be attributed to the increased solubility of chitosan in acidic medium. Thus, from a more practical point of view, the puerarin mucoadhesive microparticles can liberate substantial amounts of puerarin in acidic gastric fluid and minimize the release in the intestines, achieving the purpose of the controlled release of puerarin side-specific particles in the stomach.

**Figure 6.** Puerarin release curves in different media: SGF (pH 1.2) and SIF (pH 6.8).

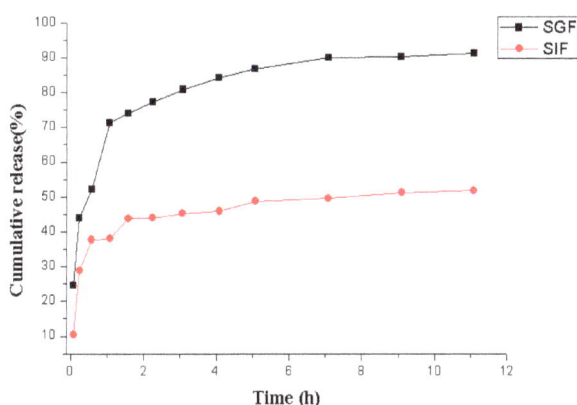

*3.4. In Vitro Evaluation of Mucoadhesiveness*

The *in vitro* adhesiveness test (Table 3) revealed that the percentage of puerarin microparticles remaining on the gastric mucosa (92.6% ± 1.7%, $n = 3$) was increased compare with the small intestinal mucosa (30.6% ± 1.7%, $n = 3$). The increased mucoadhesion of puerarin microparticles was expected to be directly related to the pH of the medium as demonstrated with chitosan. Therefore, results suggested microparticles possessed a better mucoadhesivity in stomach.

**Table 3.** Percent of Microparticles Remaining after Rinsing Mucosa of the Stomach and Small Intestine with SGF and SIF, respectively.

| Number | % of Microparticles Remaining | |
| --- | --- | --- |
| | Stomach SGF | Small Intestine SIF |
| 1 | 92.5 | 30.5 |
| 2 | 91.0 | 29.0 |
| 3 | 94.5 | 32.5 |
| Average | 92.6 ± 1.7 | 30.6 ± 1.7 |

*3.5. Fluorescence Imaging of the Gastrointestinal Tract*

We assumed that increasing gastric residence time of the microparticles is one of the key features that enhances the bioavailability of puerarin in the gastric mucosa. The gastric residence time of FITC-CS microparticles were monitored using the *In-vivo* Imaging System FX Pro (Kodak, Rochester, NY, USA) as shown in Figure 7. These results suggested that FITC-CS microparticles adhere to the gastric mucosa after intragastric administration. Even at 6 h and 8 h, the fluorescence intensities of FITC-CS microparticles on the surface of gastric mucosa were still relatively high, which indicated that the microparticles possess enhanced mucoadhesive properties; therefore, microparticles adhered to the gastric mucosa prevent gastric acid from eroding the gastric mucosa. This phenomenon may be explained by the interaction between the carboxy groups of chitosan and the gastric acid in mucin molecules, which is responsible for enhancing the permeability of gastroretentive delivery and enhancing the effective drug absorption [33,51].

*3.6. Gastro-Protective Study Results*

3.6.1. Ulcer Index and Percent Inhibition

The anti-ulcer effects of puerarin mucoadhesive microparticles on the ethanol-induced ulcer model in rats are presented in Figure 8. When rats were treated with ethanol (5 mL/kg) alone, extensive and visible gastric lesions were observed in the surface epithelial cells of gastric mucosa (Figure 8B) with an UI score of 24.72 ± 1.32. However, pre-treatment with puerarin mucoadhesive microparticles protected ethanol-induced gastric injury in a dose-dependent manner (Table 4). At a dose of 600 mg/kg, puerarin mucoadhesive microparticles significantly ($p < 0.01$) reduced the intensity of gastric mucosal damage and demonstrated increased gastroprotective activity (79.3%) compared with the control drug rebamipide (77.3%). The results of the present study demonstrated that animals pretreated with puerarin mucoadhesive microparticles (Figure 8E–H) exhibited a dose-dependent protection of mucosal layer damage and a substantial reduction in continuous gastric mucosa hyperemia (Figure 8A). Ethanol consumption is known to be one of many factors causing gastric ulcer formation owing to the generation of oxygen-derived free radicals, such as superoxide anions, lipid peroxides, and hydroxyl radicals [52]. The obtained results indicate that the puerarin mucoadhesive microparticles may exhibit strong antioxidant and radical scavenging potential, suppressing ethanol-induced depletion of gastric mucosa in rats.

**Figure 7.** The fluorescence intensity of FITC-CS microparticles in different tissues (Left→Right: Stomach, Duodenum, Jejunum and Colon) varied from 0 to 8 h.

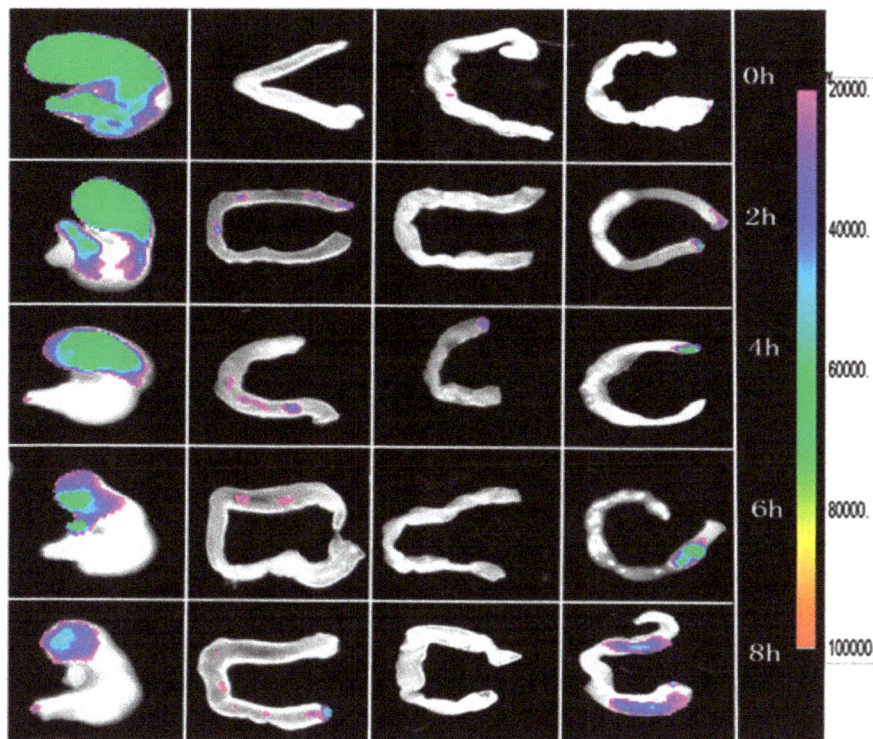

**Table 4.** The effect of puerarin microspheres on gastric ulcer index and inhibition of ethanol-induced gastric mucosal lesions in rats.

| Animal Group | Pre-Treatment | Ulcer Index (Score) (Mean ± S.E.) | Inhibition (%) |
|:---:|:---:|:---:|:---:|
| A | Normal control | -- | -- |
| B | Ulcer control | 24.72 ± 1.32 | 0 |
| C | Omeprazole (20 mg/kg) | 4.93 ± 0.36 | 80.0 |
| D | Rebamipide (100 mg/kg) | 5.61 ± 0.55 | 77.3 |
| E | Microspheres (150 mg/kg) | 19.96 ± 1.15 | 19.3 |
| F | Microspheres (300 mg/kg) | 12.53 ± 0.98 | 49.3 |
| G | Microspheres (450 mg/kg) | 7.92 ± 0.76 | 68.0 |
| H | Microspheres (600 mg/kg) | 5.87 ± 0.61 | 76.2 |

**Figure 8.** Effect of puerarin microparticles on ethanol-induced gastric ulcer in rats. (**A**) Control group; (**B**) Ethanol group, 5.0 mL/kg; (**C**) Omprazole, 20 mg/kg; (**D**) Rebamipide, 100 mg/kg; (**E**) Puerarin microparticles, 150 mg/kg; (**F**) Puerarin microparticles, 300 mg/kg; (**G**) Puerarin microparticles, 450 mg/kg; (**H**) Puerarin microparticles, 600 mg/kg. All drugs were orally administered.

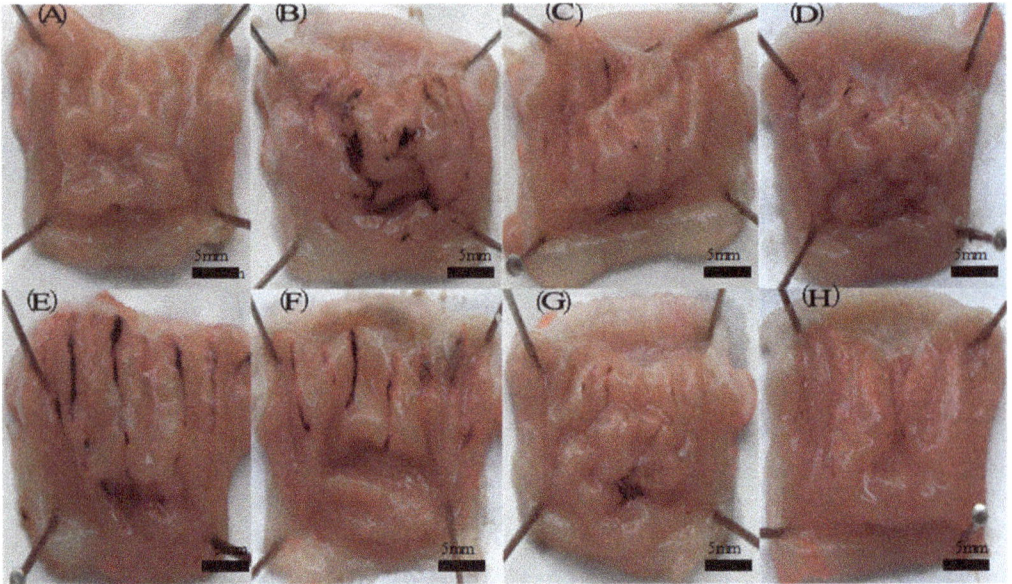

### 3.6.2. Histological Results

To confirm the results of preventing ethanol-induced gastric damage, the stomachs were evaluated by histological observation using PAS staining in the superficial layer of the gastric mucosa. The PAS staining abnormality is used to observe glycogen levels in tissues. The gastric mucosa in animals pretreated with standard drugs (omeprazole and rebamipide) (Figure 9C,D) or puerarin mucoadhesive microparticles (Figure 9E–H) exhibited substantial expansion of a continuous PAS-positive mucous gel layer that lined the entire gastric mucosal surface (magenta color), indicating an increase in the glycoprotein content of the gastric mucosa in pretreated rats. As shown in Figure 9, rats treated with absolute ethanol exhibited disrupted epithelial cells from the upper portion of fundic glands, vacuolization, necrosis and deep dilated inter-glandular spices (Figure 9B) compared with the stomach of normal animals (Figure 9A). Pre-treatment with puerarin mucoadhesive microparticles (Figure 9E–H) or standard drugs (omeprazole and rebamipide) (Figure 9C,D) afford relatively enhanced protection by decreasing gastric ulcer damage, with only slight damage observed in the superficial epithelium (Figure 9G–H). Puerarin microparticles (Figure 9H) exhibited slightly enhanced reduction in gastric ulcer damage compared with the standard drug rebamipide (Figure 9D). With regard to reducing epithelial cell damage, puerarin microparticles protected against mucosal layer damage in a dose-dependent fashion.

**Figure 9.** Effect of puerarin microparticles on gastric tissue glycoprotein-PAS staining of ethanol-induced gastric damage in rats. (**A**) Control group; (**B**) Ethanol group; 5 mL/kg; (**C**) Omprazole, 20 mg/kg; (**D**) Rebamipide, 100 mg/kg; (**E**) Puerarin microparticles, 150 mg/kg; (**F**) Puerarin microparticles, 300 mg/kg; (**G**) Puerarin microparticles, 450 mg/kg; and (**H**) Puerarin microparticles, 600 mg/kg. The black arrows indicate the glycoprotein, which appears as a magenta stain, and the red arrows indicate loss of continuity. (PAS stain 200×).

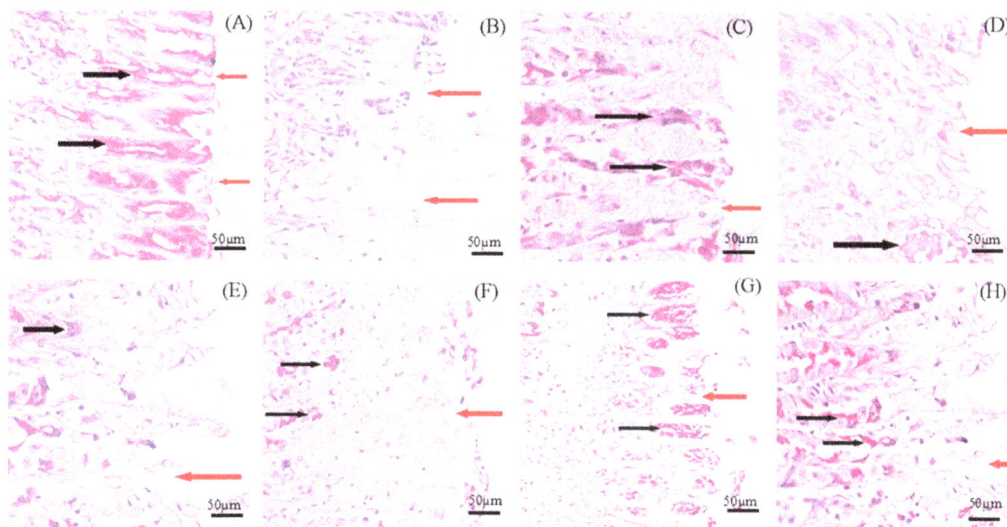

3.6.3. Measurement of TNF-α, 1L-1β, IL-6 Expression and PGE$_2$ Production

Excessive alcohol consumption can produce acute hemorrhagic gastric erosions, and even result in gastritis characterized by mucosal edema, sub-epithelial hemorrhages, cellular exfoliation, and inflammatory cell infiltration, which is an essential acute inflammatory reaction [53]. TNF-α, 1L-1β, IL-6 and PGE2, which are related to the immunopathology of acute or chronic inflammatory diseases, were considered as primary pro-inflammatory cytokines and mediators. As Figure 10 demonstrates, ethanol-induced gastric injury resulted in a burst of TNF-α (A); 1L-1β (B); IL-6 (C) expression and PGE$_2$ (D) production, whereas mice administered standard drugs (omeprazole and rebamipide) and puerarin mucoadhesive microparticles (300, 450 and 600 mg/kg) exhibited significantly reduced increased in TNF-α, 1L-1β and IL-6 ($p < 0.01$) and antagonized the reduction of PGE2 in a concentration-dependent manner.

Considering the industrial process and the possibility of clinical application in the future, we designed a novel core-shell type pH-sensitive mucoadhesive microparticle containing puerarin. This novel mucoadhesive microparticle uses a unique biomaterial combination of chitosan and sodium alginates, which are FDA approved and successfully used in a variety of biomedical applications and products. To improve the mucoadhesive properties of polymeric excipients, numerous attempts have been undertaken based on the gastric-specific delivery, such as thiolated chitosans [6] and chitosan–carboxymethylcellulose [54]; however, these matrix materials do not have FDA approval and have not been used in clinical applications. However, we design this gastric-specific delivery system using FDA-approved materials and simple technological preparations, thereby potentially allowing the realization of industrial production.

**Figure 10.** Effect of puerarin microparticles on TNF-α, IL-6, IL-1β, and PGE₂ levels in ethanol-induced gastric mucosa tissues. TNF-α (A); IL-1β (B); IL-6 (C) and PGE₂ (D) in stomach tissue were analyzed by commercially available ELISA kits. # $p < 0.05$ ($n = 6$) compared with the control group, * $p < 0.05$; ** $p < 0.01$ ($n = 6$) compared with the ethanol group.

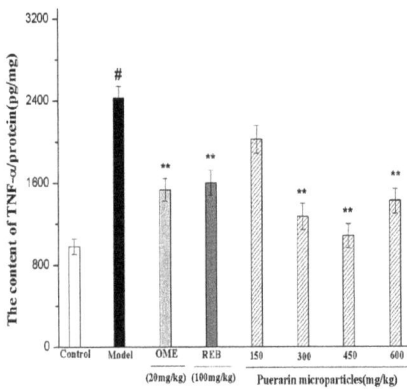

(A)

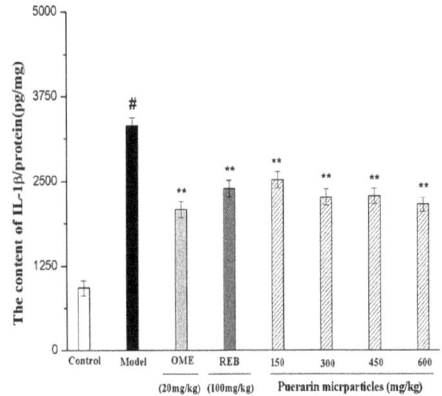

(B)

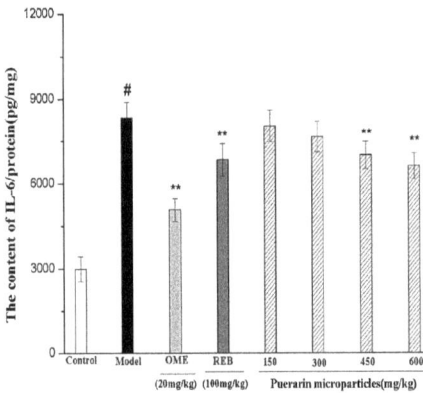

(C)

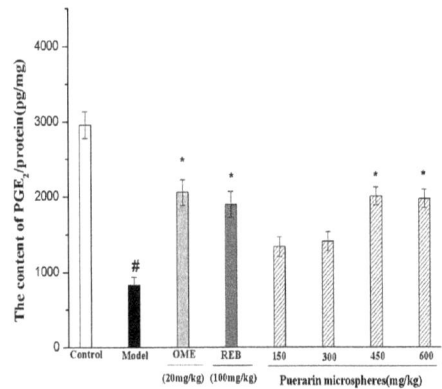

(D)

Peptic ulcers arise from imbalances between offensive factors, such as gastric acid, and protective factors, such as prostaglandins. Gastric acid plays an important role in the pathogenesis of gastric ulcers as stated by the dictum of Karl Schwartz—"no acid, no ulcer" [55]—which has been quoted for decades. Over the last century, therapies for peptic ulcers have evolved from surgery to acid suppressants along with *Helicobacter pylori* eradication [8]. Omeprazole, a benzimidazole proton pump inhibitor (H⁺/K⁺ATP-ase), has anti-inflammatory and antioxidant properties in addition to its ability to stimulate gastric mucus secretion [56]; this agent serves as one of the most effective ulcer treatment to date. Rebamipide protects the gastric mucosa and promotes the quality of ulcer healing by increasing the glycoprotein content in gastric mucus and decreasing reactive oxygen species [57]. Regarding the treatment of gastric ulcers, both omeprazole and rebamipide rely on a single or partial mechanism, which is not perfect. The developed preparation combines above-standard drug advantages. First, the volume of mucoadhesive microparticles is relatively small, whereas the specific surface area is relatively large. After administration, microparticles quickly form a layer of membrane on the surface of the gastric mucosa, protecting the gastric mucosa from erosion induced by a variety of agents, including ethanol and gastric acid. Moreover, puerarin is the main isoflavone glycoside and a major active ingredient extracted from the traditional Chinese medicine Radix Puerariae. Its many biological actions have been reported by numerous studies, including inflammation [35] and oxidation effects [58] as well as the effects on vascular smooth muscle cells [59] and endothelial cells, [60] which suggest that this compound is an effective medicine used to treat gastric ulcers. More importantly, the developed mucoadhesive microparticles increase the residence time of drugs and sustained drug release for several hours in the stomach so effective drug concentration of drugs can be achieved at the surface of the gastric mucous, eradicating *H. pylori* completely.

These puerarin mucoadhesive microparticles exhibited pH-sensitive properties and extended the drug retention time in the stomach during *in vitro* and *in vivo* evaluations. These results were attributed to the use of sodium alginate as the core bead and chitosan as the coating shell. We determined the antiulcer action of puerarin mucoadhesive microparticles using a rat model of ethanol-induced gastric ulcer. This model is commonly used to evaluate the activity of antiulcer agents. A previous study demonstrated that ethanol-induced gastritis influences the formation of experimentally induced gastric injury in rats [61]. We demonstrated the protective action of puerarin mucoadhesive microparticles against ethanol-induced gastric injury through anti-inflammatory actions accomplished via reduced levels of cytokines, such as TNF-$\alpha$, 1L-1$\beta$, IL-6 and PGE$_2$. Puerarin mucoadhesive microparticles serve as an effective approach for targeting drug release at its site of absorption, sustaining its release, improving its oral availability and promoting gastro-protective effects in the treatment of gastric ulcers.

## 4. Conclusions

In this work, pH-responsive mucoadhesive microparticles of puerarin with a core-shell structure were successfully prepared using an emulsification-internal gelatin method. The encapsulation efficiency of the optimized microparticles containing puerarin was increased compared with other agents. The *in vitro* release test and mucoadhesive tests suggest that the mucoadhesion and cumulative release of puerarin mucoadhesive microparticles were influenced by the pH of the test medium. Based on fluorescence imaging of the gastrointestinal tract, the puerarin mucoadhesive microparticles were retained in the gastrointestinal tract for an extended period of time, adhering to the surface of the gastric wall and improving puerarin bioavailability at the gastric mucosa. Puerarin mucoadhesive microparticles were clearly demonstrated to function as an antiulcer agent by enhancing the gastric mucosal defense. In the puerarin mucoadhesive microparticles-pretreated groups, the microparticles reversed the decrease in PAS staining induced by ethanol; significant increased TNF-α, IL-1β and IL-6 levels; and decreased the level of PGE$_2$.

## Acknowledgments

This work was supported by the Major National S&T Program of China (No. 2012BAI29B02), the Fundamental Research Funds for the Central Universities (NO. 2012LZD06), the Major National Program of China (2060302), the National Natural Science Foundation of China (81473542) and the Specialized Research Fund for the Doctoral Program of Higher Education of China (20131210110008).

## Author Contributions

Conceived and designed the experiments: Fan-Yun Meng and Yuan-Lu Cui. Performed the experiments: Jing-Yi Hou. Analyzed the data: Li-Na Gao. Wrote the paper: Jing-Yi Hou.

## Conflict of Interest

The authors declare no conflict of interest.

## References

1.  Yeomans, N.; Naesdal, J. Systematic review: Ulcer definition in NSAID ulcer prevention trials. *Aliment. Pharmacol. Ther.* **2008**, *27*, 465–472.
2.  Anal, A.K.; Bhopatkar, D.; Tokura, S.; Tamura, H.; Stevens, W.F. Chitosan-alginate multilayer beads for gastric passage and controlled intestinal release of protein. *Drug Dev. Ind. Pharm.* **2003**, *29*, 713–724.
3.  Arao, T.; Udayama, M.; Kinjo, J.; Nohara, T.; Funakoshi, T.; Kojima, S. Preventive effects of saponins from puerariae radix (the root of Pueraria lobata Ohwi) on *in vitro* immunological injury of rat primary hepatocyte cultures. *Biol. Pharm. Bull.* **1997**, *20*, 988–991.
4.  Artursson, P.; Lindmark, T.; Davis, S.S.; Illum, L. Effect of chitosan on the permeability of monolayers of intestinal epithelial cells (Caco-2). *Pharm. Res.* **1994**, *11*, 1358–1361.
5.  Axon, A. The role of acid inhibition in the treatment of Helicobacter pylori infection. *Scand. J. Gastroenterol.* **1994**, *29*, 16–23.
6.  Bernkop-Schnürch, A.; Guggi, D.; Pinter, Y. Thiolated chitosans: development and *in vitro* evaluation of a mucoadhesive, permeation enhancing oral drug delivery system. *J. Control. Release* **2004**, *94*, 177–186.
7.  Fontana, G.; Licciardi, M.; Mansueto, S.; Schillaci, D.; Giammona, G. Amoxicillin-loaded polyethylcyanoacrylate nanoparticles: Influence of PEG coating on the particle size, drug release rate and phagocytic uptake. *Biomaterials* **2001**, *22*, 2857–2865.
8.  Hunt, R.H.; Yuan, Y. Acid-NSAID/Aspirin Interaction in Peptic Ulcer Disease. *Dig. Dis.* **2011**, *29*, 465–468.

9.  Dhaliwal, S.; Jain, S.; Singh, H.P.; Tiwary, A. Mucoadhesive microspheres for gastroretentive delivery of acyclovir: *In vitro* and *in vivo* evaluation. *AAPS J.* **2008**, *10*, 322–330.

10. Le Bail, P.; Morin, F.G.; Marchessault, R.H. Characterization of a crosslinked high amylose starch excipient. *Int. J. Biol. Macromol.* **1999**, *26*, 193–200.

11. Hasani, S.; Pellequer, Y.; Lamprecht, A. Selective adhesion of nanoparticles to inflamed tissue in gastric ulcers. *Pharm. Res.* **2009**, *26*, 1149–1154.

12. Patel, J.K.; Chavda, J.R. Formulation and evaluation of stomach-specific amoxicillin-loaded carbopol-934P mucoadhesive microspheres for anti-Helicobacter pylori therapy. *J. Microencapsul.* **2009**, *26*, 365–376.

13. Schmidgall, J.; Hensel, A., Bioadhesive properties of polygalacturonides against colonic epithelial membranes. *Int. J. Biol. Macromol.* **2002**, *30*, 217–225.

14. Nagahara, N.; Akiyama, Y.; Nakao, M.; Tada, M.; Kitano, M.; Ogawa, Y. Mucoadhesive microspheres containing amoxicillin for clearance of Helicobacter pylori. *Antimicrob. Agents Chemother.* **1998**, *42*, 2492–2494.

15. Han, J.; Zhou, Z.; Yin, R.; Yang, D.; Nie, J. Alginate–chitosan/hydroxyapatite polyelectrolyte complex porous scaffolds: Preparation and characterization. *Int. J. Biol. Macromol.* **2010**, *46*, 199–205.

16. Patel, Y.L.; Sher, P.; Pawar, A.P. The effect of drug concentration and curing time on processing and properties of calcium alginate beads containing metronidazole by response surface methodology. *AAPS PharmSciTech* **2006**, *7*, E24–E30.

17. Yoo, S.-H.; Song, Y.-B.; Chang, P.-S.; Lee, H.G. Microencapsulation of α-tocopherol using sodium alginate and its controlled release properties. *Int. J. Biol. Macromol.* **2006**, *38*, 25–30.

18. Smrdel, P.; Bogataj, M.; Mrhar, A. The influence of selected parameters on the size and shape of alginate beads prepared by ionotropic gelation. *Sci. Pharm.* **2008**, *76*, 77.

19. Liu, Q.; Rauth, A.M.; Liu, J.; Babakhanian, K.; Wang, X.; Bendayan, R.; Wu, X.Y. Characterization of a microsphere formulation containing glucose oxidase and its *in vivo* efficacy in a murine solid tumor model. *Pharm. Res.* **2009**, *26*, 2343–2357.

20. Joshi, A.; Solanki, S.; Chaudhari, R.; Bahadur, D.; Aslam, M.; Srivastava, R. Multifunctional alginate microspheres for biosensing, drug delivery and magnetic resonance imaging. *Acta Biomater.* **2011**, *7*, 3955–3963.

21. Hua, S.; Ma, H.; Li, X.; Yang, H.; Wang, A. pH-sensitive sodium alginate/poly (vinyl alcohol) hydrogel beads prepared by combined $Ca^{2+}$ crosslinking and freeze-thawing cycles for controlled release of diclofenac sodium. *Int. J. Biol. Macromol.* **2010**, *46*, 517–523.

22. Pal, D.; Nayak, A.K. Development, optimization, and anti-diabetic activity of gliclazide-loaded alginate–methyl cellulose mucoadhesive microcapsules. *AAPS PharmSciTech* **2011**, *12*, 1431–1441.

23. Janes, K.; Calvo, P.; Alonso, M. Polysaccharide colloidal particles as delivery systems for macromolecules. *Adv. Drug Deliv. Rev.* **2001**, *47*, 83–97.

24. Guo, B.; Finne-Wistrand, A.; Albertsson, A.-C. Facile Synthesis of Degradable and Electrically Conductive Polysaccharide Hydrogels. *Biomacromolecules* **2011**, *12*, 2601–2609.

25. Whang, H.S.; Kirsch, W.; Zhu, Y.H.; Yang, C.Z.; Hudson, S.M. Hemostatic agents derived from chitin and chitosan. *J. Macromol. Sci. Polym. Rev.* **2005**, *C45*, 309–323.

26. Ji, C.; Khademhosseini, A.; Dehghani, F. Enhancing cell penetration and proliferation in chitosan hydrogels for tissue engineering applications. *Biomaterials* **2011**, *32*, 9719–9729.

27. Ong, S.-Y.; Wu, J.; Moochhala, S.M.; Tan, M.-H.; Lu, J. Development of a chitosan-based wound dressing with improved hemostatic and antimicrobial properties. *Biomaterials* **2008**, *29*, 4323–4332.

28. Tronci, G.; Ajiro, H.; Russell, S.J.; Wood, D.J.; Akashi, M. Tunable drug-loading capability of chitosan hydrogels with varied network architectures. *Acta Biomater.* **2014**, *10*, 821–830.

29. Strand, S.P.; Lelu, S.; Reitan, N.K.; Davies, C.D.L.; Artursson, P.; Varum, K.M. Molecular design of chitosan gene delivery systems with an optimized balance between polyplex stability and polyplex unpacking. *Biomaterials* **2010**, *31*, 975–987.

30. Murata, Y.; Maeda, T.; Miyamoto, E.; Kawashima, S. Preparation of chitosan-reinforced alginate gel beads—Effects of chitosan on gel matrix erosion. *Int. J. Pharm.* **1993**, *96*, 139–145.

31. Liu, L.-S.; Liu, S.-Q.; Ng, S.Y.; Froix, M.; Ohno, T.; Heller, J. Controlled release of interleukin-2 for tumour immunotherapy using alginate/chitosan porous microspheres. *J. Control. Release* **1997**, *43*, 65–74.

32. Porporatto, C.; Bianco, I.D.; Correa, S.G. Local and systemic activity of the polysaccharide chitosan at lymphoid tissues after oral administration. *J. Leukocyte Biol.* **2005**, *78*, 62–69.

33. Grabovac, V.; Guggi, D.; Bernkop-Schnürch, A. Comparison of the mucoadhesive properties of various polymers. *Adv. Drug Deliv. Rev.* **2005**, *57*, 1713–1723.

34. Wu, K.; Liang, T.; Duan, X.; Xu, L.; Zhang, K.; Li, R. Anti-diabetic effects of puerarin, isolated from *Pueraria lobata* (Willd.), on streptozotocin-diabetogenic mice through promoting insulin expression and ameliorating metabolic function. *Food Chem. Toxicol.* **2013**, *60*, 341–347.

35. Xiao, C.; Li, J.; Dong, X.; He, X.; Niu, X.; Liu, C.; Zhong, G.; Bauer, R.; Yang, D.; Lu, A. Anti-oxidative and TNF-α suppressive activities of puerarin derivative (4AC) in RAW264. 7 cells and collagen-induced arthritic rats. *Eur. J. Pharmacol.* **2011**, *666*, 242–250.

36. Cheng, Y.-F.; Zhu, G.-Q.; Wang, M.; Cheng, H.; Zhou, A.; Wang, N.; Fang, N.; Wang, X.-C.; Xiao, X.-Q.; Chen, Z.-W. Involvement of ubiquitin proteasome system in protective mechanisms of Puerarin to $MPP^+$-elicited apoptosis. *Neurosci. Res.* **2009**, *63*, 52–58.

37. Keung, W.M.; Klyosov, A.A.; Vallee, B.L. Daidzin inhibits mitochondrial aldehyde dehydrogenase and suppresses ethanol intake of Syrian golden hamsters. *Proc. Natl. Acad. Sci. USA* **1997**, *94*, 1675–1679.

38. Keung, W.-M.; Vallee, B.L. Daidzin and daidzein suppress free-choice ethanol intake by Syrian golden hamsters. *Proc. Natl. Acad. Sci. USA* **1993**, *90*, 10008–10012.

39. Zhang, S.; Ji, G.; Liu, J. Reversal of chemical-induced liver fibrosis in Wistar rats by puerarin. *J. Nutr. Biochem.* **2006**, *17*, 485–491.

40. Wang, F.; Li, J.; Hu, Z.; Xie, Y. Protective effect of puerarin on stress-induced gastric mucosal injury in rats. *China J. Chin. Mater. Med.* **2006**, *31*, 504–506.

41. Poncelet, D.; Lencki, R.; Beaulieu, C.; Halle, J.; Neufeld, R.; Fournier, A. Production of alginate beads by emulsification/internal gelation. I. Methodology. *Appl. Microbiol. Biotechnol.* **1992**, *38*, 39–45.

42. Rao, K.; Buri, P. A novel *in situ* method to test polymers and coated microparticles for bioadhesion. *Int. J. Pharm.* **1989**, *52*, 265–270.

43. Huang, M.; Khor, E.; Lim, L.-Y. Uptake and cytotoxicity of chitosan molecules and nanoparticles: Effects of molecular weight and degree of deacetylation. *Pharm. Res.* **2004**, *21*, 344–353.

44. Nwafor, P.A.; Okwuasaba, F.; Binda, L. Antidiarrhoeal and antiulcerogenic effects of methanolic extract of *Asparagus pubescens* root in rats. *J. Ethnopharmacol.* **2000**, *72*, 421–427.

45. George, M.; Abraham, T.E. Polyionic hydrocolloids for the intestinal delivery of protein drugs: Alginate and chitosan—A review. *J. Control. Release* **2006**, *114*, 1–14.

46. Peppas, N.A.; Buri, P.A. Surface, interfacial and molecular aspects of polymer bioadhesion on soft tissues. *J. Control. Release* **1985**, *2*, 257–275.

47. Torelli-Souza, R.R.; Cavalcante Bastos, L.A.; Nunes, H.G.; Camara, C.A.; Amorim, R.V.S. Sustained release of an antitumoral drug from alginate-chitosan hydrogel beads and its potential use as colonic drug delivery. *J. Appl. Polym. Sci.* **2012**, *126*, E409–E418.

48. Mortazavi, S.A.; Smart, J.D. An investigation into the role of water movement and mucus gel dehydration in mucoadhesion. *J. Control. Release* **1993**, *25*, 197–203.

49. Duchêne, D.; Ponchel, G. Principle and investigation of the bioadhesion mechanism of solid dosage forms. *Biomaterials* **1992**, *13*, 709–714.

50. Sahasathian, T.; Praphairaksit, N.; Muangsin, N. Mucoadhesive and floating chitosan-coated alginate beads for the controlled gastric release of amoxicillin. *Arch. Pharm. Res.* **2010**, *33*, 889–899.

51. Amiji, M.M. Tetracycline-containing chitosan microspheres for local treatment of Helicobacter pylori infection. *Cellulose* **2007**, *14*, 3–14.

52. Li, C.-Y.; Xu, H.-D.; Zhao, B.-T.; Chang, H.-I.; Rhee, H.-I. Gastroprotective effect of cyanidin 3-glucoside on ethanol-induced gastric lesions in rats. *Alcohol* **2008**, *42*, 683–687.

53. Ko, J.K.-S.; Cho, C.-H.; Lam, S.-K. Adaptive cytoprotection through modulation of nitric oxide in ethanol-evoked gastritis. *World J. Gastroenterol.* **2004**, *10*, 2503–2508.

54. Gómez-Burgaz, M.; García-Ochoa, B.; Torrado-Santiago, S. Chitosan–carboxymethylcellulose interpolymer complexes for gastric-specific delivery of clarithromycin. *Int. J. Pharm.* **2008**, *359*, 135–143.

55. Fatovic-Ferencic, S.; Banic, M. No Acid, No Ulcer: Dragutin (Carl) Schwarz (1868–1917), the Man Ahead of His Time. *Dig. Dis.* **2011**, *29*, 507–510.

56. Ohta, Y.; Kobayashi, T.; Inui, K.; Yoshino, J.; Nakazawa, S. Protective effect of ebselen, a seleno-organic compound, against the progression of acute gastric mucosal lesions induced by compound 48/80, a mast cell degranulator, in rats. *Jpn. J. Pharmacol.* **2002**, *90*, 295–303.

57. Kleine, A.; Kluge, S.; Peskar, B.M. Stimulation of prostaglandin biosynthesis mediates gastroprotective effect of rebamipide in rats. *Dig. Dis. Sci.* **1993**, *38*, 1441–1449.

58. Hwang, Y.P.; Choi, C.Y.; Chung, Y.C.; Jeon, S.S.; Jeong, H.G. Protective effects of puerarin on carbon tetrachloride-induced hepatotoxicity. *Arch. Pharm. Res.* **2007**, *30*, 1309–1317.

59. Zhu, L.-H.; Wang, L.; Wang, D.; Jiang, H.; Tang, Q.-Z.; Yan, L.; Bian, Z.-Y.; Wang, X.-A.; Li, H. Puerarin attenuates high-glucose-and diabetes-induced vascular smooth muscle cell proliferation by blocking PKC beta 2/Rac1-dependent signaling. *Free Radic. Biol. Med.* **2010**, *48*, 471–482.

60. Hu, W.; Zhang, Q.; Yang, X.; Wang, Y.; Sun, L. Puerarin Inhibits Adhesion Molecule Expression in TNF-alpha-Stimulated Human Endothelial Cells via Modulation of the Nuclear Factor kappa B Pathway. *Pharmacology* **2010**, *85*, 27–35.

61. Liu, E.S.L.; Cho, C.H. Relationship between ethanol-induced gastritis and gastric ulcer formation in rats. *Digestion* **2000**, *62*, 232–239.

# Glycol Chitosan-Based Fluorescent Theranostic Nanoagents for Cancer Therapy

Jin-Kyu Rhee, Ok Kyu Park, Aeju Lee, Dae Hyeok Yang and Kyeongsoon Park

**Abstract:** Theranostics is an integrated nanosystem that combines therapeutics with diagnostics in attempt to develop new personalized treatments with enhanced therapeutic efficacy and safety. As a promising therapeutic paradigm with cutting-edge technologies, theranostic agents are able to simultaneously deliver therapeutic drugs and diagnostic imaging agents and also monitor the response to therapy. Polymeric nanosystems have been intensively explored for biomedical applications to diagnose and treat various cancers. In recent years, glycol chitosan-based nanoagents have been developed as dual-purpose materials for simultaneous diagnosis and therapy. They have shown great potential in cancer therapies, such as chemotherapeutics and nucleic acid and photodynamic therapies. In this review, we summarize the recent progress and potential applications of glycol chitosan-based fluorescent theranostic nanoagents for cancer treatments and discuss their possible underlying mechanisms.

Reprinted from *Mar. Drugs*. Cite as: Rhee, J.-K.; Park, O.K.; Lee, A. Yang, D.H.; Park, K. Anticancer and Cancer Preventive Properties of Marine Polysaccharides: Some Results and Prospects. *Mar. Drugs* **2014**, *12*, 6038-6057.

## 1. Introduction

Theranostics is a system that integrates targeting, therapeutic, and diagnostic functions within an all-in-one platform [1]. Currently, diagnostic imaging and treatment processes are carried out separately in the study of the characteristics (*i.e.*, cellular phenotype, heterogenecity, *etc.*) of cancers and administration of drugs for therapy [2,3]. These separate processes require a long time period in which to evaluate drug efficacy and adjust the treatment plan accordingly, resulting in loss of opportunity for effectively treating some diseases, especially rapidly progressing cancers [4]. In contrast, integrated theranostic nanoagents can deliver diagnostic imaging agents capable of detecting and monitoring the early onset of diseases and simultaneously transport suitable therapeutic drugs over a prolonged period in order to enhance therapeutic efficacy [5]. This all-in-one theranostic approach is less time consuming and subsequently allows for a faster and more precise decision, allowing for more effective outcomes. Furthermore, theranostic technologies will radically change the way we diagnose, treat, and prevent cancer in oncology, and they show great promise in the emerging field of personalized medicine.

Advances in nanotechnology have contributed to the development of novel multifunctional nanoagents that enable specific delivery of imaging agents and therapeutic drugs to target diseased tissues for cancer imaging and therapy, and thus, they have ultimately led to the newest technology, "theranostics." Nanotheranostics involves the application and further development of various nanoparticle systems, such as polymer conjugations, dendrimers, micelles, liposomes, metal and inorganic nanoparticles, carbon nanotubes, and polymeric nanoparticles, for sustained, controlled, and targeted co-delivery of diagnostic and therapeutic agents in order to achieve improved results and fewer side effects [6]. Since these nanoparticles have nanoscale size dimensions (10–500 nm), they can navigate through microvasculatures and across various biological barriers to preferentially accumulate in tumor tissues due to the "enhanced permeability and retention" (EPR) effects, which are the hallmark of leaky vasculatures and poor lymphatic drainage [7]. Ample functional groups and easy modification with hydrophobic segments allow these nanoparticles to be modified by imaging agents and therapeutic drugs, which can either be encapsulated by or conjugated to polymeric nanoparticles. Therefore, polymeric nanoparticles have been employed to serve as diagnostic tools, therapeutic carriers, or both [4]. Additionally, polymeric nanoparticles improve the half-lives, solubility, and stability of imaging probes and therapeutic drugs while dramatically reducing potential side effects [8–10]. These features make polymeric nanoparticles preferable for customized and personalized translational medicine.

A diverse set of non-invasive imaging modalities is employed for the detection of cancer at early stages, discovery and development of new drugs, and monitoring of drug responses by offering information about biological changes and living systems, as well as visualization of the distribution of theranostic nanoagents in real time [4,11,12]. These non-invasive imaging modalities include positron-emission tomography (PET), magnetic resonance imaging (MRI), X-ray computed tomography (CT), single photon emission computed tomography (SPECT), ultrasound (US), and optical fluorescence imaging [12]. As shown in Figure 1, each imaging modality has its own unique advantages and disadvantages regarding sensitivity, spatial resolution, cost, safety, and tissue penetration [13]. Recently, near-infrared fluorescence (NIRF) imaging techniques have been used for real-time imaging in live animals. Although poor tissue penetration must be overcome with this method when applied in clinics, the NIRF imaging system is safe, highly sensitive, and capable of multicolor imaging to monitor the fate of theranostic agents in live animals without the requirement of a local cyclotron, incontinent radionuclide-labeling step, or expensive instruments [14]. Also, an optical imaging approach in the NIR window (700–900 nm) is very useful to identify the fundamental processes at the cellular and molecular levels because the absorbance and autofluorescence of hemoglobin (the main absorber in the visible region), water, and lipids (primary absorbers of infrared light) are lower in the NIR range [15].

Chitosan, a deacetylated derivative of chitin, is a copolymer that consists of two repeating units (*i.e.*, *N*-acetyl-2-amino-2-D-glucopyranose and 2-amino-2-deoxy-D-glucopyranose) linked by a β-(1→4)-glycosidic bond [16]. Chitosan is a biocompatible, biodegradable, and low-immogenic polymer that has great potential for a wide range of biomedical applications, such as drug delivery, gene delivery, cell imaging, and as a sensor in the treatment and diagnosis of some diseases [16]. However, the poor solubility of chitosan in aqueous solutions at pH > 6.0 is a major limitation to these potential uses. Glycol chitosan (GC) is a water-soluble chitosan derivative at neutral pH due to the introduction of a hydrophilic ethylene glycol group. Over the last 10 years, GC-based polymeric nanoparticles have been developed as therapeutic carriers (*i.e.*, anticancer drugs [17–19], peptides [20,21], nucleic acids [22,23], and diagnostic imaging agents [24–26]) in oncology. This review article describes the recent progress with GC-based fluorescent theranostic nanoagents as dual-purpose agents used for simultaneous diagnosis and therapy and further discusses their possible underlying mechanisms.

**Figure 1.** Non-invasive imaging modalities and their characteristics for biomedical applications. Permission from reference [13], Copyright © 2011, Royal Society of Chemistry.

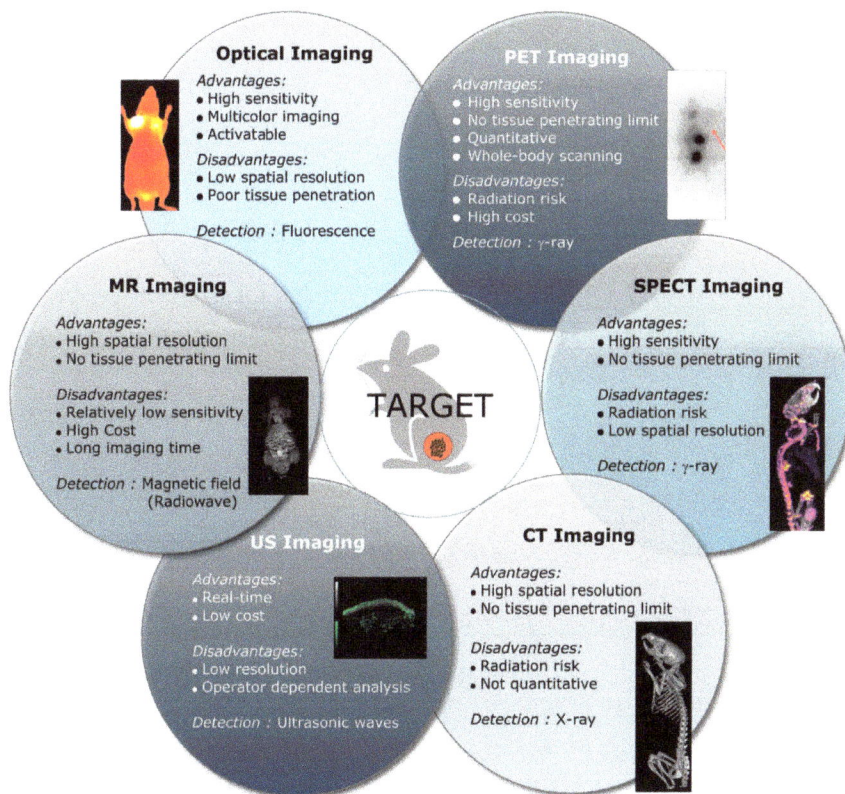

## 2. Basic Components for Manufacturing Theranostic Nanoagents

Integrated theranostic nanoagents offer multifunctional platforms for simultaneous cancer diagnosis and therapy. They provide a great deal of information for rapid disease verification and exact localization of the diseased tissues and permit the rapid delivery of therapeutic agents to the target tissues. To achieve the concept of theranostics, most theranostic nanoagents are typically designed in consideration of four basic components: signal emitter, therapeutic payload, payload carrier, and targeting ligand [4]. Representative examples of the components are shown in Figure 2 and Table 1.

**Figure 2.** Four basic components for the design of theranostic nanoagents.

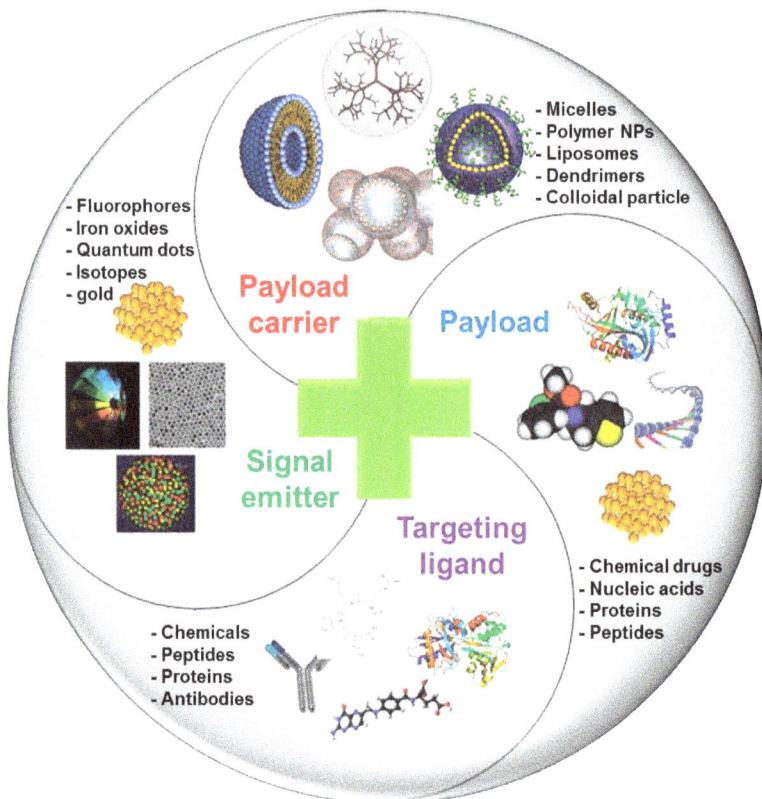

The signal emitter possesses certain unique optical, magnetic, or radioactive properties. Therapeutic drugs can be chemotherapeutic drugs, therapeutic proteins and peptides, or nucleic acids. The drug carrier is a kind of matrix comprised of polymeric materials. In general, intact and modified polymers have ample functional groups (such as $-NH_2$, $-COOH$, $-OH$, $-SH$, or $-N_3$, *etc.*) that offer flexibility in integrating multifunctionalities. Due to this flexibility, both the signal emitter and therapeutic drugs can be either non-covalently encapsulated in the carrier via hydrophobic and/or electrostatic interactions or covalently conjugated to the surface of the drug carrier [27,28]. Importantly, most of the synthetic and natural polymers used for biomedical applications are cleavable and biodegradable. Sometimes, the unique characteristics of tumor microenvironments, such as enzymes and pH, which would trigger drug release from a drug carrier, are used as another drug delivery approach. For example, enzymatic cleavage is highly specific for certain tumors where specific enzymes are overexpressed. Enzymatically-degradable drug delivery carriers showed a rapid drug release upon specific enzyme exposure, whereas minimal drug release occurs without enzymes. In case of non-enzymatic drug carriers, they showed the sustained delivery of therapeutic drugs at the target site. Finally, targeting ligands with high affinity to tumor cells or angiogenic endothelial cells are always covalently attached to the surface of the drug carriers [29]. Because passive targeting delivery of nanoparticles does not often operate effectively in poorly vascularized regions, an active targeting approach using a targeting ligand is required in order to increase accumulation of the nanoparticle in the disease tissue and to facilitate detection efficiency while reducing unwanted uptake by normal tissue, thus minimizing side effects. As described above, to meet the requirements for theranostics, the manufacturing processes of multifunctional theranostic nanoagents as a single system must be fairly complicated. However, theranostic nanoagents have promising advantages because they allow *in situ* imaging, targeted delivery, and controlled release of therapeutic drugs to diseases sites, as well as real-time monitoring of treatment responses.

**Table 1.** Examples of four basic components for the design of theranostic nanoagents.

| Components | Examples |
|---|---|
| **Signal Emitters** | **Fluorophores**: Fluorescein isothiocyanate (FITC), Alexa Fluor 488, yellow fuorescent protein (YFP), Rhodamine, tetramethylrhodamine (TRITC), cyanine 3(Cy3), red fluorescent protein (RFP), Texas Red, Cy5, Alexa Fluor 647, Cy5.5, Cy7, protoporphyrin IX (PpIX), and chlorine e6 (Ce6), *etc.*<br>**Isotopes**: $^{76}$Br, $^{124}$I, $^{94m}$Tc, $^{68}$Ga, $^{66}$Ga, $^{60}$Cu, $^{64}$Cu, $^{89}$Zr, *etc.*<br>**Magnetic resonance imaging agents**: iron oxide, iron platinum, manganese, gadolinium, *etc.*<br>**Other metals**: Quantom dots, silver and gold nanoparticles, *etc.* |
| **Payload** | **Chemical drugs**: Doxorubicin, cisplatin, paclitaxel, docetaxel, camptothecin, mitoxantrone, gemcitabin, curcumin, photosensitizers, imatinib, trastuzumab, sinutinib, cetuximab, *etc.*<br>**Protein and peptide drugs**: RGD, buserelin, gonadorelin, leuprolide, triptorelin, abarelix, cetrorelix, Tumor necrosis factor-related apoptosis-inducing ligand (TRAIL), melanoma differentiation associated-7 (MDA-7), E1A, E4ORF4, VP3 (apoptin), cytokines (interleukin-2, interferon alpha-n3, interferon beta-1, inteferon alpha-2b), monoclonal antibodies (zevalin, mylotarg, bexxar, herceptin, avastin), *etc.*<br>**Neucleic acids**: Plasmids, antisense oligonucleotides, ribozymes, DNAzymes, aptamers, small interfering RNA (siRNA), small hairpin RNA (shRNA), and microRNA, *etc.* |
| **Payload Carriers** | Macromolecular prodrugs, stealth nanoparticles, micelles, nanogels, nanocapsules, polymersomes, liposomes, dendrimers, porous silica nanoparticles, *etc.* |
| **Targeting Ligands** | **Angiogenic endothelial cell target**: RGD, vascular endothelial growth factor, TGN peptide, *etc.*<br>**Cancer cell target**: Epidermal growth factor receptor monoclonal antibody, epidermal growth factor, human epidermal receptor 2, transferrin, A10 aptamer, As1411 aptamer, cRGD, galactose, hyaluronic acid, folic acid, glycyrrhizin, *etc.* |

## 3. Glycol Chitosan-Based Theranostic Nanoagents

A variety of polymeric nanoparticles for drug delivery, diagnosis, and therapy have been developed. Among them, glycol chitosan (GC) has attracted interest because it is soluble in aqueous media, biocompatible, biodegradable, and has low immunogenicity [30]. Over the last

10 years, GC-based nanoparticles (GC NPs) have been intensively studied as drug delivery carriers for therapy and/or imaging agents for diagnosis. GC NPs are prepared by chemical conjugation of a hydrophilic GC polymer (250 kDa) with hydrophobic molecules. At the initial stage, GC NPs were developed as drug delivery carriers for cancer therapy. Due to their hydrophobic moieties and positive charge, GC NPs can non-covalently encapsulate hydrophobic cancer drugs [17–19], peptides [20], or nucleic acids [22] and still show potent therapeutic efficacy. Since 2006 when various non-invasive optical imaging modalities became widespread, optical imaging probes for the detection of various cancers (head and neck, brain, liver, colon, and metastatic cancer) were also developed by introducing a near-infrared fluorophore (Cyanine 5.5, Cy5.5) to GC NPs [24,26,31]. The constructed Cy5.5-labeled GC-5β-cholanic acid conjugates formed self-assembled nanostructures with diameters of 260 ± 30 nm and showed good colloidal stability for up to one month in PBS (pH 7.4) [24] (Figure 3A,B). To verify the superior tumor-targeting efficacy of Cy5.5-labeled GC NPs, several key factors influencing biodistribution and tumor-targeting of the nanoparticle system were investigated. Firstly, Cy5.5 (small molecule), Cy5.5-labeled GC (soluble polymer), and Cy5.5-labeled GC NPs were intravenously injected to SCC7 (squamous cell carcinoma) tumor-bearing mice. Compared to fluorescence intensities of Cy5.5 and Cy5.5-labeled GC, Cy5.5-labeled GC NPs exhibited strong fluorescence signals in the whole body and in tumor tissues for up to three days (Figure 3C), implying that the nanoparticle system has much stronger tumor-targeting characteristics than do small molecules and soluble polymer. Secondly, whole body fluorescence images of three types of Cy5.5-labeled GC NPs using different molecular weights of GC (20, 100, and 250 kDa) were performed to investigate the effects of molecular weight on tumor-targeting efficacy [24]. *In vivo* fluorescence images showed that the highest molecular weight GC NPs had a much longer circulation time in the blood stream and were more preferentially accumulated in tumor tissues than were the relatively lower molecular weight GC NPs. Thirdly, the deformability of GC NPs is also an important factor influencing tumor-targeting efficiency. As red blood cells (8 μm) of a highly flexible nature can readily pass through small micro-vessels (2.5 μm) [32], more than 95% of Cy5.5-labeled GC NPs (260 ± 30 nm) easily passed through a 200-nm pore size filter. However, 200-nm rigid Cy5.5-labeled polystyrene (PS) NPs did not easily pass through even a 450-nm pore size filter (Figure 3D). Indeed, deformable Cy5.5-labeled GC NPs showed strong NIRF signals in tumor tissues after passing through the *in vivo* filtration system of the liver and spleen [31] (Figure 3E). However, rigid and non-deformable PS NPs were primarily localized in the liver and spleen. These results suggest that the particles must be either smaller than the critical size or deformable enough to avoid *in vivo* filtration systems [33]. Finally, GC NPs have a positive surface charge and lipophilicity to facilitate rapid cellular uptake, which may improve the residence time of NPs in tumor tissues and thereby enhance the efficiency of diagnosis and therapy. These properties demonstrate the excellent tumor-targeting characteristics of GC-based theranostic NPs, making them one of the more promising of the recently developed GC-based fluorescent theranostic nanoagents that are being studied for simultaneous diagnosis and therapy.

**Figure 3.** (**A**) Chemical structure of Cy5.5-labeled glycol chitosan-5β cholanic acid conjugates and TEM image; (**B**) Colloidal stability of Cy5.5-labeled GC NPs in PBS for one month; (**C**) Time-dependent tumor targeting specificity of free Cy5.5, water soluble Cy5.5-labeled glycol chitosan polymer, and Cy5.5-labeled GC NPs in SCC7 tumor-bearing mice; (**D**) Filtration test of Cy5.5-labeled glycol chitosan polymer, Cy5.5-labeled GC NPs, and Cy5.5-labeled polystyrene beads with different pore sizes; (**E**) *Ex vivo* organ distribution of (**a**) Cy5.5-labeled GC NPs and (**b**) Cy5.5-labeled polystyrene beads. Reprinted with permission from [31] and [33], Copyright © 2011 and 2010 Elsevier.

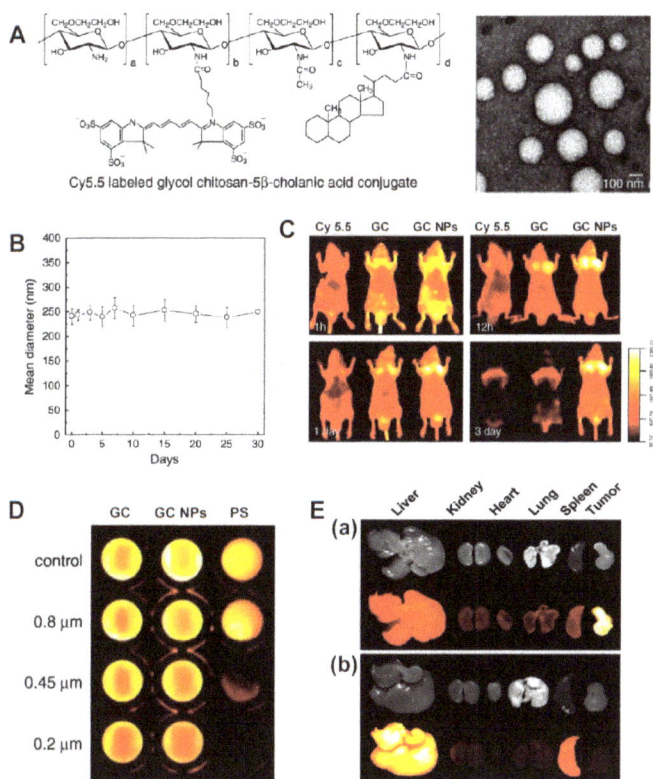

*3.1. Small Molecular Drug-Based Theranostic Nanoagents*

As previously described, GC NPs have good colloidal stability, deformability (or flexibility), and rapid cellular uptake and are very suitable as drug delivery carriers and imaging agents. To achieve the theranostic concept in an all-in-one platform, chemotherapeutic drugs are non-covalently encapsulated in Cy5.5-labeled GC NPs. Here, Cy5.5, GC NPs, and chemotherapeutic drugs act as signal emitter, payload carrier, and payload, respectively. Using several Cy5.5-labeled GC NPs constructed by conjugation of GC with 5β-cholanic acid, deoxycholic acid, or hydrotropic oligomer, chemotherapeutic drugs, such as paclitaxel [33,34], cisplatin [35], camptothecin [36], or docetaxel [37], can be readily encapsulated into the GC NPs via hydrophobic interactions. These GC NPs can be used as a Cremophor EL (polyoxyethylated caster oil)/absolute ethanol-free formulation to solubilize extremely insoluble drugs, such as paclitaxel [33,34] and docetaxel [37]. The GC NP system can also protect the drug activity of hydrolysis-labile drugs, such as camptothecin [36]. Furthermore, hydrotropic DENA (N,N-diethylnicotinamide)-based polymeric GC NPs can enhance drug-loading content (or efficiency) by almost two-fold compared to that of GC-5β-cholanic acid NPs because hydrotropic oligomers as water-soluble compounds enhance the water solubility of sparingly soluble drugs [34,38]. With the help of *in vivo* fluorescence imaging modalities, several pieces of information were confirmed: Cy5.5-labeled GC NPs containing chemotherapeutic drugs have a long circulation time (three to seven days), show specific tumor accumulation (nearly two- to four-fold) compared to that in normal tissues [33,34,37], and exhibit dose-dependent delivery efficiency to tumors. Also, the repeated injection frequency (or intervals) of theranostic nanoagents can be determined by monitoring the NIRF signal in tumor tissues. Therefore, based on the obtained important information driven by NIRF whole and *ex vivo* images, the therapeutic efficacies of the nanoagents can be greatly maximized. This evidence suggests that the use of theranostic nanoagents will play an important role in attaining more specific information, such as circulation time, biodistribution, nanoparticle injection intervals and dosages, and therapeutic response monitoring, allowing for optimized treatment protocols.

Typically, when researchers develop theranostic nanoagents, they make an effort to produce optimized systems with high targeting efficiency. However, bare nanoparticles and drug-loaded nanoparticles have quite different biodistributions and tumor-targeting characteristics [39]. In fact, the *in vivo* fate of a nanoparticle system can be altered because the physicochemical properties of nanoparticle systems, such as particle size, colloidal stability, and deformability, can be different before and after drug encapsulation into nanoparticle systems. Therefore, researchers should perform *in vivo* studies with a single platform containing both signal emitter and payload in order to obtain more accurate and precise information regarding theranostic nanosystems.

### 3.2. siRNA-Based Theranostic Glycol Chitosan Nanoagents

Nucleic acid therapy is promising for the treatment of various diseases, such as Alzheimer's disease, cancer, adenosine deaminase deficiency, and cystic fibrosis [40]. Current and potential therapeutic nucleic acids include plasmids, antisense oligonucleotides, ribozymes, DNAzymes, aptamers, and small interfering RNA (siRNA). These therapeutic nucleic acids can alter gene expression at the transcriptional or post-transcriptional level and may be effective in treating cancer and cardiovascular and inflammatory diseases. Although they are powerful therapeutic agents for the treatment of diseases, there are still obstacles to be overcome. Naked nucleic acids are highly susceptible to enzymatic degradation. Also, large and negatively-charged nucleic acids are not easily internalized by cells due to the difficult in crossing negatively-charged cell membranes. Thus, naked nucleic acid delivery requires direct injection of nucleic acids to the disease areas via physical methods, such as electroporation, gene gun, or ultrasound [41]. However, systemic delivery of naked nucleic acids is quite ineffective due to the minimal amount of intact polynucleotide reaching diseased sites because of the degradation by nucleases within the physiological fluids. Also, the direct injection approach limits efficient delivery only to anatomically accessible target sites.

Recently, among various nucleic acids, siRNA has attracted a great deal of attention as a potential therapeutic agent due to its highly sequence-specific gene silencing ability and generality in therapeutic targets. The difficulty of systemic siRNA is that its delivery is severely hindered in clinical applications due to its susceptibility to degradation by nuclease. To achieve efficient systemic delivery of therapeutic siRNA, many researchers have focused on the development of nonviral vehicles, which are nontoxic and less immunostimulatory and can have more versatile modifications for carrying different types of drug payloads. GC NPs have been tested for systemic delivery of siRNA; however, the electrostatic interaction between positively-charged GC NPs and negatively-charged siRNA is too weak to form condensed and stable siRNA/GC NP vehicles. To obtain vehicles that are more condensed and stable, GC-5β-cholanic acid and PEI-5β-cholanic acid were mixed together at a 1:1 weight ratio to yield GC-PEI NPs [23]. RFP-siRNA and GC-PEI NPs at a weight ratio of 1:5 formed more condensed and stable nano complexes (250 nm) with nearly 100% loading efficiency due to the increased positive charge caused by mixing GC NPs with PEI NPs. The RFP-siRNA/GC-PEI NPs successfully protected encapsulated RFP-siRNA from degradation by RNase A. Also, GC-PEI NPs effectively delivered RFP-siRNA to the cell cytoplasm and exerted remarkable silencing effects by suppressing RFP expression in RFP-expressing B16F10 cells. *In vivo* fluorescence images revealed that the intravenously injected Cy5.5-labeled RFP-siRNA/GC-PEI NPs were highly accumulated in tumor tissues. Due to effective delivery of RFP-siRNA into tumor tissues, the RFP signal intensity of RFP-B16F10 tumors treated with RFP-siRNA/GC-PEI NPs was 4.8-fold lower than that of the free siRNA group.

Kim and his colleagues synthesized a novel alternative siRNA, polymerized siRNA (poly-siRNA), to enhance the stability of the siRNA [42]. To polymerize siRNA, dithiol-modified siRNA (RFP- or VEGF-specific siRNA) bearing thiol groups at the 5'-ends of both sense and anti-sense strands were reacted in the presence of $N,N,N',N'$-tetramethyl-azodicarboxamide (Figure 4A). The polymerized siRNA consisted of a broad range of base pairs (50–300 bps and greater than 300 bps) through disulfide-polymerization of thiol groups at both ends of the modified siRNA. This polymerized siRNA can be converted to original mono-siRNA in the presence of a reducing agent, such as dithiothreitol (DTT) or under reductive conditions as exist in the cell cytosol. The *in vitro* serum stability test showed that mono-siRNA was degraded within 1 h, whereas most of the poly-siRNA was degraded within 12 h, suggesting that poly-siRNA is much more stable and less degradable by serum nuclease compared to mono-siRNA [43]. Although poly-siRNA is more stable than mono-siRNA, the degradation of poly-siRNA is still very susceptible to enzymatic degradation in *in vivo* physiological fluids. To overcome this problem, Kim and his colleagues synthesized a new systemic poly-siRNA delivery carrier, thiolated GC (tGC) polymer, using sulfosuccinimidyl-6-[3′(2-pyridyldithio)-propionamido] hexanoate (Sulfo-LC-SPDP) and DTT (Figure 4B) [43]. The tGC polymer formed stable nanostructures with poly-siRNA (RFP or VEGF) through enhanced electrostatic interaction and a self-crosslinking mechanism, leading to increased serum stability up to 24 h. The poly-siRNA/tGC (psi-tGC) NPs rapidly internalized and localized in the cytosol within 1 h and then showed efficient RFP gene silencing. After intravenous injection,

FPR 675-labeled poly-siRNA-tGC was preferentially accumulated in tumor tissues compared to naked FPR 675-labeled poly-siRNA or FPR 675-labeled-psi/PEI polyplexes, suggesting higher tumor selectivity of poly-siRNA-tGC NPs (Figure 4C). *In vivo* fluorescence images and therapeutic tests demonstrated that poly-siRNA(RFP)-tGC showed effective RFP gene silencing *in vivo*, and poly-siRNA(VEGF)-tGC NPs also significantly inhibited neovascularization via effective and specific VEGF gene silencing, leading to successful tumor suppression (Figure 4D,E). These results support the theory that the modified GC derivatives are suitable vehicles for siRNA delivery. However, more optimized treatment protocols for safe and effective systemic siRNA delivery carriers are still required for a wide range of clinical applications of siRNA.

**Figure 4. (A)** Scheme of polymerized siRNA (poly-siRNA) synthesis. Reprinted with permission from [42], Copyright © 2009 Elsevier B.V.; **(B)** Preparation of poly-siRNA/tGC nanoparticles for siRNA delivery; **(C)** *In vivo* real-time NIRF imaging of poly-siRNA/tGC in SCC7 tumor-bearing mice after i.v. injection of FPR675-labeled nanoparticles; **(D)** Inhibition of blood vessel formation by poly-siRNA (VEGF)/tGC; **(E)** Antitumor effects of control, poly-siRNA, poly-siRNA (scramble)/tGC, and poly-siRNA (VEGF)/tGC. Reprinted with permission from [43], Copyright © 2012 WILEY-VCH Verlag.

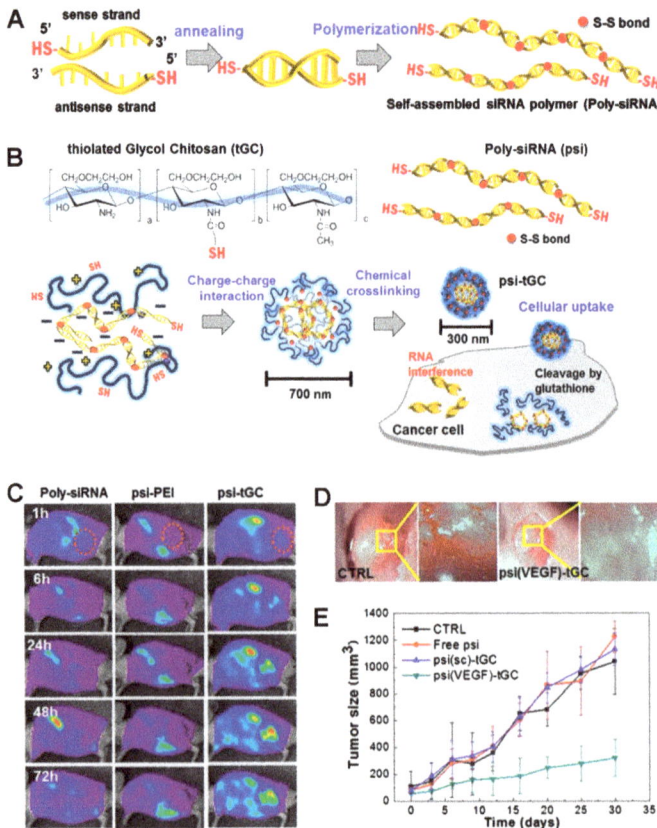

*3.3. Photosensitizer-Based Theranostic Nanoagents*

Photodynamic therapy (PDT) is a relatively new type of treatment that is attracting interest as a potential cancer treatment. PDT is a nonthermal photochemical reaction, which requires the simultaneous presence of a photosensitizing drug, oxygen, and a special type of light [44]. The photosensitizing drug alone is harmless in the absence of light and oxygen. The administered photosensitizing drug is only activated by irradiation of light to generate reactive oxygen species (ROS), including singlet oxygen ($^1O_2$), hydroxyl radicals ($\cdot OH$), and superoxide ($O^{2-}$), which subsequently trigger lethal oxidative stress and membrane damage in the treated cells, resulting in apoptosis, necrosis, or autophagy at the area of light exposure [44–48]. In addition, photosensitizing drugs show unique luminescent properties that can be useful as fluorescence imaging agents to track, visualize, and quantify the photosensitizing drugs in diseased tissues [48]. These dual features of PS, including signal emission and payload (drug) delivery, allow photosensitizing agents to act as theranostic agents for simultaneous diagnosis and image-guided therapy.

Currently, porphyrins and their derivatives are widely used as photosensitizers (PSs) in PDT. Some of these substances are already approved for use as drugs in malignant [49] or nonmalignant disease therapies [50]. However, many first- and second-generation PSs are limited in animal studies and clinical use because of non-specific skin phototoxicity, poor water solubility at physiological pH, and inefficient delivery to target tumor tissues in cancer treatment [48,51,52]. However, these limitations can be overcome by using nanoscale drug carriers. Hydrophobic PS can be encapsulated in nanoparticles or directly chemically conjugated with water-soluble polymers to enhance solubility and dispersion in an aqueous solution. Also, PS-loaded or -conjugated nanoparticles are more preferentially accumulated in tumor tissues through EPR effects [53]. The Kwon group developed protoporphyrin IX (PpIX)- and chlorin e6 (Ce6)-loaded GC NPs that are well dispersed in aqueous solution and form stable nano-structures with an average diameter around 300 nm [54,55]. These NPs also showed time-dependent release of PpIX or Ce6 from GC NPs and efficient photodynamic therapy in *in vitro* and *in vivo* studies. However, drugs physically loaded in nanoparticles showed burst drug release from nanoparticles during circulation *in vivo* [54,55]. This undesirable instability of PpIX- or Ce6-loaded GC NPs resulted in low drug delivery efficiency and decreased therapeutic effect at tumor sites as well as unintended damage to normal tissues [56]. These problems of PS-loaded nanoparticles can be overcome by chemical conjugation of PpIX or Ce6 with water soluble GC. PpIX- or Ce6-conjugated GC also formed stable and self-assembled nanoscale particles (about 250–300 nm) [55,57]. Because PpIX- or Ce6-conjugated GC NPs did not exhibit burst release from NPs due to chemical conjugation with GC, they showed less photo-toxicity compared to PpIX- or Ce6-loaded GC NPs in an *in vitro* study. However, *in vivo* imaging studies showed that they had a prolonged circulation time and accumulated more specifically in the tumor, resulting in better therapeutic efficacy. For example, Ce6-conjugated GC NPs showed a dramatic decrease of tumor volume (about 160 mm$^3$) at 20 day post-treatment, which was significantly smaller than that of Ce6-loaded GC NPs-treated mice (about 560 mm$^3$) [55]. These results suggest that the factors of burst drug release and stability of

NPs *in vivo* should be considered when constructing photoactivatable theranostic nanoagents for PDT.

The bioorthogonal chemical reporter strategy is a method for labeling and visualizing biomolecules *in vivo* without the requirement of genetic manipulation [58,59]. In this approach, metabolic labeling of the cell with azides primes the target biomolecule to be visualized by covalent attachment of an imaging probe. As a chemical reporter, azide is the most widely used because of its small size, metabolic stability, and lack of reactivity with natural biofunctionality [58,60]. The reaction of azide-alkyne cycloaddition forms an azide and a terminal alkyne (called "click chemistry"), which involves the use of a Cu catalyst [61,62]. Among various alkyne reagents, cyclooctynes react with azides without the use of copper, referred to as "Cu-free click chemistry," to achieve bioorthogonal labeling [63]. Copper-free click chemistry has been widely applied in biological and biomedical fields, such as in the labeling of proteins, nucleotides, or cells; in the analysis of metabolic pathways; and for the surface modification of nanoagents [64–67]. Recently, Lee *et al.* reported a novel two-step photoactivatable theranostic strategy *in vivo* via metabolic glycoengineering and Cu-free click chemistry (Figure 5A) [68]. To achieve this approach, they prepared two different nanoagents as follows. Firstly, for generation of azide groups on tumor tissues, the precursor (tetraacetylated *N*-azidoacetyl-D-mannosamine, Ac4ManNAz) was loaded into GC NPs with an amphiphilic structure via hydrophobic interactions. When Ac4ManNAz-loaded GC NPs were added to tumor cells or tumor-bearing mice, azide groups were site-specifically generated on tumor cells or tissues by metabolic glycoengineering after effective delivery and rapid uptake of Ac4ManNAz-loaded GC NPs into tumor cells. An *in vitro* cell study showed that Ac4ManNAz-loaded GC NPs enabled a longer lifetime for the azide groups on cells compared to free Ac4ManNAz because of the sustained release of Ac4ManNAz from GC NPs (Figure 5B). Furthermore, Ac4ManNAz-loaded GC NPs successfully generated large amounts of azide groups irrespective of the kind of tumor cells targeted (KB, A549, U87MG, MCF7, MDA-MD-468, and MDA-MD-436). Immunohistochemistry and fluorescence images also demonstrated that Ac4ManNAz-loaded GC NPs with a longer circulation time and a higher tumor-targeting efficiency effectively delivered Ac4ManNAz, resulting in much greater generation of the azide group on tumor tissues compared to normal tissues (*i.e.*, liver, lung, spleen, and kidney) (Figure 5C,D). Secondly, for specific delivery of photoactivatable agents to azide groups generated on tumor tissues by copper-free click chemistry, bicycle [6.1.0] nonyne (BCN)-PEG-NHS and Ce6 were conjugated with glycol chitosan polymer to obtain BCN-Ce6-GC NPs. Through copper-free click chemistry, BCN-Ce6-GC NPs specifically bind with azide groups generated on tumor cell membranes by Ac4ManNAz-loaded GC NPs. Compared to free Ce6 and Ce6-GC NPs, BCN-Ce6-GC NPs were more accumulated in tumor regions after azide generation caused by pretreatment with Ac4ManNAz-loaded GC NPs (Figure 5E). *In vivo* photodynamic therapy demonstrated that a two-step strategy using Ac4ManNAz-loaded GC NPs and BCN-Ce6-GC NPs showed significant black scab generation and effective tumor destruction after laser irradiation compared to use of free Ce6 or BCN-Ce6-GC NPs alone (Figure 5F). This two-step theranostic approach has great potential for the enhancement of the tumor-targeting ability of theranostic agents and their therapeutic effects in cancer therapy. However, further optimized conditions are required to more specifically generate azide groups on target-diseased sites.

**Figure 5.** (**A**) Schematic illustration of the two-step *in vivo* tumor targeting strategy for nanoparticles via metabolic glycoengineering and click chemistry; (**B**) Time-dependent lifetime of azide groups generated by free Ac4ManNAz and Ac4ManNAz-loaded GC NPs; (**C**) Intravenous injection of Ac4ManNAz-loaded GC NPs and metabolic glycoengineering on tumor tissue *in vivo*; (**D**) Western blot analysis of major organs and tumor tissue after i.v. injection of AC4ManNAz-loaded GC NPs; (**E**) Tumor targeted image of BCN-Ce6-GC NPs in tumor bearing mice after pretreatment of Ac4ManNAz-GC NPs; (**F**) *In vivo* photodynamic therapy in tumor bearing mice and tumor images of mice treated with BCN-Ce6-GC NPs and Ac4ManNAz-GC NPs at day seven and 21. Reprinted with permission from [68], Copyright © 2014 American Chemical Society.

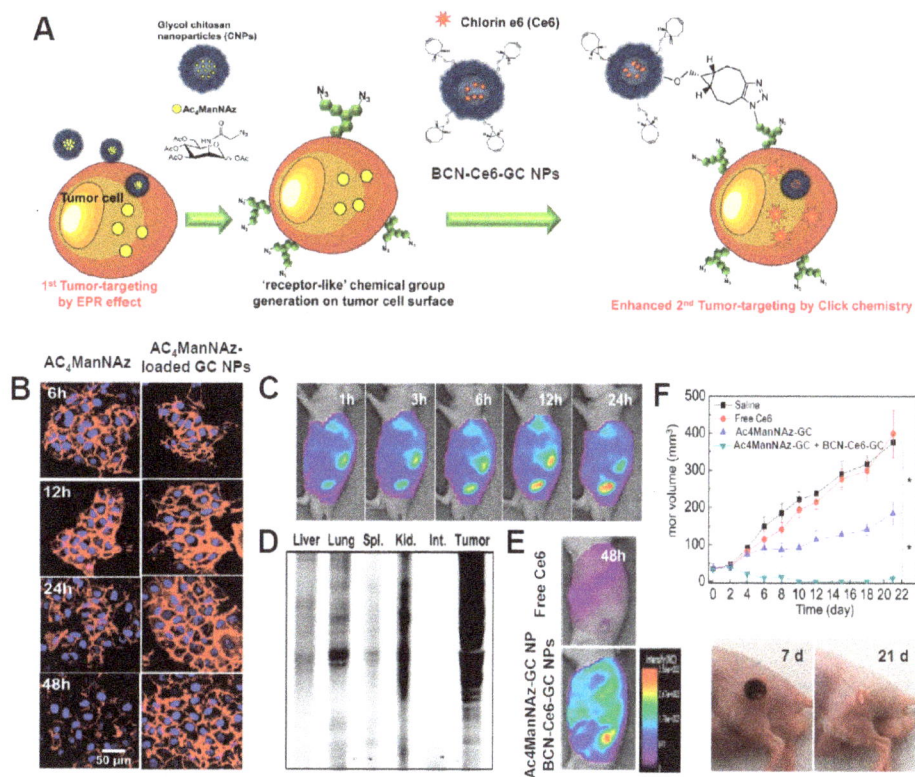

Tumor tissues have a more acidic microenvironment due to lactic acid production in hypoxic areas. Indeed, solid tumors with a pH ranging from 5.8 to 7.7 are on average 0.5 units lower than the pH of normal tissues. Thus, the use of different pH environments has been a promising avenue for cancer imaging and therapy. Recently, Park *et al.* developed a photoactivatible theranostic nanoagent that quickly switches into an aggressive molecule for tumor imaging and destruction within the acidic environment of the tumor [69]. The smart pH-sensitive photoactivatable theranostic system consists of a GC backbone, a functional 3-diethylaminopropyl isothiocyanate (DEAP, pH sensitive moiety), a Ce6 block (photosensitizer), and polyethylene glycol (PEG). This theranostic nanoagent includes an intelligent switch from self-assembly (*i.e.*, self-quenched state of photosensitizer) at physiological pH 7.4 into extended random molecules (*i.e.*, dequenched state for ROS production) at the extracellular acidic pH. At physiological pH 7.4, it forms a self-assembled molecule, 150 nm in diameter, and shows no singlet-oxygen production or noticeable cell death. However, when exposed to extracellular acidic pH (pH 6.8 or 6.4), it changes to the dequenched state, thereby emitting a strong NIRF signal and singlet-oxygen generation, resulting in higher phototoxicity and efficient tumor destruction of HeLa cells. This pH-sensitive photoactivatable smart system enables targeted high-dose cancer therapy while ensuring the safety of normal tissues.

## 3.4. Fullerene-Based Theranostic Nanoagents

Fullerene ($C_{60}$) is a soccer ball-shaped structure with 12 pentagons (due to $C_5$-$C_5$ single bonds) and 20 hexagons ($C_5$-$C_6$ double bonds). Since the discovery of $C_{60}$ in 1985, fullerene has attracted much attention and has been viewed as having great potential for a variety of applications. Due to its unique chemical structure, $C_{60}$ possesses interesting photo-physical properties and generates ROS by exposure to visible light [70] and thereby can be used as a potentially strong photoactivatable agent for PDT in biological systems [44]. However, due to its inherent extreme hydrophobicity and innate tendency to aggregate in water and biological media, $C_{60}$ has inefficient photoactivity and is less promising for application in photoactivatable drugs in biomedicine [44]. To overcome this shortcoming of $C_{60}$, it was chemically conjugated to polysaccharides, such as GC and hyaluronic acid [71–73]. Unlike pristine $C_{60}$ molecules, which rapidly aggregated within 5 min, GC-$C_{60}$ conjugates formed self-organized nanoparticles (approximately 10-23 nm in diameter) in PBS and were stable for more than one month without any precipitation [71]. Solubilization of $C_{60}$ seemed to improve the light-sensitization of $C_{60}$ molecules. When illuminated with a 670-nm laser source, GC-$C_{60}$ conjugates generated singlet oxygen and significantly induced KB cell death, whereas free $C_{60}$ conjugates did not. More recently, Kim *et al.* developed an endosomal pH-activated GC-fullerene derivative for PDT that was prepared using a simple two-step chemical reaction of (i) 2,3-dimethylmaleic acid (DMA) to free amine groups of GC and (ii) free hydroxyl groups of GC-DMA to π-π carbon bonds of $C_{60}$ [73]. The GC-DMA-$C_{60}$ conjugates formed self-assembled multi-nanogel aggregates (283 nm) at pH 7.4 due to the electrostatic interactions between pendant DMA groups and the residual free amine groups of GC. During light illumination at 670 nm, GC-DMA-$C_{60}$ nanogels showed less generation of singlet oxygen and less cytotoxicity of KB cells at pH 7.4 owing to an increased photo-interference effect between $C_{60}$ molecules close packed in multi-nanogel aggregates. However, these multi-nanogel aggregates were divided into single nanogel parts (approximately 46 nm) at endosomal pH 5.0 due to the reduction of electrostatic interactions resulting from cleavage of the DMA blocks [74]. In particular, singlet oxygen generation and phototoxicity were significantly increased at endosomal pH 5.0. Another important consideration is that the solubilized GC-fullerene derivatives enable photo-luminescent tumor imaging without labeling of any fluorophores or isotopes [71–73]. Indeed, *in vivo* fluorescence images demonstrated that GC-C$_{60}$- or GC-DMA-C$_{60}$-emitting fluorescence signals accumulated in tumor tissues in KB tumor-bearing mice. These solubilized fullerene derivatives are useful and promising for PDT. However, the fluorescence intensities of fullerene derivatives seem to be weaker than those of NIR fluorophores and other photosensitizers. These concerns should be further investigated to achieve high-resolution in fluorescence imaging.

## 4. Conclusions

This review article discusses the recent progress of GC-based fluorescent theranostic nanoagents for simultaneous diagnosis and therapy in cancer treatments. Due to their biocompatible, biodegradable, and low-immunogenic properties, GC and its derivatives have been extensively studied for use in a wide range of biomedical applications. In particular, GC polymer has a large number of amine groups on its GC backbone and so can be covalently or non-covalently modified with hydrophobic molecules (bile acid analogs), drugs (chemotherapeutic small molecular drugs, nucleic acids, photosensitizers, or fullerenes), signal emitters (NIR fluorophores, photosensitizers, or fullerenes), and other imaging tracers (isotopes) in order to yield theranostic nanosystems. These GC-based fluorescent theranostic NPs showed good colloidal stability for extended circulation in the blood stream, excellent deformability to avoid *in vivo* filtration by the liver or spleen, and/or rapid cellular uptake characteristics to facilitate delivery of theranostic agents to target sites. Due to these features, GC-based theranostic nanosystems have excellent tumor-targeting characteristics, leading to effective therapeutic results. Therefore, GC-based theranostic nanosystems will play important roles in future biomedical applications and personalized medicine. In almost all works concerning chitosan applications, chitosan and its derivatives are non-toxic, biologically compatible materials, and thus suitable for the drug delivery carriers. Sometimes, the issue for their biocompatibilities is completely disregarded due to the statement on chitosan approval by the American Food and Drug Administration (FDA) as a wound dressing material [75]. However, their biocompatibility must be addressed and considered separately, requiring specific testing in the particular conditions expected for its administration because each particular case may be quite different in several different structures, formulation, and carriers in varied conditions [76]. The manufacturing processes also needed to meet the requirements for simultaneous diagnosis and therapy of theranostic nanosystems in a single platform are generally complicated. Due to the increased complexity, the technical challenges, such as cost, colloidal stability, and reproducibility, must be considered. Future improvements should be focused on the development of innovative strategies to overcome these technical challenges.

## Acknowledgments

This research was supported in part by a Korea Basic Science Institute (KBSI) grant (T34525) to J.K. Rhee, another grant from the KBSI (D34400), and a grant of the National Research Foundation of Korea (NRF) funded by the Ministry of Education, and Science and Technology (No. 2012R1A2A2A04046108).

## Author Contributions

K. Park and D. H. Yang conceived and designed the study. J.-K. Rhee, O.K. Park, and A. Lee collected the literature and analyzed the data. J.K. Rhee, O.K. Park, K. Park and D.H. Yang wrote the manuscript.

## Conflicts of Interest

The authors declare no conflicts of interest.

## References

1.   Sumer, B.; Gao, J. Theranostic nanomedicine for cancer. *Nanomedicine* **2008**, *3*, 137–140.
2.   McCarthy, J.R. The future of theranostic nanoagents. *Nanomedicine* **2009**, *4*, 693–695.
3.   McCarthy, J.R. Multifunctional agents for concurrent imaging and therapy in cardiovascular disease. *Adv. Drug Deliv. Rev.* **2010**, *62*, 1023–1030.
4.   Fang, C.; Zhang, M. Nanoparticle-based theragnostics: Integrating diagnostic and therapeutic potentials in nanomedicine. *J. Control. Release* **2010**, *146*, 2–5.
5.   Ahmed, N.; Fessi, H.; Elaissari, A. Theranostic applications of nanoparticles in cancer. *Drug Discov. Today* **2012**, *17*, 928–934.
6.   Muthu, M.S.; Leong, D.T.; Mei, L.; Feng, S.S. Nanotheranostics—Application and further development of nanomedicine strategies for advanced theranostics. *Theranostics* **2014**, *4*, 660–677.
7.   Maeda, H.; Wu, J.; Sawa, T.; Matsumura, Y.; Hori, K. Tumor vascular permeability and the EPR effect in macromolecular therapeutics: A review. *J. Control. Release* **2000**, *65*, 271–284.
8.   Allen, T.M.; Cullis, P.R. Drug delivery systems: Entering the mainstream. *Science* **2004**, *303*, 1818–1822.
9.   Emerich, D.F.; Thanos, C.G. The pinpoint promise of nanoparticle-based drug delivery and molecular diagnosis. *Biomol. Eng.* **2006**, *23*, 171–184.
10.  Koo, Y.E.; Reddy, G.R.; Bhojani, M.; Schneider, R.; Philbert, M.A.; Rehemtulla, A.; Ross, B.D.; Kopelman, R. Brain cancer diagnosis and therapy with nanoplatforms. *Adv. Drug Deliv. Rev.* **2006**, *58*, 1556–1577.
11.  Weissleder, R. Molecular imaging in cancer. *Science* **2006**, *312*, 1168–1171.
12.  Weissleder, R.; Pittet, M.J. Imaging in the era of molecular oncology. *Nature* **2008**, *452*, 580–589.
13.  Lee, D.E.; Koo, H.; Sun, I.C.; Ryu, J.H.; Kim, K.; Kwon, I.C. Multifunctional nanoparticles for multimodal imaging and theragnosis. *Chem. Soc. Rev.* **2012**, *41*, 2656–2672.
14.  Chen, X.; Conti, P.S.; Moats, R.A. *In vivo* near-infrared fluorescence imaging of integrin alphavbeta3 in brain tumor xenografts. *Cancer Res.* **2004**, *64*, 8009–8014.
15.  Weissleder, R. A clearer vision for *in vivo* imaging. *Nat. Biotechnol.* **2001**, *19*, 316–317.
16.  Shukla, S.K.; Mishra, A.K.; Arotiba, O.A.; Mamba, B.B. Chitosan-based nanomaterials: A state-of-the-art review. *Int. J. Biol. Macromol.* **2013**, *59*, 46–58.

17. Son, Y.J.; Jang, J.S.; Cho, Y.W.; Chung, H.; Park, R.W.; Kwon, I.C.; Kim, I.S.; Park, J.Y.; Seo, S.B.; Park, C.R.; *et al*. Biodistribution and anti-tumor efficacy of doxorubicin loaded glycol-chitosan nanoaggregates by EPR effect. *J. Control. Release* **2003**, *91*, 135–145.

18. Hyung Park, J.; Kwon, S.; Lee, M.; Chung, H.; Kim, J.H.; Kim, Y.S.; Park, R.W.; Kim, I.S.; Bong Seo, S.; Kwon, I.C.; *et al*. Self-assembled nanoparticles based on glycol chitosan bearing hydrophobic moieties as carriers for doxorubicin: *In vivo* biodistribution and anti-tumor activity. *Biomaterials* **2006**, *27*, 119–126.

19. Kim, J.H.; Kim, Y.S.; Kim, S.; Park, J.H.; Kim, K.; Choi, K.; Chung, H.; Jeong, S.Y.; Park, R.W.; Kim, I.S.; *et al*. Hydrophobically modified glycol chitosan nanoparticles as carriers for paclitaxel. *J. Control. Release* **2006**, *111*, 228–234.

20. Park, J.H.; Kwon, S.; Nam, J.O.; Park, R.W.; Chung, H.; Seo, S.B.; Kim, I.S.; Kwon, I.C.; Jeong, S.Y. Self-assembled nanoparticles based on glycol chitosan bearing 5beta-cholanic acid for RGD peptide delivery. *J. Control. Release* **2004**, *95*, 579–588.

21. Kim, J.H.; Kim, Y.S.; Park, K.; Kang, E.; Lee, S.; Nam, H.Y.; Kim, K.; Park, J.H.; Chi, D.Y.; Park, R.W.; *et al*. Self-assembled glycol chitosan nanoparticles for the sustained and prolonged delivery of antiangiogenic small peptide drugs in cancer therapy. *Biomaterials* **2008**, *29*, 1920–1930.

22. Yoo, H.S.; Lee, J.E.; Chung, H.; Kwon, I.C.; Jeong, S.Y. Self-assembled nanoparticles containing hydrophobically modified glycol chitosan for gene delivery. *J. Control. Release* **2005**, *103*, 235–243.

23. Huh, M.S.; Lee, S.Y.; Park, S.; Lee, S.; Chung, H.; Lee, S.; Choi, Y.; Oh, Y.K.; Park, J.H.; Jeong, S.Y.; *et al*. Tumor-homing glycol chitosan/polyethylenimine nanoparticles for the systemic delivery of siRNA in tumor-bearing mice. *J. Control. Release* **2010**, *144*, 134–143.

24. Park, K.; Kim, J.H.; Nam, Y.S.; Lee, S.; Nam, H.Y.; Kim, K.; Park, J.H.; Kim, I.S.; Choi, K.; Kim, S.Y.; *et al*. Effect of polymer molecular weight on the tumor targeting characteristics of self-assembled glycol chitosan nanoparticles. *J. Control. Release* **2007**, *122*, 305–314.

25. Lee, S.; Ryu, J.H.; Park, K.; Lee, A.; Lee, S.Y.; Youn, I.C.; Ahn, C.H.; Yoon, S.M.; Myung, S.J.; Moon, D.H.; *et al*. Polymeric nanoparticle-based activatable near-infrared nanosensor for protease determination *in vivo*. *Nano Lett.* **2009**, *9*, 4412–4416.

26. Nam, T.; Park, S.; Lee, S.Y.; Park, K.; Choi, K.; Song, I.C.; Han, M.H.; Leary, J.J.; Yuk, S.A.; Kwon, I.C.; *et al*. Tumor targeting chitosan nanoparticles for dual-modality optical/MR cancer imaging. *Bioconjugate Chem.* **2010**, *21*, 578–582.

27. Veiseh, O.; Gunn, J.W.; Zhang, M. Design and fabrication of magnetic nanoparticles for targeted drug delivery and imaging. *Adv. Drug Deliv. Rev.* **2010**, *62*, 284–304.

28. Lewandrowski, K.U.; Gresser, J.D.; Wise, D.L.; Trantol, D.J. Bioresorbable bone graft substitutes of different osteoconductivities: A histologic evaluation of osteointegration of poly(propylene glycol-co-fumaric acid)-based cement implants in rats. *Biomaterials* **2000**, *21*, 757–764.

29. Bamrungsap, S.; Zhao, Z.; Chen, T.; Wang, L.; Li, C.; Fu, T.; Tan, W. Nanotechnology in therapeutics: A focus on nanoparticles as a drug delivery system. *Nanomedicine* **2012**, *7*, 1253–1271.

30. Zhang, Y.; Zhang, M. Calcium phosphate/chitosan composite scaffolds for controlled *in vitro* antibiotic drug release. *J. Biomed. Mater. Res.* **2002**, *62*, 378–386.

31. Na, J.H.; Koo, H.; Lee, S.; Min, K.H.; Park, K.; Yoo, H.; Lee, S.H.; Park, J.H.; Kwon, I.C.; Jeong, S.Y.; Kim, K. Real-time and non-invasive optical imaging of tumor-targeting glycol chitosan nanoparticles in various tumor models. *Biomaterials* **2011**, *32*, 5252–5261.

32. Barshtein, G.; Ben-Ami, R.; Yedgar, S. Role of red blood cell flow behavior in hemodynamics and hemostasis. *Expert Rev. Cardiovasc. Ther.* **2007**, *5*, 743–752.

33. Kim, K.; Kim, J.H.; Park, H.; Kim, Y.S.; Park, K.; Nam, H.; Lee, S.; Park, J.H.; Park, R.W.; Kim, I.S.; *et al.* Tumor-homing multifunctional nanoparticles for cancer theragnosis: Simultaneous diagnosis, drug delivery, and therapeutic monitoring. *J. Control. Release* **2010**, *146*, 219–227.

34. Saravanakumar, G.; Min, K.H.; Min, D.S.; Kim, A.Y.; Lee, C.M.; Cho, Y.W.; Lee, S.C.; Kim, K.; Jeong, S.Y.; Park, K.; *et al.* Hydrotropic oligomer-conjugated glycol chitosan as a carrier of paclitaxel: Synthesis, characterization, and *in vivo* biodistribution. *J. Control. Release* **2009**, *140*, 210–217.

35. Kim, J.H.; Kim, Y.S.; Park, K.; Lee, S.; Nam, H.Y.; Min, K.H.; Jo, H.G.; Park, J.H.; Choi, K.; Jeong, S.Y.; *et al.* Antitumor efficacy of cisplatin-loaded glycol chitosan nanoparticles in tumor-bearing mice. *J. Control. Release* **2008**, *127*, 41–49.

36. Min, K.H.; Park, K.; Kim, Y.S.; Bae, S.M.; Lee, S.; Jo, H.G.; Park, R.W.; Kim, I.S.; Jeong, S.Y.; Kim, K.; *et al.* Hydrophobically modified glycol chitosan nanoparticles-encapsulated camptothecin enhance the drug stability and tumor targeting in cancer therapy. *J. Control. Release* **2008**, *127*, 208–218.

37. Hwang, H.Y.; Kim, I.S.; Kwon, I.C.; Kim, Y.H. Tumor targetability and antitumor effect of docetaxel-loaded hydrophobically modified glycol chitosan nanoparticles. *J. Control. Release* **2008**, *128*, 23–31.

38. Rasool, A.A.; Hussain, A.A.; Dittert, L.W. Solubility enhancement of some water-insoluble drugs in the presence of nicotinamide and related compounds. *J. Pharm. Sci.* **1991**, *80*, 387–393.

39. Lee, B.S.; Park, K.; Park, S.; Kim, G.C.; Kim, H.J.; Lee, S.; Kil, H.; Oh, S.J.; Chi, D.; Kim, K.; *et al.* Tumor targeting efficiency of bare nanoparticles does not mean the efficacy of loaded anticancer drugs: Importance of radionuclide imaging for optimization of highly selective tumor targeting polymeric nanoparticles with or without drug. *J. Control. Release* **2010**, *147*, 253–260.

40. Kelkar, S.S.; Reineke, T.M. Theranostics: Combining imaging and therapy. *Bioconjugate Chem.* **2011**, *22*, 1879–1903.

41. Niidome, T.; Huang, L. Gene therapy progress and prospects: Nonviral vectors. *Gene Ther.* **2002**, *9*, 1647–1652.

42. Lee, S.Y.; Huh, M.S.; Lee, S.; Lee, S.J.; Chung, H.; Park, J.H.; Oh, Y.K.; Choi, K.; Kim, K.; Kwon, I.C. Stability and cellular uptake of polymerized siRNA (poly-siRNA)/polyethylenimine (PEI) complexes for efficient gene silencing. *J. Control. Release* **2010**, *141*, 339–346.

43. Lee, S.J.; Huh, M.S.; Lee, S.Y.; Min, S.; Lee, S.; Koo, H.; Chu, J.U.; Lee, K.E.; Jeon, H.; Choi, Y.; *et al.* Tumor-homing poly-siRNA/glycol chitosan self-cross-linked nanoparticles for systemic siRNA delivery in cancer treatment. *Angew. Chem.* **2012**, *51*, 7203–7207.

44. Sharma, S.K.; Chiang, L.Y.; Hamblin, M.R. Photodynamic therapy with fullerenes *in vivo*: Reality or a dream? *Nanomedicine* **2011**, *6*, 1813–1825.

45. Agostinis, P.; Berg, K.; Cengel, K.A.; Foster, T.H.; Girotti, A.W.; Gollnick, S.O.; Hahn, S.M.; Hamblin, M.R.; Juzeniene, A.; Kessel, D.; *et al.* Photodynamic therapy of cancer: An update. *Cancer J. Clin.* **2011**, *61*, 250–281.

46. Dolmans, D.E.; Fukumura, D.; Jain, R.K. Photodynamic therapy for cancer. *Nat. Rev. Cancer* **2003**, *3*, 380–387.

47. Henderson, B.W.; Dougherty, T.J. How does photodynamic therapy work? *Photochem. Photobiol.* **1992**, *55*, 145–157.

48. Josefsen, L.B.; Boyle, R.W. Unique diagnostic and therapeutic roles of porphyrins and phthalocyanines in photodynamic therapy, imaging and theranostics. *Theranostics* **2012**, *2*, 916–966.

49. Moore, C.M.; Pendse, D.; Emberton, M. Photodynamic therapy for prostate cancer—A review of current status and future promise. *Nat. Clin. Pract. Urol.* **2009**, *6*, 18–30.

50. Awan, M.A.; Tarin, S.A. Review of photodynamic therapy. *Surgeon* **2006**, *4*, 231–236.

51. Sun, Y.; Chen, Z.L.; Yang, X.X.; Huang, P.; Zhou, X.P.; Du, X.X. Magnetic chitosan nanoparticles as a drug delivery system for targeting photodynamic therapy. *Nanotechnology* **2009**, *20*, 135102.

52. Guillemard, V.; Saragovi, H.U. Taxane-antibody conjugates afford potent cytotoxicity, enhanced solubility, and tumor target selectivity. *Cancer Res.* **2001**, *61*, 694–699.

53. Bechet, D.; Couleaud, P.; Frochot, C.; Viriot, M.L.; Guillemin, F.; Barberi-Heyob, M. Nanoparticles as vehicles for delivery of photodynamic therapy agents. *Trends Biotechnol.* **2008**, *26*, 612–621.

54. Lee, S.J.; Park, K.; Oh, Y.K.; Kwon, S.H.; Her, S.; Kim, I.S.; Choi, K.; Lee, S.J.; Kim, H.; Lee, S.G.; *et al.* Tumor specificity and therapeutic efficacy of photosensitizer-encapsulated glycol chitosan-based nanoparticles in tumor-bearing mice. *Biomaterials* **2009**, *30*, 2929–2939.

55. Lee, S.J.; Koo, H.; Jeong, H.; Huh, M.S.; Choi, Y.; Jeong, S.Y.; Byun, Y.; Choi, K.; Kim, K.; Kwon, I.C. Comparative study of photosensitizer loaded and conjugated glycol chitosan nanoparticles for cancer therapy. *J. Control. Release* **2011**, *152*, 21–29.

56. Bae, Y.H.; Yin, H. Stability issues of polymeric micelles. *J. Control. Release* **2008**, *131*, 2–4.

57. Lee, S.J.; Koo, H.; Lee, D.E.; Min, S.; Lee, S.; Chen, X.; Choi, Y.; Leary, J.F.; Park, K.; Jeong, S.Y.; *et al.* Tumor-homing photosensitizer-conjugated glycol chitosan nanoparticles for synchronous photodynamic imaging and therapy based on cellular on/off system. *Biomaterials* **2011**, *32*, 4021–4029.

58. Baskin, J.M.; Prescher, J.A.; Laughlin, S.T.; Agard, N.J.; Chang, P.V.; Miller, I.A.; Lo, A.; Codelli, J.A.; Bertozzi, C.R. Copper-free click chemistry for dynamic *in vivo* imaging. *Proc. Natl. Acad. Sci. USA* **2007**, *104*, 16793–16797.

59. Chang, P.V.; Prescher, J.A.; Sletten, E.M.; Baskin, J.M.; Miller, I.A.; Agard, N.J.; Lo, A.; Bertozzi, C.R. Copper-free click chemistry in living animals. *Proc. Natl. Acad. Sci. USA* **2010**, *107*, 1821–1826.

60. Prescher, J.A.; Bertozzi, C.R. Chemistry in living systems. *Nat. Chem. Biol.* **2005**, *1*, 13–21.

61. Rostovtsev, V.V.; Green, L.G.; Fokin, V.V.; Sharpless, K.B. A stepwise huisgen cycloaddition process: Copper(I)-catalyzed regioselective "ligation" of azides and terminal alkynes. *Angew. Chem.* **2002**, *41*, 2596–2599.

62. Tornoe, C.W.; Christensen, C.; Meldal, M. Peptidotriazoles on solid phase: [1,2,3]-triazoles by regiospecific copper(i)-catalyzed 1,3-dipolar cycloadditions of terminal alkynes to azides. *J. Org. Chem.* **2002**, *67*, 3057–3064.

63. Agard, N.J.; Prescher, J.A.; Bertozzi, C.R. A strain-promoted [3 + 2] azide-alkyne cycloaddition for covalent modification of biomolecules in living systems. *J. Am. Chem. Soc.* **2004**, *126*, 15046–15047.

64. Ngo, J.T.; Champion, J.A.; Mahdavi, A.; Tanrikulu, I.C.; Beatty, K.E.; Connor, R.E.; Yoo, T.H.; Dieterich, D.C.; Schuman, E.M.; Tirrell, D.A. Cell-selective metabolic labeling of proteins. *Nat. Chem. Biol.* **2009**, *5*, 715–717.

65. Cheng, Z.; Al Zaki, A.; Hui, J.Z.; Muzykantov, V.R.; Tsourkas, A. Multifunctional nanoparticles: Cost *versus* benefit of adding targeting and imaging capabilities. *Science* **2012**, *338*, 903–910.

66. Gartner, Z.J.; Bertozzi, C.R. Programmed assembly of 3-dimensional microtissues with defined cellular connectivity. *Proc. Natl. Acad. Sci. USA* **2009**, *106*, 4606–4610.

67. Bertozzi, C.R.; Kiessling, L.L. Chemical glycobiology. *Science* **2001**, *291*, 2357–2364.

68. Lee, S.; Koo, H.; Na, J.H.; Han, S.J.; Min, H.S.; Lee, S.J.; Kim, S.H.; Yun, S.H.; Jeong, S.Y.; Kwon, I.C.; *et al.* Chemical tumor-targeting of nanoparticles based on metabolic glycoengineering and click chemistry. *ACS Nano* **2014**, *8*, 2048–2063.

69. Park, S.Y.; Baik, H.J.; Oh, Y.T.; Oh, K.T.; Youn, Y.S.; Lee, E.S. A smart polysaccharide/drug conjugate for photodynamic therapy. *Angew. Chem.* **2011**, *50*, 1644–1647.

70. Jensen, A.W.; Wilson, S.R.; Schuster, D.I. Biological applications of fullerenes. *Bioorg. Med. Chem.* **1996**, *4*, 767–779.

71. Kwag, D.S.; Oh, N.M.; Oh, Y.T.; Oh, K.T.; Youn, Y.S.; Lee, E.S. Photodynamic therapy using glycol chitosan grafted fullerenes. *Int. J. Pharm.* **2012**, *431*, 204–209.

72. Kwag, D.S.; Park, K.; Oh, K.T.; Lee, E.S. Hyaluronated fullerenes with photoluminescent and antitumoral activity. *Chem. Commun.* **2013**, *49*, 282–284.

73. Kim, S.; Lee, D.J.; Kwag, D.S.; Lee, U.Y.; Youn, Y.S.; Lee, E.S. Acid pH-activated glycol chitosan/fullerene nanogels for efficient tumor therapy. *Carbohydr. Polym.* **2014**, *101*, 692–698.

74. Lee, B.R.; Oh, K.T.; Baik, H.J.; Youn, Y.S.; Lee, E.S. A charge-switched nano-sized polymeric carrier for protein delivery. *Int. J. Pharm.* **2010**, *392*, 78–82.

75. Kean, T.; Thanou, M. Biodegradation, biodistribution and toxicity of chitosan. *Adv. Drug Deliv. Rev.* **2010**, *62*, 3–11.

76. Rodrigues, S.; Dionísio, M.; López, C.R.; Grenha, A. Biocompatibility of chitosan carriers with application in drug delivery. *J. Funct. Biomater.* **2012**, *3*, 615–641.

# Design of Chitosan and Its Water Soluble Derivatives-Based Drug Carriers with Polyelectrolyte Complexes

## Qing-Xi Wu, Dong-Qiang Lin and Shan-Jing Yao

**Abstract:** Chitosan, the cationic polysaccharide derived from the natural polysaccharide chitin, has been studied as a biomaterial for more than two decades. As a polycationic polymer with favorable properties, it has been widely used to form polyelectrolyte complexes with polyanions for various applications in drug delivery fields. In recent years, a growing number of studies have been focused on the preparation of polyelectrolyte complexes based on chitosan and its water soluble derivatives. They have been considered well-suited as biomaterials for a number of vital drug carriers with targeted/controlled release profiles, e.g., films, capsules, microcapsules. In this work, an overview highlights not only the favorable properties of chitosan and its water soluble derivatives but also the good performance of the polyelectrolyte complexes produced based on chitosan. Their various types of applications as drug carriers are reviewed in detail.

Reprinted from *Mar. Drugs*. Cite as: Wu, Q.-X.; Lin, D.-Q.; Yao, S.-J. Design of Chitosan and Its Water Soluble Derivatives-Based Drug Carriers with Polyelectrolyte Complexes. *Mar. Drugs* **2014**, *12*, 6236-6253.

## 1. Introduction

With nonrenewable resources running out all over the world, more and more polysaccharides from the natural world have been explored as advanced functional biomaterials and new energy resources, especially in recent years. Among them, chitin is known as the second most abundant renewable polymer in nature next only to cellulose. Chitin extensively exists in the exoskeleton of crustaceans, e.g., crab shells, lobsters, shrimp. It can also be found in mollusk radulas, cephalopod beaks, insects, fungal cell walls. Chitosan is considered a cationic polysaccharide, which is obtained from chitin following an alkaline deacetylation. With remarkable structural and functional properties, chitosan and its water soluble derivatives have been concerned by researchers in fundamental science and industry application.

Chitosan is a linear copolymer composed by glucosamine and *N*-acteyl glucosamine units, via β-(1,4) linkages, namely 2-amino-2-deoxy-β-D-glucan (GlcN) (Figure 1a). It is the product of the deacetylation reaction of chitin (2-acetamido-2-deoxy-β-D-glucan (GlcNAc)). Chitosan is able to dissolve in acidic solutions, becoming a polycationic polymer with a high density of positive charges ($-NH_3^+$ groups). It has favorable biological properties, such as no-toxicity, mucoadhesiveness, biocompatibility and, more importantly, the biodegradability, which means it could be digested by the bacteria in the human colon [1–3]. Recently, the water soluble derivatives of chitosan, hereafter water soluble chitosan (WSC), such as chitosan salts (Figure 1b), zwitterionic chitosan and chitosan oligomers, have drawn increasing attention due to their water-solubility [4–10]. WSC has the similar favorable properties with chitosan but can be dissolved in neutral aqueous media. Therefore, both of them are challenging biomaterials with potential vital applications in bioengineering and biopharmaceutical fields [11–14].

**Figure 1.** Structure of chitosan and chitosan salts.

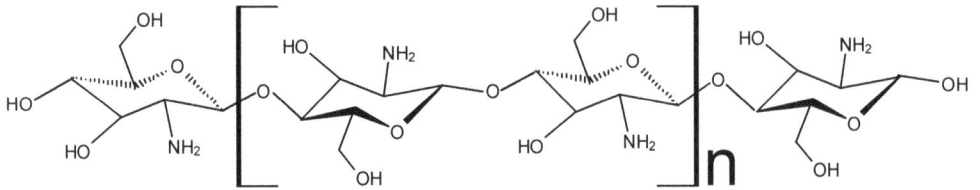

(a) Chitosan

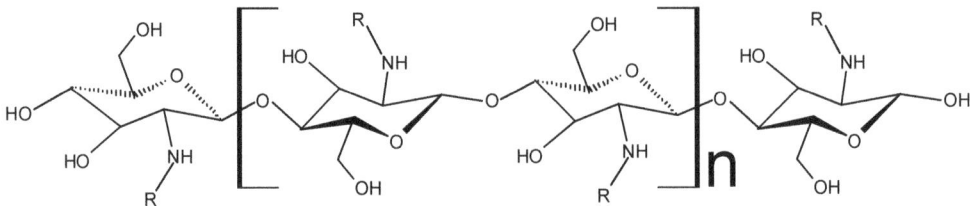

(b) Chitosan salts

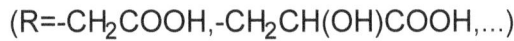

$$(R=-CH_2COOH,-CH_2CH(OH)COOH,...)$$

As a macromolecule with positive charges, chitosan and WSC can chemically conjugate with a lot of anionic substrates forming polyelectrolyte complexes (PEC). These anionic substrates include both polyanionic polymers and small molecular substances, such as sodium alginate [15,16], hyaluronic acid [17], sodium cellulose sulfate (NaCS) [18], glutaraldehyde [19], genipin [20]. Based on chitosan and WSC, the materials normally used for the preparation of PEC to design new drug delivery carriers can be seen in Table 1.

The prepared PEC based on these substances exhibit favorable biological performances, such as a definite hydrophilic and swellable character, low interfacial tension and high permeability, favorable film-forming behavior, excellent biodegradability and good biocompatibility [25]. Based on these favorable performances, PECs have received the attention of more and more researchers for the preparation of drug carriers or tissue engineering scaffolds [26–29]. The details will be presented in the next sections of this review.

**Table 1.** Materials normally used for the preparation of polyelectrolyte complexes (PEC) based on chitosan and water soluble chitosan (WSC).

| Polycationic Polyelectrolyte | Polyanionic Polyelectrolyte | Cross-Linking Agent | Preparation Method | Package Drugs | Reference |
|---|---|---|---|---|---|
| Chitosan | Sodium alginate | Calcium chloride | Coacervation | Rifampicin | [15] |
| Chitosan | Hyaluronic acid | TPP | Ionotropic gelation | Heparin | [17] |
| Chitosan | NaCS | — | Dipping-process | 5-ASA | [18] |
| Chitosan | Carrageenan | Glutaraldehyde | Complex coacervation | *Pimenta-dioica* oil | [19] |
| Chitosan | Carboxymethyl cellulose | Genipin | *In situ* synthesis | — | [20] |
| Chitosan | Pectin | — | Wet granulation | Theo-phylline | [21] |
| Chitosan | Xanthan gum | — | Hot-melt extrusion | CPM | [22] |
| Chitosan | — | Polyethylene glycol | Emulsification | 5-FU | [23] |
| WSC[a] | Poly-(L-aspartic acid) | — | Coagulation | BSA | [9] |
| WSC[b] | NaCS | PPS | Orifice-polymerization | Lactoferrin | [24] |

TPP: pentasodium tripolyphosphate; NaCS: sodium cellulose sulfate; 5-ASA: 5-aminosalicylic acid; CPM: chlorpheniramine maleate; 5-FU: 5-fluorouracil; WSC[a]: chitosan with molecular weight 6 kDa and deacetylation degree 0.93; BSA: bovine serum albumin; WSC[b]: chitosan hydrochloride; PPS: Sodium polyphosphate.

## 2. Properties of Chitosan and WSC

### 2.1. No-Toxicity

Chitosan is a well-known approved pharmaceutical excipient with no or low toxicity [30]. Chitosan has also been approved by the US Food and Drug Administration (FDA) for use in wound dressings [31] and is used as dietary additives in Japan, Italy and Finland [32]. Despite the lethal dose presented by chitosan as $LD_{50} = 16$ g/kg body weight when orally administered to mice, this level has been shown to be biodegradable [30,33]. In another study, Costa *et al.*, showed that chitosan-based mouthwash possessed no genotoxicity and lower cytotoxicity than the commercial mouthwash [34]. Meanwhile, alcohol-free mouthwash based on water-soluble chitosan has also proved to have no cytotoxicity [35]. It had also been confirmed that the toxicological side effects of chitosan are dependent on the molecular weight, degree of deacetylation and charge density of the molecule, specifically the toxicity is related to the molecular weight when at a high degree of deacetylation and it increases with increasing density [36].

## 2.2. Solubility

Chitosan is insoluble at neutral and high pH regions due to its molecular structure and $pK_a$ (6.2–7.0) [37,38]. It means that chitosan can be protonated at low pH in aqueous solutions [39]. Therefore, acidic solvents, such as diluted solutions of acetic acid (1%–3%, v/v) and citric acid (3%–4%, v/v) are usually needed to prepare chitosan solutions. However, the derivatives of chitosan, WSC can be directly dissolved in water under neutral pH conditions. It makes the process simpler while avoiding the use of acidic solvents; therefore WSC had received the attention of more and more researchers [37,40–44].

## 2.3. Biocompatibility

Chitosan has been widely used in the biomedical field, as it has already proved to be highly biocompatible [45,46]. Additionally, as a pharmaceutical excipient, WSCs like chitosan hydrochloride were approved by the European Pharmacopoeia (4th edition, 2002). Further, Marsiyana *et al.*, verified that the chitosan-bound microtubes were highly biocompatible and the experimental cells were able to survive and proliferate at a similar rate as the control [47]. Besides, the chitosan derivative named zwitterionic chitosan (ZWC), which is soluble in water at pH's below and above the p*I*, showed an excellent compatibility with the blood components and a good toleration upon an intraperitoneal (IP) injection [7]. Furthermore, the studies of Bajaj *et al.*, confirmed that ZWC could be used as a new biocompatible pharmaceutical excipient and a functional biomaterial [8].

## 2.4. Mucoadhesiveness

Chitosan is a bioadhesive substance with vital applications due to its excellent mucoadhesive properties, when in a swollen state, based on its cationic character. The mucoadhesiveness of chitosan derives from non-covalent interactions between chitosan and mucin, such as electrostatic interactions and hydrogen bonds [48,49]. As a polycationic polymer with a high density of positive charges, it can adhere to both hard and soft tissues, such as epithelial and mucosal tissues, via hydration, hydrogen bonding and ionic interactions, and has been widely explored as drug carriers, especially for colon-specific delivery [50]. For instance, in the *in vitro* mucoadhesive tests, the prednisolone loaded alginate/chitosan microparticles prepared by the one-step method exhibited excellent mucoadhesiveness, whereas their other properties were not statistically significant different [51]. Recently, a new conception has been proposed for novel applications of chitosan. Fernandes *et al.*, designed chitosan microspheres so as to serve as binders for *Helicobacter pylori* when facing a *H. pylori* gastric infection treatment [52], meaning that, after oral administration, the chitosan microspheres would remove *H. pylori* from infected patients, taking also the advantages of muco-bacterial adhesive properties.

*2.5. Biodegradability*

Chitosan is considered to be biodegradable in animal's metabolism, as it can be degraded by enzymes which hydrolyze glycosidic bonds, like -GlcN-GlcN-, -GlcN-GlcNAc-, -GlcNAc-GlcN- and -GlcNAc-GlcNAc- linkages. It could also be hydrolyzed by certain human enzymes, especially lysozyme [53]. Besides, chitosan and its WSC-derivatives are promising biomaterials whose glycosidic bonds could be hydrolyzed in the human colon [3,54,55]. Based on the specific microflora of the colon-ecosystem, WSC-derivatives may be particularly hydrolyzed by β-glucosidase secreted by the colonic bacteria [56]. Additionally, it has already been confirmed that the biodegradability of chitosan in living organisms depends on the deacetylation degree and on its molecular weight [57–59].

## 3. Performances of PEC Based on Chitosan and WSC

PECs are polymeric materials chemically formed by polyelectrolytes of opposite charges. They can be fabricated with polycationic and polyanionic macromolecules or polyelectrolytes and surfactants with opposite charges [60]. Based on the favorable properties of chitosan/WSC, the PECs formed by chitosan/WSC and anionic substrates (such as sodium alginate, hyaluronic acid, pentasodium tripolyphosphate) may present many excellent performances, as following: (1) Good hydrophilic and swellable character; (2) Low interfacial tension and high permeability; (3) Excellent biodegradability; (4) Good biocompatibility; (5) Favorable film-forming behavior.

The good hydrophilic and swellable characters of PECs are due to their ability to swell in water and biological fluids, and retain a significant fraction of water within their latticed structures [61,62]. Their low interfacial tension and higher permeability make PECs well-suited biomaterials for the preparation of targeted/controlled drug release carriers. Due to an excellent biodegradability in the colon and good biocompatibility with organisms, PECs could be good candidates for designing new oral colon-specific drug delivery systems (OCDDS). More importantly, because of their favorable film-forming behavior, the drug carriers prepared with PECs might be the base for various formulations, such as films, capsules, microcapsules, microparticles or nanoparticles.

## 4. Drug Carriers Designed with PECs Based on Chitosan and WSC

*4.1. Films*

PECs, based on chitosan and WSC, might be used as the controlled release drug carriers for designing new skin drug delivery systems [63]. As can be seen in Table 2, some cross-linking agents, like glycerol and PEG200, were used to improve the performances of PEC films which were most of the times prepared via casting but also by self-assembly methods using some proper templates [63–66].

In a previous study, Zhu *et al.*, confirmed that the PEC films based on chitosan (molecular weight of 135.3 kDa) and NaCS (molecular weight of 710.8 kDa) showed the highest susceptibility to the hydrolysis by pepsin, amylase and trypsin. In addition, the disintegration time of the PEC films along the gastrointestinal tract (GIT) was different depending on the PEC formulations (Figure 2) [59]. The mass ratios of chitosan to NaCS had great influence on the morphology of the formulations and had important effects on the swelling properties and permeability of the films (Figure 3). A study on the release of paracetamol-loaded PEC films showed that the permeability of the films was closely related to the swelling properties and significantly influenced by the mass ratios, molecular weights and pH values [64]. These results indicated that the PEC films could be used as good candidates for the GIT delivery systems, especially for designing new colon-specific drug delivery systems.

**Table 2.** Drug carriers prepared with films of polyelectrolyte complexes (PECs).

| Polycationic Polyelectrolyte | Polyanionic Polyelectrolyte | Cross-Linking Agent | Preparation Method | Package Drugs | Reference |
|---|---|---|---|---|---|
| Chitosan | Polyacrylic acid | Glycerol/ PEG200/ Hydrovance/ Trehalose | Cast | — | [63] |
| Chitosan | NaCS | — | Cast | Paracetamol /5-ASA | [59,64] |
| Chitosan | Polyalkyleneoxide -maleic acid copolymer | — | Cast | Salicylic acid/Phenol | [65] |
| Chitosan | Hyaluronic acid | — | Self-assembly | — | [66] |

**Figure 2.** *In vitro* degradation profiles of chitosan/NaCS films in simulated gastric fluid (SGF, stage I), simulated intestinal fluid (SIF, stage II) and simulated colonic fluid (SCF, stage III). Sample 1: 563.3 kDa chitosan and 169.7 kDa NaCS; sample 2: 563.3 kDa chitosan and 31.2 kDa NaCS; sample 3: 135.3 kDa chitosan and 710.8 kDa NaCS; sample 4: 563.3 kDa chitosan and 710.8 kDa NaCS. Modified and cited from Zhu *et al.* [59].

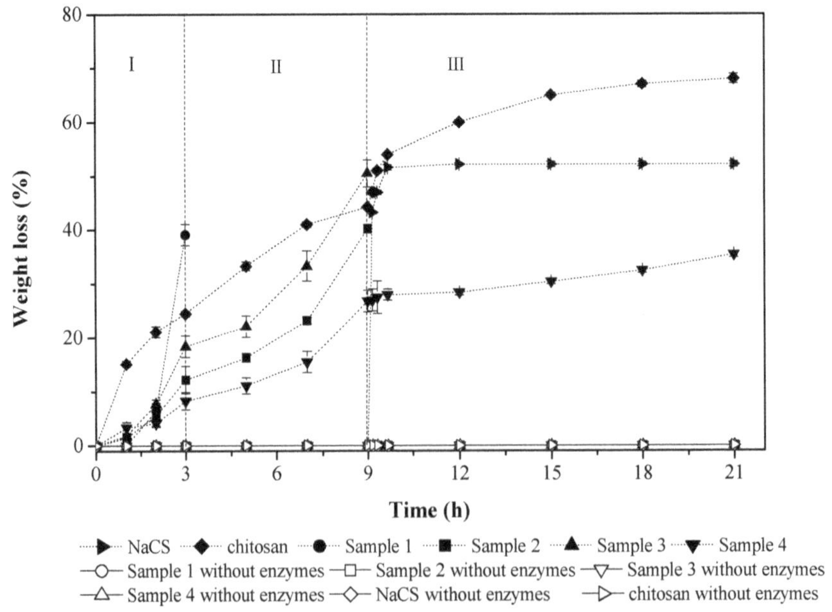

**Figure 3.** SEM morphology of chitosan/NaCS films prepared with different mass ratios. Mass ratios of chitosan to NaCS of (**a**) 1:4; (**b**) 1:2; (**c**) 3:4 and (**d**) 1:1. Chitosan with molecular weight 563.3 kDa and NaCS with molecular weight 710.8 kDa were used. Modified and cited from Zhu *et al.* [64].

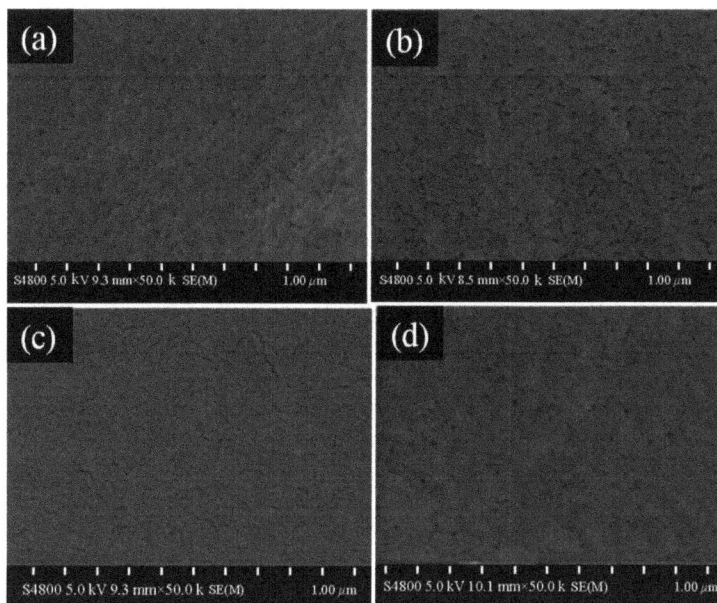

*4.2. Hard Hollow Capsules*

Hard hollow capsules made up of chitosan have been a research concern since the 1990s [55]. Due to the solubility of chitosan in acidic conditions, hard hollow capsules prepared with chitosan must be coated with enteric coatings, like hydroxypropyl methylcellulose phthalate (HPMCP), to prevent disintegration during their passage through the stomach and small intestine [67]. These kinds of chitosan capsules proved to be useful carriers for colon-specific delivery of drugs like *n*-dodecyl-β-D-maltopyranoside and rebamipide, and could increase the effects of drugs by enhancing their absorption by the intestinal membranes [68,69].

However, hard hollow capsules prepared with PEC and based on chitosan were seldom reported. In the past few years, Wang *et al.*, developed a novel PEC capsule system which was formed by chitosan and sodium cellulose sulfate (NaCS) [18]. The PEC-based hard hollow capsules had a relatively homogeneous and smooth morphology (Figure 4a). *In vitro* degradation studies showed that the PEC films could be degraded by colon microflora and hydrolyzed in simulated gastrointestinal fluids, like simulated gastric (SGF) and intestinal fluids (SIF) (Figure 4b–f). More importantly, this kind of PEC-based hard hollow capsules loaded with 5-ASA may release about 80% of the drug in the simulated colonic fluid (SCF) during 4 h, indicating an excellent microflora-activated and colon-specific performance (Figure 4g). All these results indicated that the PEC-based capsules could be good candidates for designing new colon-specific drug delivery systems [18,70].

**Figure 4.** SEM morphology of the capsules and films, and the *in vitro* drug release profiles based on NaCS-chitosan. (**a**) Hard hollow capsules; (**b**) Films at 0 h in the *in vitro* experiment; (**c**) Films at 1 h in the *in vitro* experiment (SGF); (**d**) Films at 5 h in the *in vitro* experiment (SIF); (**e**) Films at 11 h in the *in vitro* experiment (SCF); (**f**) Films at 17 h in the *in vitro* experiment (SCF); (**g**) *In vitro* drug release profiles of 5-ASA from drug-loaded capsules based on NaCS-chitosan films or not. Stage I, in the SGF for 1 h; stage II, in the SIF for 4 h; stage III, in the SCF for 7 h. Sample C1(■), sample C2(●), sample C3 (▲), sample C1 in PBS after 5 h (□), sample C2 in PBS after 5 h (○), sample C3 in PBS after 5 h (Δ), capsule without NaCS-chitosan (◊). Samples (C1, C2, C3) were prepared with NaCS-chitosan films, gelatin and carrageenan as raw materials; capsules without NaCS-chitosan were prepared with gelatin and carrageenan as raw materials by the same method. Modified and cited from Wang *et al.* [18].

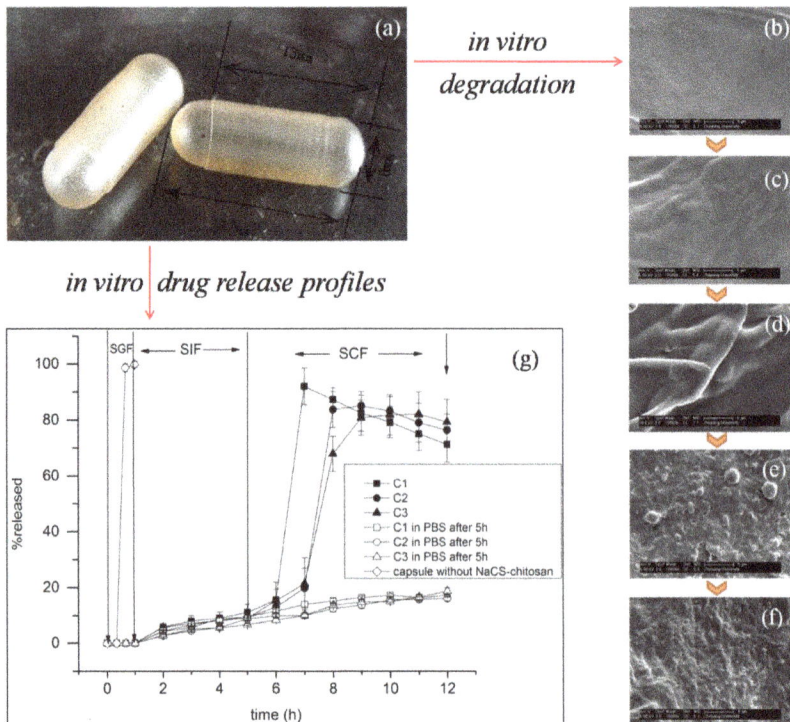

### 4.3. Microcapsules

Microcapsules of PEC based on chitosan and WSC, have gained large attention due to their potential applications (Table 3). With a large surface area, PEC microcapsules were designed in order to carry various drugs for targeted/controlled release [71–76]. Besides, they have also been widely studied in several biotechnological fields, such as fermentation with immobilized cells [77] and as vehicles for delivering probiotic bacteria [78,79].

**Table 3.** Drug carriers prepared with polyelectrolyte complexes (PEC) microcapsules.

| Polycationic Polyelectrolyte | Polyanionic Polyelectrolyte | Cross-Linking Agent | Preparation Method | Package Drugs | Reference |
|---|---|---|---|---|---|
| Chitosan | NaCS | Sodium polyphosphate | Orifice-polymerization | 5-ASA | [71] |
| Chitosan | Sodium alginate | — | Electrospray | Albumin | [72] |
| Chitosan | Sodium alginate | Calcium chloride | Modified orifice | Albendazole | [73] |
| Chitosan | NaCS | — | Self-assembly | — | [74] |
| Chitosan | kappa-carrageenan | Glutaraldehyde/ Genipin/ Tannic acid | Emulsion | Neem Seed Oil | [75] |
| WSC[b] | NaCS | Sodium polyphosphate | Orifice-polymerization | Lactoferrin | [76] |

**Figure 5.** SEM morphology of the microcapsules and pure 5-ASA, and the *in vitro* drug release profiles. (**a**) Transection image of the double-walled capsule; (**b**) Transection image of the outer coated membrane layer (outer wall) and the loaded drug of 5-ASA; (**c**) Pure 5-ASA; (**d**) *In vitro* drug release studies in SCF (pH 6.4) and PBS (pH 6.4); (**e**) Nonlinear curve fitting of accumulative drug release in SCF (pH 6.4). Microcapsules were prepared with NaCS, WSC[b] and PPS as raw materials. Modified and cited from Wu *et al.* [71].

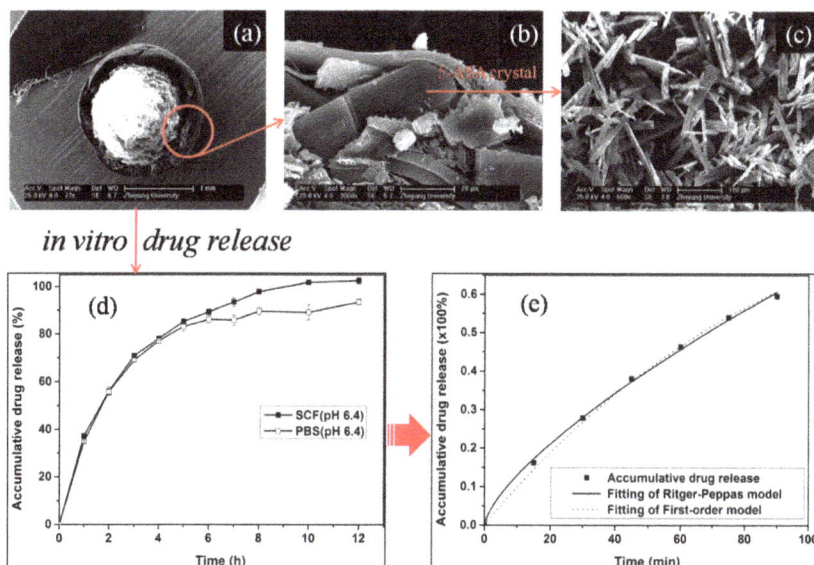

Recently, novel PEC microcapsules based on NaCS, chitosan/WSC and sodium polyphosphate (PPS) were developed following simple processes, and this type of microcapsules could be used for designing new colon-specific drug delivery systems [24,71,76]. In this system, NaCS is the polyanion with $-SO_3^-$ groups while chitosan/WSC is the polycation with $-NH_3^+$ groups, PPS was used as a cross-linking agent. Based on the PEC obtained by ionization, spherical microcapsules were prepared by the orifice-polymerization method. These materials had been successfully used to encapsulate two kinds of model drugs: 5-aminosalicylic acid (5-ASA, a small molecular drug) [71] and lactoferrin (LF, a protein drug) [24,76].

It was verified that the PEC microcapsules loaded with 5-ASA had a relatively high loading efficiency (60.77%) and encapsulation efficiency (90.03%). SEM micrographs showed that the microcapsules were involved by a double-walled structure (shell) (Figure 5a,b). SEM transection images showed that 5-ASA entrapped in the microcapsule was in a crystal form (Figure 5b,c). *In vitro* release analysis showed that the drug was completely released in the simulated colonic fluid (SCF, pH 6.4), and the drug release was under the mechanism of anomalous transport (Figure 5d,e) [71].

The microcapsules made of PEC and loaded with LF were also successfully prepared by Wu *et al.* [24,76]. SEM studies showed that the PEC microcapsules had a typical wall-capsule structure with smooth surfaces (Figure 6a,b). Fourier transform infrared spectroscopy (FT-IR) spectra analysis indicated that $-NH_3^+$ of chitosan/WSC, $-SO_3^-$ of NaCS and $-[P_2O_5^{4-}]-$ of PPS may react to form PEC. A schematic illustration of polyelectrolyte complexes formation process can be seen in Figure 6c. Drug loading and encapsulation efficiency studies also showed that the PEC microcapsules had a relatively high loading efficiency (49.06%) and encapsulation efficiency (86.3%). *In vitro* release studies showed that the microcapsules had a regular drug release behavior and the drug was released sustainably and completely in SCF (pH 5.5–7.0) [24].

**Figure 6.** SEM morphology of the LF loaded NaCS-WSC-PPS microcapsules, and its formation process. (**a**) External appearance; (**b**) Transection image; (**c**) Schematic illustration of polyelectrolyte complexes formation process. Modified and cited from Wu *et al.* [24].

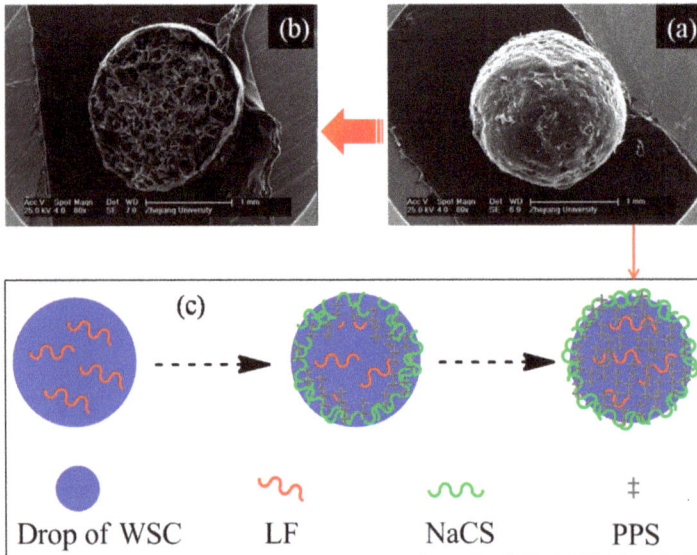

Table 4. Drug carriers prepared with microparticles or nanoparticles of polyelectrolyte complexes (PEC).

| Polycationic Polyelectrolyte | Polyanionic Polyelectrolyte | Cross-Linking Agent | Preparation Method | Package Drugs | Reference |
| --- | --- | --- | --- | --- | --- |
| Chitosan | Dextran sulfate | — | Self-assembly | Insulin | [80] |
| WSC[c] | Sodium alginate | Calcium chloride | Coaxial air-flow | Naproxen | [10] |
| Chitosan | Pectin | Tripolyphosphate | Emulsion | Gliclazide | [81] |
| Chitosan | Hyaluronan sodium salt | — | Stirring (Non-solvent) | Chloramphenicol succinate sodium salt/ Cefotaxime sodium salt | [82] |
| Chitosan | Polybetaine | — | Stirring | Chloramphenicol succinate sodium salt | [83] |
| Chitosan | Hyaluronic acid | — | Self-assembly | Paclitaxel | [84] |
| Chitosan | Carboxymethyl gum kondagogu | — | Coacervation | Ofloxacin | [85] |
| Chitosan | Sodium alginate | — | Ionic gelation | Amoxicillin | [86] |

WSC[c]: oligochitosan with deacetylation degree >85% and molecular weight around 3 kDa.

## 4.4. Microparticles/Nanoparticles

Microparticles or nanoparticles of PEC based on chitosan and WSC are also popular forms of drug carriers, as can be seen in Table 4. These are the most common strategies to improve the bioavailability of protein drugs via micro- and nanoencapsulation techniques. For example, in order to improve insulin bioavailability, Balabushevich et al., developed a kind of multifunctional protein-polymer microparticles via self-assembly method [80]. When using this multicomponent of insulin loaded microparticle system, the oral bioavailability of loaded-insulin improved due to the cumulative effect of each component, and the blood glucose level effectively lowered in the diabetic rats.

Besides, chitosan was usually used to coat hyaluronic acid-paclitaxel nanoparticles to prepare pH-responsive PEC drug-loaded-nanoparticles [84,87]. It is well-known that paclitaxel is a mitotic inhibitor used in cancer chemotherapy [88,89]. This kind of PEC nanoparticles takes several favorable advantages, such as a simple and feasible process, with a targeting and pH-sensitive release. For instance, the formulation of ofloxacin loaded nanoparticles provided a sustained drug release with 27% of the drug getting released in 12 h in the in vitro tests [90]. Guo et al., designed a kind of novel polyelectrolyte complex nanoparticles (PCNs) which are capable of associating bovine serum albumin (BSA), and in vitro studies showed that the system could keep a sustained drug release manner for 1 month without burst release [91]. Anitha et al., developed a combinatorial nanomedicine of 5-FU and curcumin (CUR) loaded nanoparticles, in vitro drug release profile showed a sustained release over a period of 4 days, further in vivo experiments in mouse verified an improved plasma concentration which could be prolonged up to 72 h [92]. Therefore, microparticles or nanoparticles of PEC based on chitosan and WSC could potentially be used in vital applications, such as designing of targeted/controlled drug delivery systems.

## 5. Conclusions

In view of the vital properties, such as no-toxicity, high biocompatibility and excellent biodegradability, chitosan and its water soluble derivatives (WSC) will be challenging biomaterials with potential applications in pharmaceutical fields, especially in the targeted/controlled release drug delivery field. Further, based on the favorable performances, such as good hydrophilic and swellable character, low interfacial tension and high permeability and favorable film-forming behavior, chitosan-based polyelectrolyte complexes, in proper forms like films, capsules and microparticles, might become important drug carriers with a promising application prospect.

## Acknowledgments

This work was supported by the Doctoral Research Start-up Fund of Anhui University, the National Natural Science Foundation of China and the Doctoral Programs Foundation of Ministry of Education of China.

## Conflicts of Interest

The authors declare no conflict of interest.

## References

1. Onishi, H.; Machida, Y. Biodegradation and distribution of water-soluble chitosan in mice. *Biomaterials* **1999**, *20*, 175–182.
2. Xia, W.S.; Liu, P.; Liu, J. Advance in chitosan hydrolysis by non-specific cellulases. *Bioresour. Technol.* **2008**, *99*, 6751–6762.
3. Zhang, H.; Alsarra, I.A.; Neau, S.H. An *in vitro* evaluation of a chitosan-containing multiparticulate system for macromolecule delivery to the colon. *Int. J. Pharm.* **2002**, *239*, 197–205.
4. Zhang, Y.Q.; Niu, Y.G.; Luo, Y.C.; Ge, M.; Yang, T.; Yu, L.L.; Wang, Q. Fabrication, characterization and antimicrobial activities of thymol-loaded zein nanoparticles stabilized by sodium caseinate-chitosan hydrochloride double layers. *Food Chem.* **2014**, *142*, 269–275.
5. Dang, Q.F.; Yan, J.Q.; Li, Y.; Cheng, X.J.; Liu, C.S.; Chen, X.G. Chitosan acetate as an active coating material and its effects on the storing of *Prunus avium* L. *J. Food Sci.* **2010**, *75*, S125–S131.
6. Parodi, B.; Russo, E.; Caviglioli, G.; Baldassari, S.; Gaglianone, N.; Schito, A.M.; Cafaggi, S. A chitosan lactate/poloxamer 407-based matrix containing Eudragit RS microparticles for vaginal delivery of econazole: Design and *in vitro* evaluation. *Drug Dev. Ind. Pharm.* **2013**, *39*, 1911–1920.
7. Xu, P.S.; Bajaj, G.; Shugg, T.; van Alstine, W.G.; Yeo, Y. Zwitterionic chitosan derivatives for pH-sensitive stealth coating. *Biomacromolecules* **2010**, *11*, 2352–2358.
8. Bajaj, G.; van Alstine, W.G.; Yeo, Y. Zwitterionic chitosan derivative, a new biocompatible pharmaceutical excipient, prevents endotoxin-mediated cytokine release. *PLoS One* **2012**, *7*, 1–10.
9. Shu, S.J.; Zhang, X.G.; Teng, D.Y.; Wang, Z.; Li, C.X. Polyelectrolyte nanoparticles based on water-soluble chitosan-poly(L-aspartic acid)-polyethylene glycol for controlled protein release. *Carbohyd. Res.* **2009**, *344*, 1197–1204.
10. Čalija, B.; Cekić, N.; Savić, S.; Daniels, R.; Marković, B.; Milić, J. pH-sensitive microparticles for oral drug delivery based on alginate/oligochitosan/Eudragit® L100–55 "sandwich" polyelectrolyte complex. *Colloid. Surf. B* **2013**, *110*, 395–402.
11. Franco, R.A.; Nguyen, T.H.; Lee, B.T. Preparation and characterization of electrospun PCL/PLGA membranes and chitosan/gelatin hydrogels for skin bioengineering applications. *J. Mater. Sci. Mater. M.* **2011**, *22*, 2207–2218.
12. Mahmoudzadeh, M.; Fassihi, A.; Emami, J.; Davies, N.M.; Dorkoosh, F. Physicochemical, pharmaceutical and biological approaches toward designing optimized and efficient hydrophobically modified chitosan-based polymeric micelles as a nanocarrier system for targeted delivery of anticancer drugs. *J. Drug Target.* **2013**, *21*, 693–709.

13. Supper, S.; Anton, N.; Seidel, N.; Riemenschnitter, M.; Curdy, C.; Vandamme, T. Thermosensitive chitosan/glycerophosphate-based hydrogel and its derivatives in pharmaceutical and biomedical applications. *Expert Opin. Drug Deliv.* **2014**, *11*, 249–267.

14. Zakhem, E.; Raghavan, S.; Bitar, K.N. Neo-innervation of a bioengineered intestinal smooth muscle construct around chitosan scaffold. *Biomaterials* **2014**, *35*, 1882–1889.

15. Lacerda, L.; Parize, A.L.; Fávere, V.; Laranjeira, M.C.M.; Stulzer, H.K. Development and evaluation of pH-sensitive sodium alginate/chitosan microparticles containing the antituberculosis drug rifampicin. *Mat. Sci. Eng. C* **2014**, *39*, 161–167.

16. Xiong, Y.; Yan, K.; Bentley, W.E.; Deng, H.B.; Du, Y.M.; Payne, G.F.; Shi, X.W. Compartmentalized Multilayer Hydrogel Formation Using a Stimulus-Responsive Self-Assembling Polysaccharide. *ACS Appl. Mater. Inter.* **2014**, *6*, 2948–2957.

17. Oyarzun-Ampuero, F.A.; Brea, J.; Loza, M.I.; Torres, D.; Alonso, M.J. Chitosan-hyaluronic acid nanoparticles loaded with heparin for the treatment of asthma. *Int. J. Pharm.* **2009**, *381*, 122–129.

18. Wang, M.J.; Xie, Y.L.; Zheng, Q.D.; Yao, S.J. A novel, potential microflora-activated carrier for a colon-specific drug delivery system and its characteristics. *Ind. Eng. Chem. Res.* **2009**, *48*, 5276–5284.

19. Dima, C.; Cotarlet, M.; Alexe, P.; Dima, S. Microencapsulation of essential oil of pimento [*Pimenta dioica (L) Merr.*] by chitosan/*k*-carrageenan complex coacervation method. *Innov. Food Sci. Emerg.* **2014**, *22*, 203–211.

20. Kaihara, S.; Suzuki, Y.; Fujimoto, K. *In situ* synthesis of polysaccharide nanoparticles via polyion complex of carboxymethyl cellulose and chitosan. *Colloid. Surf. B.* **2011**, *85*, 343–348.

21. Pandey, S.; Mishra, A.; Raval, P.; Patel, H.; Gupta, A.; Shah, D. Chitosan-pectin polyelectrolyte complex as a carrier for colon targeted drug delivery. *J. Young Pharm.* **2013**, *5*, 160–166.

22. Fukuda, M.; Peppas, N.A.; McGinity, J.W. Properties of sustained release hot-melt extruded tablets containing chitosan and xanthan gum. *Int. J. Pharm.* **2006**, *310*, 90–100.

23. Ganguly, K.; Aminabhavi, T.M.; Kulkarni, A.R. Colon targeting of 5-fluorouracil using polyethylene glycol cross-linked chitosan microspheres enteric coated with cellulose acetate phthalate. *Ind. Eng. Chem. Res.* **2011**, *50*, 11797–11807.

24. Wu, Q.X.; Zhang, Q.L.; Lin, D.Q.; Yao, S.J. Characterization of novel lactoferrin loaded capsules prepared with polyelectrolyte complexes. *Int. J. Pharm.* **2013**, *455*, 124–131.

25. Hamman, J.H. Chitosan based polyelectrolyte complexes as potential carrier materials in drug delivery systems. *Mar. Drugs* **2010**, *8*, 1305–1322.

26. Luo, Y.C.; Wang, Q. Recent development of chitosan-based polyelectrolyte complexes with natural polysaccharides for drug delivery. *Int. J. Biol. Macromol.* **2014**, *64*, 353–367.

27. Yan, S.F.; Zhang, K.X.; Liu, Z.W.; Zhang, X.; Gan, L.; Cao, B.; Chen, X.S.; Cui, L.; Yin, J.B. Fabrication of poly(L-glutamic acid)/chitosan polyelectrolyte complex porous scaffolds for tissue engineering. *J. Mater. Chem. B* **2013**, *1*, 1541–1551.

28. Ma, G.P.; Wang, Z.L.; Chen, J.; Yin, R.X.; Chen, B.L.; Nie, J. Freeze-dried chitosan-sodium hyaluronate polyelectrolyte complex fibers as tissue engineering scaffolds. *New J. Chem.* **2014**, *38*, 1211–1217.

29. Busilacchi, A.; Gigante, A.; Mattioli-Belmonte, M.; Manzotti, S.; Muzzarelli, R. Chitosan stabilizes platelet growth factors and modulates stem cell differentiation toward tissue regeneration. *Carbohyd. Polym.* **2013**, *98*, 665–676.

30. Arai, K.; Kinumaki, T.; Fujita, T. Toxicity of chitosan. *Bull. Tokai Region. Fish. Res. Lab.* **1968**, *56*, 88–94.

31. Wedmore, I.; McManus, J.G.; Pusateri, A.E.; Holcomb, J.B. A special report on the chitosan-based hemostatic dressing: Experience in current combat operations. *J. Trauma* **2006**, *60*, 655–658.

32. Illum, L. Chitosan and its use as a pharmaceutical excipient. *Pharm. Res.* **1998**, *15*, 1326–1331.

33. Singh, V.; Tiwari, M. Hydrophobic modification of chitosan and its physicochemical evaluation as sustained release tablet formulation. *Asian J. Chem.* **2011**, *23*, 2141–2150.

34. Costa, E.M.; Silva, S.; Costa, M.R.; Pereira, M.; Campos, D.A.; Odila, J.; Madureira, A.R.; Cardelle-Cobas, A.; Tavaria, F.K.; Rodrigues, A.S.; *et al.* Chitosan mouthwash: Toxicity and *in vivo* validation. *Carbohyd. Polym.* **2014**, *111*, 385–392.

35. Chen, C.Y.; Chung, Y.C. Antibacterial effect of water-soluble chitosan on representative dental pathogens *Streptococcus Mutans* and *Lactobacilli Brevis*. *J. Appl. Oral Sci.* **2012**, *20*, 620–627.

36. Kean, T.; Thanou, M. Biodegradation, biodistribution and toxicity of chitosan. *Adv. Drug Deliver. Rev.* **2010**, *62*, 3–11.

37. Hawary, D.L.; Motaleb, M.A.; Farag, H.; Guirguis, O.W.; Elsabee, M.Z. Water-soluble derivatives of chitosan as a target delivery system of Tc-99m to some organs *in vivo* for nuclear imaging and biodistribution. *J. Radioanal. Nucl. Chem.* **2011**, *290*, 557–567.

38. Hejazi, R.; Amiji, M. Chitosan-based gastrointestinal delivery systems. *J. Control. Release* **2003**, *89*, 151–165.

39. Nunthanid, J.; Huanbutta, K.; Luangtana-anan, M.; Sriamornsak, P.; Limmatvapirat, S.; Puttipipatkhachorn, S. Development of time-, pH-, and enzyme-controlled colonic drug delivery using spray-dried chitosan acetate and hydroxypropyl methylcellulose. *Eur. J. Pharm. Biopharm.* **2008**, *68*, 253–259.

40. Shu, X.Z.; Zhu, K.J. Controlled drug release properties of ionically cross-linked chitosan beads: The influence of anion structure. *Int. J. Pharm.* **2002**, *233*, 217–225.

41. Rai, G.; Jain, S.K.; Agrawal, S.; Bhadra, S.; Pancholi, S.S.; Agrawal, G.P. Chitosan hydrochloride based microspheres of albendazole for colonic drug delivery. *Pharmazie* **2005**, *60*, 131–134.

42. Sobol, M.; Bartkowiak, A.; de Haan, B.; de Vos, P. Cytotoxicity study of novel water-soluble chitosan derivatives applied as membrane material of alginate microcapsules. *J. Biomed. Mater. Res. A* **2013**, *101*, 1907–1914.

43. Xiao, C.M.; Sun, F. Fabrication of distilled water-soluble chitosan/alginate functional multilayer composite microspheres. *Carbohyd. Polym.* **2013**, *98*, 1366–1370.

44. Sheng, Y.; He, H.J.; Zou, H. Poly(lactic acid) nanoparticles coated with combined WGA and water-soluble chitosan for mucosal delivery of beta-galactosidase. *Drug Deliv.* **2014**, *21*, 370–378.

45. Keong, L.C.; Halim, A.S. *In vitro* models in biocompatibility assessment for biomedical-grade chitosan derivatives in wound management. *Int. J. Mol. Sci.* **2009**, *10*, 1300–1313.

46. Muzzarelli, R.; Baldassarre, V.; Conti, F.; Ferrara, P.; Biagini, G.; Gazzanelli, G.; Vasi, V. Biological activity of chitosan: Ultrastructural study. *Biomaterials* **1988**, *9*, 247–252.

47. Henricus, M.M.; Fath, K.R.; Menzenski, M.Z.; Banerjee, I.A. Morphology controlled growth of chitosan-bound microtubes and a study of their biocompatibility and antibacterial activity. *Macromol. Biosci.* **2009**, *9*, 317–325.

48. Bravo-Osuna, I.; Vauthier, C.; Farabollini, A.; Palmieri, G.F.; Ponchel, G. Mucoadhesion mechanism of chitosan and thiolated chitosan-poly(isobutyl cyanoacrylate) core-shell nanoparticles. *Biomaterials* **2007**, *28*, 2233–2243.

49. Meng-Lund, E.; Muff-Westergaard, C.; Sander, C.; Madelung, P.; Jacobsen, J. A mechanistic based approach for enhancing buccal mucoadhesion of chitosan. *Int. J. Pharm.* **2014**, *461*, 280–285.

50. Gulbake, A.; Jain, S.K. Chitosan: A potential polymer for colon-specific drug delivery system. *Expert Opin. Drug Deliv.* **2012**, *9*, 713–729.

51. Wittaya-areekul, S.; Kruenate, J.; Prahsarn, C. Preparation and *in vitro* evaluation of mucoadhesive properties of alginate/chitosan microparticles containing prednisolone. *Int. J. Pharm.* **2006**, *312*, 113–118.

52. Fernandes, M.; Gonçalves, I.C.; Nardecchia, S.; Amaral, I.F.; Barbosa, M.A.; Martins, M.C.L. Modulation of stability and mucoadhesive properties of chitosan microspheres for therapeutic gastric application. *Int. J. Pharm.* **2013**, *454*, 116–124.

53. Muzzarelli, R. Human enzymatic activities related to the therapeutic administration of chitin derivatives. *Cell. Mol. Life Sci.* **1997**, *53*, 131–140.

54. Sinha, V.R.; Kumria, R. Polysaccharides in colon-specific drug delivery. *Int. J. Pharm.* **2001**, *224*, 19–38.

55. Tozaki, H.; Komoike, J.; Tada, C.; Maruyama, T.; Terabe, A.; Suzuki, T.; Yamamoto, A.; Muranishi, S. Chitosan capsules for colon-specific drug delivery: Improvement of insulin absorption from the rat colon. *J. Pharm. Sci.* **1997**, *86*, 1016–1021.

56. Orienti, I.; Cerchiara, T.; Luppi, B.; Bigucci, F.; Zuccari, G.; Zecchi, V. Influence of different chitosan salts on the release of sodium diclofenac in colon-specific delivery. *Int. J. Pharm.* **2002**, *238*, 51–59.

57. Yang, Y.M.; Hu, W.; Wang, X.D.; Gu, X.S. The controlling biodegradation of chitosan fibers by *N*-acetylation *in vitro* and *in vivo*. *J. Mater. Sci.-Mater. M.* **2007**, *18*, 2117–2121.

58. Xu, J.; McCarthy, S.P.; Gross, R.A.; Kaplan, D.L. Chitosan film acylation and effects on biodegradability. *Macromolecules* **1996**, *29*, 3436–3440.

59. Zhu, L.Y.; Lin, D.Q.; Yao, S.J. Biodegradation of polyelectrolyte complex films composed of chitosan and sodium cellulose sulfate as the controllable release carrier. *Carbohyd. Polym.* **2010**, *82*, 323–328.

60. Thunemann, A.F.; Muller, M.; Dautzenberg, H.; Joanny, J.; Lowen, H. Polyelectrolytes with defined molecular architecture II polyelectrolyte complexes. *Adv. Polym. Sci.* **2004**, *166*, 113–171.

61. Ramaraj, B.; Radhakrishnan, G. Hydrogel capsules for sustained drug-release. *J. Appl. Polym. Sci.* **1994**, *51*, 979–988.

62. Il'Ina, A.V.; Varlamov, V.P. Chitosan-based polyelectrolyte complexes: A review. *Appl. Biochem. Microbiol.* **2005**, *41*, 5–11.

63. Silva, C.L.; Pereira, J.C.; Ramalho, A.; Pais, A.A.C.C.; Sousa, J.J.S. Films based on chitosan polyelectrolyte complexes for skin drug delivery: Development and characterization. *J. Membrane Sci.* **2008**, *320*, 268–279.

64. Zhu, L.Y.; Yan, X.Q.; Zhang, H.M.; Lin, D.Q.; Yao, S.J.; Jiang, L. Determination of apparent drug permeability coefficients through chitosan-sodium cellulose sulfate polyelectrolyte complex films. *Acta Phys.-Chim. Sin.* **2014**, *30*, 365–370.

65. Yoshizawa, T.; Shin-ya, Y.; Hong, K.; Kajiuchi, T. pH- and temperature-sensitive release behaviors from polyelectrolyte complex films composed of chitosan and PAOMA copolymer. *Eur. J. Pharm. Biopharm.* **2005**, *59*, 307–313.

66. Feng, Q.; Zeng, G.; Yang, P.; Wang, C.; Cai, J. Self-assembly and characterization of polyelectrolyte complex films of hyaluronic acid/chitosan. *Colloid. Surf. A* **2005**, *257–258*, 85–88.

67. Tozaki, H.; Odoriba, T.; Okada, N.; Fujita, T.; Terabe, A.; Suzuki, T.; Okabe, S.; Muranishi, S.; Yamamoto, A. Chitosan capsules for colon-specific drug delivery: enhanced localization of 5-aminosalicylic acid in the large intestine accelerates healing of TNBS-induced colitis in rats. *J. Control. Release* **2002**, *82*, 51–61.

68. Fetih, G.; Lindberg, S.; Itoh, K.; Okada, N.; Fujita, T.; Habib, F.; Artersson, P.; Attia, M.; Yamamoto, A. Improvement of absorption enhancing effects of *n*-dodecyl-β-D-maltopyranoside by its colon-specific delivery using chitosan capsules. *Int. J. Pharm.* **2005**, *293*, 127–135.

69. Huang, B.B.; Li, G.F.; Luo, J.H.; Duan, L.; Nobuaki, K.; Akira, Y. Permeabilities of rebamipide via rat intestinal membranes and its colon specific delivery using chitosan capsule as a carrier. *World J. Gastroenterol.* **2008**, *14*, 4928–4937.

70. Wang, M.J.; Xie, Y.L.; Chen, Z.J.; Yao, S.J. Optimizing preparation of NaCS-chitosan complex to form a potential material for the colon-specific drug delivery system. *J. Appl. Polym. Sci.* **2010**, *117*, 3001–3012.

71. Wu, Q.X.; Yao, S.J. Novel NaCS-CS-PPS microcapsules as a potential enzyme-triggered release carrier for highly-loading 5-ASA. *Colloid. Surf. B* **2013**, *109*, 147–153.

72. Fukui, Y.; Maruyama, T.; Iwamatsu, Y.; Fujii, A.; Tanaka, T.; Ohmukai, Y.; Matsuyama, H. Preparation of monodispersed polyelectrolyte microcapsules with high encapsulation efficiency by an electrospray technique. *Colloid. Surf. A* **2010**, *370*, 28–34.

73. Simi, S.P.; Saraswathi, R.; Sankar, C.; Krishnan, P.N.; Dilip, C.; Ameena, K. Formulation and evaluation of Albendazole microcapsules for colon delivery using chitosan. *Asian Pac. J. Trop. Med.* **2010**, *3*, 374–378.

74. Xie, Y.L.; Wang, M.J.; Yao, S.J. Preparation and characterization of biocompatible microcapsules of sodium cellulose sulfate/chitosan by means of layer-by-layer self-assembly. *Langmuir* **2009**, *25*, 8999–9005.

75. Devi, N.; Maji, T.K. Effect of crosslinking agent on Neem (*Azadirachta Indica A. Juss.*) Seed Oil (NSO) encapsulated microcapsules *kappa*-carrageenan and chitosan polyelectrolyte complex. *J. Macromol. Sci. A* **2009**, *46*, 1114–1121.

76. Wu, Q.X.; Li, M.Z.; Yao, S.J. Performances of NaCS-WSC protein drug microcapsules with different degree of substitution of NaCS using sodium polyphosphate as cross-linking agent. *Cellulose* **2014**, *21*, 1897–1908.

77. Yu, W.T.; Song, H.Y.; Zheng, G.S.; Liu, X.D.; Zhang, Y.; Ma, X.J. Study on membrane characteristics of alginate-chitosan microcapsule with cell growth. *J. Membr. Sci.* **2011**, *377*, 214–220.

78. Cook, M.T.; Tzortzis, G.; Charalampopoulos, D.; Khutoryanskiy, V.V. Production and evaluation of dry alginate-chitosan microcapsules as an enteric delivery vehicle for probiotic bacteria. *Biomacromolecules* **2011**, *12*, 2834–2840.

79. Argin, S.; Kofinas, P.; Lo, Y.M. The cell release kinetics and the swelling behavior of physically crosslinked xanthan-chitosan hydrogels in simulated gastrointestinal conditions. *Food Hydrocolloid.* **2014**, *40*, 138–144.

80. Balabushevich, N.G.; Pechenkin, M.A.; Shibanova, E.D.; Volodkin, D.V.; Mikhalchik, E.V. Multifunctional polyelectrolyte microparticles for oral insulin delivery. *Macromol. Biosci.* **2013**, *13*, 1379–1388.

81. Barakat, N.S.; Almurshedi, A.S. Preparation and characterization of chitosan microparticles for oral sustained delivery of Gliclazide: *In Vitro/In Vivo* evaluation. *Drug Dev. Res.* **2011**, *72*, 235–246.

82. Vasiliu, S.; Popa, M.; Luca, C. Evaluation of retention and release processes of two antibiotics from the biocompatible core-shell microparticles. *Eur. Polym. J.* **2008**, *44*, 3894–3898.

83. Racovita, S.; Vasiliu, S.; Vlad, C.D. New drugs delivery systems based on polyelectrolyte complexes. *Rev. Roum. Chim.* **2010**, *55*, 659–666.

84. Li, J.; Huang, P.; Chang, L.; Long, X.; Dong, A.; Liu, J.; Chu, L.; Hu, F.; Liu, J.; Deng, L. Tumor targeting and pH-responsive polyelectrolyte complex nanoparticles based on hyaluronic acid-paclitaxel conjugates and chitosan for oral delivery of paclitaxel. *Macromol. Res.* **2013**, *21*, 1331–1337.

85. Kumar, A.; Ahuja, M. Carboxymethyl gum kondagogu-chitosan polyelectrolyte complex nanoparticles: Preparation and characterization. *Int. J. Biol. Macromol.* **2013**, *62*, 80–84.

86. Arora, S.; Gupta, S.; Narang, R.K.; Budhiraja, R.D. Amoxicillin loaded chitosan-alginate polyelectrolyte complex nanoparticles as mucopenetrating delivery system for *H. Pylori.* *Sci. Pharm.* **2011**, *79*, 673–694.

87. Paliwal, R.; Paliwal, S.R.; Agrawal, G.P.; Vyas, S.P. Chitosan nanoconstructs for improved oral delivery of low molecular weight heparin: *In vitro* and *in vivo* evaluation. *Int. J. Pharm.* **2012**, *422*, 179–184.

88. Li, C.; Newman, R.A.; Wu, Q.P.; Ke, S.; Chen, W.; Hutto, T.; Kan, Z.; Brannan, M.D.; Charnsangavej, C.; Wallace, S. Biodistribution of paclitaxel and poly(L-glutamic acid)-paclitaxel conjugate in mice with ovarian OCa-1 tumor. *Cancer Chemoth. Pharm.* **2000**, *46*, 416–422.

89. Jain, A.K.; Swarnakar, N.K.; Godugu, C.; Singh, R.P.; Jain, S. The effect of the oral administration of polymeric nanoparticles on the efficacy and toxicity of tamoxifen. *Biomaterials* **2011**, *32*, 503–515.
90. Shelly; Ahuja, M.; Kumar, A. Gum ghatti-chitosan polyelectrolyte nanoparticles: Preparation and characterization. *Int. J. Biol. Macromol.* **2013**, *61*, 411–415.
91. Guo, R.; Chen, L.L.; Cai, S.S.; Liu, Z.H.; Zhu, Y.; Xue, W.; Zhang, Y.M. Novel alginate coated hydrophobically modified chitosan polyelectrolyte complex for the delivery of BSA. *J. Mater. Sci.-Mater. Med.* **2013**, *24*, 2093–2100.
92. Anitha, A.; Sreeranganathan, M.; Chennazhi, K.P.; Lakshmanan, V.; Jayakumar, R. *In vitro* combinatorial anticancer effects of 5-fluorouracil and curcumin loaded *N,O*-carboxymethyl chitosan nanoparticles toward colon cancer and *in vivo* pharmacokinetic studies. *Eur. J. Pharm. Biopharm.* **2014**, *88*, 238–251.

# Does the Use of Chitosan Contribute to Oxalate Kidney Stone Formation?

Moacir Fernandes Queiroz, Karoline Rachel Teodosio Melo, Diego Araujo Sabry, Guilherme Lanzi Sassaki and Hugo Alexandre Oliveira Rocha

**Abstract:** Chitosan is widely used in the biomedical field due its chemical and pharmacological properties. However, intake of chitosan results in renal tissue accumulation of chitosan and promotes an increase in calcium excretion. On the other hand, the effect of chitosan on the formation of calcium oxalate crystals (CaOx) has not been described. In this work, we evaluated the antioxidant capacity of chitosan and its interference in the formation of CaOx crystals *in vitro*. Here, the chitosan obtained commercially had its identity confirmed by nuclear magnetic resonance and infrared spectroscopy. In several tests, this chitosan showed low or no antioxidant activity. However, it also showed excellent copper-chelating activity. *In vitro*, chitosan acted as an inducer mainly of monohydrate CaOx crystal formation, which is more prevalent in patients with urolithiasis. We also observed that chitosan modifies the morphology and size of these crystals, as well as changes the surface charge of the crystals, making them even more positive, which can facilitate the interaction of these crystals with renal cells. Chitosan greatly influences the formation of crystals *in vitro*, and *in vivo* analyses should be conducted to assess the risk of using chitosan.

Reprinted from *Mar. Drugs*. Cite as: Queiroz, M.F.; Teodosio Melo, K.R.; Sabry, D.A.; Sassaki, G.L.; Oliveira Rocha, H.A. Does the Use of Chitosan Contribute to Oxalate Kidney Stone Formation? *Mar. Drugs* **2015**, *13*, 141-158.

## 1. Introduction

Chitin and its derivative, chitosan, are biopolymers obtained from a large number of terrestrial and marine sources. They have become increasingly important since the study of fishing tailings of crustaceans began in the 1970s. Since then, various studies have been conducted on their properties, which provided a basis for the use of these two polymers in industrial and biotechnological applications [1]. Another factor that partly explains the industrial applicability of chitin/chitosan is the fact that chitin is the second most abundant natural polymer around the world. Chitin is composed of units of D-$N$-acetyl glucosamine linked together by β-(1–4). Chitosan is obtained from chitin, which undergoes different processes that remove the acetyl groups. The process of deacetylation of chitin to form chitosan is not complete, so by controlling the reaction conditions, it is possible to obtain chitosan with different levels of acetylation. Therefore, chitosan is defined as a linear polysaccharide formed by the random distribution of two monosaccharides, D-glucosamine and D-$N$-acetyl-glucosamine, which are joined together by a β-(1–4) bond. The amine groups are positively charged under physiological conditions [2].

Currently, many of the polymers used in various areas are synthetic materials, but their biocompatibility and biodegradability are very limited. On the other hand, chitosan is well known for its biocompatibility by presenting unique characteristics, such as a pH-dependent behavior, namely regarding its molecular conformation and solubility in the environment in which it is found, namely mucoadhesivity and the ease of overcoming the epithelial junctions. Furthermore, chitosan also has many pharmacological properties, making it a strong candidate to replace synthetic polymers [3,4]. In this context, in recent years, chitosan has been widely used for nanoparticle production; by the year 2012, there were approximately 10,000 published articles that had a nanotechnology and chitosan theme, accumulating more than 119,000 citations [5], which shows the considerable interest from the scientific community in the development of compounds made from chitosan. In addition, much of this interest is generated by the fact that chitosan transfers many of its properties to the nanoparticles formed from it. This leads to a question: Can the toxicity of chitosan also be transferred to nanocomposites? Existing data currently suggest that the polysaccharide chitosan is a compound with low toxicity [6,7] and that the chitosan nanoparticle toxicity would be more related to the nanoparticle size and the presence of other compounds than to the presence of chitosan [8].

Most of the chitosan-based nanocomposites, when administered to animals or patients, release chitosan into the blood stream [9]. The chitosan reaches several organs and tends to accumulate in the kidneys 8 h after oral administration [10,11], specifically in the proximal tubule cells [12]. It was also shown that the presence of chitosan in the body increases the amount of calcium excreted in urine [13]. Nevertheless, no studies have reported the toxicity of chitosan in renal tissue nor is there evidence that this caused the calcium oxalate crystal formation and consequent urolithiasis.

Urolithiasis is the formation of kidney stones, which can lead to tissue damage. This condition is a common cause of hospitalization. It is estimated that about 122 of 100,000 hospital admissions can be assigned to it. Moreover, once a patient is diagnosed with kidney stones, it is likely that the patient will develop new stones. Some studies have shown that 50%–70% of patients with a history of urolithiasis will have another crisis over the next 10 years [14].

The process of crystal formation occurs from urinary supersaturation, which provides nucleation of crystals. This event occurs when the crystal is used as a niche for similar crystals and/or macromolecules joined together, creating bigger and bigger particles. Once nucleated, the deposition of crystals in the other niche is easy and does not require such high levels of saturation as earlier in the process. The core can grow and add other crystals or organic matrix, forming the calculus, or be eliminated in the form of crystalluria [15]. After the crystallization, aggregation can occur, which describes the connection process of the crystals, resulting in the formation of agglomerate, which can precipitate [16].

Oxidative stress is another factor related to the formation of kidney stones [17]. Studies with mice that were induced to form kidney stones of calcium oxalate (CaOx) using different agents showed a decrease in plasma activities of antioxidant enzymes superoxide dismutase (SOD), catalase, glutathione peroxidase (GPx), glucose-6-phosphate dehydrogenase and glutathione S-transferase, as well as decreased plasma levels of free radical scavengers: vitamin E, vitamin C, protein thiol and reduced glutathione (GSH). It was also demonstrated that there was an increase in plasma lipid peroxidation marker molecules [18]. Data with patients who form CaOx calculus also show similar changes, indicating a positive correlation between the decrease of antioxidant defenses and the presence of oxalate/CaOx and CaOx crystal formation [19]. On the other hand, there are studies showing that antioxidant molecules can inhibit the formation of oxalate crystals in renal tissue [20,21].

As previously stated, chitosan is accumulated in renal tissue. Furthermore, it was demonstrated that the presence of chitosan in the body increases the amount of calcium excreted in urine [13], which is a primary factor in the formation of kidney stones. Given the above, this study investigated whether chitosan is able to induce the formation of CaOx crystals *in vitro* and whether it has antioxidant activity.

## 2. Results and Discussion

### 2.1. Chitosan Characterization

Chitosan was obtained commercially, and efforts were made to confirm its identity. To check whether there was contamination of the sample by impurities that could alter our results, we performed FTIR and $^1$H RMN analyses.

### 2.1.1. Chitosan FTIR Analyses

The FTIR test was used to assess the functional groups present in the chitosan.

In Figure 1, we can observe the infrared spectrum of chitosan. A strong band in the region 3291–361 cm$^{-1}$ corresponds to N-H and O-H stretching, as well as the intramolecular hydrogen bonds. The absorption bands at around 2921 and 2877 cm$^{-1}$ can be attributed to C-H symmetric and asymmetric stretching, respectively. These bands are characteristics typical of polysaccharide and are found in other polysaccharide spectra, such as xylan [22], glucans [23] and carrageenans [24]. The presence of residual *N*-acetyl groups was confirmed by the bands at around 1645 cm$^{-1}$ (C=O stretching of amide I) and 1325 cm$^{-1}$ (C-N stretching of amide III), respectively. We did not find the small band at 1550 cm$^{-1}$ that corresponds to N-H bending of amide II. This is the third band characteristic of typical N-acetyl groups, and it was probably overlapped by other bands. A band at 1589 cm$^{-1}$ corresponds to the N-H bending of the primary amine [25]. The CH$_2$ bending and CH$_3$ symmetrical deformations were confirmed by the presence of bands at around 1423 and 1375 cm$^{-1}$, respectively. The absorption band at 1153 cm$^{-1}$ can be attributed to asymmetric stretching of the C-O-C bridge. The bands at 1066 and 1028 cm$^{-1}$ correspond to C-O stretching. All bands are found in the spectra of samples of chitosan reported by others [26,27].

Since the chitosan used in this study is from animal origin, there is always the possibility of contamination by glycosaminoglycans (GAGs), which are another type of polysaccharide found in these organisms. GAGs are sulfated, and the presence of sulfate groups covalently bonded to the polysaccharide may be confirmed in the infrared spectra by the presence of very strong bands in the region around 1260–1270 cm$^{-1}$ [28]. In the spectrum obtained from chitosan (Figure 1), the signal at 1260 cm$^{-1}$ is very small and, therefore, does not correspond to sulfate groups, thus ruling out contamination of chitosan by GAGs. This signal at 1260 cm$^{-1}$ was assigned as the bending vibrations of hydroxyls present in chitosan [27]. The signal at 896 cm$^{-1}$ corresponds to the CH bending out of the plane of the ring of monosaccharides.

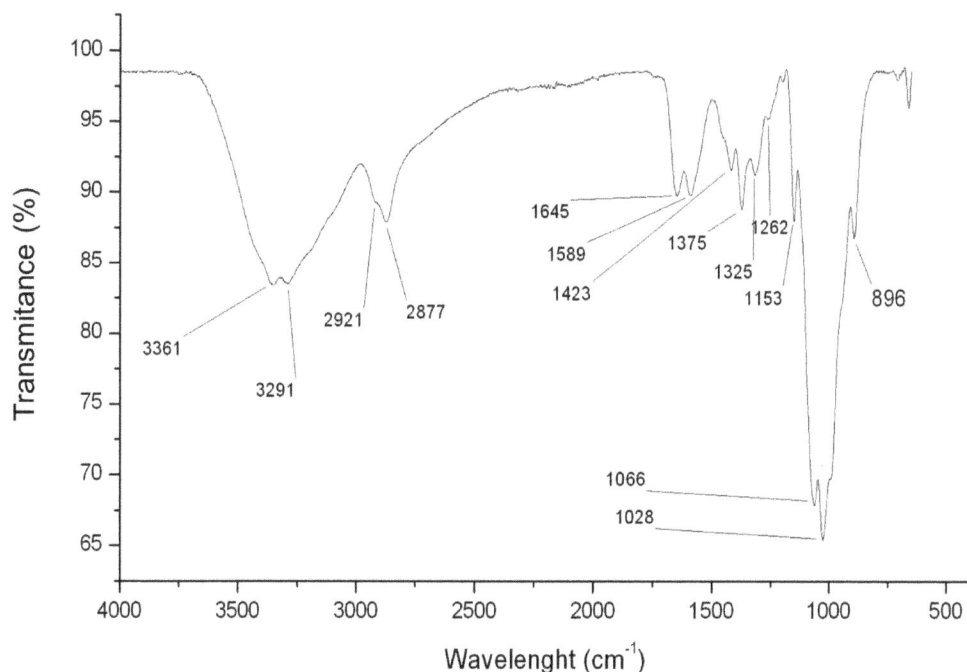

**Figure 1.** FTIR spectrum of chitosan with the characteristic signs as evidence.

2.1.2. Chitosan $^1$H NMR Analyses

In Figure 2, we can observe the $^1$H NMR spectrum of commercial chitosan. Using this technique, we can obtain a fingerprint spectrum of each molecule. For our sample, characteristic peaks of chitosan [29,30] were identified. In the region between 3.8 and 4.2 ppm are the signals of H2, H3, H4, H5 and H6 of the aldohexoses, which overlap and, thus, make evaluation difficult. Since the signals of the anomeric protons (H1) are clear at 5.25 ppm, a peak was marked as glucosamine anomeric H (H-1 (D)) and the signal at 5 ppm was assigned as anomeric H1-N acetyl glucosamine (H-1 (A)). The peak at 3.5 ppm was assigned as H2 glucosamine (H-2 (D)), and the peak at 2.5 ppm corresponded to the hydrogens of the methyl group of N-acetyl-glucosamine (H-AC). The peak at 4.75 ppm corresponded to the H of the solvent.

It is also possible to discover the degree of deacetylation (DD) of chitosan through $^1$H NMR, which is an efficient method and widely accepted in the literature for this determination. In order to determine the DD, the integral of some peaks of the $^1$H NMR spectrum of chitosan was used. There are several equations for this calculation [29]. In our case, we used equations as demonstrated by Lavertu *et al.* [30] and an average DD of 76.47% ± 4.08%, which is consistent with the range indicated by the supplier (75%–85%).

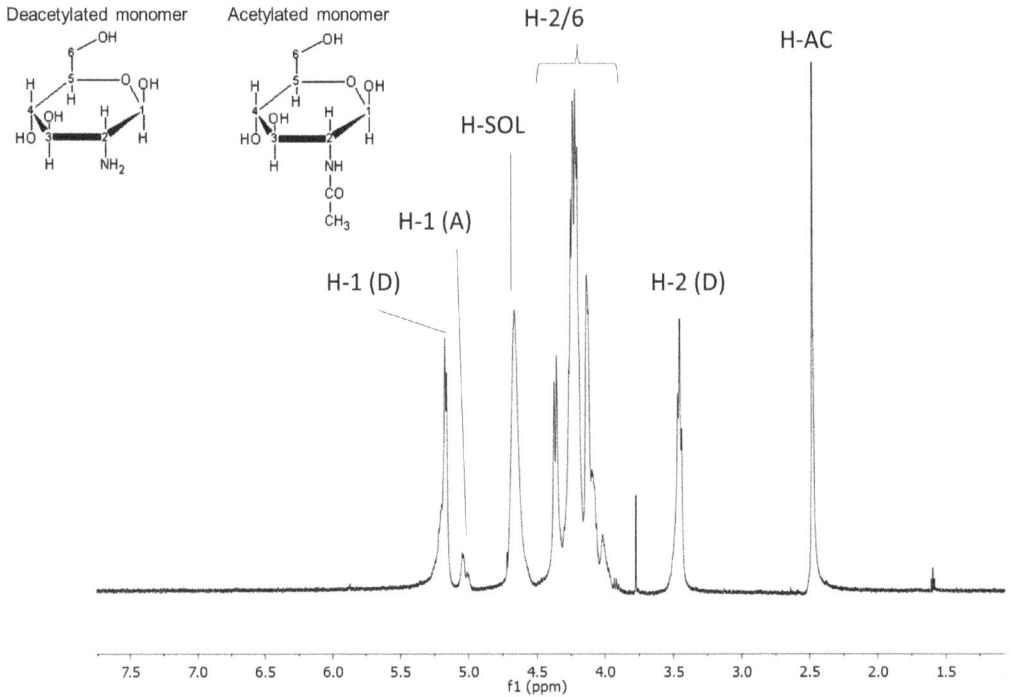

**Figure 2.** Chitosan $^1$H NMR Spectrum. AC corresponds to the acetyl group of glucosamine; D and A correspond to hydrogen of deacetylated and acetylated residues, respectively. H-SOL signaling corresponds to the solvent.

*2.2. Antioxidant Activities*

Free radicals are highly reactive molecules or ions, because they have one or more unpaired electrons in their outer shell [31]. High concentrations of these radicals can generate various physiological disorders and the onset of disease [32]. To combat free radicals, organisms use various antioxidant systems formed by enzymes and/or antioxidant molecules.

Some organs, such as the liver, heart and brain, are more affected by free radicals than others, due to several factors. In the case of kidneys, free radicals cause a specific injury: the presence of CaOx crystals induces the production of reactive species, which induce the formation of more CaOx crystals, which consequently promotes the formation of more radicals and tissue damage [17]. Therefore, the use of antioxidants may prevent crystal formation and consequent renal damage [20,21].

To evaluate the antioxidant capacity of chitosan, 5 (five) tests were performed: total antioxidant capacity, reducing power, chelation of copper, iron chelation and scavenging of the hydroxyl radical.

The total antioxidant capacity test measures the ability of the electron-donating compound in an acid medium. In this test, the polysaccharide showed low activity with 1 g of sample, an activity equivalent to 30 µg of vitamin C observed.

The reducing power test also evaluates the ability of the molecule to donate electrons. This assay was expressed as the percentage activity of ascorbic acid control at 0.1 mg/mL. In this test, the chitosan (from 0.05 to 1 mg/mL) showed maximum activity at a concentration of 1 mg/mL corresponding to 34% ± 4% of the vitamin C activity. This activity was similar to those observed with other polysaccharides obtained with sulfated fucan from seaweed *Spatoglossum schröederi* and sulfated galactans obtained from *Caulerpa cupressoides*, *Caulerpa prolifera* and *Gracilaria caudata* [33]. Furthermore, the effect observed here for chitosan as a reducing agent was superior to that reported in other studies [26,34,35].

We evaluated this activity using two different methods, neither of which demonstrated chitosan's iron-chelating activity. Several studies have shown that chitosan has iron-chelating activity, but this activity is not greater than 30% [26,34,36,37]. In addition, previous studies also reported that iron-chelating activity is dependent on both the molecular weight and the DD [36,37]. Thus, the smaller and more deacetylated the chitosan, the greater its chelating activity, as shown by Chien and colleagues [36]. These authors determined the iron-chelating activity of three different chitosans with DD of 98.5%, which possess different molecular weights (12, 95 and 318 kDa). The 95-kDa and 318-kDa chitosans (1 mg/mL) showed about 12% iron-chelating activity, whereas 12-kDa chitosan (1 mg/mL) showed about 23% iron-chelating activity. The chitosan used here has a molecular weight of 58 kDa, and its DD is about 76%, a combination of characteristics that could justify the fact that the chitosan did not exhibit iron-chelating activity.

In Figure 3, we observed the ability to chelate copper ions from chitosan; values of 90% chelation of the metal with only 0.5 mg/mL of sample were found; when this concentration was doubled, chelation of about 100% was obtained. This activity was greater than that described by Vino *et al.* [26], who showed chitosan (1 mg/mL) with a copper chelation capacity of around 88%.

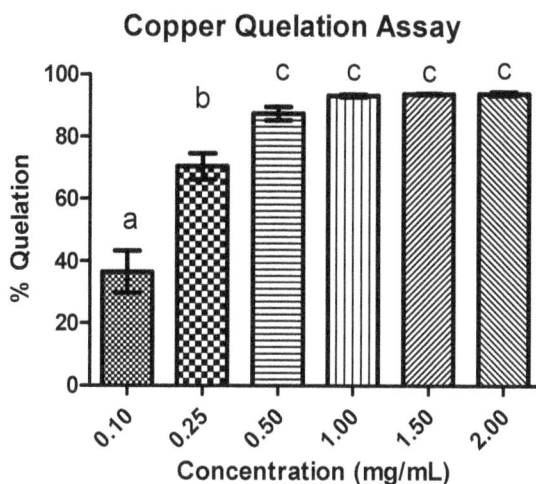

**Figure 3.** Activity of copper chelation on different chitosan concentrations. The letters indicate a significant difference between samples ($p < 0.05$).

Metals, such as iron and copper, in mobile environments can participate in reactions that ultimately produce hydroxyl radicals. This is very effective at causing lipid peroxidation. Therefore, the chitosan may indirectly inhibit lipid peroxidation. This property can be very important in avoiding the formation of CaOx kidney stones in that these crystals adhere to the surface of epithelial cells exactly where the surface is damaged due to lipid peroxidation [18]. The recent literature also shows that molecules with antioxidant capacity have demonstrated a potential to reduce crystal formation *in vitro* [38,39].

## 2.3. Crystal Formation

### 2.3.1. Crystal Formation *in Vitro*

Crystal formation consists of three events: nucleation, growth and aggregation. Nucleation is the approximation of ions of different charge, forming a nucleus from which the crystals are formed. The ions present in a solution are attracted to the nucleus, forming the first nanocrystal, which will increasingly attract ions entering the phase of crystal growth. Finally, the crystals begin to collide, merge and reach a size at which precipitation occurs by setting the stage for aggregation [40].

The test of crystal formation *in vitro* evaluates the ability of the sample to inhibit or stimulate the formation of CaOx crystals. In Figure 4a, we observe the profile of CaOx crystal formation (control). The ascending portion of the curve (I) corresponds to the phases of nucleation and crystal growth, while the descending portion (II) corresponds to the aggregation/precipitation stage. When the formation of CaOx crystals was carried out in the presence of chitosan in three different concentrations (100, 50, 25 µg/mL), this revealed a significant increase in absorbance (Figure 4b). The chitosan in all conditions showed the increased CaOx nucleation/growth to be about 1500% (15-times). It was not possible to determine how the presence of chitosan interferes with the aggregation/precipitation, because after 30 min, it was still not possible to observe the precipitation of crystals.

### 2.3.2. Crystal Morphology

The data so far show that chitosan stimulates the formation of CaOx crystals. However, we cannot say what type of crystal is being formed. Oxalate crystals morphologically differentiate into three types: monohydrate (COM), having a rectangular geometry; dihydrate (COD), present in the microscope as pyramidal or vane shapes; and trihydrate (COT), which has a complex geometry, characterized by the presence of several edges. Green and Ratan [41] showed that the COD-type crystals are found in abundance in the urine of healthy patients, and the COM type are those most commonly found in patients with urolithiasis and with a greater ability to cause cell damage. The crystals of the COD type are formed spontaneously in urine, which has different mechanisms to increase the stability of the COD crystals, which are more readily excreted. In a patient with urolithiasis, these stabilizing mechanisms are not efficient, making the COD crystals, which are not very stable, dissociate into the COM-type, which is more harmful [41]. In the renal tubule, COM crystals, positively charged, interact with cell surfaces that act as negatively charged surface. This difference in electrical charge mediates the adhesion of crystal cells. Once on the cell surface, COM crystals can reach the intracellular environment by endocytosis or other mechanisms, and when this occurs, this creates oxidative stress that promotes the release of pro-inflammatory damage and cell death [42,43].

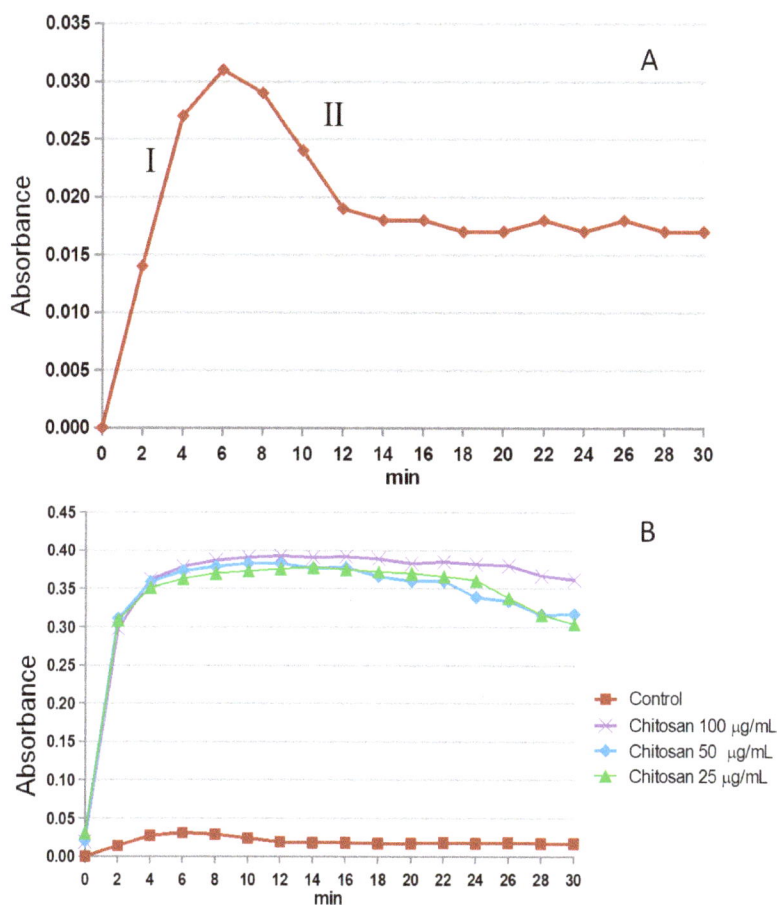

**Figure 4.** Profile of crystals forming from solutions. (**A**) Profile of the control solution formation, aggregation phases (I) and precipitation (II) are indicated with Roman numerals; (**B**) We can see the profile of crystal formation in the presence of different concentrations of chitosan.

In Figure 5, we can observe the crystals formed in CaOx control conditions (Figure 5a), in the presence of dextran (Figure 5b) and chitosan (Figure 5c). Comparing the three figures, one can clearly see that the number of crystals in Figure 5c is much greater. In fact, without the presence of chitosan (Figure 5a,b), an average of $9 \pm 0.7$ per field can be observed, whereas in the presence of chitosan, the number of crystals is increased to about $167 \pm 23$ per field. In Figure 5b,d, the morphology and size of the crystals were not changed by dextran. These data indicate that crystal formation in the presence of chitosan is specifically chitosan related and is not an unspecific colloidal effect.

These data confirmed what had been observed in the previous section and indicated that chitosan stimulates the formation of oxalate crystals. Another important factor that can be highlighted is that when these crystals were counted, it was found that in the control conditions, the ratio of COD:COM was 1:4 by field. The presence of chitosan modified the COD:COM ratio to 1.2:166 per field.

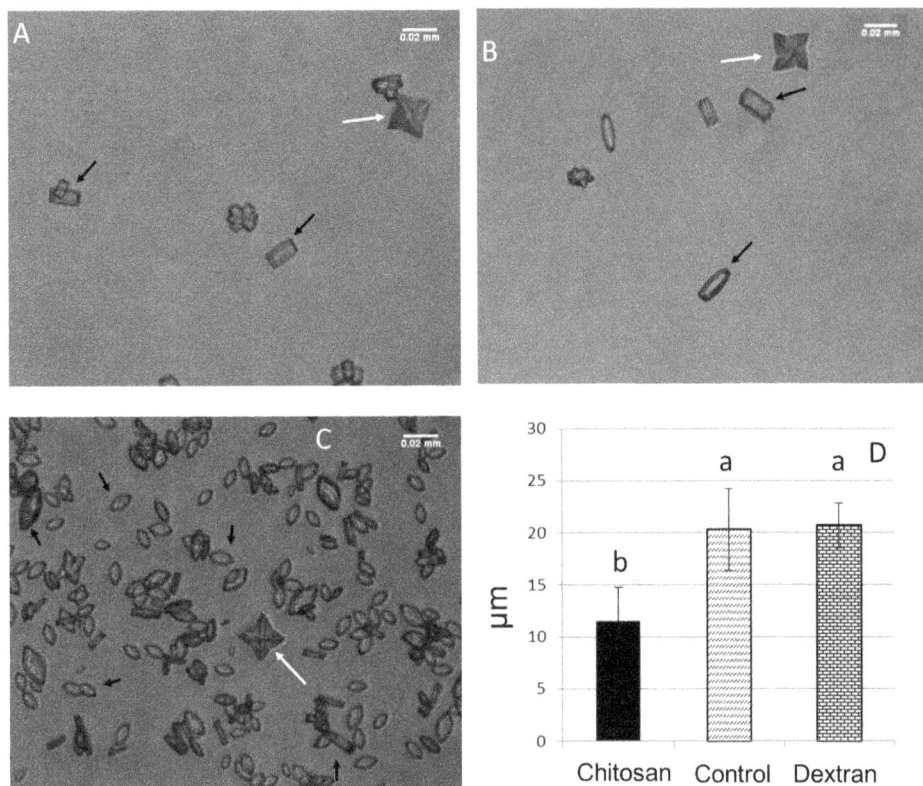

**Figure 5.** Crystal morphology analysis: comparison of the morphology of the crystals increased by 600×. (**A**) Control, with few crystals per field; (**B**) crystals formed in the presence of 100 µg/mL dextran; (**C**) crystals formed in the presence of 100 µg/mL chitosan, where we can see a large increase in the total number of crystals. White arrows indicate COD (dihydrate CaOx) and black arrows point to COM (monohydrate CaOx); (**D**) Average size with crystals formed in the presence and absence of chitosan and dextran.

Not only was the number of COM crystals altered by the presence of chitosan, but the size and morphology of these crystals were also changed. The crystals in the control group exhibited a rectangular morphology (Figure 5a) and an average particle size of $20.32 \pm 3.95$ µM (Figure 5c). In the presence of chitosan, the COM crystals had a more spheroid shape (Figure 5b), indicating that chitosan affects the crystal lattice point, preventing the formation of perfect CaOx crystals. Furthermore, with the presence of chitosan, the average size of the crystals was $11.53 \pm 3.23$ µM (Figure 5c).

2.3.3. Zeta Potential ($\zeta$)

The crystals are formed spontaneously from the nearest compatible ions and have a residual charge. This charge allows them to attract or repel, thus interfering with crystal growth [44]. COM crystals are different: the positive side is rich in $Ca^{2+}$, and the other side is rich in oxalate, which is negative. Recently, we have shown that negatively-charged polysaccharides (fucans and sulfated glucans) can associate with the positive faces of the CaOx crystals, thus reducing the surface charge of the crystals and, therefore, being able to alter the morphology of the crystals, as well as to decrease the size of the COM crystals [38]. Our question was whether the chitosan would also be associated with the surface of COM crystals. In order to answer this question, we measured the zeta potential of the crystals.

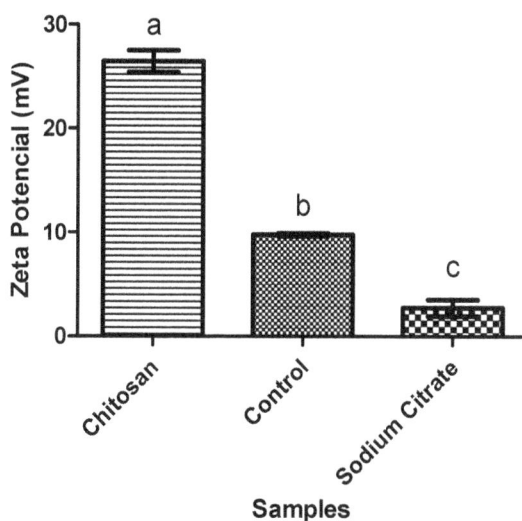

**Figure 6.** Zeta potential of the CaOx crystal samples without (control) or with chitosan or sodium citrate. Each letter indicates a statistically different group ($p < 0.05$).

The zeta potential ($\zeta$) reflects the surface charge of particulate matter in relation to the load of the solution in which it lies. In Figure 6, we can see the total load of CaOx crystals in the presence or absence (control) of chitosan and citrate. It was observed that the crystals of the control group showed a positive $\zeta$ due to the presence of $Ca^{2+}$. When citrate, an inhibitor of CaOx crystals, was present, the $\zeta$ decreased, due to the negative charges of citrate. Nevertheless, the opposite effect was observed in the presence of chitosan; the $\zeta$ crystals increased nearly 2.5-fold compared to $\zeta$ presented by the crystals in the control group. This increased $\zeta$ indicates that the crests of chitosan are associated with the crystals formed, since chitosan has a positive charge and is therefore able to increase the $\zeta$ CaOx crystals.

The data presented here leads us to suggest that the formation of CaOx crystals in the presence of chitosan starts with nucleation, but during the following process, chitosan starts to associate itself with the surface of the growing crystal, interfering with the crystal morphology. Furthermore, due to its positive character, chitosan by electrostatic repulsion prevents ions of $Ca^{2+}$ from binding to the growing crystal until it reaches a point that the crystal stops growing. The calcium that does not react remains available for new crystals to be formed, which would explain the greater number of crystals formed in the presence of this polysaccharide in comparison to the control. It is worth noting that the presence of chitosan on the surface of the crystals, also by electrostatic repulsion, prevents the aggregation phase from occurring, which explains the smaller size of the crystals formed in the presence of chitosan compared to the control, as well as the fact that we did not identify the stage of aggregation/precipitation after 30 min (Section 2.3.1).

It has been shown that the presence of adverse polymers, including polysaccharides, decreases $\zeta$ crystal formation and increases the stability of COD crystals, preventing these from transforming into COM crystals [38,45]. However, with the presence of chitosan, the proportion of COM crystals, which are more damaging, compared to the COD, increased, which indicates that the chitosan was not able to stabilize the COD crystals.

Chitosan is gaining more acceptance in daily activities, since it is generally known to be a molecule without toxic effects, and its uses range from food supplement for weight loss [10,46] to even raw material for the production of nanoparticles and hydrogel drug carriers [8,47]. In 2013 alone, more than 350 articles on the use of chitosan nanoparticles as drug and/or carriers of drugs were published. Therefore, understanding the possible toxic effects of this molecule is needed. What we found here was that the literature has examples that show that chitosan has an affinity for renal tissue [10,11] and that it increases the concentration of urinary calcium [13]. Furthermore, our data show that chitosan increases the formation of CaOx crystals *in vitro*, mainly COM crystals, and it also increases the positive character of COM crystals, leaving them, in theory, more likely to interact with the negative charges on the cell surface and, thus, more likely to cause damage and urolithiasis. Therefore, we conclude that chitosan may be an inducer of renal stone formation. However, it is still too early to say for certain, because *in vivo* tests are needed to confirm the data obtained here *in vitro*. Such *in vivo* tests are currently in progress.

## 3. Experimental

### 3.1. Chitosan

The chitosan was purchased from Sigma-Aldrich (Ref: 448869–250 g; Lot: 61496MJ, St. Louis, MO, USA).

### 3.2. Fourier Transformed Infrared Spectroscopy (FTIR)

The chitosan (5 mg) was thoroughly mixed with dry potassium bromide. The infrared spectra between 500 and 4000 $cm^{-1}$ were obtained with a tablet containing KBr and chitosan using a Thermo Nicolet Nexus 470 ESP FTIR spectrometer (Thermo Nicolet, Madison, WI, USA). Thirty-two scans at a resolution of 4 $cm^{-1}$ were evaluated and referenced against air.

*3.3. Nuclear Magnetic Resonance (NMR) Spectroscopy*

The chitosan (50 mg) was dissolved in 800 μL of deuterium oxide ($D_2O$). NMR spectra ($^1H$) were obtained in a Bruker Avance III 400 MHz spectrometer (Bruker BioSpin Corporation, Billerica, MA, USA) with an inverse 5-mm broadband probe head (BBI) at 70 °C. The chemical shifts were expressed in δ relative to acetone at δ 2.21, based on sodium 2,2-dimethyl-2-silapentane-3,3,4,4,5,5-$d_6$-5-sulfonate (DSS) at δ = 0.00 in accordance with IUPAC recommendations.

Determination of Deacetylation Degree

For determining the DD sample, we used the integrals of the peaks observed in the anomeric region of $^1H$ NMR as demonstrated by Lavertu *et al.* [30], which applied to our chitosan. The formula used was:

$$DD(\%) = \left( \frac{H1D}{H1D + H1A} \right) \times 100 \qquad (1)$$

*3.4. Determination of Chitosan Molecular Weight*

The molecular weight of chitosan was determined by high performance size exclusion chromatography (HPSEC) (GE Healthcare Bio-Sciences, Pittsburgh, PA, USA) on TSK-Gel® 3000 (30 cm × 0.75 cm), with a column temperature of 60 °C. The chitosan was eluted with 0.2 M NaCl in 0.05 M acetate buffer, pH 5.0, at a flow rate of 1.0 mL/min and detected by a refractive index detector. The column was calibrated using different dextrans (10; 47; 74; 147 kDa) purchased from Sigma (St. Louis, MO, USA).

*3.5. Antioxidant Activity*

3.5.1. Determination of Total Antioxidant Capacity

This assay is based on the reduction of Mo (VI) Mo (V) by chitosan and subsequent formation of a phosphate green complex/Mo (V) with acid pH. Tubes containing chitosan and reagent solution (0.6 M sulfuric acid, 28 mM sodium phosphate and 4 mM ammonium molybdate) were incubated at 95 °C for 90 min. After the mixture had cooled to room temperature, the absorbance of each solution was measured at 695 nm against a blank. Total antioxidant capacity was expressed as ascorbic acid equivalent.

3.5.2. Reducing Power

The reducing power was quantified according to the methodology described by Costa *et al.* [33]. The test samples (4 mL) in different concentrations (0.25–1 mg/mL) were mixed in a phosphate buffer (0.2 M, pH 6.6) with potassium ferricyanide (1%) and incubated for 20 min at 50 °C. The reaction was interrupted by the addition of TCA (trichloroacetic acid) to 10%. Subsequently, distilled water and ferric chloride (0.1%) were added to the samples. Readings were taken at 700 nm. The data were expressed as a percentage of the activity shown by 0.1 mg/mL of vitamin C, which corresponds to 100%.

### 3.5.3. Hydroxyl Radical Scavenging Activity Assay

The scavenging assay of the hydroxyl radical was based on the Fenton reaction ($Fe^{2+} + H_2O_2 \rightarrow Fe^{3+} + OH^- + OH$). The results were expressed as inhibition rates. The hydroxyl radicals were generated using 3 mL of sodium phosphate buffer (150 mM, pH 7.4) containing 10 mM $FeSO_4 \cdot 7H_2O$, 10 mM EDTA, 2 mM of sodium salicylate 30% $H_2O_2$ (200 mL) and different concentrations of chitosan. In the control, sodium phosphate buffer replaced $H_2O_2$. The solutions were incubated at 37 °C for 1 h, and the presence of the hydroxyl radical was detected through the monitoring of the absorbance at 510 nm. Gallic acid was used as a positive control.

### 3.5.4. Ferrous Chelating

Both methods used the ferrozine and $FeCl_2$ complex to determine the antioxidant capacity.

In the first method, chitosan at different concentrations (0.01–2 mg/mL) was added to a reaction mixture containing $FeCl_2$ (0.05 mL, 2 mM) and ferrozine (0.2 mL, 5 mM). The mixture was stirred and incubated for 10 min at room temperature, and the absorbance of the mixture was measured at 562 nm against a blank. EDTA was used as standard.

In the second method, chitosan at different concentrations (0.5–2 mg/mL) was mixed with 3.7 mL of methanol and 0.01 mL of 2 mM $FeCl_2$, then 0.2 mL of 5 mM ferrozine were added to initiate the reaction. The mixture was shaken vigorously and kept at room temperature for 10 min. Absorbance was determined at 562 nm against a blank, and EDTA was used as the standard.

For both methods, the chelating effect was calculated using the corresponding absorbance (A) in the formula given below, where control is the condition in the absence of chelating agents:

$$Chelating\ effect(\%) = \left( \frac{A_{control} - A_{sample}}{A_{control}} \right) \times 100 \tag{2}$$

### 3.5.5. Copper Chelating

The ability to chelate the copper ion from the extracts was determined by the method described by Anton [48]. Pyrocatechol violet, the reagent used in this assay, has the ability to associate with certain cations, such as aluminum, copper, bismuth and thorium. In the presence of chelating agents, this combination is not formed, resulting in decreased staining. The test is performed in 96-well microplates with a reaction mixture containing different concentrations of samples (0.1–2 mg/mL), pyrocatechol violet (4 mM) and copper II sulfate pentahydrate (50 mg/mL). All wells were homogenized with the aid of a micropipette, and the solution absorbance was measured at 632 nm. The ability of the samples to chelate the copper ion was calculated using the corresponding absorbance (A) in the following formula, where control is the condition in the absence of chelating agents:

$$Copper\ chelation(\%) = \left(\frac{A_{control} - A_{sample}}{A_{control}}\right) \times 100 \qquad (3)$$

### 3.6. Calcium Oxalate Crystallization Assay

The effect of polysaccharide in the crystallization of calcium oxalate was spectrophotometrically measured for 30 min at 620 nm, as described by Zhang *et al.* [39]. This assay is based on quantification by the optical density of metastable solutions of $Ca^{2+}$ and oxalate, by means of a mixture of calcium chloride (8 mmol/L) and sodium oxalate (1 mmol/L), 200 mmol/L of sodium chloride and 10 mmol/L of sodium acetate. The concentrations of compounds present in this mixture are close to the physiological urinary concentrations. The $CaCl_2$ (1.0 mmol/L) solution was constantly stirred at 37 °C, either in the absence or the presence of different concentrations of chitosan (100, 50 and 25 µg/mL). After obtaining a stable baseline, crystallization was induced by the addition of a solution of $Na_2C_2O_4$ (1.0 mmol/L) to achieve final concentrations of 4 mmol/L of calcium and 0.5 mmol/L of oxalate. The data is presented as absorbance × time (min).

### 3.7. Image Analysis Crystal Morphology

The crystals were induced to take shape in the presence or the absence of chitosan or dextran (100 µg/mL). After 30 min, the solutions were centrifuged (5000× g), and the supernatant was discarded. The crystals were then suspended in 0.5 mL of water and a part of 0.1 mL was put on a histological blade and taken to a microscope. The crystal morphology was analyzed in 10 randomly selected fields at 60× magnification. Images were captured from different fields. Three different experiments were performed.

### 3.8. Zeta Potential ($\zeta$) Measurements

The crystals were induced to form in the presence or absence of chitosan or sodium citrate (0.25 mM). After 30 min, the solutions were centrifuged (5000× g). The crystal concentrate was then suspended in 1.5 mL of water, and the zeta potential of the $\zeta$ samples was obtained using a Zeta Plus® analyzer (Brookhaven instruments, Holtsville, NY, USA).

### 3.9. Statistical Analysis

All of the data are expressed as the mean ± standard deviation ($n = 3$). To test the difference between results, the ANOVA test was performed. The Student–Newman–Keuls test ($p < 0.05$) was used to solve similarities found by the ANOVA. All tests were performed in GraphPad Prism 5 (GraphPad Softwares, La Jolla, CA, USA).

## 4. Conclusions

The $^1$H NMR and FTIR data show that the commercial chitosan exhibited the characteristic signals of the polymer.

The commercial chitosan sigma showed low or no antioxidant activity for TAC, reducing power, hydroxyl radical scavenge and iron chelation tests; on the other hand, it showed excellent activity in the chelation of copper, reaching 100% in a concentration of 1 mg/mL.

The presence of chitosan increased the number of CaOx crystals formed, especially COM crystals, without affecting the number of COD crystals. This polymer also changed the size and morphology of crystals formed, which, due to the presence of chitosan, became more rounded. Chitosan also changes the surface charge of the crystals, making them much more positive.

## Acknowledgments

The authors wish to thank Conselho Nacional de Desenvolvimento Científico e Tecnológico (CNPq), Coordenacão de Aperfeiçoamento Pessoal de Nível Superior (CAPES) and also Ministerio de Ciencia, tecnologia e informação (MCTI) for the financial support. Hugo Alexandre Oliveira Rocha and Guilherme Lanzi Sassaki are CNPq fellowship honored researchers. Moacir Queiroz and Karoline Melo had a master scholarship from CAPES. Diego de Araujo Sabry has a Ph.D. scholarship from CNPq. We wish to thank Centro de Ressonância Magnética Nuclear at Universidade Federal do Parana.

## Author Contributions

Moacir Fernandes Queiroz and Karoline Rachel Teodosio Melo performed the major part of experimental work. Diego Araujo Sabry and Guilherme Lanzi Sassaki performed the NMR analyses. Moacir Fernandes Queiroz and Hugo Alexandre Oliveira Rocha prepared experimental design and wrote the manuscript.

## Conflicts of Interest

The authors declare no conflict of interest.

## References

1. Hayes, M. Chitin, Chitosan and their Derivatives from Marine Rest Raw Materials: Potential Food and Pharmaceutical Applications. In *Marine Bioactive Compounds*; Springer: New York, NY, USA, 2012; pp. 115–128.
2. Jayakumara, R.; Menon, D.; Manzoor, K.; Nair, S.V.; Tamura, H. Biomedical applications of chitin and chitosan based nanomaterials—A short review. *Carbohydr. Polym.* **2010**, *82*, 227–232.
3. Laurienzo, P. Marine Polysaccharides in Pharmaceutical Applications: An Overview. *Mar. Drugs* **2010**, *8*, 2435–2465.
4. Casettari, L.; Vllasaliu, D.; Lam, J.K.; Soliman, M.; Illum, L. Biomedical applications of amino acid-modified chitosans: A review. *Biomaterials* **2012**, *33*, 7565–7583.
5. Melo-Silveira, R.F.; Almeida-Lima, J.; Rocha, H.A.O.; Pomin, V.H. *Marine Medicinal Glycomics*, 1st ed.; Nova Science: New York, NY, USA, 2013; pp. 454–463.

6. Kean, T.; Thanou, M. Biodegradation, biodistribution and toxicity of chitosan. *Adv. Drug. Deliv. Rev.* **2010**, *62*, 3–11.

7. Baldrick, P. The safety of chitosan as a pharmaceutical excipient. *Regul. Toxicol. Pharmacol.* **2010**, *56*, 290–299.

8. Garcia-Fuentes, M.; Alonso, M.J. Chitosan-based drug nanocarriers: Where do we stand? *J. Control. Release* **2012**, *161*, 496–504.

9. Wang, J.J.; Zeng, Z.W.; Xiao, R.Z.; Xie, T.; Zhou, G.L.; Zhan, X.R.; Wang, S.L. Recent advances of chitosan nanoparticles as drug carriers. *Int. J. Nanomed.* **2011**, *6*, 765–774.

10. Zhang, H.L.; Tao, Y.; Guo, J.; Hu, Y.M.; Su, Z.Q. Hypolipidemic effects of chitosan nanoparticles in hyperlipidemia rats induced by high fat diet. *Int. Immunopharmacol.* **2011**, *11*, 457–461.

11. Xia, W.; Liu, P.; Zhang, J.; Chen, J. Biological activities of chitosan and chitooligosaccharides. *Food Hydrocoll.* **2011**, *25*, 170–179.

12. Yuan, Z.X.; Zhang, Z.R.; Zhu, D.; Sun, X.; Gong, T.; Liu, J.; Luan, C.T. Specific renal uptake of randomly 50% N-acetylated low molecular weight chitosan. *Mol. Pharm.* **2009**, *6*, 305–314.

13. Wada, M.; Nishimura, Y.; Watanabe, Y.; Takita, T.; Innami, S. Accelerating effect of chitosan Intake on Urinary calcium excretion by rats. *Biosci. Biotech. Biochem.* **1997**, *61*, 1206–1208.

14. Mahmood, A.; Silbergleit, A.; Olson, R.; Cotant, M. Urolithiasis: The influence of stone size on management. *Nat. Clin. Pract. Urol.* **2007**, *4*, 570–573.

15. Finlayson, B. Phisicochemical aspects of urolithiasis. *Kidney Int.* **1978**, *13*, 344–360.

16. Ogawa, Y.; Miyazato, T.; Hatano, T. Oxalate and Urinary Stones. *World J. Surg.* **2000**, *24*, 1154–1159.

17. Thamilselvan, S.; Hackett, R.L.; Khan, S.R. Lipid peroxidation in ethylene glycol induced hyperoxaluria and calcium oxalate nephrolithiasis. *J. Urol.* **1997**, *157*, 1059–1063.

18. Selvam, R. Calcium oxalate stone disease: Role of lipid peroxidation and antioxidants. *Urol. Res.* **2002**, *30*, 35–47.

19. Anbazhagan, M.; Hariprasad, C.; Samudram, P.; Latha, P.; Latha, M.; Selvam, R. Effect of oral supplementation of vitamin E in hyperoxaluric patients on urinary risk factors. *J. Clin. Biochem. Nutr.* **1999**, *27*, 37–47.

20. Davalos, M.; Konno, S.; Eshghi, M.; Choudhury, M. Oxidative renal cell injury induced by calcium oxalate crystal and renoprotection with antioxidants: A possible role of oxidative stress in nephrolithiasis. *J. Endourol.* **2010**, *24*, 339–345.

21. Holoch, P.A.; Tracy, C.R. Antioxidants and self-reported history of kidney stones: The National Health and Nutrition Examination Survey. *J. Endourol.* **2011**, *25*, 1903–1908.

22. Melo-Silveira, R.F.; Fidelis, G.P.; Costa, M.S.S.P.; Telles, C.B.S.; Dantas-Santos, N.; Elias, S.O.; Ribeiro, V.B.; Barth, A.L.; Macedo, A.J.; Leite, E.L.; *et al. In Vitro* Antioxidant, Anticoagulant and Antimicrobial Activity and in Inhibition of Cancer Cell Proliferation by Xylan Extracted from Corn Cobs. *Int. J. Mol. Sci.* **2012**, *13*, 409–426.

23. Wolkers, W.F.; Oliver, A.E.; Tablina, F.; Crowea, J.H. A Fourier-transform infrared spectroscopy study of sugar glasses. *Carbohydr. Res.* **2004**, *339*, 1077–1085.

24. Silva, F.R.F.; Dore, C.M.P.G.; Marques, C.T.; Nascimento, M.S.; Benevides, N.M.B.; Rocha, H.A.O.; Chavante, S.F.; Leite, E.L. Anticoagulant activity, paw edema and pleurisy induced carrageenan: Action of major types of commercial carrageenans. *Carbohydr. Polym.* **2010**, *79*, 26–33.

25. Lim, S.H.; Hudson, S.M. Synthesis and antimicrobial activity of a water-soluble chitosan derivative with a fiber-reactive group. *Carbohydr. Res.* **2004**, *339*, 313–319.

26. Vino, A.B.; Ramasamy, P.; Shanmugam, V.; Shanmugam, A. Extraction, characterization and *in vitro* antioxidative potential of chitosan and sulfated chitosan from Cuttlebone of *Sepia aculeata Orbigny*, 1848. *Asian. Pac. J. Trop. Biomed.* **2012**, *2*, S334–S341.

27. Song, C.; Yu, H.; Zhang, M.; Yang, Y.; Zhang, G. Physicochemical properties and antioxidant activity of chitosan from the blowfly *Chrysomya megacephala larvae*. *Int. J. Biol. Macromol.* **2013**, *60*, 347–354.

28. Costa, M.S.S.P.; Costa, L.S.; Cordeiro, S.L.; Almeida-Lima, J.; Dantas-Santos, N.; Magalhães, K.D.; Sabry, D.A.; Albuquerque, I.R.L.; Pereira, M.R.; Leite, E.L.; *et al.* Evaluating the possible anticoagulant and antioxidant effects of sulfated polysaccharides from the tropical green alga *Caulerpa cupressoides var. flabellate*. *J. Appl. Phycol.* **2012**, *24*, 1159–1167.

29. Czechowska-Biskup, R.; Jarosińska, D.; Rokita, B.; Ulański, P.; Rosiak, J.M. Determination of Degree of Deacetylation of Chitosan-Comparision of Methods. *Prog. Chem. Appl. Chitin Deriv.* **2012**, *XVII*, 5–20.

30. Lavertu, M.; Xia, Z.; Serreqi, A.; Berrada, M.; Rodrrigues, A.; Wang, D.; Buschmann, M.; Gupta, A. A validated H NMR method for the determination of the degree of deacetylation of chitosan. *J. Pharm. Biomed. Anal.* **2003**, *32*, 1149–1158.

31. Wickens, A.P. Ageing and the free radical theory. *Respir. Physiol.* **2001**, *128*, 379–391.

32. Cuzzocrea, S.; McDonald, M.C.; Mazzon, E.; Filipe, H.M.; Centorrino, T.; Lepore, V.; Terranova, M.L.; Ciccolo, A.; Caputi, A.P.; Thiemermann, C. Beneficial effects of tempol, a membrane-permeable radical scavenger, on the multiple organ failure induced by zymosan in the rat. *Crit. Care Med.* **2001**, *29*, 102–111.

33. Costa, L.S.; Fidelis, G.P.; Cordeiro, S.L.; Oliveira, R.M.; de Sabry, D.A.; Camara, R.B.G.; Nobre, L.T.D.B.; da Costa, M.S.S.P.; de Lima, J.A.; de Farias, E.H.C.; *et al.* Biological activities of sulfated polysaccharides from tropical seaweeds. *Biomed. Pharmacother.* **2010**, *64*, 21–28.

34. Prabu, K.; Natarajan, E. *In Vitro* Antimicrobial and Antioxidant Activity of Chitosan Isolated from *Podophthalmus vigil*. *J. App. Pharm. Sci.* **2012**, *9*, 075–082.

35. Kuppusamy, S.K.; Karuppaiah, J. *In Vitro* evaluation of free radical scavenging activity of chitosan. *Int. J. Pharm. Life Sci.* **2013**, *4*, 2685–2690.

36. Chien, P.-J.; Sheu, F.; Huang, W.-T.; Su, M.-S. Effect of molecular weight of chitosans on their antioxidative activities in apple juice. *Food Chem.* **2007**, *155*, 221–226.

37. Xing, R.; Liu, S.; Guo, Z.; Yu, H.; Wang, P.; Lia, L.Z.; Lia, P. Relevance of molecular weight of chitosan and its derivatives and their antioxidant activities *in vitro*. *Bioorg. Med. Chem.* **2005**, *13*, 1573–1577.

38. Melo, K.R.T.; Câmara, R.B.G.; Queiroz, M.F.; Vidal, A.A.J.; Lima, C.R.M.; Melo-Silveira, R.F.; Almeida-Lima, J.; Rocha, H.A.O. Evaluation of Sulfated Polysaccharides from the Brown Seaweed *Dictyopteris Justii* as Antioxidant Agents and as Inhibitors of the Formation of Calcium Oxalate Crystals. *Molecules* **2013**, *18*, 14543–14563.

39. Zhang, C.Y.; Wu, W.H.; Wang, J.; Lan, M.B. Antioxidant properties of polysaccharide from the brown seaweed *Sargassum graminifolium* (Turn.), and its effects on calcium oxalate crystallization. *Mar. Drugs* **2012**, *10*, 119–130.

40. Kulaksizoglu, S.; Sofikerim, M.; Cevik, C. *In vitro* effect of lemon and orange juices on calcium oxalate crystallization. *Int. Urol. Nephrol.* **2008**, *40*, 589–594.

41. Green, W.; Ratan, H. Molecular mechanisms of urolithiasis. *Urology* **2013**, *81*, 701–704.

42. Lieske, J.C.; Deganello, S.; Toback, F.G. Cell-crystal interactions and kidney stone formation. *Nephron* **1999**, *81*, 8–17.

43. Yuen, J.W.; Gohel, M.D.; Poon, N.W.; Shum, D.K.; Tam, P.C.; Au, D.W. The initial and subsequent inflammatory events during calcium oxalate lithiasis. *Clin. Chim. Acta* **2010**, *411*, 1018–1026.

44. Banþeld, J.F.; Welch, S.A.; Zhang, H.; Ebert, T.T.; Penn, R.L. Aggregation-Based Crystal Growth and Microstructure Development in Natural Iron Oxyhydroxide Biomineralization Products. *Science* **2000**, *289*, 751–754.

45. Escobar, C.; Neira-Carrillo, A.; Fernández, M.S.; Arias, J.L. *Biomineralization: From Paleontology to Materials Science*; Arias, J.L., Fernández, M.S., Eds.; Editorial Universitaria: Santiago, Chile, 2007; pp. 343–358.

46. Gades, M.D.; Stern, J.S. Chitosan supplementation and fat absorption in men and women. *J. Am. Diet. Assoc.* **2005**, *105*, 72–77.

47. Giri, T.K.; Thakur, A.; Alexander, A.; Ajazuddin; Badwaik, H.; Tripathi, D.K. Modified chitosan hydrogels as drug delivery and tissue engineering systems: Present status and applications. *Acta Pharm. Sin. B* **2012**, *2*, 439–449.

48. Anton, A. Colorimetric Estimation of Aluminum with Pyrocatechol Violet. *Anal. Chem.* **1960**, *32*, 725–726.

# Chitosan in Mucoadhesive Drug Delivery: Focus on Local Vaginal Therapy

Toril Andersen, Stefan Bleher, Gøril Eide Flaten, Ingunn Tho, Sofia Mattsson and Nataša Škalko-Basnet

**Abstract:** Mucoadhesive drug therapy destined for localized drug treatment is gaining increasing importance in today's drug development. Chitosan, due to its known biodegradability, bioadhesiveness and excellent safety profile offers means to improve mucosal drug therapy. We have used chitosan as mucoadhesive polymer to develop liposomes able to ensure prolonged residence time at vaginal site. Two types of mucoadhesive liposomes, namely the chitosan-coated liposomes and chitosan-containing liposomes, where chitosan is both embedded and surface-available, were made of soy phosphatidylcholine with entrapped fluorescence markers of two molecular weights, FITC-dextran 4000 and 20,000, respectively. Both liposomal types were characterized for their size distribution, zeta potential, entrapment efficiency and the *in vitro* release profile, and compared to plain liposomes. The proof of chitosan being both surface-available as well as embedded into the liposomes in the chitosan-containing liposomes was found. The capability of the surface-available chitosan to interact with the model porcine mucin was confirmed for both chitosan-containing and chitosan-coated liposomes implying potential mucoadhesive behavior. Chitosan-containing liposomes were shown to be superior in respect to the simplicity of preparation, FITC-dextran load, mucoadhesiveness and *in vitro* release and are expected to ensure prolonged residence time on the vaginal mucosa providing localized sustained release of entrapped model substances.

Reprinted from *Mar. Drugs*. Cite as: Andersen, T.; Bleher, S.; Flaten, G.E.; Tho, I.; Mattsson, S.; Škalko-Basnet, N. Chitosan in Mucoadhesive Drug Delivery: Focus on Local Vaginal Therapy. *Mar. Drugs* **2015**, *13*, 222-236.

## 1. Introduction

Chitosan is a linear polysaccharide that is composed of copolymers of β(1-4)-linked *N*-acetylglucosamide and glucosamine. It is obtained by deacetylation of chitin, a natural polymer obtained from various sources, such as crustacean shells, fungi and bacteria; as a pharmaceutical raw material it is mostly obtained as a waste product of the shell fish industry, and is interesting as an affordable, renewable and sustainable product [1–4]. Chitosan can be obtained exhibiting various degrees of deacetylation (DD) and molecular weights, which determine its physicochemical and biological properties. The DD, as well as molecular weight, are directly proportional to physical properties, such as the solubility and viscosity. The mucoadhesiveness, antimicrobial effects and other biological properties are also related to the DD [5]. Although chitosan exhibits toxic effects on several bacteria, fungi and parasites, it is regarded safe for use in humans [6]. Chitosan is biodegradable and has been proven to be a safe and non-toxic excipient in pharmaceutical formulations such as a dressing in wound healing, in tissue engineering, and for surface modification of implantable devices [2,7,8]. In addition, it can be easily manufactured into nanofiber, beads, micro- and nanoparticles, among other delivery systems [9].

Chitosan can be used as mucoadhesive polymer for drug delivery via various mucosal surfaces. The positive charge of chitosan molecule is considered to be the main factor responsible for its mucoadhesive properties; the electrostatic interactions between the mucus layer containing negatively charged mucin and positively charged chitosan are considered the reason for its good adhesion on the mucosal surfaces [10]. In addition to the electrostatic forces there are other possible contributing factors to its mucoadhesivness, such as its wettability, entanglement, possible interactions with the mucin from the weaker Van der Waal's forces, and hydrogen bonding, as well as the hydrophobic interactions between the hydrophobic segments of the molecules. This enhanced bioadhesiveness will lead to increased retention time at the administration site, ensuring localized drug release and improved therapy. The use of chitosan in drug delivery systems has been extensive, both for systemic and localized drug delivery [4,11]; it has been shown to be a valuable excipient in tablets, emulsions, powders and gels providing a controlled release of the incorporated drug. On the smaller end of the scale chitosan has also been used in the development of chitosan-based nanoparticles, nanoemulsions and as a coating material for liposomes [12–18].

Local treatment with mucoadhesive drug delivery systems can offer several advantages, such as reduced administration frequencies, prolonged residence time and avoidance of disadvantages of systemic treatment. Additional advantage of chitosan as a mucoadhesive polymer is that it does not inactivate upon contact with mucin and its mucoadhesiveness does not weaken with time [19].

In respect to vaginal drug delivery systems, the main obstacles that need to be overcome for successful localized therapy are the great variations in the local pH and epithelial thickness depending on the age and hormone status, and a highly folded epithelial surface. Nanomedicine, particularly mucoadhesive nanopharmaceuticals, offers means of achieving a uniform distribution throughout the vaginal site [16,20]. Our group has been extensively studying the delivery systems able to improve local vaginal drug therapy. The mucoadhesiveness of chitosan is pH-dependent and stronger at the acidic pH providing an additional reason why we believe that chitosan has a great potential in vaginal delivery. We have recently developed several chitosan-based mucoadhesive drug delivery systems for local vaginal treatment [17,21,22]. The methods used to include/attach chitosan to the delivery systems varied from a simple one-pot preparation method, where chitosan was included in the first preparation step [21], to chitosan coating of the surface of preformed liposomes [17] or chitosan used as an excipient in pre-liposome tablets [22].

In respect to simplicity of the manufacturing conditions, the one-pot preparation method for production of chitosan-containing liposomes is particularly interesting [21]. The preparation process resulted in an *in situ* coating of the liposomes where it was hypothesized that the polymer is found both as a coating on the surface of the chitosan-containing liposomes and embedded in the aqueous compartment within the liposomes. In this study we wanted to further characterize this novel delivery system, particularly focusing on the mucoadhesiveness of the system and its ability to incorporate larger drug molecules, like biologicals. For that purpose we prepared chitosan-containing liposomes with two different model substances (fluorescein isothiocyanate dextran of Mw 4000 and 20,000 Da, FITC-dextran 4 and FITC-dextran 20, respectively). The ability of this type of liposomes to interact with mucin and, at the same time, provide sustained release of entrapped fluorescent substances was compared with the non-mucoadhesive (plain) and chitosan-coated liposomes containing the same dextran.

## 2. Results and Discussion

In order to achieve optimal treatment in local vaginal drug delivery it is important to provide a sufficient amount of the drug at the vaginal site for a sufficient amount of time [23]. Moreover, lower doses, drug targeting to the vaginal site, lower administration frequency may also lead to cost reduction of the therapy [24]. The important features of a drug delivery system directly contributing to the efficacy of the therapy are the drug load (entrapment of the drug within the carrier) and the mucoadhesion of the system, which will both ensure the increased concentration of the drug at the active site and its prolonged residence time [20]. In addition, the mucoadhesive delivery system needs to exhibit a predictable release of the entrapped/incorporated drug and be of a size that allows the system to reach the target tissue within the vaginal cavity [25]. These important characteristics were therefore the focus of this study.

### 2.1. Characterization of Liposomes

The entrapment of the model substances in three types of liposomes is presented in Figure 1. Both the low and high molecular weight FITC-dextrans were entrapped to the highest extent within chitosan-containing liposomes. The entrapment within the chitosan-coated and plain liposomes was similar for each type of FITC-dextran, and the pattern was consistent for both the low and high molecular weight FITC-dextrans. This may be explained by the fact that the liposomes that are the basis of the chitosan-coated liposomes are the same as the plain liposomes, except for the additional chitosan coating on their surface, and that the FITC-dextrans have been entrapped into the liposomes prior to the coating. The chitosan-containing liposomes are entirely different types of liposomes as they are formed in the presence of both chitosan and drug, in this case the model FITC-dextran. The presence of chitosan inside as well as outside the liposomes probably contributes to pulling more of the substance into the aqueous compartments of the liposomes. Both FITC-dextran and chitosan have a high number of hydrogen-bonding capable groups, which may contribute positively to pulling more FITC-dextrans into the liposomes; in addition, the chitosan embedded in the liposomal structure may disorganize the structure of the lipid bilayers and provide more room for the FITC-dextran inside the aqueous compartments of the chitosan-containing liposomes. As expected, the entrapment of FITC-dextran 20 was less than FITC-dextran 4 for all types of vesicles, which can be attributed to its larger molecular weight. However, both model substances were entrapped with rather high efficiencies indicating that the chitosan-containing liposomes can entrap sufficient amounts of larger molecules, such as biologicals, within their structure.

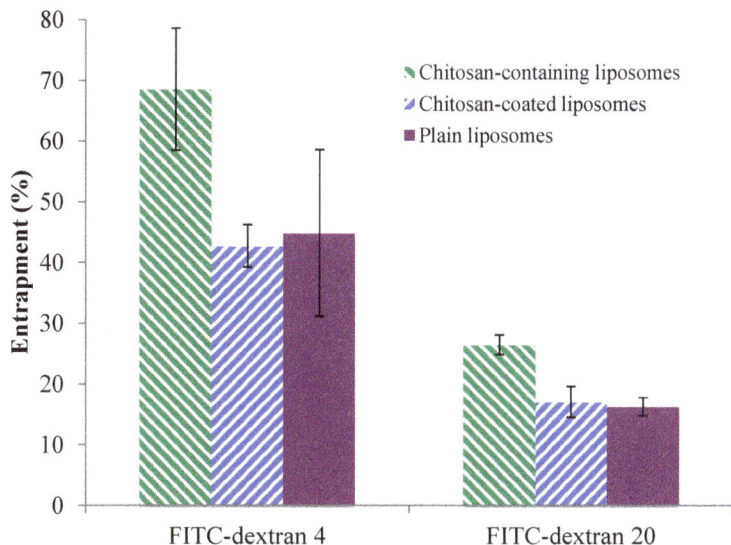

**Figure 1.** Entrapment of two FITC-dextrans in chitosan-containing liposomes, chitosan-coated liposomes, and plain liposomes. All values represent the mean $\pm$ SD ($n = 3$).

The liposomes prepared by the one-pot method are known to be larger than 1 micron with rather high polydispersity index (PI). They were also clearly of multilamellar nature [21]. To gain more control over the polydispersity of the samples, since this is expected to influence both the distribution of liposomes within vaginal cavity and the drug release rate, the sonication was applied. The sizes of the sonicated liposomes are best described by bimodal distributions where similarly sized liposomes are grouped in populations and the volume-weighted percentage of particles with a specific mean are calculated (Table 1). Chitosan-coated liposomes were the smallest of tested formulations, whereas the plain liposomes were the largest. Interestingly, liposomes containing FITC-dextran 20 were of smaller sizes than the same liposomes containing FITC-dextran 4. The smaller size of the liposomes containing FITC-dextran 20 can also be seen as a contributing factor to why the larger model substance was entrapped to a lower extent as compared to the FITC-dextran 4; smaller liposomes have less available aqueous part for accommodation of hydrophilic molecules. Rather unexpected results were the size distributions of plain liposomes. However, similar findings that polymer-coated liposomes were smaller than non-coated liposomes were reported earlier [26,27]. The reason behind this observation could be that chitosan is known to form a cage-like steric barrier that protects liposomes from aggregation, whereas in the case of non-coated liposomes the agglomeration can occur [26].

**Table 1.** Size distributions of liposomes. All values represent the mean size ± SD, and are volume-weighted (%) bimodal distribution ($n = 3$).

| Type of Liposomes | Peak 1 * | | Peak 2 * | | PI |
|---|---|---|---|---|---|
| | Size (nm) | % | Size (nm) | % | |
| *FITC-dextran 4* | | | | | |
| Chitosan-containing | 76 ± 40 | 20 ± 7 | 287 ± 48 | 79 ± 9 | 0.30 ± 0.01 |
| Chitosan-coated | 48 ± 25 | 69 ± 3 | 197 ± 27 | 21 ± 3 | 0.35 ± 0.15 |
| Plain | 56 ± 20 | 16 ± 13 | 337 ± 53 | 85 ± 13 | 0.36 ± 0.08 |
| *FITC-dextran 20* | | | | | |
| Chitosan-containing | 50 ± 19 | 29 ± 7 | 257 ± 42 | 64 ± 8 | 0.33 ± 0.01 |
| Chitosan-coated | 27 ± 4 | 26 ± 9 | 99 ± 18 | 74 ± 9 | 0.34 ± 0.01 |
| Plain | 51 ± 3 | 39 ± 2 | 219 ± 3 | 54 ± 24 | 0.37 ± 0.05 |

* The values are shown as a Nicomp distribution, which gave the best fit for the measured data (Fit error <1.5; residual error <10).

The zeta potential of the plain liposomes, regardless of the type of the entrapped FITC-dextran, was close to neutral (0.93 mV), which is expected since the lipid used to form vesicles is neutral. The chitosan containing formulations, chitosan-containing and chitosan-coated liposomes, exhibited a positive zeta potentials (2.45 and 6.73 mV, respectively) reflecting the positive charge of the surface-available chitosan.

## 2.2. Surface-Available Chitosan

Although the zeta potentials indicated the presence of chitosan on the liposomal surface for both the chitosan-containing and chitosan-coated liposomes, we wanted to confirm that chitosan is indeed available to interact with mucin and thus ensure the system's bioadhesiveness. In the case of the chitosan-containing liposomes, where chitosan was present during the formation of the liposomes, it is expected that a proportion of the polymer is lodged inside the lamellar structure of the liposomes. Therefore, to prove this hypothesis, the availability of chitosan on the surfaces of all liposomes was evaluated. As can be seen in Figure 2, the plain liposomes did not exhibit any (or in a negligent amount) surface-available chitosan. The small percentage detected can be due to a limitation of the test. The chitosan-containing and chitosan-coated liposomes exhibited a high degree of surface-available chitosan; the chitosan-coated vesicles contained significantly ($p < 0.01$) more chitosan on their surface (80%) as compared to the chitosan-containing liposomes (approx. 65%). Considering that for the chitosan-coated liposomes all, or most of the chitosan, should be surface-available, this finding was as expected. The fact that about 35% of chitosan was not surface-available in the chitosan-containing liposomes indicated that parts of chitosan are indeed embedded within this type of liposomes, and proved our initial hypothesis. These findings are also in agreement with the zeta potentials measured on liposomal surfaces where the chitosan-coated liposomes exhibited higher zeta potential.

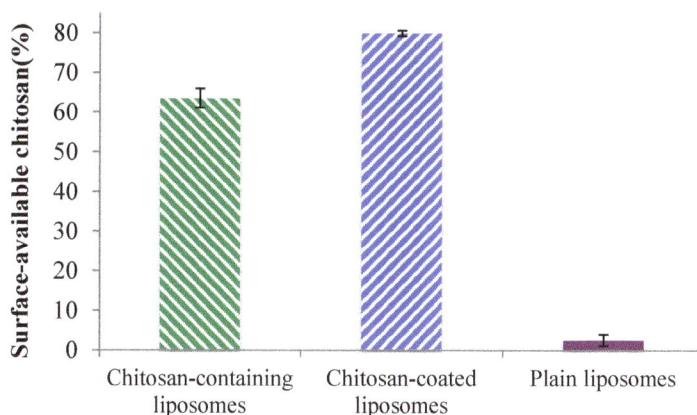

**Figure 2.** Percentage of surface-available chitosan determined in chitosan-containing, chitosan-coated liposomes, and plain liposomes. All values represent the mean $\pm$ SD ($n = 3$).

## 2.3. Mucin-Binding Properties of Liposomes

After confirming that there are high amounts of surface-oriented chitosan available for possible interaction with mucin, both on the surface of the chitosan-containing and chitosan-coated liposomes, an *in vitro* mucin test was applied to confirm the system's adhesiveness. The binding efficiency of the liposomes to the model porcine mucin (PM) was used to demonstrate the mucin-binding capability of the formulations and to estimate the mucoadhesive behavior. The chitosan-coated liposomes exhibited the highest PM binding efficiency, closely followed by the chitosan-containing liposomes, while the plain liposomes, as expected, exhibiting lower mucoadhesiveness (Figure 3). These findings were in direct agreement with the chitosan surface availability data (Figure 2) where the chitosan-coated liposomes were shown to have more available chitosan on the surface. However, even though the chitosan-containing and chitosan-coated liposomal formulations were significantly different ($p < 0.05$) regarding the mucin-binding capacity, this was less pronounced than the difference in the amount of surface available chitosan. The plain liposomes exhibited the PM binding efficiency of about 50%, which is significantly less ($p < 0.001$) than the other two liposomal formulations. One can argue that plain liposomes should have negligible mucin-binding capacity; however due to the ultracentrifugation applied to separate liposomes from bound mucin, it is possible that some plain liposomes interacted physically with the mucin without the actual electrostatic interactions that were targeted in the test. It is also possible that there is a hydrophobic interaction between the liposomes and mucin that leads to the findings in Figure 3. Our findings are also comparable to the results reported earlier for the sonicated plain liposomes [27].

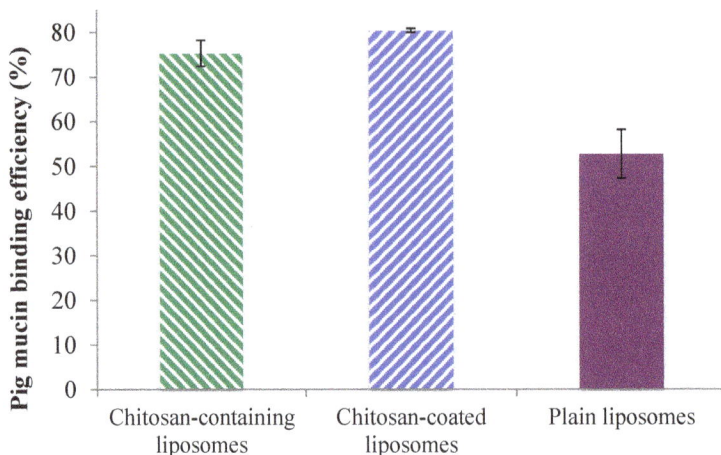

**Figure 3.** Binding efficacy of the liposomes to porcine mucin. All values represent the mean ± SD ($n$ = 3).

## 2.4. In Vitro Release of FITC-Dextrans from Liposomes

Cumulative release of FITC-dextran 4 and FITC-dextran 20 from all three liposomal formulations is shown in Figures 4 and 5, respectively. All three types of delivery systems released FITC-dextran 4 in a sustained manner as compared to the FITC-dextran 4 solution (Figure 4). The chitosan-containing liposomes were found to sustain the initial release to a greater extent than the chitosan-coated liposomes, however after 2 h the release of FITC-dextran 4 was slower from the chitosan-coated compared to chitosan-containing liposomes although not on significant level. The release of the high molecular weight FITC-dextran 20 (Figure 5) was found to be faster than the release of low molecular FITC-dextran 4. Again the control (FITC-dextran 20 solution) exhibited the highest cumulative release; however in this case the chitosan-containing liposomes sustained the release of FITC-dextran 20 to the greatest extent among the tested formulations. Interestingly, the chitosan-coated liposomes released more FITC-dextran 20 than the plain liposomes (Figure 5), which is exactly the opposite behavior as found for the low molecular weight FITC-dextran 4. Another interesting observation was the fast initial release of FITC-dextran from all liposomal formulations. It seems that the chitosan-coated liposomes provided an initial burst release of the high molecular weight fluorescent marker. One possible explanation can be that the rather large molecule of FITC-dextran 20 (20,000 Da) was not only entrapped but also embedded between the vesicle bilayers close to the outer bilayer and was released by a rapid diffusion at the start of the release study. In addition, the smaller liposomal size, and thus the larger total surface area of liposomes containing FITC-dextran 20 could facilitate its faster release as compared to the release of FITC-dextran 4.

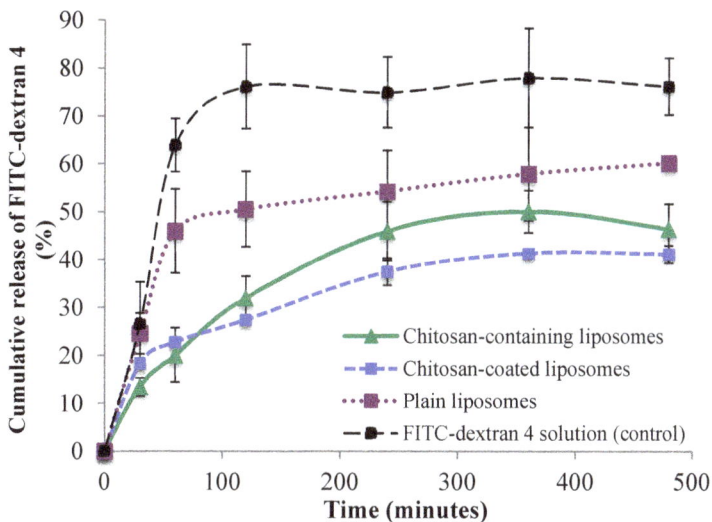

**Figure 4.** Cumulative release of FITC-dextran 4 from chitosan-containing liposomes, chitosan-coated liposomes, and plain liposomes. All values represent the mean ± SD ($n = 3$).

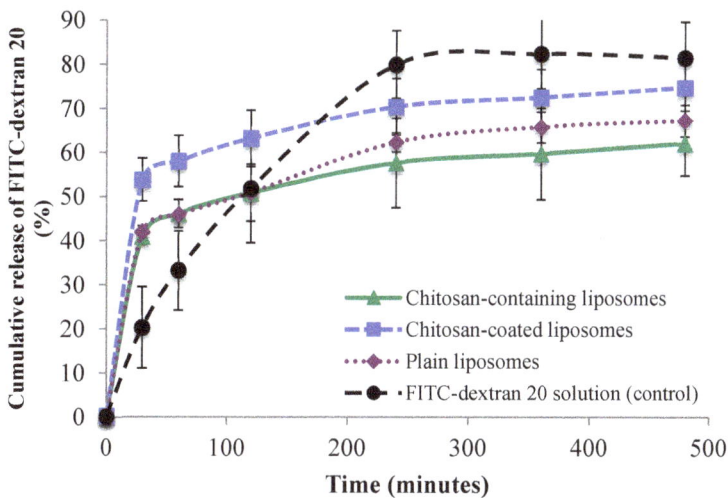

**Figure 5.** Cumulative release of FITC-dextran 20 from chitosan-containing liposomes, chitosan-coated liposomes, and plain liposomes. All values represent the mean ± SD ($n = 3$).

Based on the surface availability of chitosan on the chitosan-containing liposomes, and the ability to bind to mucin, this type of liposomes offers the potential to adhere to the vaginal mucosa and reside at the vaginal site for a prolonged period of time to ensure sufficiently high amounts of the drug at the site of action. The entrapment of large molecular weight model substances in the chitosan-containing liposomes was superior to entrapment of the same substances in the chitosan-coated liposomes. Moreover, the release of incorporated model substances of higher molecular weights (4000 and 20,000 Da) indicates that the chitosan-containing liposomes will release the incorporated material (e.g., drug) in a sustained manner. The fate of intravaginally administered drugs can be seen as a multi-compartment interactive event where the effects of the delivery system, the amount and viscosity of vaginal fluid, the presence of semen, the epithelium conditions and disease state need to be considered when optimizing the formulation [28]. Additional advantage of chitosan is its non-toxicity, as it is expected that chitosan-based delivery systems will not cause vaginal irritation. Very recently, the indications that chitosan can disrupt the bacterial biofilms in bacterial vaginosis have been reported, which would strengthen the potentials of chitosan as vaginal mucoadhesive delivery system [29].

## 3. Experimental Section

### 3.1. Materials

Soy phosphatidylcholine (Lipoid S100, Lipoid GmbH, Ludwigshafen, Germany) was a generous gift by Lipoid GmbH. Chitosan (60,000 Da; 77% degree of deacetylation (DD)), two types of fluorescein isothiocyanate dextran (FITC-dextran 4 and FITC-dextran 20 corresponding Mw 4000 and 20,000, respectively), mucin from porcine stomach type II, Triton X, methanol and n-propanol were all products of Sigma Aldrich Inc. (Steinheim, Germany). Cibacron Brilliant Red 3B-A was purchased from Santa Cruz Biotechnology Inc. (Santa Cruz, CA, USA). Sepharose CL-4B gel was ordered from Pharmacia Bioteck AB (Uppsala, Sweden). All other chemicals used in the experiments were of analytical grade.

### 3.2. Preparation of Vesicles

#### 3.2.1. Preparation of Chitosan-Containing Liposomes

Chitosan-containing liposomes were prepared by the one-pot preparation method previously developed in our research group [21]. Briefly, Lipoid S100 (SPC, 200 mg) was dissolved in an adequate amount of methanol. The solvent was evaporated using a rotoevaporator system (Büchi rotavapor R-124, with vacuum controller B-721, Büchi vac V-500, Büchi Labortechnik, Flawil, Switzerland) under a vacuum at 45 °C. The resulting film was redispersed with 100 μL of n-propanol by help of a micro syringe pipette (Hamilton, Bonaduz, Switzerland). The dispersion was needle-injected into 2 mL of aqueous media containing 0.17% (w/w) chitosan in 0.1% (v/v) acetic acid and either FITC-dextran 4 or FITC-dextran 20 (42.0 mg) and stirred for 2 h at room temperature (23 °C). The dispersion was left in a refrigerator overnight prior to vesicle size reduction and characterization.

### 3.2.2. Plain Liposomes

Plain, non-mucoadhesive liposomes, were prepared under the same conditions using the same lipid composition to prepare the film, which was subsequently redispersed and injected into aqueous solution of either FITC-dextran 4 or FITC-dextran 20. The dispersion was left in a refrigerator overnight prior to vesicle size reduction and characterization.

### 3.2.3. Vesicle Size Reduction

The chitosan-containing and plain (non-mucoadhesive) liposomes were reduced to a smaller size by sonication using a Sonics High Ultrasonic Processor (Sigma-Aldrich Chemie GmbH, Steinheim, Germany). Prior to sonication, the samples were diluted to a suitable volume (5 mL) with distilled water and sonicated for 45 s using an ice bath to prevent heating of the samples.

### 3.2.4. Chitosan-Coated Liposomes

Coating of sonicated plain FITC-dextran containing liposomes was performed by a previously reported method [17]. In brief, the chitosan solution (0.1% w/v) in glacial acetic acid (0.1% v/v) was added drop-wise to an equal volume of liposomes under the controlled magnetic stirring at room temperature for 1 h. Upon completion of stirring, the dispersion was left in a refrigerator overnight.

### 3.3. Entrapment Efficiency

In order to remove the unentrapped FITC-dextrans from liposomes two different separation methods were used, depending of the molecular weight of the model substance. For the liposomes containing FITC-dextran 4, dialysis in a dialysis membrane (Mw cut off: 12–14,000 Daltons; Medicell International Ltd., London, UK) against distilled water was applied for 24 h at room temperature. For liposomes containing FITC-dextran 20, a column separation on a Sepharose CL-4B gel was used.

The entrapment efficiency of the liposomal formulations was determined by fluorescence measurements using a Polarstar flourimeter (Fluostar, BMG Technologies, Offenburg, Germany) on excitation and emission wavelengths of 485 and 520 nm, respectively. To dissolve lipid, liposomal samples were pretreated by addition of 10% (v/v) of Triton X in a volume ratio of 1:1. Standard curves for both FITC-dextrans in water and FITC-dextrans in aqueous Triton X solutions were prepared and used for the fluorescence determination.

### 3.4. Particle Size Analysis

The size distributions were measured by photon correlation spectroscopy using a Submicron Particle-sizer (Model 360, Nicomp, Santa Barbara, CA, USA). To avoid possible interference caused by dust particles, test tubes were pre-rinsed with distilled water and bath-sonicated for 10 min. In addition, all sample preparations were performed in a laminar airflow bench. The liposomal samples were diluted with filtered (0.2 μm Milipore filters) distilled water to provide appropriate count intensity (approx. 250–350 kHz) and measured in three parallels (run time 10 min at 23 °C).

Both Gausssian and Nicomp algorithms were fitted to the experimental data to find the distribution that best describes the particle population [30]. As the fit error was found to be smaller than 1.5, and the residual error was smaller than 10, Nicomp distribution was selected. The volume-weighted distribution was used to determine the mean diameter and PI of all samples.

## 3.5. Zeta Potential Determination

The zeta potential of all liposomes was measured on a Malvern Zetasizer Nano ZS (Malvern Instruments Ltd, Oxford, UK). The instrument was calibrated throughout the measurements using the Malvern zeta potential transfer standard ($-50 \pm 5$ mV). The samples were diluted in filtered water until an appropriate count rate was achieved and measured in a measuring cell. All measurements were performed at 23 °C and the results represent an average of at least three independent measurements [16].

## 3.6. Determination of Surface-Available Chitosan

To determine the surface-available chitosan the colorimetric method originally reported by Muzzarelli [31] was applied. Glycine buffer (pH 3.2) was prepared by dissolving 1.87 g of glycine and 1.46 g of NaCl in 250 mL of distilled water; an aliquot of 81 mL was further diluted with 0.1 M HCl to a final volume of 100 mL. Cibacron Brilliant Red 3B-A (150 mg) was dissolved in 100 mL of distilled water. The dye solution (5 mL) was further diluted to 100 mL with the glycine buffer. Liposomal suspensions were diluted with distilled water to desirable concentration (1:2, v/v) before 3 mL of the final dye solution was added. UV absorbance was measured photometrically at 575 nm (Agilent Technologies, Santa Clara, CA, USA). The surface-available chitosan was calculated using the following equation:

$$Surface - available\ chitosan = \frac{C_s}{C_C} \times 100$$

where Cs is the concentration of surface-available chitosan in the sample and Cc is the concentration of chitosan used to prepare the liposomal formulations.

A standard curve was made by suspending chitosan powder (0.5 g) in 50 mL of distilled water. After 30 min at room temperature, 2.0 mL of glacial acetic acid (99.8% w/w) was added. An additional 50 mL of distilled water was added to acidic chitosan solution, before the final dilution with distilled water provided a final concentration of 0.5 g/L. Standard solutions were made by diluting the chitosan solution with glycine buffer to desired concentrations.

## 3.7. Mucin-Binding Test as Indicator of Mucoadhesiveness

The mucoadhesive properties were determined by the method developed by Pawar et al. [32] and modified in our group [27]. The porcine mucin (PM; 400 µg/mL) was hydrated in the phosphate buffer (0.05 M, pH 7.4), the suspension mixed with the vesicle suspension (1:1, v/v) and the mixture incubated at room temperature (23 °C) for 2 h prior to centrifugation for 60 min at 216,000× g and 10 °C (Optima LE-80; Beckman Instruments, Palo Alto, CA, USA). Absorbance of the remaining free PM in the supernatants was measured by UV spectrophotometry (Microtitre plate reader; Spectra Max 190 Microplate, Spectrophotometer Molecular Devices, Sunnyvale, CA, USA) at 251 nm. The mucoadhesiveness was expressed as PM binding efficiency calculated by the following equation:

$$PM\ binding\ eff. = \left(\frac{C_0 - C_S}{C_0}\right) \times 100$$

where $C_0$ is the initial concentration of PM used for incubation (400 μg/mL) and $C_S$ is the measured concentration of free PM in the supernatant after removal of the liposome-bound PM. The standard curve was determined from the standard PM solutions in the phosphate buffer made by diluting the PM stock solution to 40, 80, 120, 160, 200, 240, 280, and 320 μg/mL, respectively.

### 3.8. In Vitro Release Studies

Release studies were performed using the Franz diffusion cells (PermeGear, Hellertown, PA, USA) with the heating circulator (Julabo Labortechnik F12-ED, Seelback, Germany) maintaining the temperature at 37 °C. The cells with 12 mL volume acceptor chambers and a diffusion area of 1.77 cm² were used in *in vitro* studies based on the method by Hurler *et al.* [33] Polyamide membranes (0.2 μm pore size, Sartorius polyamide membrane; Sartorius AG, Gröttingen, Germany) were used. The formulations were added to the donor compartment in a volume of 600 μL. The acceptor chambers were filled with distilled water, and kept at 37 °C. Samples (500 μL) from the acceptor medium were taken at 30, 60, 120, 240, 360 and 480 min, and replaced with the fresh medium. Both the sampling port and the donor chamber were covered with quadruple layers of parafilm to prevent evaporation. Quantification of released fluorescent markers was determined based on the flourimetric measurements at excitation and emission wavelengths of 485 and 520 nm, respectively. All experiments were carried out in triplicate.

### 3.9. Statistical Evaluation

The student's *t*-test was used for comparison of two means. A significance level of $p < 0.05$ was considered to be appropriate.

## 4. Conclusions

The mucoadhesive nanosize delivery systems, the chitosan-containing liposomes, were shown to entrap/incorporate higher amounts of the fluorescent model substances of different molecular weight (4000 and 20,000 Da) as compared to conventional plain and chitosan-coated liposomes. The higher entrapment can be explained by the embedding of chitosan also within the lamellar structure of the liposomes and not only on the surface as proven in the surface-availability tests. The chitosan-containing liposomes were also able to ensure sustained release of entrapped material. The ability of surface-available chitosan to interact with mucus was confirmed indicating system's potential to prolong the residence time at the vaginal site.

## Acknowledgments

The authors are grateful to Lipoid GmbH, Ludwigshafen, Germany for a continuous support in supplying the lipids.

## Author Contributions

T.A., G.E.F., I.T., S.M. and N.S-B. designed and planned the experiments. T.A. and S.B. conducted the experiments. All authors contributed to the manuscript preparation. N. S-B. is a senior author and project leader.

## Conflict of Interests

The authors declare no conflict of interests.

## References

1. Prashant, K.V.H.; Tharanathan, R.N. Chitin/chitosan: Modifications and their unlimited application potential- an overview. *Trends Food Sci. Technol.* **2007**, *18*, 117–131.
2. Pal, K.; Behera, B.; Roy, S.; Ray, S.S.; Thakur, G. Chitosan based delivery systems on a length scale: Nano to macro. *Soft Mater.* **2013**, *11*, 125–142.
3. Bernkop-Schnuerch, A.; Duennhaupt, S. Chitosan-based drug delivery systems. *Eur. J. Pharm. Biopharm.* **2012**, *81*, 463–469.
4. Uchgebu, I.F.; Carlos, M.; McKay, C.; Hou, X.; Schaetzlein, A.G. Chitosan amphiphiles provide new drug delivery opportunities. *Polym. Int.* **2014**, *63*, 1145–1153.
5. Dash, M.; Chiellini, F.; Ottenbrite, R.M.; Chiellini, E. Chitosan-A versatile semisynthetic polymer in biomedical applications. *Prog. Polym. Sci.* **2011**, *36*, 981–1014.
6. Kean, T.; Thanou, M. Biodegradation, biodistribution and toxicity of chitosan. *Adv. Drug Deliv. Rev.* **2010**, *62*, 3–11.
7. Kim, I.-Y.; Seo, S.-J.; Moon, H-S.; Yoo, M.-K.; Park, I.-Y.; Kim, B.-C.; Cho, C.-S. Chitosan and its derivatives for tissue engineering applications. *Biotechnol. Adv.* **2008**, *26*, 1–21.
8. Bhattarai, N.; Gunn, J.; Zhang, M. Chitosan-based hydrogels for controlled, localized drug delivery. *Adv. Drug Deliv. Rev.* **2010**, *62*, 83–99.
9. Jayakumar, R.; Menon, D.; Manzoor, K.; Nair, S.V.; Tamura, H. Biomedical applications of chitin and chitosan based nanomaterials—A short review. *Carbohyd. Polym.* **2010**, *82*, 227–232.
10. Singla, A.K.; Chawla, M. Chitosan: Some pharmaceutical and biological aspects—An update. *J. Pharm. Pharmacol.* **2001**, *53*, 1047–1067.
11. Perioli, L.; Ambrogi, V.; Venezia, L.; Pagano, C.; Ricci, M.; Rossi, C. Chitosan and modified chitosan as agents to improve performances of mucoadhesive vaginal gels. *Colloids Surf. B Biointerfaces* **2008**, *66*, 141–145.
12. Li, N.; Zhuang, C.; Wang, M.; Sun, X.; Nie, S.; Pan, W. Liposomes coated with low molecular weight chitosan and its potential use in ocular drug delivery. *Int. J. Pharm.* **2009**, *379*, 131–139.

13. Zaru, M.; Manca, M.-L.; Fadda, A.M.; Antimisiaris, S.G. Chitosan-coated liposomes for delivery to lungs by nebulization. *Colloids Surf. B Biointerfaces* **2009**, *71*, 88–95.

14. Calderon, L.; Harris, R.; Cordoba-Diaz, M.; Elorza, M.; Elorza, B.; Lenoir, J.; Andriaens, E.; Remon, J.P.; Heras, A.; Cordoba-Diaz, D. Nano and microparticulate chitosan-based systems for antiviral topical delivery. *Eur. J. Pharm. Sci.* **2013**, *48*, 216–222.

15. Casettari, L.; Illum, L. Chitosan in nasal delivery systems for therapeutic drugs. *J. Control. Release* **2014**, *190*, 189–200.

16. Vanić, Ž.; Škalko-Basnet, N. Mucosal nanosystems for improved topical drug delivery: Vaginal route of administration. *J. Drug. Del. Sci. Technol.* **2014**, *24*, 435–444.

17. Jøraholmen, M.W.; Vanić, Ž.; Tho, I.; Škalko-Basnet, N. Chitosan-coated liposomes for topical vaginal therapy: Assuring localized drug effect. *Int. J. Pharm.* **2014**, *472*, 94–101.

18. Berginc, K.; Suljaković, S.; Škalko-Basnet, N.; Kristl, A. Mucoadhesive liposomes as new formulations for vaginal delivery of curcumin. *Eur. J. Pharm. Biopharm.* **2014**, *87*, 40–46.

19. Valenta, C. The use of mucoadhesive polymers in vaginal delivery. *Adv. Drug Delivery Rev.* **2005**, *57*, 1692–1712.

20. Vanić, Ž.; Škalko-Basnet, N. Nanopharmaceuticals for improved topical vaginal therapy: Can they deliver? *Eur. J. Pharm. Sci.* **2013**, *50*, 29–41.

21. Andersen, T.; Vanić, Ž.; Flaten, G.E.; Mattsson, S.; Tho, I.; Škalko-Basnet, N. Pectosomes and chitosomes as delivery systems for metronidazole: The one-pot preparation method. *Pharmaceutics* **2013**, *5*, 445–456.

22. Vanić, Ž.; Planinšek, O.; Škalko-Basnet, N.; Tho, I. Tablets of pre-liposomes govern *in situ* formation of liposomes: Concept and potential of the novel drug delivery system. *Eur. J. Pharm. Biopharm.* **2014**, *88*, 443–454.

23. Hainer, B.L.; Gibson, M.V. Vaginitis: Diagnosis and treatment. *Am. Fam. Physician* **2011**, *83*, 807–825.

24. Andrews, G.P.; Laverty, T.P.; Jones, D.S. Mucoadhesive polymeric platforms for controlled drug delivery. *Eur. J. Pharm. Biopharm.* **2009**; *71*, 505–518.

25. Das Neves, J.; Bahia, M.F.; Amiji, M.M; Sarmento, B. Mucoadhesive nanomedicines: Characterization and modulation of mucoadhesion at the nanoscale. *Expert Opin. Drug Deliv.* **2011**, *8*, 1085–1104.

26. Tan, H.W.; Mishran, M. Characterization of fatty acid liposome coated with low molecular-weight chitosan. *J. Liposome Res.* **2012**; *22*, 329–335.

27. Naderkhani, E.; Erber, A.; Škalko-Basnet, N.; Flaten, G.E. Improved permeability of acyclovir: Optimization of mucoadhesive liposomes using the Phospholipid Vesicle-Based Permeation Assay. *J. Pharm. Sci.* **2014**, *103*, 661–668.

28. Katz, D.F.; Gao, Y.; Kang, M. Using modeling to help understand vaginal microbicide functionality and create better products. *Drug Deliv. Transl. Res.* **2011**, *1*, 256–276.

29. Kandimalla, K.K.; Borden, E.; Omtri, R.S., Boyapati, S.P.; Smith, M.; Lebby, K.; Mulpuru, M.; Gadde, M. Ability of chitosan gels to disrupt bacterial biofilms and their applications in the treatment of bacterial vaginosis. *J. Pharm. Sci.* **2013**, *102*, 2096–2101.

30. Di Cagno, M.; Styskala, J.; Hlavac, J.; Brandl, M.; Bauer-Brandl, A.; Škalko-Basnet, N. Liposomal solubilization of new 3-hydroxy-quinolinone derivatives with promising anticancer activity: A screening method to identify maximum incorporation capacity. *J. Liposome Res.* **2011**, *21*, 272–278.

31. Muzzarelli, R.A.A. Colorimetric determination of chitosan. *Anal. Biochem.* **1998**, *260*, 255–257.

32. Pawar, H.; Douroumis, D.; Boateng, J.S. Preparation and optimization of PMAA-chitosan-PEG nanoparticles for oral drug delivery. *Colloids Surf. B Biointerfaces* **2012**, *90*, 102–108.

33. Hurler, J.; Berg, O.A.; Skar, M.; Conradi, A.H.; Johnsen, P.J.; Škalko-Basnet, N. Improved burns therapy: Liposomes-in-hydrogel delivery system for mupirocin. *J. Pharm. Sci.* **2012**, *101*, 3906–3915.

# Chitin and Chitosan as Direct Compression Excipients in Pharmaceutical Applications

Adnan A. Badwan, Iyad Rashid, Mahmoud M.H. Al Omari and Fouad H. Darras

**Abstract:** Despite the numerous uses of chitin and chitosan as new functional materials of high potential in various fields, they are still behind several directly compressible excipients already dominating pharmaceutical applications. There are, however, new attempts to exploit chitin and chitosan in co-processing techniques that provide a product with potential to act as a direct compression (DC) excipient. This review outlines the compression properties of chitin and chitosan in the context of DC pharmaceutical applications.

Reprinted from *Mar. Drugs*. Cite as: Badwan, A.A.; Rashid, I.; Al Omari, M.M.H.; Darras, F.H. Chitin and Chitosan as Direct Compression Excipients in Pharmaceutical Applications. *Mar. Drugs* **2015**, *13*, 1519-1547.

## 1. Introduction

The exploitation of new techniques in pharmaceutical processing has given preferential emphasis to the use of DC over wet granulation approaches to tablet production. Apart from the simplicity of formulation and manufacture, the key advantages of DC include reduced capital, labor, and energy costs, and the avoidance of water of granulation for water-sensitive drugs [1].

There exist two aspects that are necessary for DC processing to stand as a real industrial operation. The first one is the properties and functionalities of the inactive pharmaceutical ingredients (*i.e.*, excipients). As a general rule, it is industrially desirable to minimize the number of additives through the use of multifunctional excipients, typically needed to act as a diluent, filler, binder, glidant, disintegrant, or lubricant. The second one is the complexity of the powder modification process for the excipient to be successful as a DC excipient. Some processes represent highly effective techniques for powder modification that suit DC applications, e.g., spray drying [2]. However, the level of complexity of these processes with regard to operation and unit control is high and they may impose high costs and investment of time. Consequently, it is industrially desirable to utilize, for example, roll compaction for powder consolidation as an effective approach for dry granulation [3].

On the other hand, the choice of suitable excipients for DC is a critical decision. In addition, knowledge and understanding of the behavior of these excipients are important to avoid potential problems during manufacturing [4]. However, few excipients can be directly compressed into tablets, owing to detrimental physical properties such as poor compactibility, flowability, and compressibility [5]. Therefore, there is a need to improve such properties by physical or chemical co-processing modifications [6].

*1.1. Chitin and Chitosan Production*

Preparation of chitin and its derivatives, such as chitosan, was fully described by Daraghmeh *et al.*, in addition to its physico–chemical properties and methods of analysis [7]. Chitins are usually isolated from the shells of marine crustaceans, which are highly abundant as a waste product from seafood processing. Crustacean shells contain 30%–40% proteins, 30%–50% calcium carbonate, and 20%–30% chitin in addition to lipidic pigments such as carotenoids (astaxanthin, astathin, canthaxanthin, lutein, and β-carotene). The proportion of each component varies with species and with season. Upon extraction, chitin is subjected to acid treatment to remove calcium carbonate, followed by alkaline treatment to remove proteins and a depigmentation step to remove the coloring agents, in particular astaxanthin [8,9].

Chitosan is prepared by hydrolysis of chitin using severe alkaline treatment. When thermal treatments of chitin under strong aqueous alkali are used, partial deacetylation takes place (degree of acetylation (DA) lower than 30%), transforming chitin into chitosan. The foregoing can be achieved with sodium or potassium hydroxides at a concentration of 30–50% *w/v* at high temperature (100 °C) [8,9].

The DA and molecular weight (MW) are important parameters to be examined because they affect the physical and chemical properties of chitin and chitosan [8,10]. The acetylated units prevail in chitin (DA typically > 90%), while chitosan has a typical DA of less than 35%.

Different techniques have been used to measure the DA including IR, near IR, and NMR ($^{1}$H NMR, $^{13}$C NMR) spectroscopy, in addition to pyrolysis gas chromatography, gel permeation chromatography, zero- and first-order derivative UV spectrophotometry, thermogravimetric analysis, potentiometric titration, acid hydrolysis and HPLC, separation spectrometry methods, and, more recently, near-IR spectroscopy [8,11,12].

*1.2. Chitin and Chitosan: Physical and Chemical Properties*

After cellulose, chitin is the second most abundant polysaccharide found in nature. Its chemical structure is similar to cellulose (Figure 1) which lacks the amine groups (thus chitin and chitosan are heteropolymers, while cellulose is a homopolymer) [8]. The presence of amino and hydroxyl groups in chitin and chitosan may offer opportunities to modify their chemical structures, subsequently improving their physical, chemical, and biological properties, including solubility [13].

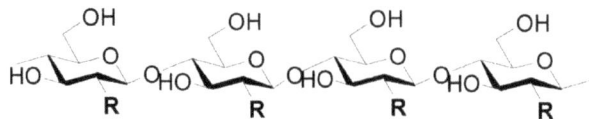

**Figure 1.** Chemical structures of cellulose (R = OH), chitin (R = NHCOCH₃), and chitosan (R = NH₂).

As a result of extensive hydrogen bonding that promotes the semi-crystalline nature of chitin as well as its cohesive energy, chitin solubility is limited in all of the typical solvents, including aqueous and most organic solvents [13,14]. For example, chitin is considered soluble in hexafluoroacetone, hexafluoroisopropanol, and chloroalcohols when these solvents are mixed with mineral acids and dimethylacetamide in solutions containing 5% lithium chloride [14]. Strong polar protic solvents such as trichloroacetic acid and dichloroacetic acid in halogenated hydrocarbons were found to dissolve chitin. Furthermore, a mixture of calcium chloride and methanol acts as a good solvent combination for chitin [13].

On the other hand, chitosan is readily soluble in dilute acidic solutions below pH 6.0 (average pKa = 6.30) [13], which makes it a water-soluble cationic polyelectrolyte. As the pH increases above 6, chitosan loses its charge and becomes insoluble. The following salt forms of chitosan are considered soluble: acetate, formate, lactate, citrate, malate, glyoxylate, pyruvate, glycolate, and ascorbate [13]. However, the presence of glycerol 2-phosphate at a neutral pH of 7–7.1 offered an aqueous-based solution of chitosan at room temperature [15].

The presence of the reactive amino groups and the primary hydroxyl groups allow chitin and chitosan to be complexed or derivatized readily [16]. The chemical modifications may improve their physico-chemical properties, including solubility. The presence of water-soluble entities, hydrophilic moieties, and bulky and hydrocarbon groups extend their applications in various fields [13–15,17].

*1.3. Applications of Chitin and Chitosan*

The chelating ability of chitin and its derivatives facilitates their use as chromatographic and industrial adsorbents for the collection of industrial pollutants such as trace metals from aqueous and organic solutions, sea water, silver thiosulfate, and actinides [18–20]. In pharmacological applications, it was found that chitin activates peritoneal macrophages *in vivo*, whereas it suppresses the growth of tumor cells in mice, and stimulates nonspecific host resistance against *Escherichia coli* infection [21]. In addition, chitin accelerates wound healing [21,22]. Chitin derivatives are widely used to immobilize enzymes in the food industry and in other areas such as biosensors [21], and to immobilize antibodies in the presence of alginate [23]. They are also used as binders in the paper-making process [15]. Furthermore, chitin film and fiber are used in medical and pharmaceutical applications as wound-dressing material [22,24,25]. Recently, chitin has been involved in the conversion of biomass into a value-added, renewable nitrogen-containing furan derivative [26,27].

Chitosan has shown promise for use in different biomedical applications because of its high specific surface area and high porosity. For example, chitosan has been used in surgical sutures, dental implants, renewable artificial skin, bone rebuilding, contact lenses, controlled release of drugs for animals and humans, and as encapsulating material [15,28–38]. In addition, it has applications in agriculture, water and waste treatment, food and beverages, cosmetics and toiletries, and biopharmaceutical products [15,39].

## 2. Chitin and Chitosan for Direct Compression Processing

The suitability of chitosan for use in biomedical and pharmaceutical formulations is attributed to its inherent properties such as biodegradability, low toxicity, and good biocompatibility [40]. Among numerous pharmaceutical applications, it has been widely used as a vehicle for directly compressed tablets, a binder, a disintegrant, a granulating agent, and a carrier for sustained release preparations [17]. In solid dosage form preparations, chitosan has been used as a co-grinding diluent for the enhancement of the dissolution rate and bioavailability of water-insoluble drugs and as a penetration enhancer for peptide drugs [40].

Chitin and chitosan have been widely acknowledged as effective tablet disintegrants due to their high water absorption capacity. Such functionality was observed in tablets at chitin/chitosan concentrations below 70% [41]. Nonetheless, within the industrial framework, chitosan is not a common pharmaceutical additive in large-scale formulations. This is due to the fact that chitosan lacks good flow properties and compressibility [42]. Previous studies showed their limited use as fillers in directly compressed tablets [43,44], mainly due to their apparent low density, poor flow, and inadequate compressibility, resulting in tablets with very low mechanical strength. Even granulation or the inclusion of dry binders seemed to fail to induce the required mechanical strength.

For chitin, early attempts at its utilization as a pharmaceutical excipient were thoroughly investigated by Sawayanagi *et al.* [45]. They used physical mixing to produce binary mixtures of chitin with microcrystalline cellulose (Avicel PH 101®), lactose, or potato starch. They concluded that the flowability and tablet hardness when using the combined powders were greater than that when using microcrystalline cellulose, lactose, or potato starch as an individual excipient. The improvement of powder flow by the addition of chitin to microcrystalline cellulose (Avicel PH 102®) and co-processed lactose composed of a spray-dried mixture of 75% α-lactose monohydrate and 25% cellulose powder (Cellactose®) was recently confirmed by Mir *et al.* [46]. The bulk and tapped densities and the powder flow measured by the Carr Index (CI) and the angle of repose were all seen to increase upon the addition of chitin. The authors further pointed out that the highest CI was achieved with chitin alone, with a CI of 13.1% and a flow rate of 5.48 $g/cm^2$ s. However, the inclusion of chitin in Avicel PH 102® and Cellactose® mixtures lubricated with magnesium stearate at a concentration of 0.5% *w/w* resulted in tablets with impaired mechanical properties. These results contradict the early findings of Sawayanagi *et al.* [45], probably due to the method of compression they were using. In the later work, a hydraulic tablet press with a compression duration time of 30 s was used for tablet compression whereas in the former work [46] a single station tableting machine was used with a dwell time generally estimated to be less than 0.1 s [47].

In studies carried out by Aucamp [43], Buys [48], and de Kock [44], it could be seen that chitosan could not be compressed into tablets on an eccentric tablet press. Aucamp came to the conclusion that even if combining chitosan with fillers such as Avicel PH 200® or Prosolv® SMC 90 (co-processed microcrystalline cellulose and colloidal silicon dioxide) the tablet strength was still weak. The combination of chitosan with the filler in the ratio 70:30 gave the best results. The conclusion was that the filler improved the flowability of the powder blend, resulting in better die filling and an increase in the tablet strength. The foregoing was correlated to the high surface area available for particle bonding resulting in decreased interparticular spaces (voids) [43]. Buys and de Kock compressed chitosan into mini-tablets. De Kock could not compress chitosan powder into tablets with desirable tablet strength; however, with the combination of binders and fillers chitosan mini-tablets could be obtained. Buys found that chitosan could only be compressed at high compression forces. It would be difficult to obtain these high compression forces needed to compress the powder when using an eccentric tablet press. The force exerted on the powder was achieved by adjusting the distance between the upper and lower punches. The problem of obtaining these higher compression forces was solved when a sufficient amount of chitosan powder filled the die before compressing the powder. These results concluded that although more chitosan powder could be filled into the die, the tablet weight was still relatively small.

As a rule of thumb, bulk density is an indicator of a powder's ability to undergo compression and compaction. Filler-binders or diluents generally provide the bulk of the tablet and are also responsible for flow and compaction properties. The bulk and tapped density of chitin and chitosan rank lowest when compared to other common filler binders and diluents (Figure 2) [9,46]. Such low density is attributed to their high particulate irregularities, which bring about a highly porous structure and a high specific surface area. In this regard, chitosan presents the highest specific surface area and pore volume among some common excipients presented in Table 1. Chitosan structure typically has significant internal void space in the form of pores and channels [49]. Moreover, the fibrous nature of chitin with irregular and some threaded surface will give rise to randomly sized but large voids (spaces between particles) between chitin/chitosan particles [50,51]. This can be justified by the big difference between bulk (0.15 g/mL) and tapped (0.40 g/mL) densities of chitosan powder (Figure 2), unlike the bulk (0.33 g/mL) and tapped (0.41 g/mL) densities of the almost spherically shaped particles of polyvinyl pyrrolidine (PVP K30). Similar conclusions can apply to microcrystalline cellulose due to its fibrous irregular particle shape.

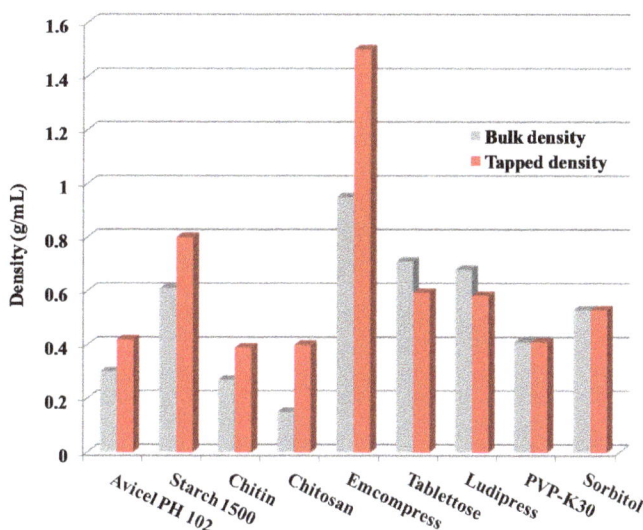

**Figure 2.** Bulk and tapped densities of chitin and chitosan in comparison with other common filler-binder excipients. Data were obtained from Mir *et al.* [46], Rojas *et al.* [52], and Sonnekus [53].

**Table 1.** Specific surface area and pore volume of chitosan and some common excipients.

| Excipient | Specific Surface Area (m²/g) | Pore Volume (cm³/g) | References |
|---|---|---|---|
| Lactose H₂O | 0.26 | 0.090 | [54] |
| Microcrystalline cellulose | 0.42 | 1.67 | [55,56] |
| Maize starch | 0.58 | 0.0012 | [57] |
| Synthesized CaHPO₄ | 3.31 | 0.0065 | [58] |
| Chitosan | 330 | 15 | [59] |

Microcrystalline cellulose: Avicel® PH 101.

## 2.2. Powder Flow

The flow properties of the powder mixture are important to ensure mass uniformity of a tablet and thus prevent unacceptable variation in thickness, disintegration time, and strength [60]. On the basis of bulk and tapped densities, the powder flowability can be measured. For example, the CI is an indication of the flowability, and indirectly the compressibility, of the powder, as calculated according to Equation (1):

$$Carr's\ Index\ (CI) = Compressibility\ (\%) = \frac{Tapped\ densit - Bulk\ density}{Tapped\ density} \times 100\% \qquad (1)$$

CI values of 5–10, 12–16, 18–21, and 23–28 indicate excellent, good, fair, and poor flow properties of the material, respectively [61]. Therefore, it is clear that chitosan is not a free-flowing powder, and problems with filling a small die in a tablet press can be expected. Its compressibility is reported to be poor when compared to that of common DC excipients (Figure 3).

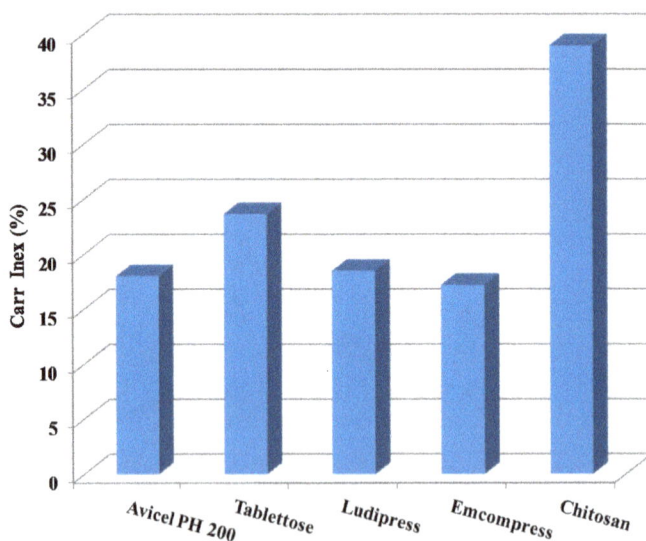

**Figure 3.** Carr Index (CI) of chitosan and some common direct compression excipients. Data were obtained from García Mir *et al.* [46], Rojas *et al.* [52], and Sonnekus [53].

Generally, studies indicate that the flowability of powders containing spherical particles is much better than that of those containing elongated or irregular particles [62]. In this context, it was proposed that elongated or irregular particles obstruct powder flow and reduce flowability, as they tend to mechanically interlock or entangle with each other [63]. Thus the CI of chitosan was expected to be high because of its fibrous structure, which facilitates entanglements between particles, in addition to its cohesive nature resulting in adverse mechanical interlocking of powders with irregular shapes; consequently, poor flow properties are displayed [64].

The flowability of chitosan is affected by its moisture content and distribution at the time it is expected to flow. High moisture content negatively affects the flow of chitosan [65]. An increase in the relative humidity from 11% to 75% results in an increase in the CI from 30.7% to 36.1%. Moreover, chitosan's flowability is affected by its particle size. The bigger the particle size, the better the flowability of chitosan. The smallest fraction (<90 μm) has a very poor flowability with a composite CI of 40.7%, while the fraction with a particle size of more than 212 μm has a CI of 29.7% [66].

## 2.3. Tensile Strength

The mechanical strength of tablets produced upon compression is the most essential requirement of DC excipients. With respect to chitin, their tablets manifest acceptable mechanical properties (Figure 4). This can be attributed to the irregular particle shape, the external surface area, and the rough surface texture of chitin; all contribute to the high surface bonding between the particles [67]. The tensile strength of chitosan tablets can be correlated with the plastic deformation nature of chitosan or with its volume reduction on compression. The volume reduction is associated with the elimination of pores. Generally, reducing compact pores results in a higher tensile strength of the tablets [68].

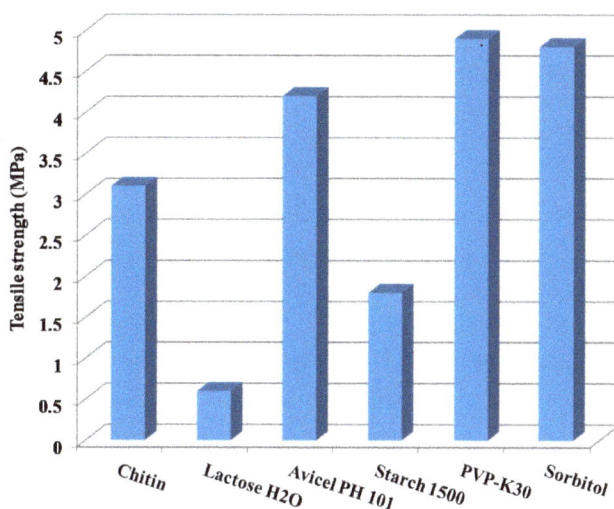

**Figure 4.** Tensile strength of chitin and some common direct compression excipients. Data were obtained from Rojas *et al.* [52,69].

2.3.1. Effect of Moisture Content

Moisture content plays a significant role in the consolidation and compaction of pharmaceutical powders [70–74]. The foregoing is attributed to the beneficial plasticizing effect of water on the polymer matrix or to the detrimental formation of stable hydrogen bonding bridges, resulting in an anti-plasticizing effect. [75]. These changes are a result of the combined effect of moisture on the inter-particle and intermolecular forces [72]. Accordingly, chemical or physical association between water and a polymer takes place, leading to a change in the behavior of water and of the polymer [76,77]. However, the extent of such association can alter the moisture action from that of a good tablet binder to a factor responsible for the weak tensile strength of tablets [73].

For chitosan, the tensile strength of the tablets compressed with dried chitosan powder were less at each of the compression forces used, when compared to that of tablets compressed with powder that was stored under atmospheric conditions containing 9.39% and 11.86% moisture [66]. In an attempt to elucidate the moisture-tensile strength effect, García Mir et al. attributed the effect, generally, to the ability of chitosan to hold a relatively large amount of water in its internal structure [78], and specifically to externally adsorbed water, which allows for the formation of hydrogen bonding between particles, thus preventing elastic recovery and/or increasing the interparticulate van der Waal's forces. Consequently, the effects of surface micro-irregularities and inter-particle separation become reduced. On the other hand, excessive moisture provokes a disruption of the binding force between particles, resulting in a decrease in the tensile strength of tablets due to high absorbed water within the particle or condensed water in the surface [72]. Chitin, as a disintegrant, acts to enhance porosity and provide these pathways into the tablet. Liquid is drawn up or "wicked" into these pathways, replacing the air between the tablet particles, and thus weakening the intermolecular bonds [79].

2.3.2. Effect of Degree of Deacetylation

The contribution of the degree of deacetylation (DDA) on the tensile strength has been previously studied by Gupta and Kumar. They pointed out that the hardness of chitin tablets was greater than that of chitosan tablets [80]. They attributed the difference in hardness to the structural rigidity of chitin due to its acetylamino groups and to the higher degree of polymerization typically found in chitin. The degree of polymerization of chitin would be reduced during the deacetylation of chitin with a strong alkali to prepare chitosan. The results of Rojas et al. confirm the aforementioned finding [52]. They pointed out that chitosan of low DDA has better mechanical properties compared to chitosan of a higher DDA. They contributed this phenomenon to the fact that chitin's rigid structure is attributed to intra-sheet hydrogen bonds dominated by strong C–O⋯N–H hydrogen bonds, and to strong inter-molecular hydrogen bonds dominated by the amide groups, which undergo dramatic change into a less rigid orientation. The foregoing is a result when chitin is subjected to high NaOH concentrations and high reaction temperatures. Such hard conditions lead to a chitin with a low DA, low yield, and high crystallinity, which, in turn, forms weak compacts and has rapid disintegration times [52].

2.3.3. Effect of Molecular Weight

The total length of the chitosan polymer is an important characteristic of the molecule. Hence, the MW is a key feature for its functional properties [81]. The first investigation of the effect of chitosan's MW on tensile strength was carried out using chitosan films [82]. An increase in the MW of chitosan increased the tensile strength of the membrane because of intra- and inter-molecular hydrogen bonding [83].

Rege *et al.* investigated tablet properties when using chitosan samples of different MW [42]. They demonstrated that a lower MW provides a higher tensile strength to a chitosan tablet (Figure 5). Consequently, low MW chitosans can be used to modify drug release to a greater extent than can high MW chitosana.

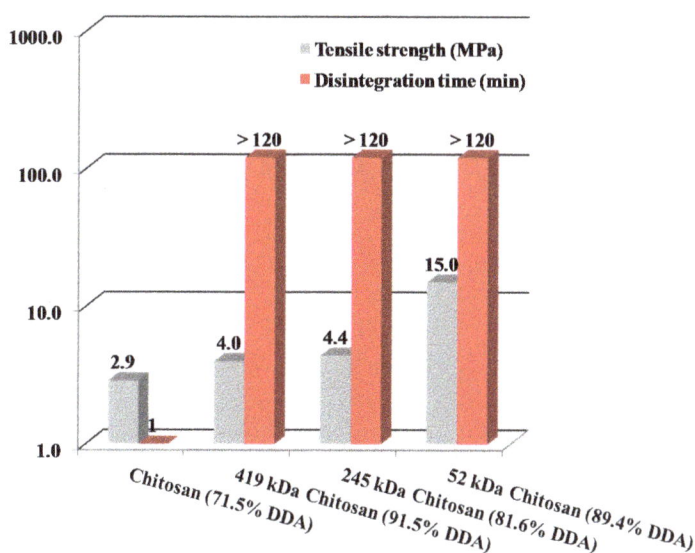

**Figure 5.** Tensile strength (MPa) and disintegration time (min) of chitin and chitosan with different molecular weights. Data were obtained from Rege *et al.* [42].

Rashid *et al.* confirmed the aforementioned tensile strength dependency on MW; however, they used chitosan samples of much lower MW and lower compression pressures [6]. In their results, the highest MW chitosan (100 kDa) showed the highest compact tensile strength (Figure 6) at compression loads > 300 kg. They correlated such findings to the plastic deformation of chitosan, which was highest at 100 kDa, as indicated by its lowest yield pressure. Plastically deforming materials expose new surfaces upon compression and which are ready to provide further binding of the particles. On the other hand, the lowest MW chitosan samples (8 kDa) exhibited less plastic behavior or more brittle-fracture upon compression, in addition to lower elastic recovery. Such new fragments give rise to more binding surfaces and thereby high tensile strength. Therefore, Figure 6 illustrates the high tensile strength of chitosan when it is of a highly plastically deforming or a high

318

brittle-fracture nature upon compression. Chitosans of MW between 100 and 8 kDa exhibit tensile strength values that are almost between that of the highest and lowest MW.

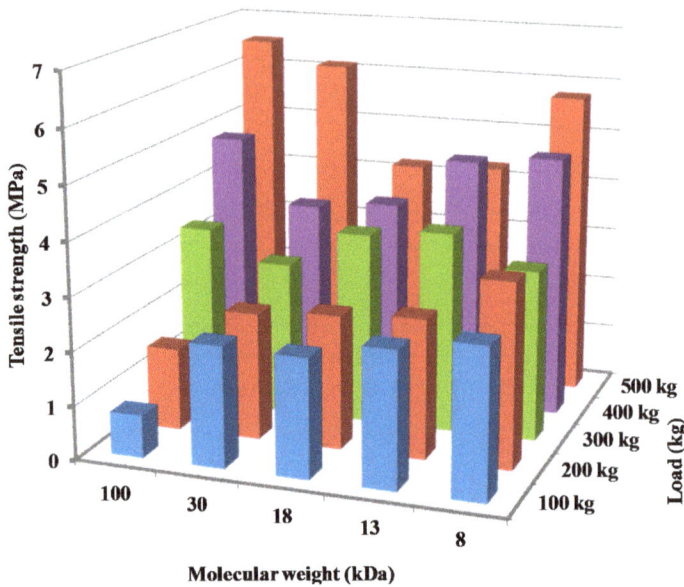

**Figure 6.** Effect of compression pressure on the tensile strength of tablets using chitosan samples of different molecular weights. Data were obtained from Rashid *et al.* [6].

## 2.3.4. Effect of Lubricant

In general, hydrophobic lubricants such as magnesium stearate have a negative effect on the crushing strength of plastically deforming constituents of tablets (e.g., microcrystalline cellulose) than on brittle ones (e.g., CaHPO₄) [84]. As brittle materials are more likely to fracture and fragment during compaction, more fresh surfaces, not covered by lubricant particles, are generated. These new surface areas tend to bond together and thus the effect of lubricants is minimized. On the other hand, film formation by lubricants on plastically deforming particles weakens the bonding of the granules as there are fewer fresh surfaces formed during compaction. In general, hydrophobic lubricants provide efficient coating to the surface of particles and prevent the formation of hard compacts. This effect was more pronounced in highly plastic materials that had a smooth surface, such as pregelatinized starch. For chitin, despite its highly porous structure and its ability to undergo plastic deformation upon compression, its particle surface is highly irregular. Therefore, chitin's external surface area dominates over other interparticulate bonding mechanisms upon compaction [67,85]. After Rojas *et al.* summarized common plastic and brittle excipient sensitivity to 1% lubricant [52], they concluded that because chitin was the material least sensitive to lubrication, it had better compactibility than pregelatinized starch, calcium diphosphate, and lactose monohydrate when lubricated (Figure 7).

The amount of magnesium stearate appeared to greatly affect the mechanical strength of chitin-containing tablets [46]. Tablets with a magnesium stearate concentration of 0.1% *w/w* exhibited a clearly higher crushing strength and lower friability than those compressed with a magnesium stearate concentration of 0.5% *w/w*. Picker-Freyer and Brink correlated the lubricant effect on tensile strength to the disruption of the microstructure of chitin [86]. Mir *et al.* attributed this effect to the reduction of interparticle bonding associated with chitin or a result of physical and chemical interaction between chitin and magnesium stearate [46]. Rashid *et al.* have shown that, upon mixing chitin with magnesium stearate, the specific surface area is considerably decreased while the particle size distribution remains unchanged [84]. On mixing with lubricant, microcrystalline cellulose undergoes a reduction in specific surface area followed by an increase in the particle size distribution, which has been correlated to agglomeration. Therefore, chitin exhibits high surface coverage by the lubricant, whereas microcrystalline cellulose exhibits particle agglomeration [84].

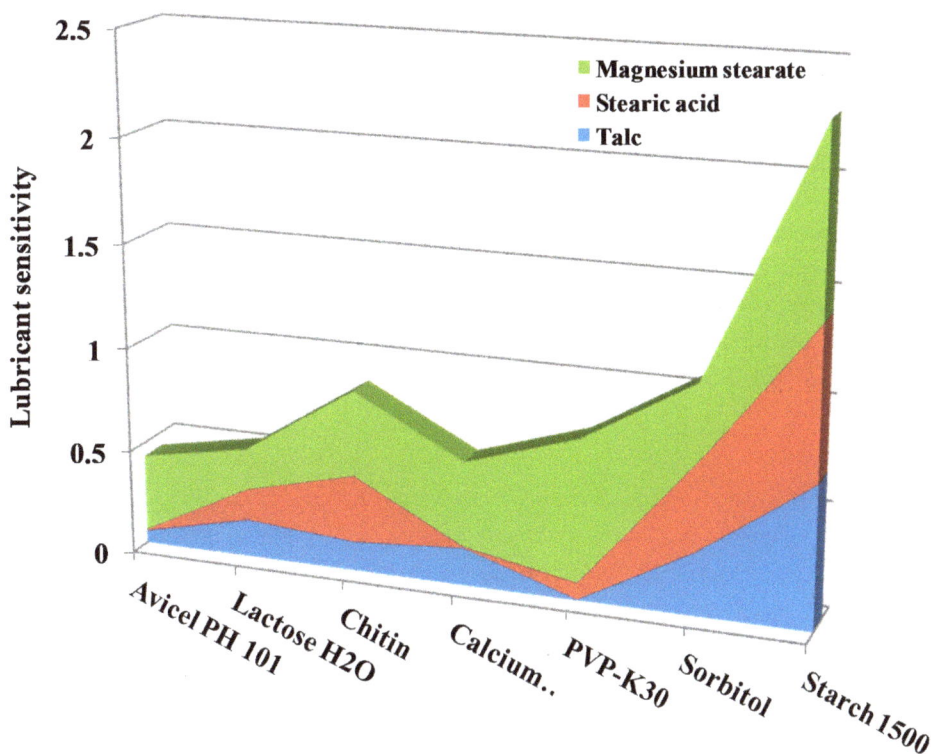

**Figure 7.** Lubricant sensitivity of chitin and common excipients in the presence of different lubricant types. Data were obtained from Rojas *et al.* [52,69].

## 2.4. Compressibility of Chitin and Chitosan

Previous studies by Aucamp reveal poor compression characteristics for the pure chitosan raw material on an eccentric tablet press [43]. The unsuccessful attempt to produce tablets from pure chitosan with an average particle size of 215.6 µm was attributed to its poor compressibility and flow properties. From the results of a study by Buys [48], it was concluded that the poor compressibility of chitosan, resulting in tablets with low crushing strength and relative high friability, was due to the high porosity of chitosan. Therefore, the mass of chitosan filling the die was relatively low and, during compression, the tablet press could not sufficiently accomplish the necessary volume reduction of the material even at the highest compression setting.

Another drawback to the compression properties for chitosan is the relatively thin compacts produced to achieve an acceptable mechanical tablet strength and friability. Perioli *et al.* prepared tablets made from chitosan and PVP K90 or Polycarbophil, NOVEON® AA-1 (PCP AA-1) and noted that the tablets' width increased as the synthetic polymer content rose (PVP K90 > PCP AA-1), while it was inversely proportional to the amount of chitosan [87].

### 2.4.1. Heckel Analysis

Compression properties determine the ability of powders to be compressed into tablets. These properties impart the tablet shape, porosity, and hardness, as well as the powder die-filling extent whereby the tablet weight is established. A number of mathematical models are available to analyze powder compression properties. Heckel analysis still remains the most powerful model in describing powder compressibility.

The Heckel equation (Equation (2)) is used for powder densification, where it describes the change of powder porosity as a function of the applied pressure [88]:

$$\ln \frac{1}{1-D} = kP + A \tag{2}$$

where $D$ is the density of a powder compact at pressure $P$, and $k$ is the slope of the data when presented as in Equation (1). The value of $k$ is a measure of the plasticity of a compacted material. The inverse of the slope is the yield pressure of the materials ($P_y$) [89], which describes the tendency of the material to deform either by plastic deformation or by brittle fracture. $P_y$ is inversely related to the ability of the material to deform plastically under pressure.

$A$ is a constant related to the die filling and particle rearrangement before deformation and bonding of the discrete particles.

Two main parameters, $D_A$, and $D_B$, derived using the Heckel equation are helpful to assess the densification process. The relative density, $D_A$, represents the total degree of densification, and the relative density, $D_B$, describes particle rearrangement during the initial stages of compression. The two parameters are calculated from Equations (3) and (4):

$$D_A = 1 - e^{-A} \tag{3}$$

$$D_B = D_A - D_o \tag{4}$$

where $D_0$ represents the relative density of powder at the point when the applied pressure is equal to zero.

When Heckel analysis is carried out for chitin in comparison with other common plastic and brittle excipients, the Heckel parameters can be summarized in Table 2. The yield pressure, which is a measure of the ductility of the materials, demonstrates that the plastic deformation of chitin is lower than that of PVP K30, which represented the highest plastically deforming excipient, followed by sorbitol, pregelatinized starch (Starch 1500), and Avicel PH® 101. Calcium diphosphate as a brittle excipient presented the highest $P_y$ value or the lowest ductility, followed by lactose monohydrate [52].

**Table 2.** The Heckel parameters for chitin and different common DC excipients. Data were extracted from Rojas *et al.* [52,69].

| Parameter | Calcium Diphosphate | Chitin | Lactose H₂O | Avicel PH 101 | Starch 1500 | PVP K30 | Sorbitol |
|---|---|---|---|---|---|---|---|
| $P_Y$ | 250.1 | 122 | 150 | 62.5 | 75.1 | 35.7 | 48.4 |
| $D_0$ | 0.36 | 0.12 | 0.38 | 0.23 | 0.33 | 0.27 | 0.39 |
| $D_A$ | 0.49 | 0.52 | 0.69 | 0.44 | 0.48 | 0.72 | 0.79 |
| $D_B$ | 0.13 | 0.31 | 0.31 | 0.21 | 0.15 | 0.46 | 0.4 |

Starch 1500: pregelatinized starch, Avicel PH® 101: microcrystalline cellulose.

Moreover, $D_A$, $D_B$, and $D_0$, which represent the total degree of densification, the phase of rearrangement of particles during the initial stages of compression, and the relative density of powder when the applied pressure is equal to zero, are further presented in Figure 8. Sorbitol had the largest densification during die filling ($D_0$); Avicel® PH 101, along with chitin, had the lowest values. The low densification during die filling resulted in the thin compacts produced using chitosan-PVP K90 with high chitosan content [87]. On the other hand, PVP K30 and sorbitol presented the largest total particle densification ($D_A$) and the largest rearrangement ($D_B$) upon densification. Conversely, pregelatinized starch and calcium diphosphate presented the lowest rearrangement at initial compression pressures ($D_B$). This is attributed to their initial large bulk densities and low porosity, causing small volume reduction at low pressures [52].

The low bulk density and low densification upon die filling of chitin or chitosan powders encouraged Buys to use a double filling cycle on a modified tablet press for the processing of chitosan in mini-tablets [48]. This has resulted in promising compression profiles for the material when the powder volume in the die cavity was increased through a double filling cycle. It was therefore postulated that if enough powder could be filled into the die cavity of a tablet press to increase the packing density of the material, then efficient particle bonding during compression should be able to produce tablets of acceptable mechanical strength.

322

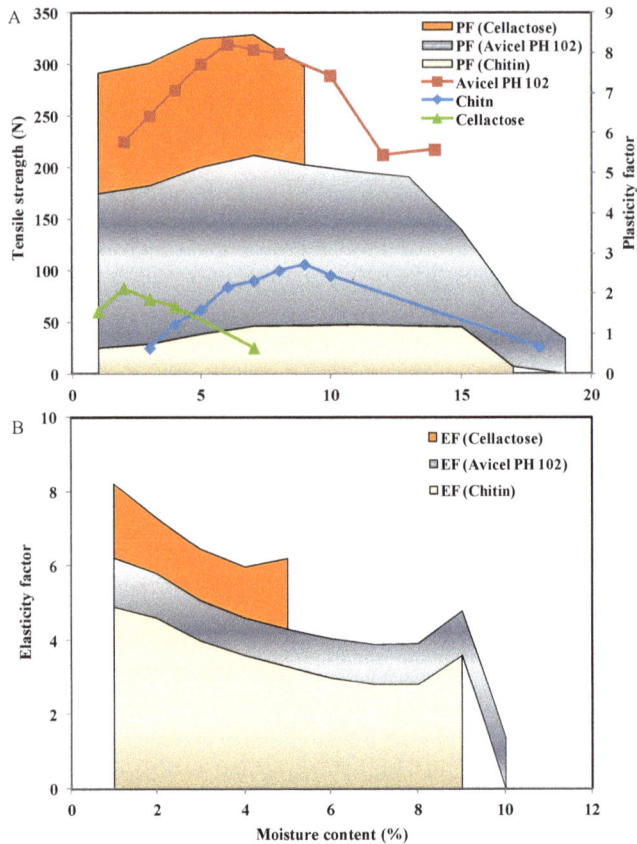

**Figure 8. (A)** Tensile strength and plasticity factor (PF) and **(B)** elasticity factor (EF) for chitin, microcrystalline cellulose (Avicel® PH 102), and co-processed spray dried lactose (Cellactose®) as a function of moisture content. Data were obtained from Khan and Pilpel [71], and García Mir *et al.* [78].

## 2.4.2. Kawakita Analysis

The compression behavior of the powder can also be evaluated using Kawakita analysis (Equation (5)). This model is dependent on the bulk density of the powder, unlike the true density, on which the Heckel model is dependent. The Kawakita equation is used to study powder compression via the degree of volume reduction:

$$\frac{P}{C} = \frac{P}{a} + \frac{1}{ab} \tag{5}$$

where $C$ is the degree of volume reduction of the powder column under the applied pressure $P$. The constant $a$ is the minimum porosity of the material before compression. The constant $b$ relates to the amount of plasticity of the material. The reciprocal of $b$ ($1/b$), known as $P_k$, defines the pressure required to reduce the powder bed by 50% [90,91]. It is worth noting that $P_k$ values are an inverse measure of the amount of plastic deformation occurring during compression [92].

## 2.4.3. The Gurnham Equation

The Gurnham equation can be used to study the compression process in pharmaceutical powders [93]. In this model, any increase in pressure, expressed as a fractional increase over the existing pressure, is expected to result in a proportional increase in the apparent density of powder mass. According to Gurnham's equation:

$$\varepsilon\,(\%) = -cln\sigma_c + d \tag{6}$$

where $c$ (the negative of the slope obtained by plotting $\varepsilon$ (%) vs. $ln\sigma_c$ and $d$ (the y-intercept) are constants. The constant $c$ provides a good representation of material compressibility. Higher $c$ values indicate better compressibility.

## 2.4.4. Plasticity/Elasticity Factors

Upon compression, the plasticity and elasticity of materials can be measured using the force-distance curve near the maximum force by a method described by Antikainen and Yliruusi [94]. The plasticity factor (PF) determines the extent of plastic deformation at a certain compression force, as described in Equation (7):

$$PF = \left(\frac{W_1}{W_1 + W_2}\right) \times 100\% \tag{7}$$

where $W_1$ and $W_2$ are calculated from the force–displacement curve [94]. The elasticity factor (EF) can be calculated using Equation (8):

$$EF = \left(\frac{S_{max} - S_{od}}{S_{max} - S_o}\right) \times 100 \tag{8}$$

where $S_{max}$ is the maximum upper punch displacement, $S_o$ is the displacement of the upper punch at first detection of force, and $S_{od}$ is the displacement of the upper punch in the decompression phase [94].

Without the need for double die filling, Braja and Subrata have managed to prepare metoprolol tartarate tablets comprising the drug and chitosan through DC [95]. The contribution of chitosan to the compression properties was compared to that of tablets made with Eudragit RL-100, ethyl cellulose, hydroxyethyl cellulose (HEC), and hydroxypropylmethyl cellulose (HPMC) K-100. When $P_Y$ and "$a$" of the Heckel and Kawakita equations were used to estimate the compressibility parameters, the plasticity appeared to follow the order chitosan > Eudragit RL 100 > ethyl cellulose > HPMC K100 > HEC. However, estimation of powder properties upon compression was carried out using a hydraulic tablet press with one minute dwelling time. Ching et al. emphasized that the tabletability and compressibility of plastic and brittle pharmaceutical powders are speed-dependent [96].

The plasto-elasticity behavior of chitin was quantified (Figure 8) along with Avicel® PH 102 and Cellactose® from the force distance curve using Antikainen and Yliruusi's method [94]. Avicel® PH 102 and chitin mainly undergo plastic deformation during compression [94,97]. Higher plasticity, in general, would lead to more contact points for interparticulate bonding [98]. This justifies the highest tensile strength displayed by Avicel® PH 102 tablets, followed by chitin and

Cellactose® (Figure 8). For Cellactose®, despite its low cellulose content, the binding between lactose particles is mediated by cellulose [97,99].

On the other hand, elastic deformation causes a profound decrease in the tensile strength of tablets. This is due to disruption of interparticulate bonds when the compaction pressure is released. As a material exhibiting high plastic deformation, Avicel® PH 102 has a minimal tendency to encounter a reversible deformation behavior. Of the values for excipients' elasticity factor in Figure 8, chitin's elasticity is the highest, followed by Cellactose® and Avicel® PH 102. This higher elasticity therefore contributes to the lowest tensile strength observed with chitin tablets.

## 2.5. Factors Contributing to the Powder Compressibility Properties of Chitin/Chitosan

### 2.5.1. Moisture Content

It is generally accepted that moisture content has the largest impact on powder compressibility [70,71]. Increasing the moisture content decreases the granule porosity and fragmentation propensity and hence increases granule strength [100]. As seen in Figure 8, the values for the plasticity factor (PF) initially increased for chitin, Cellactose®, and Avicel® PH 102, reaching the maximum at 1.5%–2.5%, 3%–5%, and 7%–10% $w/w$ moisture, respectively. The highest values of PF (4.4%) were obtained for Avicel® PH 102, whereupon the PF value was clearly decreased as the moisture content was increased up to 14% (at 95% RH) as a consequence of free water effect.

### 2.5.2. Degree of Deacetylation

At present, there is no solid data on the effect of chitosan's degree of deacetylation on powder behavior upon compression. However, Picker-Freyer et al. noted that according to the DDA no order in powder compressibility could be set up [86].

### 2.5.3. Molecular Weight

Heckel and Kawakita analyses were investigated by Rashid et al. and Qandil et al. on different MW chitosan powders of the same DDA [6,16]. With regard to the Kawakita parameter $a$, Table 3 shows the highest porosity is obtained for the highest MW chitosan, whereas the lowest porosity is obtained for the lowest MW chitosan. On the other hand, the amount of plastic deformation decreases (higher $1/b$ values) for the lower MW chitosan samples. The foregoing was further verified by the yield pressure parameter ($P_Y$) of Heckel analysis, which revealed that the higher the chitosan MW the higher its plastic deformation upon compression. This explains the increase in tensile strength for lower MW chitosan samples (presented in Figure 6), especially at low compression loads (<300 kg). It has to be noted that the extent of die filling and particle rearrangement before compression ($A$) for all samples is nearly the same (Table 3), probably due to similar particle size distribution of each of the chitosan samples.

**Table 3.** The Kawakita and Heckel parameters of chitin and chitosan of different molecular weights. Data were obtained from Rashid *et al.* [6].

| Material/MW (kDa) | Kawakita Parameter | | | | | |
|---|---|---|---|---|---|---|
| | *a* | *ab* | *b* | *1/b* | $P_Y$ | *A* |
| Chitin | 0.818 | 0.077 | 0.094 | 10.57 | - | - |
| Chitosan/100 | 0.75 | 0.092 | 0.12 | 8.15 | 72.5 | 0.42 |
| Chitosan/30 | 0.54 | 0.066 | 0.12 | 8.14 | 98.0 | 0.46 |
| Chitosan/18 | 0.63 | 0.084 | 0.13 | 25.55 | 106.4 | 0.47 |
| Chitosan/8 | 0.52 | 0.024 | 0.046 | 21.55 | 153.9 | 0.60 |

Kawakita *a, ab* and 1/b parameters represent porosity, extent of fragmentation, and plastic deformation, respectively. Heckel $P_Y$ and A parameters represent yield pressure and particle rearrangement, respectively. MW represents molecular weight.

In a related study presented by Katharina *et al.* wherein they investigated the slope of the Heckel function for different MW chitosans, chitosan with a MW of 87.2 kDa behaves in a manner similar to Avicel® PH 102, and the others with 173.3 and 210.5 kDa showed a lower Heckel slope and thus higher resistance against deformation [86]. They suggested that the higher Heckel slope is the result of the lower MW of the chitosan. These results contradict the findings by Rashid *et al.* on chitosan plasticity [6]. It can be postulated that such inconsistency is related to the differences in the physical characteristics of the chitosans used. For example, the 173.3, 210.5, and 87.2 kDa chitosans differ in DDA, bulk density, and particle size. Each of these differences affects the extent of packing and deformation extents upon compression. In addition, the determination of the Heckel slopes includes plastic and elastic deformation, and therefore the contribution of the undetermined elastic recovery might have contributed to the Heckel slope.

A clearer judgment on the plasticity-MW relationship of chitosan can be drawn from the results presented by Chen and Hwa, who explored the effect of MW of chitosans with the same DDA on the elasticity (elongation at break) and tensile strength of chitosan films [101]. These films would have lost the contributions of particle size and size distribution to these parameters. Both parameters of the membranes prepared from high MW chitosan were higher than those of low MW chitosan.

## 2.6. Compressibility Changes upon Formulation and/or Modification of Chitosan

There are numerous applications of chitosan described in the literature, especially when it was used in solid dosage form. However, few studies have investigated the powder compression properties and tabletability of chitosan in relation to its physical and/or chemical modification or even to its simple role as an additive.

### 2.6.1. Physical Mixing

A combination of chitosan with other polymers has been used either to provide a desired function for controlled or immediate release products or to improve the compressibility of chitosan. For example, Knapczyk showed that chitosan of 66% DDA, when used as a filler or binder in DC processing, produced tablets that suffer from low mechanical resistance but did not affect mass flow nor undermine rapid tablet disintegration [102].

In the preparation of sustained release DC tablets of ciprofloxacin HCl with a 1:1 ratio of chitosan and gum kondagogu, the powder's and tablets' physical properties were evaluated [103]. The powder mixtures comprising the drug, the polymeric matrix, and starch have recorded bulk densities of 0.43–0.48 g/mL. In other words, the drug (bulk density of 0.2 g/mL) has been formulated into a compressible powder by physical mixing, reaching double its own bulk density. Furthermore, a CI of 3.4%–6.16% was achieved. It is clear that the contribution of the bulk densities and the improvement in the flow of the preparations are more likely attributed to starch (~0.55 g/mL), which is present at a high level, and to gum kondagogu (CI of 16% and bulk density of 0.704 g/mL) [103].

A similar approach involving chitosan physically mixed with other hydrophilic polymers was utilized to produce sustained release DC terbutaline sulfate tablets [104], employing chitosan and xanthan gum mixed at a 1:1 mass ratio with sodium bicarbonate as a release-modifying agent. Although the properties of the physically mixed powders were not recorded, results of drug content, friability, weight variation, and tablet hardness from the three batches' reproducibility data indicated batch-to-batch reproducibility, and no significant differences were noticed. Accordingly, the requisite powder's flow properties are achieved with such a polymeric combination. Such improvement in flow is anticipated by the high bulk density of sodium bicarbonate (~1.0 g/mL), which should ultimately improve the extent of die filling.

The effect of chitosan on powder compressibility when present with other polymeric excipients (e.g., xanthan gum) was described by Eftaiha *et al.* [105]. They correlated the compression to the relative bulk and tapped density of chitosan and xanthan gum, from which the porosity was determined according to Equation (9):

$$\varepsilon = 1 - \rho \tag{9}$$

where $\varepsilon$ is porosity and $\rho$ is the relative density. Accordingly, the porosity of the bulk and the tapped powder for chitosan is 0.879 and 0.842, while for xanthan gum it is 0.571 and 0.510, respectively. Based on the porosity values, chitosan is more porous than xanthan gum, giving rise to a higher extent of volume reduction upon compression for chitosan than for xanthan gum. The foregoing was verified using force-displacement curves, whereby chitosan showed a high displacement when compared to xanthan upon compression. Furthermore, the Gurnham equation (Equation (6)) was used to investigate different mixtures of chitosan and xanthan gum. Since ductile and brittle materials demonstrate large or little amounts of plastic deformation before fracture, respectively [106], according to Gurnham's model and Zhao's classification, xanthan gum is a brittle material, whereas chitosan is a ductile material (Figure 9). Furthermore, plasticity increases as the mass fraction of chitosan is increased and the 1:1 chitosan:xanthan gum mass ratio represents a reasonably ductile combination of sufficient tensile strength. The foregoing ratio was estimated to present a percolation threshold that generally takes place between plastic and elastic materials at specific concentrations.

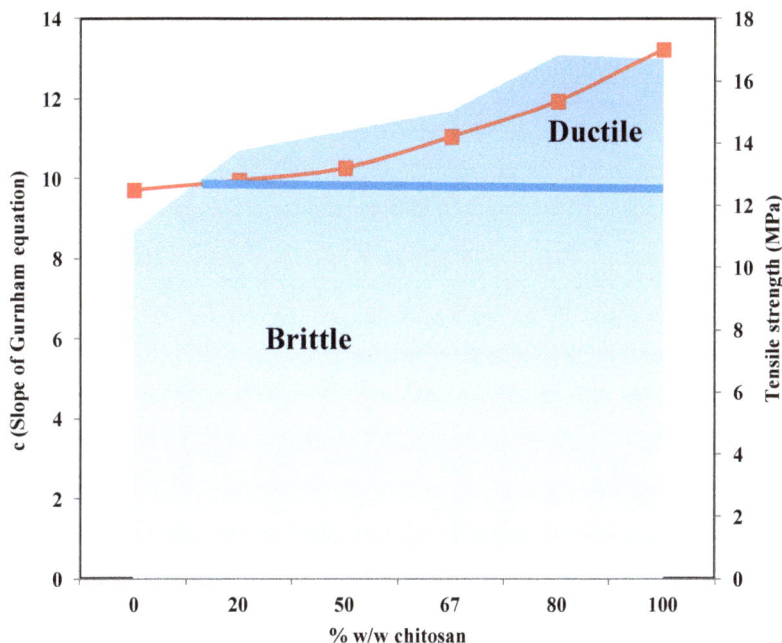

**Figure 9.** The effect of chitosan content on the plasticity of a chitosan–xanthan mixture. Data were obtained from Eftaiha *et al.* [107].

## 2.6.2. Spray-Drying

Due to the fact that spray-drying offers a means of obtaining powders of predetermined particle size and shape [108], most spray-drying processing of chitosan was carried out mainly to improve powder flow. Thus powder compressibility and in most instances powder compactibility are improved. The use of spray-dried chitosan as an excipient for directly compressible tablet formulations has been reported earlier [109]. The suitability of chitosan in the formulation of sustained release dosage forms of a few drugs has been disclosed [110–112]. Although chitosan is insoluble in water, its solubility in weakly acidic media makes it available for processing by spray-drying. On the other hand, once dissolved, it forms protonated chitosan amines. The acquired positive charges can result in precipitation of complexes or insoluble salt forms of chitosan upon addition of negatively charged molecules during processing [113].

Rege *et al.* spray-dried chitosans of different MW and compared these products with tray-dried chitosans of equivalent MW [109]. The bulk density of spray-dried chitosan, in general, was higher than tray-dried chitosan. The foregoing is correlated to the powder packing characteristics, where the small, spherical, spray-dried particles are expressed to closely pack together and thus lower the volume-to-mass ratio; consequently, a higher bulk density is obtained. On the contrary, the large, irregular, tray-dried particles showed poor packing characteristics with a lower bulk density. With regard to compressibility, spray-dried chitosans, in general, exhibited a lower percentage of compressibility in contrast to tray-dried chitosans. This difference corresponds to the improved flow property of the spray-dried material [114]. Such behavior is attributed to the fact that spray-dried particles, in general, are hollow spheres, with lower particle density than the relatively solid tray-dried particles. With regard to the effect of MW on the properties of spray-dried chitosan, although the tablets' tensile strength was not measured, Rege *et al.* highlighted that, upon preparation, tray-drying invariably resulted in hard tenacious masses that needed vigorous milling, whereas spray-dried granules did not require additional milling [109,115]. Nevertheless, in a separate study, Rege *et al.* managed to test the tensile strength of tetracycline-chitosan tablets prepared by spray- and tray-drying techniques [109]. They concluded that the tensile strength of tablets containing spray-dried chitosan was generally higher than in those containing tray-dried chitosan at each MW. Furthermore, the tensile strength of low MW chitosan tablets (2–16.6 kDa) was higher than that of tablets containing chitosans of MW 280–519 kDa.

Similar conclusions regarding powder flow and compressibility properties were drawn when a naproxen sodium–chitosan complex was spray- and tray-dried [116]. The significant result in this work is the disappearance of the crystalline structure of the naproxen–chitosan complex upon spray-drying, as naproxen and chitosan have highly and partially crystalline structures, respectively. Such crystallographic modification is further confirmed upon spray-drying of theophylline–chitosan complexes [110]. Theoretically, as the percent relative crystallinity increases, the crushing strength of tablets also increases [117]. Crystalline regions have a highly ordered arrangement of molecules in their structure. Upon compression of crystalline materials, the crystalline regions are forced to become closely packed. The tighter molecular arrangement, in combination with the high plastic deforming ability of e.g., microcrystalline cellulose and starch, facilitates the formation of hydrogen bonding upon compression, resulting in the formation of strong compacts [6,117]. The aforementioned fact contradicts with the reported high tensile strength of chitosan complexes, which became amorphous after being subjected to spray-drying. Upon compression of spray-dried chitosan, more particle–particle contact occurs, either by plastic or brittle deformation, as the next examples elucidate.

Figure 10 presents the powder and tablet characteristics of spray-dried mixtures of chitosan and hydrolyzed gelatin. Initially, at all concentrations of chitosan, the powders show better flow characteristics, with higher tensile strength, than hydrolyzed gelatin itself. Increasing the content of chitosan favors an increase in the yield pressure, which implies that plasticity decreases with an increase in the concentration of chitosan. However, a decrease in plasticity results in lower contact surface area and therefore lower tensile strength of the compacts. This contravenes the trend toward an increase in tensile strength as the chitosan content is increased (Figure 10). Suruchi *et al.* suggest that this could be attributed to the formation of low-strength granules that fracture readily, resulting in a significant increase in particle–particle contact surface area, which leads to enhanced bonding between adjacent particles [118].

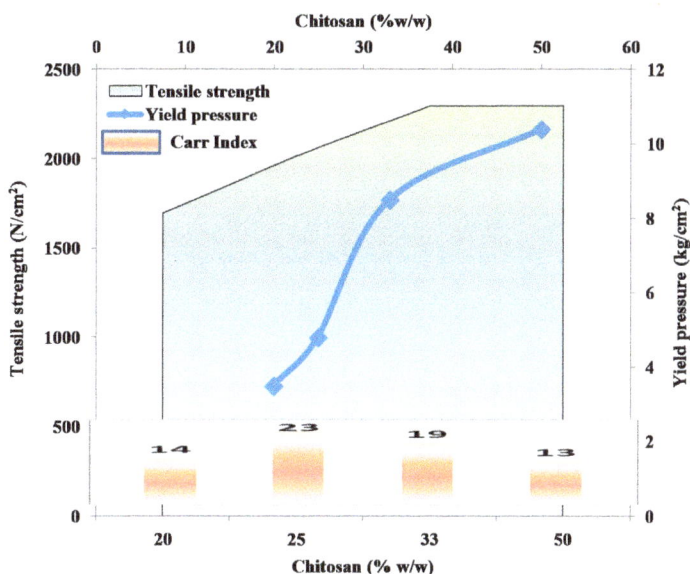

**Figure 10.** Effect of chitosan content on powder and tablet characteristics of spray-dried mixtures of chitosan and hydrolyzed gelatin. Data were obtained from Kokil *et al.* [118].

### 2.6.3. Co-Precipitation of Silicon Derivatives on Chitin/Chitosan

In the search for new multifunctional excipients with strong binding, good flow, and fast disintegration characteristics, there has been a focus on silicon derivatives. Initially, silicon dioxide was co-precipitated onto chitosan and chitin at a 1:1 mass ratio [10,50,51,119]. In addition to enhanced binding and disintegration properties, the compressibility improved in comparison to their initial properties. For example, the 0.27 g/mL bulk densities of chitin increased to 0.45 g/mL for a chitin–silicon dioxide co-precipitate and the powder compressibility is 7.3% for a chitosan–silicon dioxide co-precipitate (Table 4). Consequently, the powder flow has earned an "Excellent" rank under the CI criteria. Furthermore, as evidenced by the $D_A$ and $D_B$ values, the chitin–silica co-precipitate undergoes a high extent of packing and rearrangement in comparison to Avicel® 200 (microcrystalline cellulose of particle size 180 µm). With regard to powder deformation under compression, both Avicel® 200 and the co-processed excipients undergo plastic deformation to a similar extent when their yield pressure ($P_Y$) values are considered. However, a faster onset of plastic deformation ($1/b$) takes place by individual (unprocessed) excipients due to their higher compressibility ($a$) and high particle rearrangement ($ab$).

The change in powder compressibility due to formation of the co-precipitates can be attributed to the dramatic change in chitin or chitosan structures, from thin flat surfaces, some with irregular folded edges, to three-dimensional compacts of chitin–silica. The aforementioned was evidenced by an almost 40% reduction in the measured specific surface areas for the co-precipitates when compared to their native excipients. However, the partially crystalline nature of chitin was still intact. Ultimately, co-processing of silicon dioxide/silicate onto chitin or chitosan brings about freely flowing and denser packing particles without significantly affecting the plasticity of the native excipient or its crystalline structure, unlike what is observed with spray-drying.

**Table 4.** The powder properties of chitin and chitosan mixtures with silicate excipients, in comparison with co-processed microcrystalline cellulose (Avicel® PH 200). Data were obtained from El-Barghouthi *et al.* [119] and Rashid *et al.* [50,51].

| Mixture | BD | TD | % Comp. | Heckel Parameters | | | Kawakita Parameters | | | |
|---|---|---|---|---|---|---|---|---|---|---|
| | | | | $P_Y$ | $D_A$ | $D_B$ | $a$ | $b$ | $1/b$ | $ab$ |
| Chitosan–silica (50% chitosan) | 0.38 | 0.41 | 7.32 | – | – | – | – | – | – | – |
| Chitin–silica (50% chitin) | 0.45 | 0.5 | 10 | 98 | 0.165 | 0.588 | – | – | – | – |
| Chitin–Mg silicate (68% chitin) | – | – | – | – | – | – | 0.75 | – | 17.37 | 0.043 |
| Chitin | 0.27 | 0.39 | 30.77 | – | – | – | 0.82 | 1.67 | 0.6 | 0.077 |
| Avicel® 200 | – | – | – | 81.3 | 0.09 | 0.611 | – | – | – | – |

Kawakita $a$, $ab$, and $1/b$ parameters represent porosity, extent of fragmentation, and plastic deformation, respectively. Heckel $P_Y$, $D_A$, and $D_B$ parameters represent yield pressure, the total degree of densification, and the phase rearrangement of particles during the initial stages of compression, respectively. BD and TD represent the bulk and tapped densities, respectively.

The interaction of co-processed chitin–metal silicate excipients with model drugs was investigated in aqueous slurry and in the solid state [120]. When cefotaxime sodium was chosen as a model drug that exhibits acid or base catalysis, chitin–aluminum silicate showed minimum drug instability in the solid state, close to where the maximum drug stability in the slurry was observed. This was attributed to the catalytic properties of chitin–aluminum silicate. Generally, catalytic activities are associated with oxidation/reduction and acid/base reactions of the metal cation on the silica surface. Such activity depends on the polarizing power of the metal, which is a function of the effective nuclear charge and size of the cation. On the other hand, the slurry method did not efficiently predict the solid-state surface acidity and stability of cefotaxime sodium. Moreover, the solid-state chemical stability might be influenced by factors other than the solid-state acidity. The stability of cefotaxime sodium was achieved with chitin–magnesium silicate when the surface pH was almost neutral.

2.6.4. Co-Processing of Chitin/Chitosan by Compaction

Roll compaction is a continuous dry granulation process that is widely employed in the pharmaceutical industry to manufacture free flowing agglomerates. In this technique, compacted ribbons or flakes are produced and then milled to form granules of desired size. Such mechanical densification results in an increase in the bulk density, thus producing high-quality tablets with high dose uniformity and low weight variation [3].

Compaction of chitosan was carried out for the purpose of characterizing the compaction properties of chitin samples of different MW (listed previously in Table 3) [121]. With respect to granules' deformation mode, compacted chitin undergoes plastic deformation to a greater extent (lower $P_Y$) than does native chitin or even any or the co-precipitated excipients listed in Table 4. Such high plasticity was confirmed when chitin was compacted with mannitol at a 20:80 (mannitol:chitin) mass ratio. The plasticity was identified from the low Kawakita parameter ($1/b$) of the compacted mixture, 7.8, compared to that of the individual components (10.6 for chitin and 10.3 for mannitol). Such high plasticity is responsible for the high tensile strength of tablets made from the co-processed excipient. Compressibility ($a$) of the compacted mixture is nearly the same for chitin and is relatively low for mannitol ($a = 0.576$). Therefore, co-processing of chitin with mannitol provides no substantial increase in the compressibility of chitin. At 20% level, mannitol occupies only a limited area of the large surface pores of chitin. These pores are responsible for the decrease in the volume of chitin powder upon compression [122].

## 3. Conclusions

Pharmaceutical applications of chitin and chitosan and their derivatives as effective excipients can be aligned for DC processing. The diversity of physico-chemical properties of semi-crystalline nature, DDA, and MW enhance beneficial use as such and as a co-processed excipient in pharmaceutical preparations. Moreover, their high surface area, porous structure, and plastic deforming nature enhance necessary particle bonding and tabletability in the DC mode with low sensitivity upon lubrication. Optimal use as a single multifunctional excipient can be established when chitin and chitosan are co-processed with other excipients.

## Author Contributions

Adnan A. Badwan contributed to the concept of the review and its preparation; Iyad Rashid and Mahmoud M.H. Al Omari drafted and wrote the review; Fouad H. Darras provided a significant contribution in writing the review. All authors approved the final version of the review.

## Conflicts of Interest

The authors declare no conflict of interest.

## References

1.  Gohel, M.C.; Jogani, P.D. A review of co-processed directly compressible excipients. *J. Pharm. Pharm. Sci.* **2005**, *8*, 76–93.
2.  Michoel, A.; Rombaut, P.; Verhoye, A. Comparative evaluation of co-processed lactose and microcrystalline cellulose with their physical mixtures in the formulation of folic acid tablets. *Pharm. Dev. Technol.* **2002**, *7*, 79–87.
3.  Bindhumadhavan, G.; Seville, J.P.K.; Adams, M.J.; Greenwood, R.W.; Fitzpatrick, S. Roll compaction of a pharmaceutical excipient: Experimental validation of rolling theory for granular solids. *Chem. Eng. Sci.* **2005**, *60*, 3891–3897.

4.  Pingali, K.; Mendez, R.; Lewis, D.; Michniak-Kohn, B.; Cuitino, A.; Muzzio, F. Mixing order of glidant and lubricant—Influence on powder and tablet properties. *Int. J. Pharm.* **2011**, *409*, 269–277.

5.  Haware, R.V.; Tho, I.; Bauer-Brandl, A. Evaluation of a rapid approximation method for the elastic recovery of tablets. *Powder Technol.* **2010**, *202*, 71–77.

6.  Rashid, I.; al Omari, M.M. H.; Badwan, A.A. From native to multifunctional starch-based excipients designed for direct compression formulation. *Starch Stärke* **2013**, *65*, 552–571.

7.  Daraghmeh, N.H.; Chowdhry, B.Z.; Leharne, S.A.; al Omari, M.M.; Badwan, A.A. Chapter 2—Chitin. In *Profiles of Drug Substances Excipients, and Related Methodology*; Harry, G.B., Ed.; Academic Press: Waltham, MA, USA, 2011; Volume 36, pp. 35–102.

8.  Ravi Kumar, M.N.V. A review of chitin and chitosan applications. *React. Funct. Polym.* **2000**, *46*, 1–27.

9.  Aranaz, I.; Mengibar, M.; Harris, R.; Panos, I.; Miralles, B.; Acosta, N.; Galed, G.; Heras, A. Functional characterization of chitin and chitosan. *Curr. Chem. Biol.* **2009**, *3*, 203–230.

10. Hamid, R.A.; Al-Akayleh, F.; Shubair, M.; Rashid, I.; Remawi, M.A.; Badwan, A. Evaluation of three chitin metal silicate co-precipitates as a potential multifunctional single excipient in tablet formulations. *Mar. Drugs* **2010**, *8*, 1699–1715.

11. Zhang, Y.; Xue, C.; Xue, Y.; Gao, R.; Zhang, X. Determination of the degree of deacetylation of chitin and chitosan by X-ray powder diffraction. *Carbohydr. Res.* **2005**, *340*, 1914–1917.

12. Sweidan, K.; Jaber, A.M.; Al-jbour, N.; Obaidat, R.; Al-Remawi, M.; Badwan, A. Further investigation on the degree of deacetylation of chitosan determined by potentiometric titration. *J. Excip. Food Chem.* **2011**, *2*, 16–25.

13. Pillai, C.K.S.; Paul, W.; Sharma, C.P. Chitin and chitosan polymers: Chemistry, solubility and fiber formation. *Prog. Polym. Sci.* **2009**, *34*, 641–678.

14. Dutta, P.K.; Dutta, J.; Tripathi, V.S. Chitin and chitosan: Chemistry, properties and applications. *J. Sci. Ind. Res.* **2004**, *63*, 20–31.

15. Rinaudo, M. Chitin and chitosan: Properties and applications. *Prog. Polym. Sci.* **2006**, *31*, 603–632.

16. Qandil, A.; Obaidat, A.; Ali, M.M.; Al-Taani, B.; Tashtoush, B.; Al-Jbour, N.; al Remawi, M.; Al-Sou'od, K.; Badwan, A. Investigation of the interactions in complexes of low molecular weight chitosan with ibuprofen. *J. Sol. Chem.* **2009**, *38*, 695–712.

17. Kumar, M.N.; Muzzarelli, R.A.; Muzzarelli, C.; Sashiwa, H.; Domb, A.J. Chitosan chemistry and pharmaceutical perspectives. *Chem. Rev.* **2004**, *104*, 6017–6084.

18. Muzzarelli, R.A.; Tubertini, O. Chitin and chitosan as chromatographic supports and adsorbents for collection of metal ions from organic and aqueous solutions and sea-water. *Talanta* **1969**, *16*, 1571–1577.

19. Datta, P.K.; Basu, P.S.; Datta, T.K. Isolation and characterization of *Vicia faba* lectin affinity purified on chitin column. *Prep. Biochem.* **1984**, *14*, 373–387.

20. Songkroah, C.; Nakbanpote, W.; Thiravetyan, P. Recovery of silver-thiosulphate complexes with chitin. *Proc. Biochem.* **2004**, *39*, 1553–1559.

21. Krajewska, B. Application of chitin- and chitosan-based materials for enzyme immobilizations: A review. *Enzyme Microb. Technol.* **2004**, *35*, 126–139.

22. Lim, S.H.; Hudson, S.M. Synthesis and antimicrobial activity of a water-soluble chitosan derivative with a fiber-reactive group. *Carbohydr. Res.* **2004**, *339*, 313–319.

23. Albarghouthi, M.; Fara, D.A.; Saleem, M.; el-Thaher, T.; Matalka, K.; Badwan, A. Immobilization of antibodies on alginate-chitosan beads. *Int. J. Pharm.* **2000**, *206*, 23–34.

24. Yusof, N.L.; Wee, A.; Lim, L.Y.; Khor, E. Flexible chitin films as potential wound-dressing materials: Wound model studies. *J. Biomed. Mater. Res. A* **2003**, *66*, 224–232.

25. Rathke, T.D.; Hudson, S.M. Review of chitin and chitosan as fiber and film formers. *J. Macromol. Sci. C* **1994**, *34*, 375–437.

26. Pierson, Y.; Chen, X.; Bobbink, F.D.; Zhang, J.; Yan, N. Acid-catalyzed chitin liquefaction in ethylene glycol. *ACS Sustain. Chem. Eng.* **2014**, *2*, 2081–2089.

27. Chen, X.; Chew, S.L.; Kerton, F.M.; Yan, N. Direct conversion of chitin into a *N*-containing furan derivative. *Green Chem.* **2014**, *16*, 2204–2212.

28. Muzzarelli, R.A.; Barontini, G.; Rocchetti, R. Immobilized enzymes on chitosan columns: α-chymotrypsin and acid phosphatase. *Biotechnol. Bioeng.* **1976**, *18*, 1445–1454.

29. Muzzarelli, R.; Baldassarre, V.; Conti, F.; Ferrara, P.; Biagini, G.; Gazzanelli, G.; Vasi, V. Biological activity of chitosan: Ultrastructural study. *Biomaterials* **1988**, *9*, 247–252.

30. Muzzarelli, R.; Tarsi, R.; Filippini, O.; Giovanetti, E.; Biagini, G.; Varaldo, P.E. Antimicrobial properties of *N*-carboxybutyl chitosan. *Antimicrob. Agents Chemother.* **1990**, *34*, 2019–2023.

31. Muzzarelli, R.A.A.; Mattioli-Belmonte, M.; Tietz, C.; Biagini, R.; Ferioli, G.; Brunelli, M.A.; Fini, M.; Giardino, R.; Ilari, P.; Biagini, G. Stimulatory effect on bone formation exerted by a modified chitosan. *Biomaterials* **1994**, *15*, 1075–1081.

32. Muzzarelli, C.; Stanic, V.; Gobbi, L.; Tosi, G.; Muzzarelli, R.A.A. Spray-drying of solutions containing chitosan together with polyuronans and characterisation of the microspheres. *Carbohydr. Polym.* **2004**, *57*, 73–82.

33. Sabnis, S.; Rege, P.; Block, L.H. Use of chitosan in compressed tablets of diclofenac sodium: Inhibition of drug release in an acidic environment. *Pharm. Dev. Technol.* **1997**, *2*, 243–255.

34. Remuñán-López, C.; Portero, A.; Vila-Jato, J.L.; Alonso, M.A.J. Design and evaluation of chitosan/ethylcellulose mucoadhesive bilayered devices for buccal drug delivery. *J. Control. Release* **1998**, *55*, 143–152.

35. Giunchedi, P.; Juliano, C.; Gavini, E.; Cossu, M.; Sorrenti, M. Formulation and *in vivo* evaluation of chlorhexidine buccal tablets prepared using drug-loaded chitosan microspheres. *Eur. J. Pharm. Biopharm.* **2002**, *53*, 233–239.

36. Athamneh, N.A.; Tashtoush, B.M.; Qandil, A.M.; Al-Tanni, B.M.; Obaidat, A.A.; Al-Jbour, N.D.; Qinna, N.A.; Al-Sou'od, K.; Al-Remawi, M.M.; Badwan, A.A. A new controlled-release liquid delivery system based on diclofenac potassium and low molecular weight chitosan complex solubilized in polysorbates. *Drug Dev. Ind. Pharm.* **2013**, *39*, 1217–1229.

37. Elsayed, A.; Al-Remawi, M.; Qinna, N.; Farouk, A.; Al-Sou'od, K.A.; Badwan, A.A. Chitosan-sodium lauryl sulfate nanoparticles as a carrier system for the *in vivo* delivery of oral insulin. *AAPS PharmSciTech* **2011**, *12*, 958–964.

38. Assaf, S.M.; al-Jbour, N.D.; Eftaiha, A.A.F.; Elsayed, A.M.; al-Remawi, M.M.; Qinna, N.A.; Chowdhry, B.; Leharne, S.; Badwan, A.A. Factors involved in formulation of oily delivery system for proteins based on PEG-8 caprylic/capric glycerides and polyglyceryl-6 dioleate in a mixture of oleic acid with chitosan. *J. Dispers. Sci. Technol.* **2011**, *32*, 623–633.

39. Qinna, N.A.; Akayleh, F.T.; al Remawi, M.M.; Kamona, B.S.; Taha, H.; Badwan, A.A. Evaluation of a functional food preparation based on chitosan as a meal replacement diet. *J. Funct. Foods* **2013**, *5*, 1125–1134.

40. Sinha, V.R.; Singla, A.K.; Wadhawan, S.; Kaushik, R.; Kumria, R.; Bansal, K.; Dhawan, S. Chitosan microspheres as a potential carrier for drugs. *Int. J. Pharm.* **2004**, *274*, 1–33.

41. Kumar, V.; de la Luz Reus-Medina, M.; Yang, D. Preparation, characterization, and tabletting properties of a new cellulose-based pharmaceutical aid. *Int. J. Pharm.* **2002**, *235*, 129–140.

42. Rege, P.R.; Shukla, D.J.; Block, L.H. Chitinosans as tableting excipients for modified release delivery systems. *Int. J. Pharm.* **1999**, *181*, 49–60.

43. Aucamp, M.E.; Campus, N.W.U.P. Assessment of the Tableting Properties of Chitosan Through Wet Granulation and Direct Compression Formulations. M.Sc. thesis, North-West University, Potchefstroom Campus, South Africa, 2004.

44. De Kock, J.M. Chitosan as a Multipurose Excipien in Directly Compressed Minitablets. Ph.D. thesis, North-West University, Potchefsroom Campus, South Africa, 2005.

45. Sawayanagi, Y.; Nambu, N.; Nagai, T. Directly compressed tablets containing chitin or chitosan in addition to lactose or potato starch. *Chem. Pharm. Bull. (Tokyo)* **1982**, *30*, 2935–2940.

46. Mir, V.G.; Heinamaki, J.; Antikainen, O.; Sandler, N.; Revoredo, O.B.; Colarte, A.I.; Nieto, O.M.; Yliruusi, J. Application of crustacean chitin as a co-diluent in direct compression of tablets. *AAPS PharmSciTech* **2010**, *11*, 409–415.

47. Charlton, B.; Newton, J.M. Theoretical estimation of punch velocities and displacements of single-punch and rotary tablet machines. *J. Pharm. Pharmacol.* **1984**, *36*, 645–651.

48. Buys, G.M.; Campus, N.W.U.P. Formulation of a Chitosan Multi-Unit Dosage Form for Drug Delivery to the Colon. Ph.D. thesis, North-West University, Potchefstroom Campus, South Africa, 2006.

49. Krasilnikova, O.K.; Solovtsova, O.V.; Khozina, E.V.; Grankina, T.Y. *Porous Structure and Adsorption Behaviours of Chitosan*; Nova Science Publisher, Inc.: Hauppauge, NY, USA, 2011.

50. Rashid, I.; Al-Remawi, M.; Eftaiha, A.A.; Badwan, A. Chitin–silicon dioxide coprecipitate as a novel superdisintegrant. *J. Pharm. Sci.* **2008**, *97*, 4955–4969.

51. Rashid, I.; Daraghmeh, N.; Al-Remawi, M.; Leharne, S.A.; Chowdhry, B.Z.; Badwan, A. Characterization of chitin-metal silicates as binding superdisintegrants. *J. Pharm. Sci.* **2009**, *98*, 4887–4901.

52. Rojas, J.; Hernandez, C.; Trujillo, D. Effect of the alkaline treatment conditions on the tableting performance of chitin obtained from shrimp. *Afr. J. Pharm. Pharmacol.* **2014**, *8*, 211–219.

53. Sonnekus, J. Characterization of the flow and compression properties of chitosan. M.Sc. thesis, North-West University, Potchefstroom Campus, South Africa, 2008.

54. De Boer, A.H.; Vromans, H.; Leur, C.F.; Bolhuis, G.K.; Kussendrager, K.D.; Bosch, H. Studies on tableting properties of lactose. *Pharm. Weekbl. Sci. Ed.* **1986**, *8*, 145–150.

55. Gustafsson, C. *Solid State Characterisation and Compaction Behaviour of Pharmaceutical Materials*; Uppsala University/Acta Universitatis Uppsaliensis: Uppsala, Sweden, 2000.

56. Koo, O.M.; Heng, P.W. The influence of microcrystalline cellulose grade on shape and shape distributions of pellets produced by extrusion-spheronization. *Chem. Pharm. Bull. (Tokyo)* **2001**, *49*, 1383–1387.

57. Sujka, M.; Jamroz, J. α-Amylolysis of native potato and corn starches—SEM, AFM, nitrogen and iodine sorption investigations. *LWT Food Sci. Technol.* **2009**, *42*, 1219–1224.

58. Luna-Zaragoza, D.; Romero-Guzmán, E.; Reyes-Gutiérrez, L. Surface and physicochemical characterization of phosphates vivianite, $Fe_2(PO_4)_3$ and hydroxyapatite, $Ca_5(PO_4)_3OH$. *J. Min. Mater. Charact. Eng.* **2009**, *8*, 591–609.

59. Quingnard, F.; di Renzo, F.; Gubal, E. From natural polysacharide to materials from catalysis, adsorption, and remediation. In *Carbohydrates in Sustainable Development I*; Springer-Verlag Berlin Heidelberg: Heidelberg, Germany, 2010, pp. 165–197.

60. Lindberg, N.O.; Palsson, M.; Pihl, A.C.; Freeman, R.; Freeman, T.; Zetzener, H.; Enstad, G. Flowability measurements of pharmaceutical powder mixtures with poor flow using five different techniques. *Drug. Dev. Ind. Pharm.* **2004**, *30*, 785–791.

61. Carr, R.L. Evaluating flow properties of solids. *Chem. Eng.* **1965**, *72*, 163–168.

62. Iida, K.; Aoki, K.; Danjo, K.; Otsuka, A.; Chen, C.Y.; Horisawa, E. A comparative evaluation of the mechanical properties of various celluloses. *Chem. Parm. Bull.* **1997**, *45*, 217–220.

63. Zainuddin, I.M.; Yasuda, M.; Horio, T.; Matsusaka, S. Experimental study on powder flowability using vibration shear tube method. *Part. Part. Syst. Charact.* **2012**, *29*, 8–15.

64. Alonso, M.J.; Sanchez, A. The potential of chitosan in ocular drug delivery. *J. Pharm. Pharmacol.* **2003**, *55*, 1451–1463.

65. Velasco, M.V.; Munoz-Ruiz, A.; Monedero, M.C.; Jiménez-Castellanos, M.R. Study of flowability of powders. effect of the addition of lubricants. *Drug Dev. Ind. Pharm.* **1995**, *21*, 2385–2391.

66. Buys, G.M.; du Plessis, L.H.; Marais, A.F.; Kotze, A.F.; Hamman, J.H. Direct compression of chitosan: Process and formulation factors to improve powder flow and tablet performance. *Curr. Drug. Deliv.* **2013**, *10*, 348–356.

67. Karehill, P.G.; Glazer, M.; Nyström, C. Studies on direct compression of tablets. XXIII. The importance of surface roughness for the compactability of some directly compressible materials with different bonding and volume reduction properties. *Int. J. Pharm.* **1990**, *64*, 35–43.

68. Mohammed, H.; Briscoe, B.J.; Pitt, K.G. The interrelationship between the compaction behaviour and the mechanical strength of pure pharmaceutical tablets. *Chem. Eng. Sci.* **2005**, *60*, 3941–3947.

69. Rojas, J.; Ciro, Y.; Correa, L. Functionality of chitin as a direct compression excipient: An acetaminophen comparative study. *Carbohydr. Polym.* **2014**, *103*, 134–139.

70. Garr, J.S.M.; Rubinstein, M.H. The influence of moisture content on the consolidation and compaction properties of paracetamol. *Int. J. Pharm.* **1992**, *81*, 187–192.

71. Khan, F.; Pilpel, N. The effect of particle size and moisture on the tensile strength of microcrystalline cellulose powder. *Powder Technol.* **1986**, *48*, 145–150.

72. Malamataris, S.; Goidas, P.; Dimitriou, A. Moisture sorption and tensile strength of some tableted direct compression excipients. *Int. J. Pharm.* **1991**, *68*, 51–60.

73. Nokhodchi, A.; Rubinstein, M.H.; Larhrib, H.; Guyot, J.C. The effect of moisture on the properties of ibuprofen tablets. *Int. J. Pharm.* **1995**, *118*, 191–197.

74. Shukla, A.J.; Price, J.C. Effect of moisture content on compression properties of two dextrose-based directly compressible diluents. *Pharm. Res.* **1991**, *8*, 336–340.

75. Ahlneck, C.; Alderborn, G. Moisture adsorption and tabletting. I. Effect on volume reduction properties and tablet strength for some crystalline materials. *Int. J. Pharm.* **1989**, *54*, 131–141.

76. Agrawal, A.M.; Manek, R.V.; Kolling, W.M.; Neau, S.H. Water distribution studies within microcrystalline cellulose and chitosan using differential scanning calorimetry and dynamic vapor sorption analysis. *J. Pharm. Sci.* **2004**, *93*, 1766–1779.

77. Hatakeyama, H.; Hatakeyama, T. Interaction between water and hydrophilic polymers. *Thermochimica Acta* **1998**, *308*, 3–22.

78. García Mir, V.; Heinämäki, J.; Antikainen, O.; Iraizoz Colarte, A.; Airaksinen, S.; Karjalainen, M.; Bilbao Revoredo, O.; Nieto, O.M.; Yliruusi, J. Effects of moisture on tablet compression of chitin. *Carbohydr. Polym.* **2011**, *86*, 477–483.

79. Ferrari, F.; Bertoni, M.; Bonferoni, M.C.; Rossi, S.; Caramella, C.; Nyström, C. Investigation on bonding and disintegration properties of pharmaceutical materials. *Int. J. Pharm.* **1996**, *136*, 71–79.

80. Kumar, G.; Ravi, M. Trends in controlled drug release formulations using chitin and chitosan. *J. Sci. Ind. Res.* **2000**, *59*, 201–213.

81. Hwang, K.T.; Jung, S.T.; Lee, G.D.; Chinnan, M.S.; Park, Y.S.; Park, H.J. Controlling molecular weight and degree of deacetylation of chitosan by response surface methodology. *J. Agric. Food Chem.* **2002**, *50*, 1876–1882.

82. Nunthanid, J.; Puttipipatkhachorn, S.; Yamamoto, K.; Peck, G.E. Physical properties and molecular behavior of chitosan films. *Drug Dev. Ind. Pharm.* **2001**, *27*, 143–157.

83. Cervera, M.F.; Heinämäki, J.; Krogars, K.; Jörgensen, A.C.; Karjalainen, M.; Colarte, A.I.; Yliruusi, J. Solid-state and mechanical properties of aqueous chitosan-amylose starch films plasticized with polyols. *AAPS PharmSciTech* **2004**, *5*, 109–114.

84. Rashid, I.; Daraghmeh, N.; Al-Remawi, M.; Leharne, S.A.; Chowdhry, B.Z.; Badwan, A. Characterization of the impact of magnesium stearate lubrication on the tableting properties of chitin-Mg silicate as a superdisintegrating binder when compared to Avicel® 200. *Powder Technol.* **2010**, *203*, 609–619.

85. Nyström, C.; Alderborn, G.; Duberg, M.; Karehill, P.G. Bonding surface area and bonding mechanism—Two important factors for the understanding of powder compactibility. *Drug Dev. Ind. Pharm.* **1993**, *19*, 2143–2196.

86. Picker-Freyer, K.M.; Brink, D. Evaluation of powder and tableting properties of chitosan. *AAPS PharmSciTech* **2006**, *7*, E152–E161.

87. Perioli, L.; Ambrogi, V.; Pagano, C.; Scuota, S.; Rossi, C. FG90 chitosan as a new polymer for metronidazole mucoadhesive tablets for vaginal administration. *Int. J. Pharm.* **2009**, *377*, 120–127.

88. Heckel, R.W. Density-pressure relationships in powder compaction. *Trans. Metall. Soc.* **1961**, *221*, 671–675.

89. Krycer, I.; Pope, D.G.; Hersey, J.A. An evaluation of the techniques employed to investigate powder compaction behaviour. *Int. J. Pharm.* **1982**, *12*, 113–134.

90. Shivanand, P.; Sprockel, O.L. Compaction behavior of cellulose polymers. *Powder Technol.* **1992**, *69*, 177–184.

91. Lin, C.W.; Cham, T.M. Compression behavior and tensile strength of heat-treated polyethylene glycols. *Int. J. Pharm.* **1995**, *118*, 169–179.

92. Nordstrom, J.; Klevan, I.; Alderborn, G. A particle rearrangement index based on the Kawakita powder compression equation. *J. Pharm. Sci.* **2009**, *98*, 1053–1063.

93. Zhao, J.; Burt, H.M.; Miller, R.A. The Gurnham equation in characterizing the compressibility of pharmaceutical materials. *Int. J. Pharm.* **2006**, *317*, 109–113.

94. Antikainen, O.; Yliruusi, J. Determining the compression behaviour of pharmaceutical powders from the force–distance compression profile. *Int. J. Pharm.* **2003**, *252*, 253–261.

95. Panda, B.; Mallick, S. Correlation between compaction and dissolution of metoprolol tartarate tablets prepared by direct compression using different polymers. *Int. J. Pharm. Pharma. Sci.* **2012**, *4*, 77–88.

96. Tye, C.K.; Sun, C.C.; Amidon, G.E. Evaluation of the effects of tableting speed on the relationships between compaction pressure, tablet tensile strength, and tablet solid fraction. *J. Pharm. Sci.* **2005**, *94*, 465–472.

97. Roberts, R.J.; Rowe, R.C. Brittle/ductile behaviour in pharmaceutical materials used in tabletting. *Int. J. Pharm.* **1987**, *36*, 205–209.

98. Akin-Ajani, O.D.; Itiola, O.A.; Odeku, O.A. Effects of plantain and corn starches on the mechanical and disintegration properties of paracetamol tablets. *AAPS PharmSciTech* **2005**, *6*, E458–E463.

99. Belda, P.M.; Mielck, J.B. The tabletting machine as an analytical instrument: consequences of uncertainties in punch force and punch separation data on some parameters describing the course of the tabletting process. *Eur. J. Pharm. Biopharm.* **1999**, *48*, 157–170.

100. Davies, W.L.; Gloor, W.T. Batch production of pharmaceutical granulations in a fluidized bed I: Effects of process variables on physical properties of final granulation. *J. Pharm. Sci.* **1971**, *60*, 1869–1874.

101. Rong Huei, C.; Hwa, H.D. Effect of molecular weight of chitosan with the same degree of deacetylation on the thermal, mechanical, and permeability properties of the prepared membrane. *Carbohydr. Polym.* **1996**, *29*, 353–358.

102. Knapczyk, J. Excipient ability of chitosan for direct tableting. *Int. J. Pharm.* **1993**, *89*, 1–7.

103. Seetharaman, S.; Balya, H.; Abdul Ahad, H. Formulation and evaluation of sustained release matrix tablets of ciprofloxacin HCL using gum kondagogu and chitosan as matrix forming polymers. *Int. J. Pharm. Sci. Rev. Res.* **2014**, *24*, 115–119.

104. Al-Akayleh, F.; Al Remawi, M.; Rashid, I.; Badwan, A. Formulation and *in vitro* assessment of sustained release terbutaline sulfate tablet made from binary hydrophilic polymer mixtures. *Pharm. Dev. Technol.* **2013**, *18*, 1204–1212.

105. Eftaiha, A.A.F.; Qinna, N.; Rashid, I.S.; Al Remawi, M.M.; Al Shami, M.R.; Arafat, T.A.; Badwan, A.A. Bioadhesive controlled metronidazole release matrix based on chitosan and xanthan gum. *Mar. Drugs* **2010**, *8*, 1716–1730.

106. Eissens, A.C.; Bolhuis, G.K.; Hinrichs, W.L.J.; Frijlink, H.W. Inulin as filler-binder for tablets prepared by direct compaction. *Eur. J. Pharm. Sci.* **2002**, *15*, 31–38.

107. Eftaiha, A.A.F.; El-Barghouthi, M.I.; Rashid, I.S.; Al-Remawi, M.M.; Saleh, A.I.; Badwan, A.A. Compressibility and compactibility studies of chitosan, xanthan gum, and their mixtures. *J. Mater. Sci.* **2009**, *44*, 1054–1062.

108. Broadhead, J.; Edmond Rouan, S.K.; Rhodes, C.T. The spray drying of pharmaceuticals. *Drug Dev. Ind. Pharm.* **1992**, *18*, 1169–1206.

109. Rege, P.R.; Garmise, R.J.; Block, L.H. Spray-dried chitinosans: Part II: *In vitro* drug release from tablets made from spray-dried chitinosans. *Int. J. Pharm.* **2003**, *252*, 53–59.

110. Asada, M.; Takahashi, H.; Okamoto, H.; Tanino, H.; Danjo, K. Theophylline particle design using chitosan by the spray drying. *Int. J. Pharm.* **2004**, *270*, 167–174.

111. Hiorth, M.; Tho, I.; Sande, S.A. The formation and permeability of drugs across free pectin and chitosan films prepared by a spraying method. *Eur. J. Pharm. Biopharm.* **2003**, *56*, 175–181.

112. Steckel, H.; Mindermann-Nogly, F. Production of chitosan pellets by extrusion/spheronization. *Eur. J. Pharm. Biopharm.* **2004**, *57*, 107–114.

113. Hugerth, A.; Caram-Lelham, N.; Sundelöf, L.O. The effect of charge density and conformation on the polyelectrolyte complex formation between carrageenan and chitosan. *Carbohydr. Polym.* **1997**, *34*, 149–156.

114. Tingstad, J.E. The theory and practice of industrial pharmacy. Second Ed. L. Lachman, H.A. Lieberman, and J.L. Kanig. Lea & Febiger, 600 Washington Square, Philadelphia. **1976**, *65*, 10.1002/jps.2600650840.

115. Rege, P.R.; Garmise, R.J.; Block, L.H. Spray-dried chitinosans. Part I: Preparation and characterization. *Int. J. Pharm.* **2003**, *252*, 41–51.

116. Bhise, K.S.; Dhumal, R.S.; Paradkar, A.R.; Kadam, S.S. Effect of drying methods on swelling, erosion and drug release from chitosan-naproxen sodium complexes. *AAPS PharmSciTech* **2008**, *9*, 1–12.

117. Rojas, J. Effect of Polymorphism on the Particle and Compaction Properties of Microcrystalline Cellulose. In *Cellulose-Medical, Pharmaceutical and Electronic Applications*; van de Ven, T., Godbout, L., Eds.; InTech: Rijeka, Croatia, 2013.

118. Kokil, S.; Patil, P.; Mahadik, K.; Paradkar, A. Studies on spray-dried mixtures of chitosan and hydrolyzed gelatin as tablet binder: A technical note. *AAPS PharmSciTech* **2005**, *6*, E437–E443.

119. El-Barghouthi, M.; Eftaiha, A.; Rashid, I.; al-Remawi, M.; Badwan, A. A novel superdisintegrating agent made from physically modified chitosan with silicon dioxide. *Drug Dev. Ind. Pharm.* **2008**, *34*, 373–383.

120. Gana, F.Z.; Rashid, I.; Badwan, A.; Alkhamis, K.A. Determination of solid-state acidity of chitin-metal silicates and their effect on the degradation of cephalosporin antibiotics. *J. Pharm. Sci.* **2012**, *101*, 2398–2407.

121. Rashid, I.; Alkhamis, K.A.; Hassan, H.A.; Altalafha, T.H.; Badwan, A.A. *Characterization of the Compression Properties of Compacted Chitosan as a Function of Molecular Weight*; 5th Granulation Workshop: Sheffield, UK, 2013.

122. Paronen, P.; Ilkka, J. Porosity-pressure functions. In *Pharmaceutical Powder Compaction Technology. Drugs and the Pharmaceutical Sciences Series*; Alderborn, G., Nystrom, C., Eds.; Marcel Dekker: New York, NY, USA, 1996; pp. 55–75.

# Influence of Molecular Weight and Degree of Deacetylation of Low Molecular Weight Chitosan on the Bioactivity of Oral Insulin Preparations

Nidal A. Qinna, Qutuba G. Karwi, Nawzat Al-Jbour, Mayyas A. Al-Remawi,
Tawfiq M. Alhussainy, Khaldoun A. Al-So'ud, Mahmoud M. H. Al Omari and
Adnan A. Badwan

**Abstract:** The objective of the present study was to prepare and characterize low molecular weight chitosan (LMWC) with different molecular weight and degrees of deacetylation (DDA) and to optimize their use in oral insulin nano delivery systems. Water in oil nanosized systems containing LMWC-insulin polyelectrolyte complexes were constructed and their ability to reduce blood glucose was assessed *in vivo* on diabetic rats. Upon acid depolymerization and testing by viscosity method, three molecular weights of LMWC namely, 1.3, 13 and 18 kDa were obtained. As for the DDA, three LMWCs of 55%, 80% and 100% DDA were prepared and characterized by spectroscopic methods for each molecular weight. The obtained LMWCs showed different morphological and *in silico* patterns. Following complexation of LMWCs with insulin, different aggregation sizes were obtained. Moreover, the *in vivo* tested formulations showed different activities of blood glucose reduction. The highest glucose reduction was achieved with 1.3 kDa LMWC of 55% DDA. The current study emphasizes the importance of optimizing the molecular weight along with the DDA of the incorporated LMWC in oral insulin delivery preparations in order to ensure the highest performance of such delivery systems.

Reprinted from *Mar. Drugs*. Cite as: Qinna, N.A.; Karwi, Q.G.; Al-Jbour, N.; Al-Remawi, M.A.; Alhussainy, T.M.; Al-So'ud, K.A.; Al Omari, M.M.H.; Badwan, A.A. Influence of Molecular Weight and Degree of Deacetylation of Low Molecular Weight Chitosan on the Bioactivity of Oral Insulin Preparations. *Mar. Drugs* **2015**, *13*, 1710-1725.

## 1. Introduction

Different formulation strategies have been investigated to overcome the gastrointestinal tract (GIT) barriers for the delivery of proteins via the oral route. These different delivery systems included microemulsions, nanoparticles and coated liposomes [1]. By using these delivery forms, it has been found that nanosized systems may offer a reasonable solution for oral protein administration [2].

The nanosized particles can be obtained either by ultra homogenization, which may expose protein to mechanical stress leading to instability, or by facilitating the formation of nano vesicles using self-emulsifying surface active agents. Among these surface active agents are caprylocaproyl macrogolglycerides and polyglyceryl-6 dioleate. These surfactants are self-emulsifying in aqueous media and form reversible micelles when dispersed in oils. In previous work however, we have confirmed that the addition of low molecular weight chitosan (LMWC) of different molecular weights to a dispersion of the two surfactants mixed in 1:1 ratio in oleic acid had resulted in the formation of reversed micelles that were shrinked to nano size vesicles [3].

Indeed, a wide range of biodegradable and conventional polymers has been investigated in forming nanosized particles. Among these polymers is chitosan, which is well established as a safe food and drug additive [4,5]. Chitosan chemically is a linear co-polymer consisting of β (1-4)-linked 2-amino-2-deoxy-D-glucose (D-glucosamine) and 2-acetamido-2-deoxy-D-glucose (N-acetyl-D-glucosamine) units. Chitosan is mainly identified and characterized by three parameters; molecular weight, DDA, and polydispersity. It is unfortunate that in most protein delivery studies high molecular weight chitosans (HMWC)s were used. In many cases, the molecular weights of the used chitosans were not predetermined. Furthermore, using the insoluble HMWCs limited their application in liquid protein delivery dosage forms. This makes using LMWCs in such preparations more flexible.

LMWCs can be mainly prepared from the HMWCs using the acidic depolymerization, oxidative, enzymatic, or ultrasonic degradation [6]. Naturally, the process of deacetylation of chitosan involves the removal of acetyl groups from the molecular chain of the polymer, leaving behind an exposed amino group (–NH$_2$) [7,8]. This positively charged group facilitates the chitosan involvement in forming more electrostatic complexes with the negatively charged molecules such as insulin amino acids. Consequently, these polyelectrolyte complexes (PECs) could be loaded with proteins resulting in micro or nano-carrier systems [9,10]. On the other hand, reducing the DDA of chitosan can be achieved by the addition of acetyl groups to the chains of the polymer by reacting chitosan solution with acetic anhydride [11]. These added groups could also influence PEC formation, and therefore, must be investigated.

Previously, a delivery system based on preparing a PEC between LMWC (13 kDa, 80 DDA%) and insulin was reported [12]. A mixture of caprylocaproyl macrogol-8-glycerides, polyglyceryl-6 dioleate and oleic acid was used to prepare the reverse micelles. This delivery system showed a reduction in glucose level in diabetic rats [13]. Furthermore, this delivery system was tested in more than 50 healthy volunteers using euglycemic technique and results showed a successful reduction in their blood glucose levels [14].

Although the used chitosans in these previous studies were purified and characterized, the impact of selecting different molecular weights and DDAs of chitosan in such nanosized preparations was not investigated. Consequently, the main aim of this study was to explore the influence of LMWCs of different DDAs on the formation of nanosized vesicles for protein delivery and its impact on insulin's *in vivo* absorption.

## 2. Results and Discussion

Many approaches have been employed to deliver proteins orally including the use of specific excipients, such as absorption enhancers, enzyme inhibitors and mucoadhesive polymers. Despite these various attempts, however, no clinically useful oral formulations have been developed until now [15].

Chitosan is a biocompatible and biodegradable polymer that has permeability enhancing and mucoadhesive properties [16,17]. These properties made the chitosan be a polymer of choice for protein delivery. While chitosan shows important functional properties, nevertheless, the high molecular weight, high viscosity and insolubility at physiological pH of chitosan restrict its use *in vivo* [18]. Indeed, the intestinal absorption of LMWC can be significantly better than that of HMWC [19]. Therefore, nanocarriers research is currently directed towards using LMWCs in drug delivery [20].

## 2.1. Preparation and Characterization of LMWCs with Different DDA

LMWCs with different molecular weights (1.3, 13, and 20 kDa) and DDA (55%, 80%, and 100%) were prepared from HMWC (250 kDa, 93% DDA). Initially, fully acetylated LMWCs were prepared by the acid depolymerization method. Table 1 shows their corresponding molecular weights as a result of changing the reaction time from 2, 3.2, to 24 h. The molecular weights, as determined by viscosity measurements, were 1.25, 12.75 and 18.2 kDa. For convenience, these molecular weights were named 1.3, 13 and 18 kDa.

To prepare LMWCs with different DDA (55%, 80% and 100%), the obtained fully deacetylated LMWCs (1.3, 13 and 18 kDa) were reacted with acetic anhydride using different molar ratio (Table 1). DDAs (55%, 80% and 100%) of each LMWC were determined by UV/visible spectrophotometry and verified using the $^1$H-NMR spectrometry. The DDA values obtained by both methods were comparable (Table 1).

**Table 1.** Experimental data of molecular weight (MW) and degree of deacetylation (DDA) determinations for low molecular weight chitosans (LMWCs).

| Molecular Weight | | | | | | | | |
|---|---|---|---|---|---|---|---|---|
| LMWC MW (kDa) | | 1.3 | | | 13 | | | 18 |
| Depolymerization time (h) | | 24 | | | 3.2 | | | 2.0 |
| Experimental MW (kDa) | | 1.25 | | | 12.75 | | | 18.20 |
| **Degree of Deacetylation (DDA)** | | | | | | | | |
| DDA % | | 55 | | | 80 | | | 100 |
| Molar ratio of chitosan:Ac$_2$O | | 1:0.60 | | | 1:0.15 | | | 1:0 |
| LMWC MW (kDa) | 1.3 | 13 | 18 | 1.3 | 13 | 18 | 1.3 | 13 | 18 |
| Experimental DDA% | | | | | | | | |
| By UV/visible | 54.9 | 54.8 | 55.1 | 79.8 | 80.3 | 80.2 | 99.6 | 99.4 | 100.3 |
| By $^1$H-NMR | 55.0 | 55.4 | 56.6 | 79.6 | 79.1 | 80.6 | 100.0 | 100.0 | 100.0 |

The FT-IR spectra of chitosan, in general, show a broad absorption band in the range 3000–3500 cm$^{-1}$ attributed to O–H and N–H stretching vibrations, while the peaks around 2885, 1650, 1589, 1326 and 1080 cm$^{-1}$ are due to the stretching vibrations of aliphatic C–H, C=O stretching in secondary amide (Amide I), free amino –NH (Amide II) and C–N–stretching in secondary amide (Amide III) and C–O–C, bonds, respectively [21]. In the present work, however, the formation of fully deacetylated LMWC was confirmed by FT-IR with the absence of Amide I peak at 1650 cm$^{-1}$ (Figure 1a), while the peak corresponding to free amino band (Amide II) appeared at 1574 cm$^{-1}$. This result is in agreement with that reported by Heux *et al.* [22]. It is worth mentioning that neither the acid hydrolysis nor the acetylation reactions altered the skeleton structures of the obtained LMWCs (Figure 1a,b).

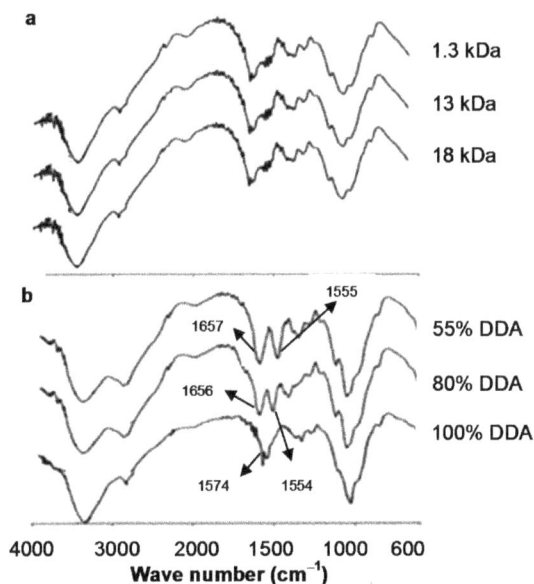

**Figure 1.** FT-IR spectra over the frequency range 4000–400 cm⁻¹: (**a**) different molecular weight chitosans (LMWCs) of fully deacetylated and (**b**) 13 kDa LMWC of different degree of deacetylation (DDA).

The acetylation of LMWC was monitored by ¹H-NMR spectroscopy, as shown in Figure 2. It was observed that the integral of the peak of the three protons of acetyl group (H-Ac) at 2.8 ppm increases by decreasing the DDA values (Figure 2).

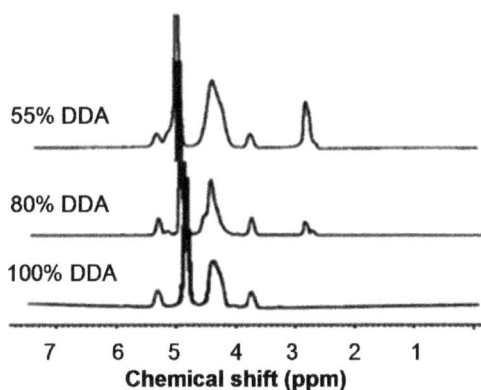

**Figure 2.** ¹H-NMR spectra for 13k Da low molecular weight chitosan (LMWC) of different degree of deacetylation (DDA).

*2.2. Surface Morphology*

The prepared LMWCs showed variations in their surface morphology as shown by the photos of their thin films (Figure 3). The crystallization and the trend of film formation were increased as long as the DDA decreased. At the lowest DDA (55%), chitosan was arranged in the form of fibers that differ in their thickness and flexibility. Furthermore, the higher molecular weights had thicker and more rigid fibers compared with the lower molecular weights that had thin and fragile fibers.

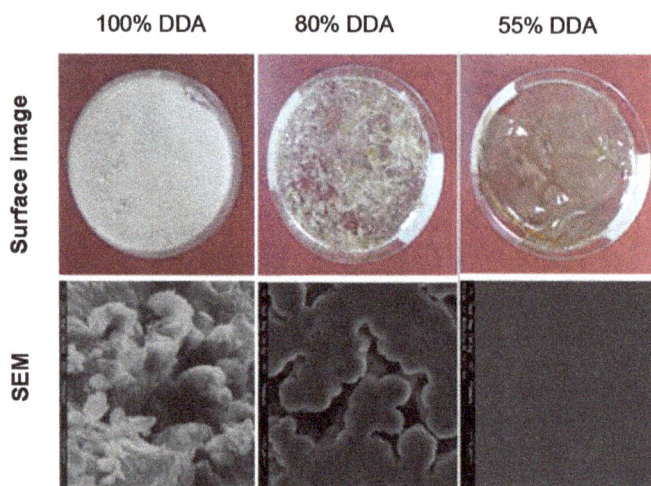

**Figure 3.** Surface images and scanning electron microscope captures of dry films of 13 kDa low molecular weight chitosan (LMWC) of different degree of deacetylation (DDA), 4000× magnification.

The Scanning Electron Microscope images of different LMWCs (Figure 3) showed that all fully deacetylated LMWCs had rough and irregular surfaces. At the DDA around 80%, the $N$-substituted polymer chains were in good morphological sphericity and aggregated to each other like rosaries. At the DDA decreased (55%), the surface shape of the LMWCs was regular, smooth, stretched and looked like a continuous flat section.

*2.3. In Silico Characterization*

The *in silico* simulations (Figure 4) showed that the best orientation of the deacetylated LMWC occurred when the constructed chitosan oligomers had been arranged as spheres bound together. When the DDA was decreased to 80%, the mode of binding between the polymer chains became helical in shape. However, chitosan oligomers with the least DDA (55%) arranged themselves in small aggregates each containing 4–5 chains constructed from glucosamine units. The best orientation of LMWC polymer with DDA of 55% incorporated only four chains while the number of chains reached up to 10 for higher DDA (>80%). It was also noted that as the DDA decreases, the intermolecular forces between the polymer chains also decrease and produce more flexible chains. Therefore, it can be predicted while constructing the PEC that the number of binding sites between insulin and LMWC would increase as the DDA decreases.

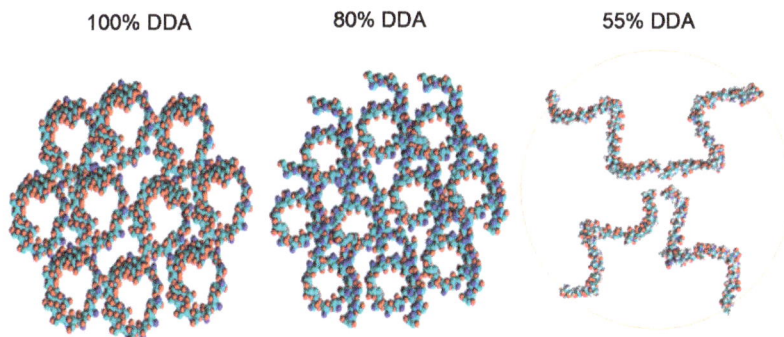

100% DDA          80% DDA          55% DDA

**Figure 4.** *In silico* arrangements of low molecular weight chitosans (LMWCs) each constructed from 50 units of D-glucosamine (10 kDa) having different degree of deacetylation (DDA).

## 2.4. Oral Insulin Formulation and Aggregation Size of the Reverse Micelle

The tested nanoparticle system can be described as a w/o microemulsion constructed by mixing LMWC with insulin to form a PEC (aqueous phase) which was then solubilized in a mixture made from Labrasol® and Plurol Oleique® dissolved in oleic acid (Figure 5). The surfactant-cosurfactant system namely, Labrasol and Plurol, was prepared at 1:1 mass ratio as previously reported [3] despite the fact that many researchers often use the 4:1 mixing ratio as delivery vehicles [23,24].

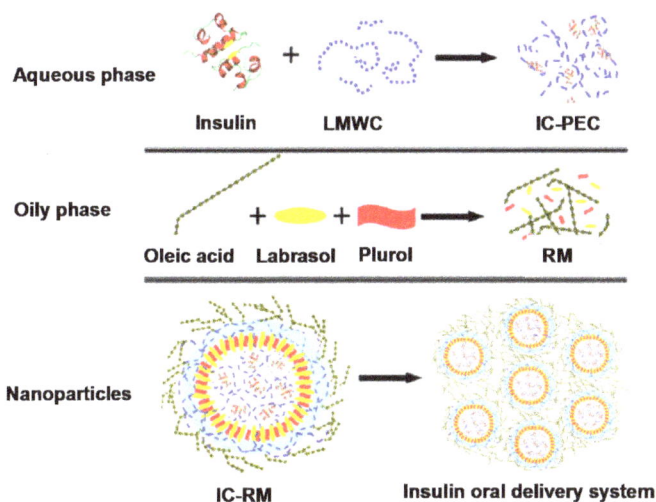

Aqueous phase

Insulin          LMWC          IC-PEC

Oily phase

Oleic acid   Labrasol   Plurol          RM

Nanoparticles

IC-RM          Insulin oral delivery system

**Figure 5.** Illustration of the essential components of the prepared insulin-chitosan polyelectrolyte complex (IC-PEC) and its revised micelles (IC-RM). LMWC represents low molecular weight chitosan.

Chitosan, as a polyelectrolyte, can form electrostatic complexes under acidic conditions. Two different types of complexes are considered, electrostatic complexes with an oppositely charged surfactant and PECs [25]. In fact, protein-PEC are not new and have been used extensively in biology over many years for protein purification, immobilization and stabilization of enzymes [26].

The relationship between the particle diameter and the amount of the aqueous phase loaded in the reverse micelle system was established for each LMWC. Figure 6 clearly shows that loading of insulin-chitosan PEC in the oleic acid and surfactant/cosurfatant mixture increased the diameter of the nanoparticles. When using 1.3 KDa LMWC with different DDA in the preparations (Figure 6a), large particle sizes of more than 2000 nm were obtained. However, increasing the molecular weight of the LMWC significantly reduced the particle size of the formed nanoparticles (Figure 6c). For all LMWCs, it can also be noted that the fully deacetylated LMWCs failed to maintain small particle sizes when the amount of the aqueous phase was increased. For example, the particle size of the reverse micelle (RM), prepared by 13 kDa LMWC of 80% DDA, decreased to be in the vicinity of 150 nm, while it reached around 700 nm when the fully deacetylated LMWC (100% DDA) was used in the RM preparation.

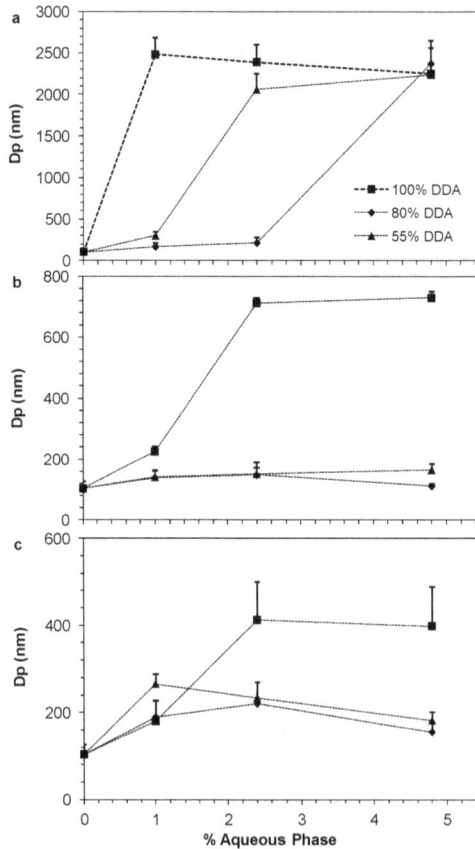

**Figure 6.** Effect of changing the percentage of aqueous phase on the aggregation size of oral insulin preparations loaded with different degree of deacetylation (DDA) of low molecular weight chitosan (LMWC): (**a**) 1.3 kDa; (**b**) 13 kDa; and (**c**) 18 kDa. Data are presented as mean ± SD ($n = 8$).

Therefore, the DDA of the incorporated LMWC in oral insulin preparations can have a large influence on the formation and properties of stable solubilized reverse micellar systems as chitosan was found to possess certain surface activity in the presence of oleic acid as previously reported by Assaf *et al.* [3].

## 2.5. In Vivo Pharmacological Activity of the Nano Dispersion System

The effect of different preparations of LMWCs with different DDA on blood glucose levels of streptozotocin induced diabetic Sprague Dawley rats are presented in Figure 7. Rats subcutaneously injected with insulin (1 IU/kg) showed an intense response of glucose reduction while the placebo preparations did not reduce blood glucose levels. Weak response to insulin was obtained when using the 1.3 kDa LMWC in IC-RM preparations. The glucose reduction was not significant in the 100% DDA preparations while better efficacy patterns, though still weak, were obtained with 80% DDA and 55% DDA (Figure 7a). Such weak response might be attributed to the larger particle size obtained when using the 1.3 kDa LMWC in the preparations as described in Figure 6a.

As for using the 13 kDa LMWC in the preparations (Figure 7b), the best reduction of glucose level was achieved with the 80% DDA where a maximum and significant decrease of 63% ± 3.9% was obtained after 8 h post administration ($p < 0.05$). In Figure 7c, the preparation containing 18 kDa LMWC/55% DDA showed the best efficacy among the other formulas where the maximum reduction in blood glucose level was achieved after 4 h of the oral dose administration and reached 65% ± 4.2%. This reduction was considered efficient as no statistical significant difference was seen when compared to the subcutaneous (S.C.) group ($p = 0.142$). Moreover, in the case of 13 and 18 kDa LMWCs, two way analysis of variance for repeated measures revealed that glucose levels were significantly changed when different DDA were used ($p < 0.01$). Such effect of DDA was not statistically significant in the case of 1.3 kDa ($p = 0.289$).

The above tested oral insulin dispersions (Figure 7) were prepared by including a fixed molar concentration (4.8 μmol/mL) of each LMWC in the preparation. However, in order to exclude the variability in the amount of LMWC incorporated in the preparation of IC-PECs in, the three formulae that showed the best extent of insulin release in the above studies were formulated to contain equal and sufficient amounts of LMWC (62.5 mg/mL) that is enough to form PEC with the whole amount of insulin in the formulae. *In vivo* results for these preparations showed that all preparations reduced significantly blood glucose levels compared to the placebo group. The formula of 1.3 kDa LMWC/80% DDA had a unique linear but rather none statistically significant pattern of glucose reduction as compared with other formulas (Figure 8). The maximum limit of blood glucose reduction (66% ± 5.9%) was obtained after 4 h of oral administration of the formula. Moreover, when comparing the formula of 13 kDa LMWC/80% DDA with the 18 kDa LMWC/55% DDA formula, Tukey's post-test revealed a significant difference in the activity between the 4th and 6th hour sampling intervals ($p < 0.05$). Therefore, other than the molecular weight and the DDA of chitosan, it seems also necessary to optimize the amount of chitosan that should be included in the formation of insulin nanoparticles. Such amount should be sufficient to interact with its counterpart electrolye during PEC formation and sufficient for protecting the outer layer of the formed aqueous nano sized droplets.

348

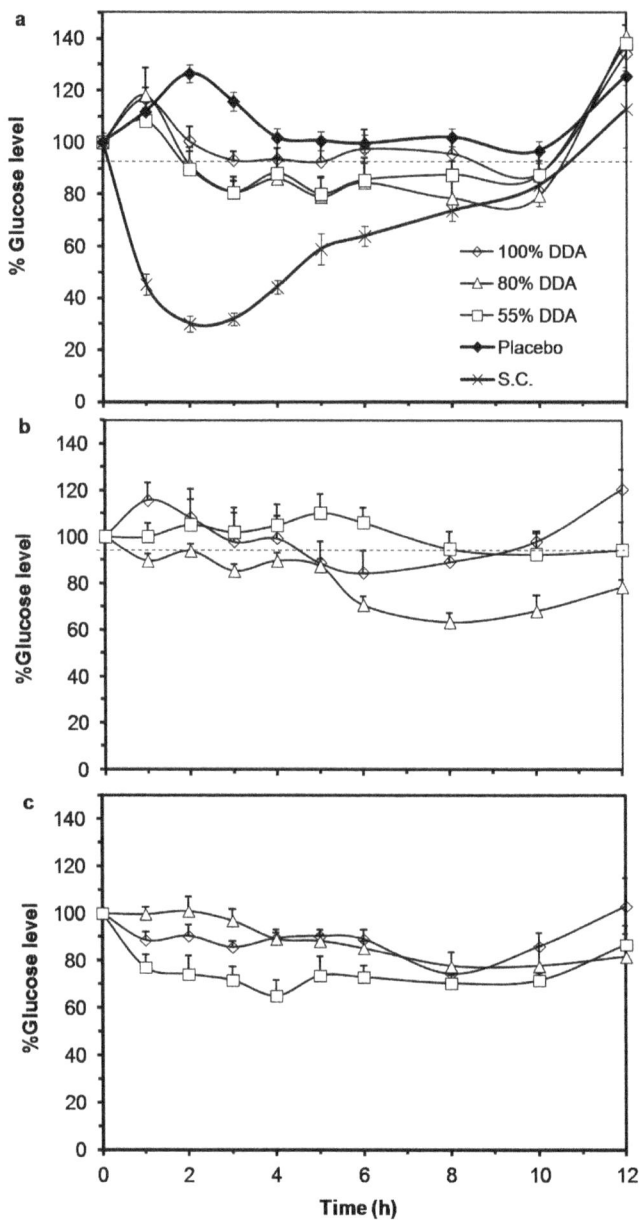

**Figure 7.** Percentage change of blood glucose levels of diabetic rats administered oral insulin (50 IU/kg) preparations loaded with different degree of deacetylation (DDA) of low molecular chitosans (LMWCs): (**a**) 1.3 kDa along with a S.C. insulin (1 IU/kg) and a placebo group; (**b**) 13 kDa and (**c**) 18 kDa. Data points are represented as mean ± SEM ($n = 10$). The chitosan concentration was fixed at 4.8 μmol/mL in all oral insulin preparations.

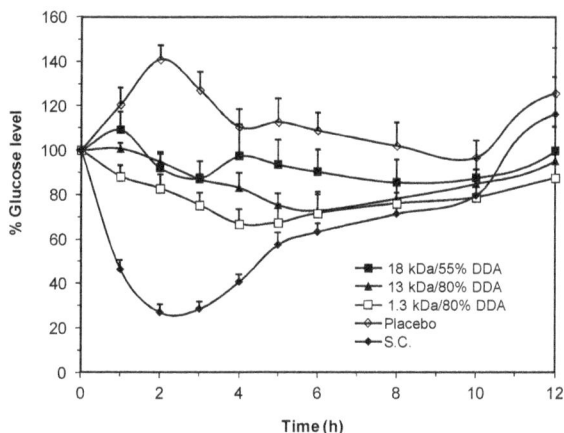

**Figure 8.** Percentage change of blood glucose levels of diabetic rats administered oral insulin (50 IU/kg) preparations loaded with LMWCs of 1.3 kDa/80%DDA; 13 kDa/80%DDA and 18 kDa/55%DDA and subcontenous (S.C.) insulin (1 IU/kg) compared to a placebo group. The chitosan concentration was fixed at 62.4 mg/mL in all oral insulin preparations. Data points are represented as mean ± SEM ($n = 10$).

## 3. Experimental Section

### 3.1. Materials

Recombinant human (rh-)insulin (99.4%) was obtained from Biocon Limited (Electronic City, Bangalore, India). Calbiochem® Streptozotocin (STZ) and oleic acid vegetable were obtained from Merck KGaA (Darmstadt, Germany). Labrasol® (PEG-8 caprylic/capric glycerides, HLB 14) and Plurol® Oleique CG (Polyglycerol-6-dioleate, HLB 6) were obtained from Gattefosse (Saint-Priest, Lyon, France). Chitosan (Molecular weight ~250 kDa and DDA ~93%) was obtained from Xiamen Xing (Shanghi, China). Purified water was obtained from the Jordanian Pharmaceutical Manufacturing (JPM) company (Naor, Jordan), which was double distilled (Conductivity < 2 µs/cm) prior its use. All other chemicals were of analytical grade.

### 3.2. Preparation of Fully Deacetylated LMWCs

Different LMWCs (1.3, 13, and 18 kDa) were prepared by acid depolymerization as reported earlier [5,27]. Chitosan (250 kDa, 93% DDA) solutions (1% in 2 M HCl) were refluxed for 2, 3.5 and 24 h to get LMWCs of 18, 13 and 1.3 kDa, respectively. At the end of the reaction, chitosan solution was added to 96% ethanol (1:2 $v/v$ aqueous to ethanol ratio). After cooling, the precipitate was filtered and washed several times with ethanol, followed by centrifugation at 4000 rpm for 5 min (accuSpin™ 3 centrifuge, Fisher Scientific, Schwerte, Germany) to get neutral pH (6.8–7) filtrate. The obtained LMWCs as HCl salt were then freeze dried for 24 h (Hetopower dry PL 9000 freeze drier, Thermo Fisher Scientific, Inc., Waltham, MA, USA).

350

## 3.3. Preparation of LMWCs with Different DDAs

LMWCs with DDA of 55% and 80% were prepared by reacting fully deacetylated LMWC with acetic anhydride at molar ratios of 1:0.15 and 1:0.6, respectively. LMWC solution (1% in water) was initially prepared and the pH was adjusted to 6.5 by drop wise addition of 6 M NaOH. Acetic anhydride was then added (1 and 2 portions for 55% and 80%, respectively) with magnetic stirring (500 rpm) at room temperature for 10 min [28]. The pH of the solution was maintained at 6.25 after the addition of each portion of acetic anhydride. The chitosan solution was then dialyzed against 4 L of distilled water under gentle stirring at room temperature for 24 h using dialysis tubes having 1000 Da molecular weight cut-off used for 1.3 KDa LMWC and 12,000–14,000 Da cut-off tubes used to dialyze 13 and 18 kDa LMWCs (Medicell International Ltd., London, UK). Finally, the dialyzed chitosan solution was poured in Petri dishes and dried overnight in an oven at 40 °C, then transferred to an amber-airtight glass bottle and stored at room temperature until used.

## 3.4. Determination of the Molecular Weight of LMWCs

The average molecular weight of the prepared LMWCs was calculated from the measured intrinsic viscosity (Vibro-viscometer SV-10, A&D Company, Tokyo, Japan) using a previously reported method [13].

## 3.5. Determination of the DDA

The DDA of the prepared LMWCs was determined by a UV-spectrophotometric method (Beckman Coulter spectrophotometer, DU 640i, Brea, CA, USA) adapted in the European Pharmacopeia (2012). The first derivative at 202 nm was measured for each LMWC dissolved in water (50 µg/mL). The pH of the solution was then measured and the DDA was determined using N-acetylglucosamine as a reference to construct a calibration curve with concentrations of 1.0, 5.0, 15.0 and 35.0 µg/mL in water. $^1$H-NMR (Bruker Avance Ultra Shield 300 MHz Spectrometer, Billerica, MA, USA) was used to confirm the obtained results as reported earlier [29]. At least 64 scans were acquired for each LMWC sample (30 mg/mL in D$_2$O). The DDA was calculated using integrals of the peak of proton H1 of deacetylated monomer (H1-D) at 5.2 ppm and the peak of the three protons of the acetyl group (H-Ac) at 2.8 ppm.

## 3.6. FT-IR Spectroscopy

The prepared LMWCs were characterized by FT-IR (Thermo scientific Nicolet Avatar 360 FT-IR ESP Spectrometer, Madison, WI, USA) using KBr pellet method.

## 3.7. Surface Morphology

The films of LMWCs, obtained after freeze drying on glass Petri dishes for 24 h, were visually examined and photographed using a digital camera (Sony Cybershot, Tokyo, Japan). Furthermore, the morphological differences of LMWCs were observed using Scanning Electron Microscopy (FEI

Quanta 200, Hillsboro, OR, USA) equipped with EDAX for X-ray microanalysis. The photomicrographs were taken at the same magnifications to facilitate comparison between them.

### 3.8. In Silico Molecular Mechanic Modeling

LMWC was built up from 50 units of D-glucosamine (10 kDa) using Hyperchem software (release 8.06) (Hypercube Inc., Gainesville, FL, USA). Three different kinds of LMWCs were built up with different DDA namely 100, 80 and 55%. Several trials were carried out to find the most suitable interaction between the constructed LMWCs.

### 3.9. Formulation of the Oral Insulin Nanoparticle Dispersion System

The oral insulin reverse micelles were prepared according to a method described by Elsayed *et al.* [13]. For the PEC preparation, a predetermined amount of each of the LMWCs was dissolved in 2 mL water. The pH of each solution was adjusted to 6.25 using 2 M NaOH, and the final volume was completed to 4 mL with water reaching a final LMWC concentration of 4.8 µmol/mL. Insulin solution was prepared by dissolving 100 mg of rh-insulin in 1 mL of 0.1 N HCl by gentle shaking. The pH was adjusted to about 8.5 by 0.1 M NaOH, followed by completing the final volume to 4 mL with water reaching a final insulin concentration of 2.15 µmol/mL. The IC-PEC (aqueous phase) was prepared by mixing the insulin and the prepared PEC solutions at room temperature by gentle stirring. The RM system was prepared by mixing Labrasol®–Plurol Oleique® (1:1 molar ratio) and oleic acid in a ratio of 20:80 ($w/w$) by mixing using a vortex.

For particle size investigations, different amounts of the aqueous phase (0.02, 0.05, 0.1, 0.15 g) were placed in tubes containing 2 g of the RM mixture in order to obtain the maximum loading capacity of the two phases. Subsequently, the tubes were vortexed for 30 s and held on a rack for 15 min at room temperature to equilibrate before measuring their aggregation sizes.

### 3.10. Aggregation Size Determinations of the Nanoparticle Dispersion System

The size of each prepared dispersion system was assessed by dynamic light scattering using a Malvern Zetasizer Nano-ZS series (Malvern Instruments, Worcestershire, UK) at 25 °C with a detection angle of 173. Eight measurements were conducted as the instrument automatically determines the number of runs in each measurement. The instrument built-in software also calculated the average and standard deviations of aggregation size measurements for each percent of loading.

### 3.11. In vivo Studies on Streptozotocine (STZ) Diabetic Rats

### 3.11.1. Animal Handling

Adult male Sprague Dawley rats with an average weight of $220 \pm 20$ g were purchased from Yarmouk University (Irbid, Jordan) and accommodated at Petra University Animal House Unit under standard temperature, humidity and photoperiod light cycles. All rats were acclimatized for ten days before experimenting day and received standard chow and tap water. All experiments were carried out in accordance with the guidelines of the Federation of European Laboratory Animal Sciences

Association (FELASA). The study protocol was approved (Approval No. PHARM3/11/2012, 3 November 2012) by the Ethical Committee of the Higher Research Council at the Faculty of Pharmacy, University of Petra (Amman, Jordan).

3.11.2. Induction of Diabetes using Streptozotocin

Diabetes was induced in male S.D. rats by intraperitoneal injection of two doses of 80 mg/kg streptozotocin (STZ) over two days. STZ was freshly dissolved in 0.1 M citrate buffer (pH 4.5). Blood glucose level was monitored by measuring glucose concentration in blood samples obtained from the tail vein of rats using a blood glucose meter (GluChec®, KMH Co. Ltd., Gyeonggi-do, Koria). Only rats with a basal blood glucose level above 200 mg/dL were considered diabetic.

3.11.3. Pharmacological Activity Evaluations of the Insulin-Loaded Dispersions

Overnight fasted STZ diabetic rats were divided randomly into five groups where each group contained ten diabetic rats. The first three groups received 50 IU/kg oral insulin preparations using oral gavage needle. The fourth group was injected subcutaneously with 1 IU/kg rh insulin solution while another group served as a control and given an oral placebo preparation (nanoparticles dispersion without insulin) through oral gavage. The blood sampling for blood glucose concentration measurement proceeded along the experiment at specific time intervals (0, 1, 2, 3, 4, 5, 6, 8, 10 and 12 h). The zero-time intervals represented the baseline glucose level for the subsequent time intervals.

*3.12. Statistical Evaluation*

One-way analysis of variance (ANOVA) followed by the Tukey's post-test was used to analyze the differences between groups and differences between time intervals amongst groups using SPSS 17 statistical package, USA. Two-way analysis of variance test for repeated measures was also used to analyze changes in glucose levels. A probability value $<0.05$ was considered the minimum level of statistical significance. The average aggregation sizes (in nM) are expressed as means $\pm$ SD (standard deviation) while blood glucose levels are presented as a percentage of control and expressed as means $\pm$ SEM (standard error of means).

# 4. Conclusions

The current investigation showed that the prepared different LMWC had different physicochemical characteristics. Such characteristics are known to influence the stability and strength of the formed polyelectrolyte complexes when react with oppositely charged molecules such as proteins [30]. However, changing the molecular weight or the DDA of the utilized LMWC can also influence the characteristics of the formed nanoparticle system. Some acetylation degree was seen essential to achieve better reduction in the particle size of the formed nanoparticles. On the other hand, when the 1.3 kDa LMWC was used in the preparations, the activity of insulin was only attractive when the amount of chitosan was increased. Such an increase in the incorporated amount of LMWC in the preparation would allow a sufficient level of interaction with insulin while protecting the outer layer of the formed nanoparticle. Therefore, the current study emphasizes the importance of optimizing the molecular weight along with the DDA and concentration of the incorporated LMWC in oral insulin delivery preparations in order to ensure the highest performance such systems.

## Acknowledgments

The authors would like to thank the Deanship of Scientific Research, University of Petra (Amman, Jordan) and the Jordanian Pharmaceutical Manufacturing Company (Amman, Jordan) for supporting this project.

## Author Contributions

Nidal A. Qinna and Qutuba G. Karwi conducted the experiments and analyzed the data and draftd the manuscript. Mayyas A. Al-Remawi and Nawzat Al-Jbour contributed in the formulation of the nanoparticles. Khaldoun A. Al-So'ud participated in the in silico experiments. Mahmoud M.H. Al Omari participated in the preparation and characterization of low molecular weight chitosans and helped in preparing the manuscript. Tawfiq M. Alhussainy participated in the design of the *in vivo* experiments. Adnan A. Badwan contributed to the conception and design of the study and aproved the final draft.

## Conflicts of Interest

The authors declare no conflict of interest.

## References

1. Gupta, S.; Jain, A.; Chakraborty, M.; Sahni, J.K.; Ali, J.; Dang, S. Oral delivery of therapeutic proteins and peptides: A review on recent developments. *Drug Deliv.* **2013**, *20*, 237–246.
2. Des Rieux, A.; Fievez, V.; Garinot, M.; Schneider, Y.-J.; Préat, V. Nanoparticles as potential oral delivery systems of proteins and vaccines: A mechanistic approach. *J. Control. Release* **2006**, *116*, 1–27.
3. Assaf, S.; Al-Jbour, N.; Eftaiha, A.; Elsayed, A.; Al-Remawi, M.; Qinna, N.; Badwan, A. Factors involved in formulation of oily delivery system for proteins based on peg-8 caprylic/capric glycerides and polyglyceryl-6 dioleate in a mixture of oleic acid with chitosan. *J. Dispers. Sci. Technol.* **2011**, *32*, 623–633.
4. Muzzarelli, R.A. Chitins and chitosans as immunoadjuvants and non-allergenic drug carriers. *Mar. Drugs* **2010**, *8*, 292–312.
5. Qinna, N.A.; Akayleh, F.T.; Al Remawi, M.M.; Kamona, B.S.; Taha, H.; Badwan, A.A. Evaluation of a functional food preparation based on chitosan as a meal replacement diet. *J. Funct. Foods* **2013**, *5*, 1125–1134.

6. Wu, T.; Zivanovic, S.; Hayes, D.G.; Weiss, J. Efficient reduction of chitosan molecular weight by high-intensity ultrasound: Underlying mechanism and effect of process parameters. *J. Agric. Food Chem.* **2008**, *56*, 5112–5119.

7. Einbu, A.; Grasdalen, H.; Varum, K.M. Kinetics of hydrolysis of chitin/chitosan oligomers in concentrated hydrochloric acid. *Carbohydr. Res.* **2007**, *342*, 1055–1062.

8. Vårum, K.M.; Ottøy, M.H.; Smidsrød, O. Acid hydrolysis of chitosans. *Carbohydr. Polym.* **2001**, *46*, 89–98.

9. Sadeghi, A.M.; Dorkoosh, F.A.; Avadi, M.R.; Saadat, P.; Rafiee-Tehrani, M.; Junginger, H.E. Preparation, characterization and antibacterial activities of chitosan, *N*-trimethyl chitosan (TMC) and *N*-diethylmethyl chitosan (DEMC) nanoparticles loaded with insulin using both the ionotropic gelation and polyelectrolyte complexation methods. *Int. J. Pharm.* **2008**, *355*, 299–306.

10. Sajeesh, S.; Bouchemal, K.; Marsaud, V.; Vauthier, C.; Sharma, C.P. Cyclodextrin complexed insulin encapsulated hydrogel microparticles: An oral delivery system for insulin. *J. Control. Release* **2010**, *147*, 377–384.

11. Wang, Q.Z.; Chen, X.G.; Liu, N.; Wang, S.X.; Liu, C.S.; Meng, X.H.; Liu, C.G. Protonation constants of chitosan with different molecular weight and degree of deacetylation. *Carbohydr. Polym.* **2006**, *65*, 194–201.

12. Badwan, A.; Al-Remawi, M.; Qinna, N.; Elsayed, A. Nanocapsules for oral delivery of proteins. EP2042166 (A1). Available online: https://data.epo.org/gpi/EP2042166A1-Nanocapsules-for-oral-delivery-of-proteins (accessed on 20 January 2015).

13. Elsayed, A.; Remawi, M.A.; Qinna, N.; Farouk, A.; Badwan, A. Formulation and characterization of an oily-based system for oral delivery of insulin. *Eur. J. Pharm. Biopharm.* **2009**, *73*, 269–279.

14. Badwan, A.; Remawi, M.; Qinna, N.; Elsayed, A.; Arafat, T.; Melhim, M.; Hijleh, O.A.; Idkaidek, N.M. Enhancement of oral bioavailability of insulin in humans. *Neuro Endocrinol. Lett.* **2009**, *30*, 74–78.

15. Park, K.; Kwon, I.C.; Park, K. Oral protein delivery: Current status and future prospect. *React. Funct. Polym.* **2011**, *71*, 280–287.

16. Muzzarelli, R.A. Human enzymatic activities related to the therapeutic administration of chitin derivatives. *Cell. Mol. Life Sci.* **1997**, *53*, 131–140.

17. Pedro, A.S.; Cabral-Albuquerque, E.; Ferreira, D.; Sarmento, B. Chitosan: An option for development of essential oil delivery systems for oral cavity care? *Carbohydr. Polym.* **2009**, *76*, 501–508.

18. Tommeraas, K.; Koping-Hoggard, M.; Varum, K.M.; Christensen, B.E.; Artursson, P.; Smidsrod, O. Preparation and characterisation of chitosans with oligosaccharide branches. *Carbohydr. Res.* **2002**, *337*, 2455–2462.

19. Chae, S.Y.; Jang, M.K.; Nah, J.W. Influence of molecular weight on oral absorption of water soluble chitosans. *J. Control. Release* **2005**, *102*, 383–394.

20. Huang, X.; Du, Y.Z.; Yuan, H.; Hu, F.Q. Preparation and pharmacodynamics of low-molecular-weight chitosan nanoparticles containing insulin. *Carbohydr. Polym.* **2009**, *76*, 368–373.

21. Palpandi, C.; Shanmugam, V.; Shanmugam, A. Extraction of chitin and chitosan from shell and operculum of mangrove gastropod nerita (dostia) crepidularia lamarck. *Int. J. Med. Med. Sci.* **2009**, *1*, 198–205.

22. Heux, L.; Brugnerotto, J.; Desbrieres, J.; Versali, M.F.; Rinaudo, M. Solid state NMR for determination of degree of acetylation of chitin and chitosan. *Biomacromolecules* **2000**, *1*, 746–751.

23. Djordjevic, L.; Primorac, M.; Stupar, M.; Krajisnik, D. Characterization of caprylocaproyl macrogolglycerides based microemulsion drug delivery vehicles for an amphiphilic drug. *Int. J. Pharm.* **2004**, *271*, 11–19.

24. Graf, A.; Jack, K.S.; Whittaker, A.K.; Hook, S.M.; Rades, T. Protein delivery using nanoparticles based on microemulsions with different structure-types. *Eur. J. Pharm. Sci.* **2008**, *33*, 434–444.

25. Rinaudo, M. Chitin and chitosan: Properties and applications. *Prog. Polym. Sci.* **2006**, *31*, 603–632.

26. Morawetz, H.; Sage, H. The effect of poly(acrylic acid) on the tryptic digestion of hemoglobin. *Arch. Biochem. Biophys.* **1955**, *56*, 103–109.

27. Obaidat, R.; Al-Jbour, N.; Al-Sou'd, K.; Sweidan, K.; Al-Remawi, M.; Badwan, A. Some physico-chemical properties of low molecular weight chitosans and their relationship to conformation in aqueous solution. *J. Solut. Chem.* **2010**, *39*, 575–588.

28. Kubota, N.; Tatsumoto, N.; Sano, T.; Toya, K. A simple preparation of half *N*-acetylated chitosan highly soluble in water and aqueous organic solvents. *Carbohydr. Res.* **2000**, *324*, 268–274.

29. Qandil, A.; Obaidat, A.; Ali, M.; Al-Taani, B.; Tashtoush, B.; Al-Jbour, N.; Al Remawi, M.; Al-Sou'od, K.; Badwan, A. Investigation of the interactions in complexes of low molecular weight chitosan with ibuprofen. *J. Solut. Chem.* **2009**, *38*, 695–712.

30. Hamman, J.H. Chitosan based polyelectrolyte complexes as potential carrier materials in drug delivery systems. *Mar. Drugs* **2010**, *8*, 1305–1322.

# Low Molecular Weight Chitosan–Insulin Polyelectrolyte Complex: Characterization and Stability Studies

Zakieh I. Al-Kurdi, Babur Z. Chowdhry, Stephen A. Leharne, Mahmoud M. H. Al Omari and Adnan A. Badwan

**Abstract:** The aim of the work reported herein was to investigate the effect of various low molecular weight chitosans (LMWCs) on the stability of insulin using USP HPLC methods. Insulin was found to be stable in a polyelectrolyte complex (PEC) consisting of insulin and LMWC in the presence of a Tris-buffer at pH 6.5. In the presence of LMWC, the stability of insulin increased with decreasing molecular weight of LMWC; 13 kDa LMWC was the most efficient molecular weight for enhancing the physical and chemical stability of insulin. Solubilization of insulin-LMWC polyelectrolyte complex (I-LMWC PEC) in a reverse micelle (RM) system, administered to diabetic rats, results in an oral delivery system for insulin with acceptable bioactivity.

Reprinted from *Mar. Drugs*. Cite as: Al-Kurdi, Z.I.; Chowdhry, B.Z.; Leharne, S.A.; Al Omari, M.M.H.; Badwan, A.A. Low Molecular Weight Chitosan–Insulin Polyelectrolyte Complex: Characterization and Stability Studies. *Mar. Drugs* **2015**, *13*, 1765-1784.

## 1. Introduction

One of the most challenging problems in the development of liquid peptide/protein pharmaceuticals is their physical and chemical instability. Most peptides and proteins are formulated so that they can be administered clinically by parenteral injections, as this is the fastest route towards commercialization. However, stabilization of peptides and proteins in a designated delivery system against degradation, particularly in the gastrointestinal tract (GIT), is a prerequisite for oral delivery. This can be carried out by using several excipients such as salts, amino acids, surfactants, polyhydric alcohols, and carbohydrates [1]. The latter include chitosans, which are composed of β-(1-4)-linked D-glucosamine and *N*-acetyl-D-glucosamine units [2]. Chitosans are non-toxic, degradable, and biocompatible polymers that exhibit different characteristics. This allows them to be used as excipients for protein formulations intended for *in vivo* delivery of biopharmaceuticals [3].

The presence of free $NH_2$ groups allows chitosan to form polyelectrolyte complexes (PECs) with negatively charged moieties. For example, PECs containing chitosan, alkyl-chitosan, and PEG-grafted alkyl-chitosan have been shown to improve insulin delivery [4,5]. Such PEC nanoparticles showed a pH-dependent stabilization of insulin [6].

Schatz *et al.* synthesized a partially *N*-sulfated chitosan. Upon acidification, nanoparticles were formed by electrostatic interactions between the non-sulfated protonated amine groups of chitosan and the negatively charged *N*-sulfated chitosan amines. These PECs can be used for encapsulation of macromolecules [7].

However, the main function of such PECs is to increase protein stability towards harsh conditions in the GIT or unfavorable storage conditions and to protect them against physical and chemical instabilities. PEC nanoparticles prepared by Mao *et al.* using chitosan, trimethyl-chitosan,

PEGylated-trimethyl-chitosan, and insulin were unaffected by lyophilization and PECs were shown to protect insulin from degradation even at temperatures as high as 50 °C for 6 h [8]. LMWCs have been used to prepare the PECs employing poly-γ-glutamic acid, which was used as a carrier for insulin, followed by enteric coating or layering with calcium alginate in order to allow oral administration [9]. Jintapattanakit *et al.* found that PECs prepared using trimethyl-chitosan (100 kDa) and PEG-graft-trimethyl-chitosan copolymer improve the stability of oral insulin [10]. Also, Song *et al.* reported an oral insulin delivery system based upon ultrathin nanofilm encapsulation technology. The proposed system can be used to load a high amount of insulin (90%) using chitosan (150–190 kDa, 75% deacetylation) [11]. Additionally, it has also been reported that the inclusion of chitosan in lipid nanoparticles enhances the physical stability of insulin by protecting against proteolysis [12].

A novel system based on solubilization of the insulin–chitosan PEC in RM system made from PEG-8 caprylic/capric glycerides and glycerol-6-dioleate as emulsifying agents and dispersed in oleic acid, has been patented by Badwan *et al.* [13,14]. The function of this solubilized PEC is to reduce the size of particles intended for oral delivery of insulin [15].

Generally, studies have been undertaken by using high molecular weight chitosans, and in the vast majority of cases the chemical stability of insulin was not evaluated in term of insulin degradation and formation of its degradation products. The objective of the work reported herein was to investigate the influence of complexing LMWCs of different molecular weights (1.3–30 kDa) with insulin on its physicochemical and biological stabilities. Insulin content was monitored and examined as well as the formation of high molecular weight proteins (HMWPs) of insulin. Furthermore, the system was evaluated for bioactivity.

## 2. Results and Discussion

### 2.1. HPLC Methods Verification

Insulin (I), A-21 desamido insulin, and HMWPs were determined by using the assay and limit of HMWP tests as stated in the human insulin USP monograph [16]. The insulin assay method was adopted for evaluating insulin stability in bulk insulin powder and in injectables [17]. Additionally, the method was found to be convenient for evaluating the stability of insulin in other delivery systems [18].

In the present work, the suitability of USP HPLC methods for the determination of insulin and HMWP in I-LMWC PEC systems was examined. Practically, insulin may be recovered either by an extraction-based method with organic solvents or by hydrolysis of the carriers (PEC or RM) with an alkaline reagent [19]. In the current work, different extraction solvents and procedures to extract insulin were evaluated. Aqueous solutions (0.01 or 0.1 N HCl) and methanol at different ratios (1/1, 2/1, 1/2, 2/3, and 3/2 v/v) were used to obtain the optimal ratio of the extraction solvent mixtures. Extraction of insulin from I-LMWC PEC preparations with a mixture of 0.01 M HCl and methanol at a ratio of 2/3 (v/v) gave acceptable recoveries for insulin (>98%); moreover, the stability of insulin in such a mixture was retained for 24 h.

Furthermore, the USP HPLC method parameters used for the assessment of the stability of bulk insulin, such as the ratio of mobile phase components and temperature [16], were evaluated for the PEC and RM systems. The ratio of mobile phase components (aqueous to acetonitrile) was found to be critical as a high acetonitrile content and a decrease in column temperature (e.g., to 35 °C) led to the precipitation of sulfate salt and subsequently affected the HPLC system parameters (e.g., retention time of insulin and resolution).

Verification of the USP HPLC method for insulin showed a linear response for signal output *versus* insulin concentration over the concentration range of 0.9–10 mg insulin/mL with an $R^2$ value >0.995; such results are in line with the acceptable verification limits [20]. The intra- and inter-day relative standard deviation (RSD) values were less than 2%, indicating good precision. No interfering peaks from the components of the delivery systems were detected. The resolution factor between insulin and A-21 desamido insulin was >2.0, indicating that the method is specific. The method sensitivity was proved by low detection limit (DL) (0.02 mg/mL) and quantitation limit (QL) (0.08 mg/mL) values. Thus, the isocratic HPLC method developed herein is, analytically, advantageous in comparison with the published gradient methods [21,22]. The results of verification of the HPLC method confirmed the applicability of the USP HPLC method for the analysis of preparations other than injectables, such as polyelectrolyte systems. Consequently, the USP method can be considered as stability indicating method for the analysis of PEC and RM delivery systems.

The data in Figure 1 shows representative HPLC outputs for both assay and limit of HMWP tests, where the peaks corresponding to insulin, A-21 desamido insulin (Figure 1A), and HMWPs (Figure 1B) are well resolved. The results of HPLC method verification are summarized in Table 1; all the verification parameters are within acceptable limits [20].

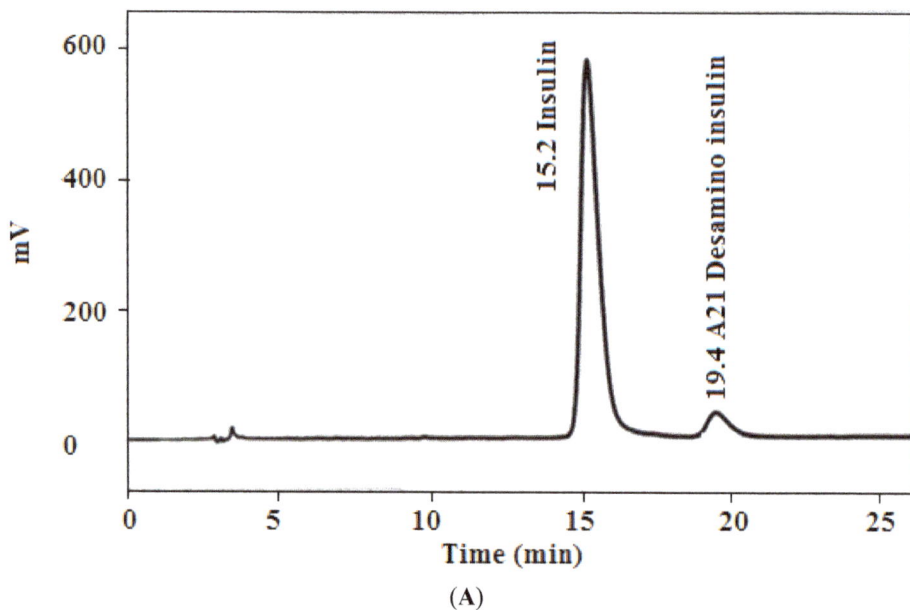

(A)

Figure 1. *Cont.*

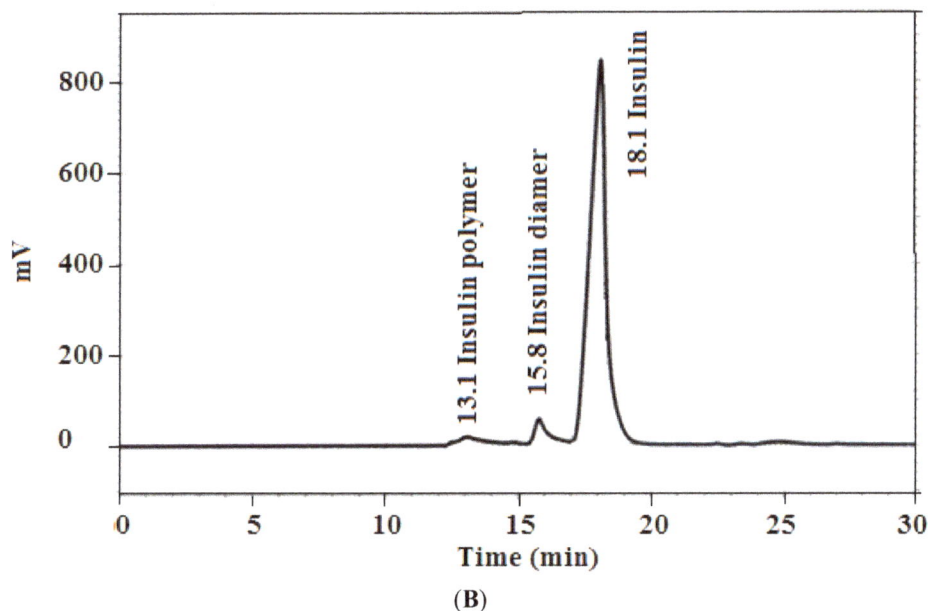

Figure 1. Representative HPLC chromatograms for (A) insulin assay (1.5 mg/mL) and (B) high molecular weight proteins (HMWPs) limit test (4.0 mg/mL).

Table 1. HPLC method verification results for insulin assay.

| Analytical Parameter | Result |
|---|---|
| Linearity Range | |
| - 0.9–10.0 mg/mL | $R^2 = 0.9998$ |
| Specificity | |
| - Interference | No interference from formulation components and related compounds |
| Precision (%) | |
| - Inter-day RSD ($n = 3 \times 3$) | 0.8–1.1 |
| - Intra-day RSD ($n = 5$) | 0.7–0.9 |
| Recovery (%) | $98.3 \pm 0.9$ |
| DL (mg/mL) | 0.02 |
| QL (mg/mL) | 0.08 |
| Stability of Solution | |
| - Decrease in assay at ambient condition | 2.5% decrease in assay after 24 h |
| System Suitability | |
| - Resolution between insulin and A-21 desamido insulin | 3.7 |
| - Tailing factor for insulin peak | <1.8 |
| - RSD of replicate injections | <1.6% |

DL and QL: detection and quantitation limits, RSD: relative standard deviation.

*2.2. Effect of the Molecular Weight and Concentration of LMWC on Insulin Stability*

Prior to studying the effect of the molecular weight of LMWC on the stability of insulin, different parameters including insulin concentration (0.9–10.0 mg/mL) and solvent (water, phosphate buffer pH 6.5, and Tris-buffer of pH 6.5), were investigated at 50 °C for 72 h. It was found that the stability of insulin increases when the concentration of insulin is increased; these results agree well with reported data [23–26]. However, it appears from the results of the present study that a concentration of 7 mg/mL is sufficient for maintaining insulin stability at pH ≈ 6.0. Furthermore, Tris-buffer (an organic buffer) improved the stability of insulin even at low concentrations of insulin (0.9 and 1.75 mg/mL) by inhibiting the re-aggregation and precipitation of insulin. Also, at neutral pH, the conversion of monomeric insulin to form dimeric, tetrameric, and eventually hexameric insulin seems to stabilize insulin [27]. At insulin concentrations of 0.9–10 mg/mL, the fractional content of the degradation products A-21 desamido insulin and dimer did not exceed 0.4% after incubation at 50 °C for 72 h. On the other hand, other HMWPs were not detected over the investigated range of insulin concentration. In neutral solutions, the insulin molecules are associated mainly into non-covalent, $Zn^{2+}$-containing hexamers [28]. The observation that dimer formation is independent of insulin concentration indicates that the intermolecular chemical reaction occurs mainly within the hexameric units and not between the hexamers in solution [29]. This might be due to the fact that hexamers are less susceptible to degradation [23].

The stability of I-LMWC PECs prepared by using LMWCs of different molecular weights (1.3–30 kDa) at 50 °C is shown in Figure 2A. The kinetic parameters for insulin degradation, as shown in Table 2, indicate a noticeable effect of molecular weight of LMWC on the extent of insulin degradation in the I-LMWC PEC preparations (*i.e.*, stability decreases with increasing molecular weight of LMWC).

The effect of 13 kDa LMWC concentration on the stability of I-LMWC PECs at 50 °C is shown in the data in Figure 2B. The results revealed a noticeable effect of increasing LMWC concentration on the degradation of insulin (Table 2).

In addition, monitoring the physical stability of I-LMWC PEC indicated that the formation of a physically stable system depends upon the molecular weight of LMWC. For example, LMWCs of shorter chains formed soluble complexes, while turbidity and precipitation were observed with higher molecular weight LMWCs (e.g., 30 kDa). This can be explained by the fact that complex formation between insulin and LMWC is mainly governed by kinetic factors which leads to preferential binding with the shorter chains due to their flexibility [8]. On the other hand, the chemical stability of insulin was affected to the same extent in the presence of different molecular weight LMWCs (Figure 2A). This may be attributed to the ratio of ionized groups of insulin ($7.0 \times 10^{20}$) to chitosan ($5.3 \times 10^{21}$), which was fixed at about 1/8 in the preparation of different I-LMWC PECs by changing the molar ratio of insulin: LMWC 1/0.2–1/4.5 (Table 2). The number of ionizable groups was calculated on the basis of previously published work [15].

Furthermore, changing the concentration of 13 kDa LMWC showed a significant effect on insulin stability (Figure 2B). Insulin instability was observed mainly at high concentrations (3.5 mg/mL), while at lower concentrations the effect is less. This may be explained by the changes in LMWC structure and particle size with concentration. With increasing concentration of LMWC, the structure becomes more helical, leading to the formation of aggregates and a concomitant increase in particle size (see Section 2.4). At high concentration, such aggregates may prevent LMWC from protecting insulin (Figure 2B).

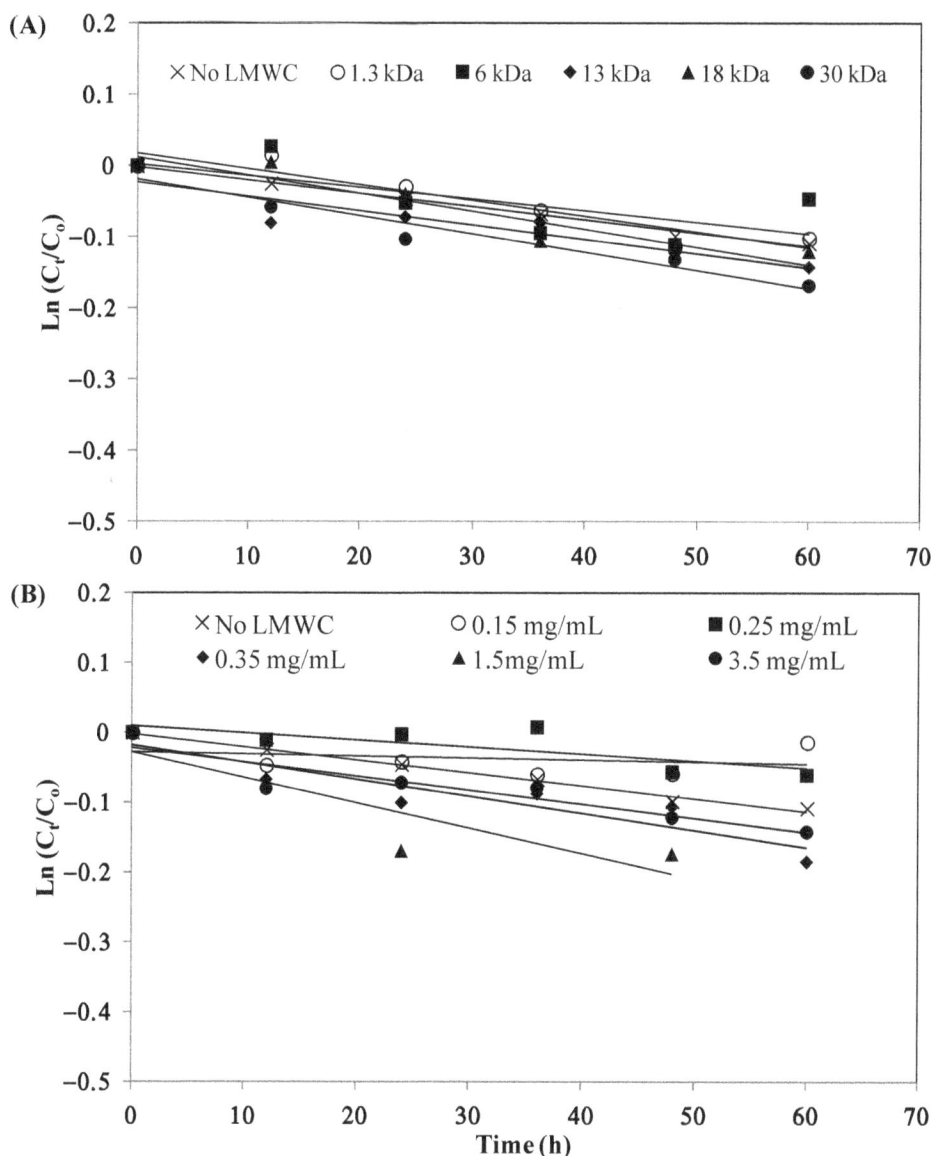

**Figure 2.** Stability of insulin in the presence of (**A**) different LMWCs (1.5 mg/mL) and (**B**) different concentrations of 13 kDa LMWC at 50 °C. $C_0$ is the initial insulin concentration and $C_t$ is the insulin concentration at different periods of incubation time. The values of Ln ($C_t/C_0$) are the mean of 3 replicates for each experiment (RSDs < 5%).

**Table 2.** First-order kinetic parameters for insulin–LMWC polyelectrolyte complex (I-LMWC PEC) degradation in the presence of different LMWCs and different concentrations of 13 kDa LMWC at 50 °C.

| LMWC Molecular Weight (kDa) [*,+] | Insulin/LMWC Molar Ratio | $k$ (h$^{-1}$) × 10$^3$ | $t_{90}$ (h) | $t_{50}$ (h) | $R^2$ |
|---|---|---|---|---|---|
| 0.0 | - | 1.2 | 88 | 587 | 0.2065 |
| 1.3 | 1/4.5 | 2.2 | 48 | 315 | 0.8780 |
| 6 | 1/1 | 1.6 | 64 | 423 | 0.4835 |
| 13 | 1/0.45 | 2.0 | 52 | 344 | 0.8428 |
| 18 | 1/0.3 | 2.5 | 42 | 274 | 0.8831 |
| 30 | 1/0.2 | 2.6 | 41 | 272 | 0.9388 |
| **[13 kDa LMWC] (mg/mL) [+]** | | | | | |
| 0.0 | - | 1.2 | 88 | 587 | 0.2065 |
| 0.15 | 1/0.02 | 1.3 | 81 | 533 | 0.9200 |
| 0.25 | 1/0.03 | 1.0 | 102 | 675 | 0.5871 |
| 0.35 | 1/0.045 | 2.4 | 43 | 283 | 0.8388 |
| 1.5 | 1/0.2 | 3.6 | 29 | 191 | 0.7704 |
| 3.5 | 1/0.45 | 2.0 | 52 | 344 | 0.8428 |

$k$: 1st order rate constant, $t_{90}$ and $t_{50}$: shelf-life for 90% and 50% intact potencies. [+] [Insulin] is 3.5 mg/mL, [*] [LMWC] is 3.5 mg/mL.

By monitoring the degradation of insulin as a function of molecular weight of LMWC, the fraction of A-21 desamido insulin (0.2% initial) increases when the molecular weight of LMWC is increased after 72 h incubation at 50°C (0.9, 1.1, 1.2, 1.4, and 1.6% for 1.3, 6, 13, 18, and 30 kDa LMWC, respectively). While the results showed an increase in the content of insulin dimer (from 0.1% to 0.6%–0.7%) regardless of the molecular weight of LMWC. This may be attributed to the fixed ratio of ionized groups of insulin to LMWC. The amino groups of LMWC have the capacity to react with insulin by intermolecular aminolysis, resulting in transamidation between the molecules. Such a reaction can result in dimer formation [29].

However, the formation of other HMWPs increases as the molecular weight of the LMWCs increases (1% for 1.3 kDa and 3%–4% for 6–30 kDa LMWCs). The formation of dimers and polymers can be explained by the ability of free NH$_2$ groups to react with the carbonyl groups of insulin (available in Asn at A-21 and B-2, and Gln available at A-5, A-15, and B-4) by intermolecular aminolysis, resulting in transamidation or Schiff base-mediated reactions between molecules forming HMWPs and, in parallel, dimer formation, probably as a result of disulfide interchange [29]. It is worth mentioning that the impact of HMWP formation on the quality and therapeutic usefulness of the pharmaceutical preparation is attributed to safety rather than efficacy. Preparation efficacy will not be affected by a decrease in the content of insulin. However, some of the immunological side effects associated with insulin therapy may be due to the presence of covalent aggregates of insulin in the therapeutic preparations, and specific antibodies against dimers have been identified in 30% of insulin-treated diabetic patients [30]. Dimer levels of 2% generated a highly hypersensitive response [31]. Accordingly, the content of HMWPs should be kept as low as possible. The acceptable

USP limit does not allow more than 3.0% HMWPs in insulin pharmaceutical preparations. This indicates that during the development of insulin delivery systems, optimization of the system is essential to prevent the formation of HMWPs.

*2.3. Effect of the Molecular Weight of LMWC on Immunological Bioactivity of Insulin*

The ELISA method used for insulin determination was found to be linear in the range of 0–100 μIU/mL with an $R^2$ value of 0.868 and DL of 0.26 μIU/mL. Method recovery at the recommended concentration (by the kit supplier), 50 μIU/mL, was carried out; the fraction recovered was 92.7%, with an RSD of 6.1% (average of 3 samples). Monitoring of insulin solutions incubated at 50 °C indicated a loss in bioactivity of 40% after an 8 h incubation, which indicates that the method is specific and loss in bioactivity of insulin can be detected using ELISA. The ELISA results indicated that insulin in the different I-LMWC-PECs prepared with LMWC of different molecular weights (1.3–30 kDa) retained its bioactivity (assay > 85%) (Table 3). The ELISA method has very high sensitivity and specificity as it depends on the reaction of the predominant protein with a specific antibody to form a complex [32]. Therefore, ELISA antigenicity is considered to be an appropriate means for detection of changes of insulin antigenic activity [33]. The surface structure of insulin was assessed by antibodies that bind to the epitopes on the insulin. The ELISA results indicated that insulin in the PEC had retained its bioactivity. ELISA results were comparable with HPLC results, which were used to assess the integrity of insulin and confirmed that the receptor-binding epitopes on insulin were maintained after complexation with LMWC [34].

**Table 3.** The immunological bioactivity of insulin-LMWC polyelectrolyte (I-LMWC PEC) of different molecular weight after incubation at 50 °C for 72 h.

| LMWC Molecular Weight (kDa) | Bioactivity (%) | RSD |
|---|---|---|
| No LMWC | 58.9 * | 10.3 |
| 1.3 | 91.1 | 3.1 |
| 6 | 92.3 | 4.7 |
| 13 | 102.9 | 6.7 |
| 18 | 94.6 | 6.1 |
| 30 | 97.1 | 5.7 |

* After 8 h of incubation, RSD: relative standard deviation.

The aforementioned stability results show a profound impact of molecular weight (*i.e.*, chain length), concentration (*i.e.*, charge ratio), pH, and buffer type of the LMWC on the development of a stable oral delivery systems for insulin. In the present work, the 13 kDa LMWC can be considered a suitable candidate to prepare the PEC and the RM systems. It showed an optimal formulation with respect to chemical and physical stability. Furthermore, it produced a suitable vehicle with optimal interfacial surface tension and nano-size particles [15], in addition to the absence of precipitation [8]. Subsequently, characterization and further *in vitro* and *in vivo* investigation of the bioactivity study were undertaken for the delivery systems prepared using the 13 kDa LMWC.

## 2.4. Characterization of I-LMWC PEC and I-LMWC RM Systems

The particle size results for I-LMWC PECs prepared using the same insulin concentration (3.5 mg/mL) and different concentrations of 13 kDa LMWC (1–5 mg/mL) were compared with the particle size results for insulin and LMWC alone. The particle size of insulin in solution was found to be around 5.0 nm, which indicates that it is present in its hexameric form [35]. However, the particle size of LMWC is concentration dependent. When the LMWC concentration is low, LMWC particles are present in a more extended form; however, above a certain concentration aggregates start to form and the particle size starts to increase; similar results have been previously reported [36].

At low concentration of LMWC (1 mg/mL) the size distribution intensity of I-LMWC PECs was $6.38 \pm 0.26$ nm (higher than the size of insulin), and only one peak was present when measuring particle size. This means that all the LMWC molecules interact with insulin molecules to form a particle larger than insulin. Increasing the LMWC concentration to 3.5 and 5 mg/mL resulted in a particle size of $6.9 \pm 0.17$ nm; however, another peak started to appear in the region of around $100 \pm 20$ nm, which represents the size of the free LMWC and aggregated LMWC in the sample (*i.e.*, LMWC un-reacted with insulin). The results of mean particle size are shown in Figure 3A. Since LMWC will react with insulin at one site only, an excess amount of LMWC will be free in the sample that may also aggregate and give a particle size of around 100 nm. The mean particle size of the RMs was $300 \pm 19$ nm.

The effect of LMWC concentration on the zeta potential of I-LMWC PEC (3.5 mg insulin/mL) was investigated. LMWC (1–5 mg/mL) without associated insulin shows a positive zeta-potential of +15–+25 mV (Figure 3A). On the other hand, the presence of insulin (with a zeta-potential of −27 mV) decreases the zeta-potential value to about +5 mV. The ionized groups of amino acid residues of insulin will be attracted to the positively charged LMWC via coulombic forces [37]. The zeta potential of the complex is positive, which means that insulin is encapsulated in the polymer, projecting positively charged chains towards the external aqueous medium. Although the zeta potential value of the complex is positive, the surface charge of the complex will be decreased when compared to LMWC alone, which is expected. This facilitates absorption of the PEC to the biolipid membranes of the GIT [38].

The data for the effect of 13 kDa LMWC concentration and pH of the I-LMWC PEC on insulin association efficiency (AE) are presented in Table 4. It is well known that the formation of PEC is pH dependent [8,39]. The investigated pH range (6.5–7.0) in the present work is close to the $pK_a$ of chitosan (about 6.5) and to the isoelectric point (pI) of insulin (about 6.4). In this pH range, electrostatic, hydrophobic interactions as well as hydrogen bonding may be involved in PEC formation, as neutral and ionized chitosan species exist in an almost equal proportion [40].

In the present work, the PEC using 13 kDa LMWC was prepared at different pH values of 6.5, 6.7, and 7.0. However, lower and high pH values were not considered ($8 < pH < 5$), where insulin degrades rapidly [8,41]. A change in pH from 6.5 to 7.0 results in a significant decrease in the value of the AE (from 76.5% to 8.6%) (Table 4). This may indicate that the PEC begins to precipitate at pH values higher than 6.5 as a result of a decrease in the solubility of the 13 kDa LMWC above its $pk_a$ value (about 6.5) [8,42]. Such precipitation was observed for aqueous solutions of 13 kDa LMWC following pH adjustment to 7.0. This noticeable precipitation is probably due to the formation of neutral LMWC. However, the AE was improved by using higher concentrations of LMWC. Such behavior was previously observed by Wu *et al.* [43].

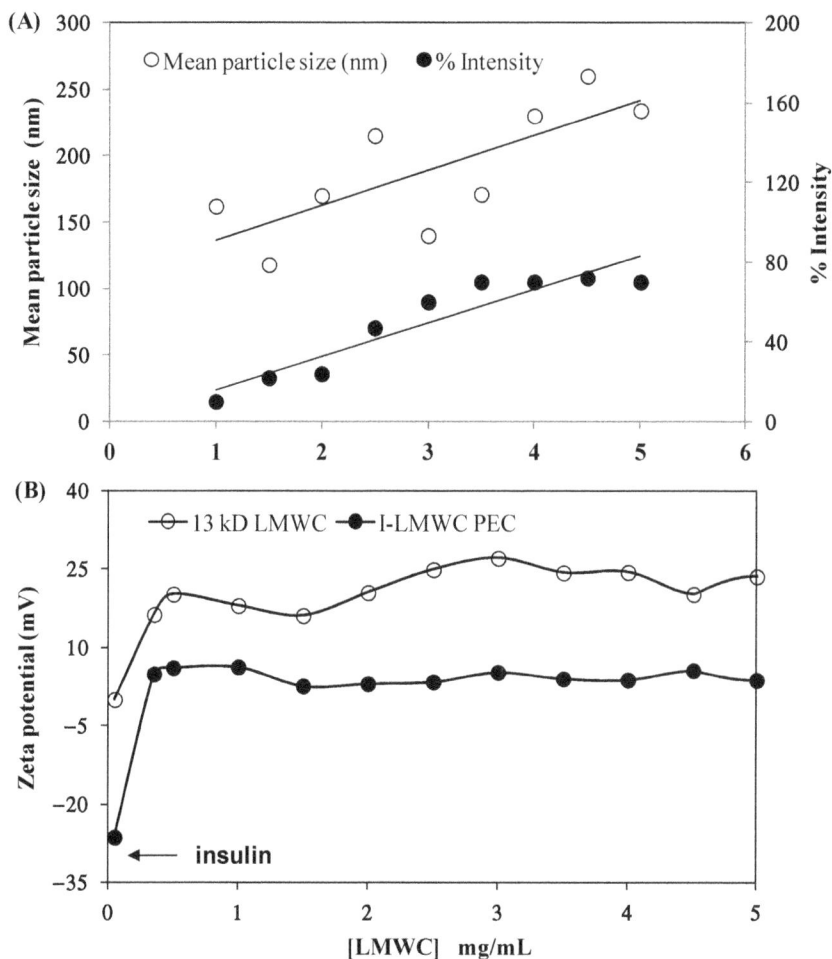

**Figure 3.** Effect of 13 kDa LMWC concentration on (**A**) the particle size of major peaks at 100–250 nm and (**B**) the zeta potential of the insulin–LMWC polyelectrolyte (I-LMWC PEC). The number of replicates is 6 and 3, respectively.

**Table 4.** Effect of 13 kDa LMWC concentration and pH on insulin association efficiency (AE).

| LMWC Concentration (mg/mL) | $pH_f$ | AE ± RSD (%) |
|---|---|---|
| 0.7 | 6.5 | 63.8 ± 2.1 |
| 3.0 | 6.5 | 76.2 ± 3.2 |
| 0.7 | 6.7 | 22.7 ± 2.8 |
| 3.0 | 7.0 | 8.6 ± 4.6 |

Number of replicates is 3 for each experiment.

## 2.5. In Vitro Evaluation of I-LMWC PEC and I-LMWC RM

### 2.5.1. In Vitro Release

The results for the *in vitro* release of insulin from the I-LMWC RM system showed a negligible release at pH 1.2 (<10% at 6 h), while at pH 6.8 the release is markedly increased (80% of the encapsulated amount at 6 h). Furthermore, the release profile at pH 6.8 was gradual and free of any detectable burst effects, as shown in the data in Figure 4.

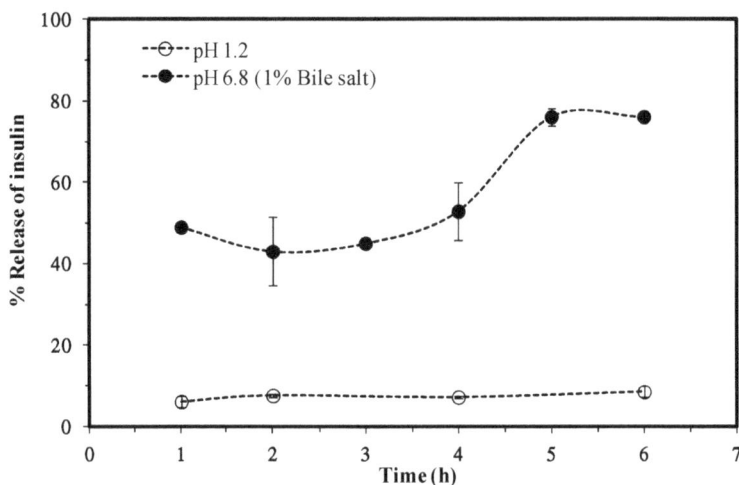

**Figure 4.** A cumulative release of insulin from insulin–LMWC reverse micelles (I-LMWC RMs) using 13 kDa LMWC.

### 2.5.2. In Vitro Evaluation of the Protective Effect

The protective ability of the RMs under conditions simulating the gastric environment was evaluated and compared with free insulin and I-LMWC PEC. Free insulin and I-LMWC PEC were found to be completely degraded during incubation with pepsin, while in the RM about 90% of insulin was recovered after incubation with simulated gastric fluid with pepsin. These results emphasize the importance of the RM system in the protection of insulin from degradation by pepsin.

### 2.6. Biological Activity

The data in Figure 5 illustrate the changes in blood glucose levels of rats after oral administration of I-LMWC PEC after solubilization in the reverse micelles. A decrease in plasma glucose level was observed. The results are significantly different when compared to a blank control ($p < 0.05$). The reverse micelle preparation resulted in minimum glucose levels, about 70% after 3 h, and the reduction in glucose levels was maintained over a prolonged period of time. It is worth mentioning that insulin and I-LMWC PEC are completely degraded under conditions simulating the gastric environment, as reported previously [14]. However, the decrease in blood glucose levels (Figure 5) may be attributed to the improved stability of insulin in the reverse micelle preparation against degradation at gastric pH values and in the presence of enzymes in the GIT system.

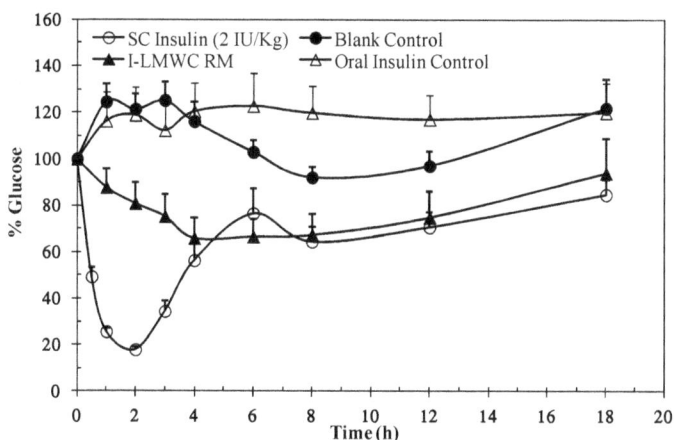

**Figure 5.** Blood glucose levels *versus* time profile after a single oral administration of 50 IU/kg insulin-LMWC reverse micelle (I-LMWC RM) and a subcutaneous administration (SC) of 2 IU/kg insulin to STZ-diabetic rats The results are expressed as mean ± SD (*n* = 10 for each group).

## 3. Experimental Section

### 3.1. Materials

USP human insulin RS (26.4 USP insulin human units/mg, lot No. J0J250) was purchased from USP Convention (Rockville, MD, USA). Recombinant human (rh) insulin of pharmaceutical grade standardized by using USP insulin human RS (potency 99.4%) was purchased from Biocon (Bangalore, India). Purified water and LMWCs of different molecular weights (1.3, 6, 13, 18, and 30 kDa) with >95% degree of deacetylation (DDA) were provided by the Jordanian Pharmaceutical Manufacturing Company (Naor, Jordan). LMWCs may be considered as derivative of chitosan with lower molecular weight, obtained by depolymerization of high molecular weight chitosan HCl (≈250 kDa and DDA 95%, Xiamen Xing, Shanghi, China). Oleic acid of pharmaceutical grade (purity >99%) was purchased from Merck (Darmstadt, Germany). Labrasol® (PEG-8 caprylic/capric glycerides) and Plurol®Oleique CG (polyglycerol-6-dioleate) were purchased from Gattefosse (Saint-Priest, Lyon, France). Streptozotocin was purchased from Sigma-Aldrich (St. Louis, MO, USA). All other chemicals were of analytical/HPLC grade and purchased from Merck.

### 3.2. Determination of Molecular Weight of LMWCs

The average molecular weight of LMWCs was determined by viscosity measurements (Vibro viscometer, SV-10 Japan) in water. The viscosity average molecular weight was obtained using the Mark–Houwink's equation, $[\eta] = k \cdot M^a$, where $[\eta]$ is the intrinsic viscosity, M is the viscosity average molecular weight, and the k and a values were 0.00058 and 0.69, respectively, based on a previous study [44].

## 3.3. Preparation of I-LMWC PEC

LMWC (1.3, 6, 13, 18, and 30 kDa) solutions of the required concentration (0.3–7 mg/mL) were prepared by dissolving LMWC powder in water, adjusting the pH to 5.5 with 0.1 N NaOH, and then making up to the required volume with water.

Insulin solutions (7 mg insulin/mL) were prepared by dissolving insulin powder in 1 mL of 0.1 N HCl, neutralized with 0.1 N NaOH and made up to a volume of 10 mL with water or 1 M Tris (hydroxylmethyl-aminomethane) buffer, pH 6.5.

I-LMWC PEC was prepared by mixing equal volumes of LMWC and insulin solutions in a glass vial under gentle magnetic stirring and incubating for 10 min at room temperature. I-LMWC PEC preparations contained 3.5 mg insulin/mL and different concentrations of LMWC (0.0–3.5 mg/mL).

## 3.4. Preparation of I-LMWC RM

An RM system was prepared based on a previous study [13]. A surfactant mixture of Labrasol® and Plurol® Oleique CG was prepared at a 1/1 (w/w) ratio by mixing the constituents using magnetic stirring for 5 min. Oleic acid (80 g) and surfactant mixture (20 g) were mixed together for 5 min; 8 mL of I-LMWC PEC (3.5/1.5), which contained 3.5 mg insulin and 1.5 mg 13 kDa LMWC/mL, was added to the mixture and mixed using a magnetic stirrer (250 rpm for 5 min).

## 3.5. Extraction Procedures

For the I-LMWC PEC system, equal volumes of the sample and a solvent mixture of 0.01 N HCl and methanol (2/3, v/v) were mixed together.

For the reverse micelle system, 2 g of the sample and 4 mL of the solvent mixture were vortexed vigorously for 2 min, centrifuged at 4000 rpm for 15 min, and the aqueous phase collected. The samples were then analyzed by HPLC to determine the insulin, A-21 desamido insulin, and HMWP content (3 replicates); the RSD values were <5%, <0.5%, and <3%, respectively.

## 3.6. HPLC Determination of Insulin

Quantitative determination of insulin was based on the USP assay method [16]. The HPLC system consisted of a TSP 1000 pump system, a TSP 1000 UV-VIS detector, and a TSP AS 3000 auto-sampler (TSP, USA). A C18 (L1) column (particle size 5 μm), dimensions of 4.6 × 150 mm (Thermo column from Thermo Fisher Scientific Inc., Rockford, IL, USA), maintained at 40 °C during analysis, was used as the stationary phase, together with a Lichrospher 100 RP-18, 5 μm particle size guard column (Merck, Germany). Elution was performed isocratically (flow rate 1 mL/min) using sulfate buffer pH 2.3-acetonitrile (73/27, v/v) as the mobile phase and UV detection at 214 nm. The injection volume was 20 μL. The resolution, R, between insulin and A-21 desamido insulin was >2, the tailing factor for insulin peak was <1.8, and RSD was <1.6%.

The resolution solution was prepared by dissolving 1.5 mg of insulin in 1 mL of 0.01 N HCl, followed by incubation of the solution at room temperature for not less than 3 days. Equipment control, data acquisition, and integration were undertaken using a ChromQuest work station.

## 3.7. Size Exclusion HPLC Determination of High Molecular Weight Proteins (HMWPs)

The method used was based on the USP limit test for HMWPs [16]. A column containing dihdroxypropane bound to silica packing material (L20) with a particle size of 5 μm and dimensions of 7.8 × 300 mm was used as the stationary phase (Waters insulin HMWP column, Dublin, Ireland). Elution was performed isocratically (flow rate 0.5 mL/min) using a mixture of an arginine solution (1 mg/mL), acetonitrile, and glacial acetic acid (65/20/15, v/v) as the mobile phase and UV detection at 276 nm. The injection volume was 100 μL.

Resolution solution was prepared by dissolving 4 mg of insulin containing not less than 0.4% HMWPs in 1 mL of 0.01 N HCl (insulin containing the indicated fraction of HMWPs was prepared by allowing insulin powder to stand at room temperature for about 5 days) [16].

## 3.8. HPLC Method Verification

The two USP HPLC methods (insulin assay and limit test for HMWPs) were verified according to USP [45] and the International Conference of Harmonization (ICH) guidelines [46]. Standard insulin solutions of different concentrations (0.9, 1.75, 3.5, 7.0, and 10.0 mg/mL) were used to assess the linearity of the calibration plot (3 replicates). The precision of the assay was determined by analyzing samples of I-LMWC PEC preparations at three different insulin concentrations (1.0, 3.5, and 10.0 mg/mL). For the assessment of the inter-day variation, samples were analyzed in triplicate ($n = 3$) on three different days. For the intra-day variation, they were analyzed 5 times ($n = 5$) on the same day. Accuracy was assessed by analyzing samples of I-CCS PEC preparations at the target concentrations of insulin of 3.5 mg/mL. Specificity was verified by analyzing the matrix, i.e., LMWC PEC, in the absence of insulin using the extraction method stated above. Additionally, a resolution solution containing insulin and A-21 desamido insulin was prepared and injected. The detection limit (DL) and quantitation limit (QL) for the HPLC method were determined based on the standard deviation of the response and the slope of the calibration curve, respectively. The stability of solutions of insulin (0.9 mg/mL) was analyzed by HPLC at 0, 12, and 24 h of storage at room temperature.

## 3.9. Stability of I-LMWC PEC

The initial experiments were designed to incubate the I-LMWC PEC samples at 40 °C; however, as long periods of time (>2 months) were required to obtain indicative results, the experimental design was changed and the samples were incubated at a higher temperature (50 °C). Samples of I-LMWC PEC preparations, using LMWCs of different molecular weights and concentrations, were incubated at 50 °C for different periods of time. Samples were withdrawn at pre-determined intervals (0, 12, 24, 36, 48, and 72 h) and tested for insulin, A-21 desamido insulin, and HMWP content and the physical stability of I-LMWC PEC preparations. In addition, the stability of insulin at different concentrations (0.9–10 mg/mL) in water and Tris-buffer at pH 6.5 was investigated at 50 °C.

## 3.10. Immunological Bioactivity of Insulin

Enzyme-linked immunosorbent assay (ELISA) was used to assess the immunological stability of insulin following formulation. Active insulin ELISA DSL-10-1600 micro-titration kits (Diagnostic Systems Laboratories Inc., Webster, TX, USA) were used. Insulin concentration was measured using an enzymatically amplified "one-step" sandwich–type immunoassay. The samples were incubated with an anti-insulin antibody in micro-titration wells that had been coated with another anti-insulin antibody. Insulin was extracted from the I-LMWC PEC (3.5/1.5 mg/mL) preparations of different molecular weight (1.3, 6, 13, 18, and 30 kDa), as described above, and then assayed according to the instructions of the manufacturer. The results were obtained by reading the optical density at 450 nm with background wavelength correction at 620 nm using a Bio-Rad microplate reader (Bio-Rad, Hercules, CA, USA).

## 3.11. Characterization of I-LMWC PEC

Particle size measurements were undertaken by dynamic light scattering using a Zetasizer Nano ZS instrument (Malvern, UK). Replicate measurements ($n = 6$) were carried out at 25 °C using a detection angle of 90°.

Zeta potential measurements ($n = 3$) were also carried out using the Zetasizer Nano ZS instrument at 25 °C using folded capillary cells integrated with gold electrodes.

I-LMWC PECs were centrifuged at 14,000 rpm for 30 min at room temperature. The quantity of insulin in the supernatants was measured using HPLC and the insulin association efficiency was calculated accordingly [14]. The number of replicates was 3 for each experiment.

## 3.12. In Vitro Evaluation of I-LMWC PEC and I-LMWC RM

### 3.12.1. In Vitro Release

The in vitro release studies of insulin from I-LMWC RM were performed by incubating in a simulated gastric medium at pH 1.2 and a simulated intestinal medium, pH 6.8, (1% bile salt v/w) at 37 °C under continuous shaking at 50 rpm. Samples were withdrawn at specific time intervals (1, 2, 3, 4, 5, and 6 h), centrifuged, and analyzed for insulin release using the USP HPLC method [16].

### 3.12.2. In Vitro Evaluation of the Protective Effect

A sample of 5 mL simulated gastric fluid (SGF) with pepsin (pH 1.2) was added to a 1 mL sample of free insulin solution, I-LMWC PEC solution, and a 2.0 g sample of I-LMWC PEC solubilized in the RM system. The samples were incubated for 1 h at 37 °C while shaking at 100 strokes/min. A 1.5 g sample of the RM was mixed with 5 mL of extraction solution of 0.010 M HCl and methanol (2/3, v/v), vortexed for 3 min, and a 100 µL sample of the aqueous layer was analyzed for insulin content by HPLC [16]. For insulin and I-LMWC PEC solutions, 100 μL samples were withdrawn after 1 h and analyzed for insulin content.

## 3.13. In Vivo Pharmacological Activity

Animal studies were conducted using adult male Sprague Dawley rats (body weight range 250–300 g) randomized into groups ($n = 10$). The animals were housed in air conditioned quarters under a photoperiod schedule of 12 h light/12 h dark cycles. The rats received standard laboratory chow and tap water 3 weeks prior to the experiments. Animal care and use was performed in compliance with the guidelines of the Federation of European Laboratory Animal Science Association and European Union (Council Directive 86/609/EEC). The study protocol was approved by the Ethical Committee of the Jordanian Pharmaceutical Manufacturing Company (JPM), Naor, Jordan. Diabetes was induced in male Sprague Dawley rats by intraperitoneal injection of two doses of 80 mg/kg streptozotocin (STZ) over two days. STZ was freshly prepared by dissolving in 0.1 M citrate buffer, pH 4.5. Blood glucose levels were monitored by measuring the glucose concentrations in blood samples obtained from the tail vein of rats using a blood glucose meter (Gluco Dr. All Medicus, Korea, range 112–444 mg/dL). Only rats with a basal blood glucose level above 200 mg/dL were considered diabetic.

STZ diabetic rats ($n = 10$) were randomized into different groups. Following initial blood glucose determinations, one group was injected with 2 IU/kg insulin and served as a positive control for insulin bioactivity. The other groups were given single an oral dose administration (50 IU/kg) of a blank control (same RM components, but without insulin), oral insulin solution, and I-LMWC RM. Blood sampling for glucose measurements proceeded during the experiments at specific time intervals (1, 2, 3, 4, 5, 6, 8, 12, and 18 h) post insulin administration.

## 4. Conclusions

The insulin USP compendium method for insulin analysis and HMWPs can be used to evaluate insulin stability in a delivery system containing insulin as well as I-LMWC PEC. Insulin stability was evaluated for insulin content, formation of HMWPs, and biological activity. In the literature, minimal studies are available covering these three elements, especially formation of HMWPs, which are very important in evaluating the suitability of the delivery system. Extraction procedures must be carefully carried out in order not to affect insulin results. Retention time optimization is important and currently insulin analysis can be executed within 20–30 min with such a convenient HPLC method. Based on stability studies, solutions of 3.5 mg/mL insulin and 1.5 mg/mL 13 kDa LMWC constitute the optimum stability formulation of the I-LMWC PEC for orally delivered insulin. Our experimental design allowed for the optimization of insulin formulation by determining parameters that affect the chemical and physical stability of insulin. The I-LMWC PEC preparation method has the advantage of not necessitating sonication and use of organic solvents during preparation, thereby minimizing possible degradation of insulin. The I-LMWC PEC system has been characterized in terms of insulin stability, where the study revealed that complexation with LMWC improves the stability of insulin. Both ELISA and *in vivo* studies confirmed the bioactivity of loaded insulin in the delivery system examined.

**Acknowledgments**

The animal work was conducted by Nidal A. Qinna form Petra University/Jordan.

**Author Contributions**

Adnan A. Badwan, Babur Z. Chowdhry and Stephen A. Leharne conceived and designed the experiments; Zakieh I. Al-Kurdi performed the experiments; Zakieh I. Al-Kurdi and Mahmoud M.H. Al Omari analyzed the data; Adnan A. Badwan contributed reagents/materials/analysis tools; Zakieh I. Al-Kurdi and Mahmoud M.H. Al Omari wrote the paper.

**Conflicts of Interest**

The authors declare no conflict of interest.

**References**

1.  Hiroyuki, H.; Tsutomu, A.; Kentaro, S. Effect of additives on protein aggregation. *Curr. Pharm. Biotechnol.* **2009**, *19*, 400–407.
2.  Aranaz, I.; Harris, R.; Heras, A. Chitosan amphiphilic derivatives chemistry and applications. *Curr. Org. Chem.* **2010**, *14*, 308–330.
3.  Junginger, H.E. Polymeric permeation enhancers. In *Oral Delivery of Macromolecular Drugs*; Bernkop-Schnürch, A., Ed.; Springer Dordrecht Heidelberg: New York, NY, USA, 2009; pp. 103–136.
4.  Mao, S.; Germershaus, O.; Fischer, D.; Linn, T.; Schnepf, R.; Kissel, T. Uptake and transport of PEG-graft-trimethyl-chitosan copolymer-insulin nanocomplexes by epithelial cells. *Pharm. Res.* **2005**, *22*, 2058–2068.
5.  Sadeghi, A.M.; Dorkoosh, F.A.; Avadi, M.R.; Saadat, P.; Rafiee-Tehrani, M.; Junginger, H.E. Preparation, characterization and antibacterial activities of chitosan, *N*-trimethyl chitosan (TMC) and *N*-diethylmethyl chitosan (DEMC) nanoparticles loaded with insulin using both the ionotropic gelation and polyelectrolyte complexation methods. *Int. J. Pharm.* **2008**, *355*, 299–306.
6.  Berger, J.; Reist, M.; Mayer, J.; Flet, O.; Gurny, R. Structure and interactions in chitosan hydrogels formed by complexation or aggregation for biomedical application, *Eur. J. Pharm. Biopharm.* **2004**, 57, 35–52.
7.  Schatz, C.; Bionaz, A.; Lucas, J.M.; Pichot, C.; Viton, C.; Domard, A.; Delair, T. Formation of polyelectrolyte complex particles from self-complexation of N-sulfated chitosan. *Biomacromolecules* **2009**, *10*, 1402–1409.

8. Mao, S.; Bakowsky, U.; Jintapattanakit, A.; Kissel, T. Self-assembled polyelectrolyte nanocomplexes between chitosan derivatives and insulin. *J. Pharm. Sci.* **2006**, *95*, 1035–1048.

9. Lin, Y.H.; Mi, F.L.; Chen, C.T.; Chang, W.C.; Peng, S.F.; Liang, H.F.; Sung, H.W.Y. Preparation and characterization of nanoparticles shelled with chitosan for oral insulin delivery. *Biomacromolecules* **2007**, *8*, 146–152.

10. Jintapattanakit, A.; Junyaprasert, V.B.; Mao, S.; Sitterberg, J.; Bakowsky, U.; Kissel, T. Peroral delivery of insulin using chitosan derivatives: A comparative study of polyelectrolyte nanocomplexes and nanoparticles. *Int. J. Pharm.* **2007**, *342*, 240–249.

11. Song, L.; Zhi, Z.L.; Pickup, J.C. Nanolayer encapsulation of insulin-chitosan complexes improves efficiency of oral insulin delivery. *Int. J. Nanomedicine* **2014**, *9*, 2127–2136.

12. Tozaki, H.; Komoike, J.; Tada, C.; Maruyama, T.; Terabe, A.; Suzuki, T.; Yamamoto, A.; Muranishi, S. Chitosan capsules for colon-specific drug delivery: Improvement of insulin absorption from the rat colon. *J. Pharm. Sci.* **1997**, *86*, 1016–1021.

13. Badwan, A.A.; Al-Remawi, M.; El-Thaher, T.; Elsayed, A. Oral delivery of protein drugs using microemulsion. EP1797870, 20 June 2007.

14. Elsayed, A.; Remawi, M.A.; Qinna, N.; Farouk, A.; Badwan, A. Formulation and characterization of an oily-based system for oral delivery of insulin. *Eur. J. Pharm. Biopharm.* **2009**, *73*, 269–279.

15. Assaf, S.M.; Al Jbour, N.D.; Eftaiha, A.F.; Elsayed, A.M.; Al Remawi, M.M.; Qinna, N.A.; Chowdhry, B.; Leharne, S.; Badwan, A.A. Factors involved in formulation for proteins based on PEG-8 caprylic/capric glycerides and polyglyceryl-6-diolate in a mixture of oleic acid with chitosan. *J. Dispers. Sci. Technol.* **2011**, *32*, 623–633.

16. Insulin Human Monograph. In *United States Pharmacopeia*; Unites States Pharmacopeia Convention: Rockville, MD, USA, 2013; pp. 3913–3914.

17. Smith, D.J.; Venable, R.M.; Collins, J. Separation and quantitation of insulins and related substances in bulk insulin crystals and in injectables by reversed-phase high performance liquid chromatography and the effect of temperature on the separation. *J. Chromatogr. Sci.* **1985**, *23*, 81–88.

18. Zhang, K.; Quan, C.; Huang, H.; Taulier, N.; Wu, X.Y. On the stability of insulin delivered through a new glucose-responsive polymeric composite membrane. *J. Pharm. Pharmacol.* **2004**, *56*, 611–620.

19. Bilati. U.; Allemann, E.; Doelker, E. Strategic approaches for overcoming peptide and protein instability within biodegradable nano- and microparticles. *Eur. J. Pharm. Biopharm.* **2005**, *59*, 375–388.

20. ORA Laboratory Procedure. USFDA. Available online: http://www.fda.gov/ScienceResearch/FieldScience/ucm171877.htm (accessed on 6 August 2013).

21. Sarmento, B.; Ribeiro, A.; Veiga, F.; Ferreira, D. Development and validation of a rapid reversed-phase HPLC method for the determination of insulin from nanoparticulate systems. *Biomed. Chromatogr.* **2006**, *20*, 898–903.

22. Iwasa, S.; Enomoto, A.; Onoue, S.; Nakai, M.; Yajima, T.; Fukushima, T. Chromatographic analysis of conformationally changed insulin and its cytotoxic effect on PC12 cells. *J. Health Sci.* **2009**, *55*, 825–831.

23. Hansen, J.F. The self-association of zinc-free human insulin and insulin analogue B13-glutamine. *Biophys. Chem.* **1991**, *39*, 107–110.

24. Hvidt, S. Insulin association in neutral solution studied by light scattering. *Biophys. Chem.* **1991**, *39*, 205–213.

25. Sluzky, V.; Klibanov, A.M.; Langer, R. Mechanism of insulin aggregation and stabilization in agitated aqueous solutions. *Biotechnol. Bioeng.* **1992**, *40*, 895–903.

26. Dathe, M.; Gast, K.; Zirwer, D.; Welfle, H.; Mehlis, B. Insulin aggregation in solution. *Int. J. Pept. Protein Res.* **1990**, *36*, 344–349.

27. Ugwu, S.O.; Apte, S.P. The effect of buffers on protein conformational stability. *Pharm. Technol.* **2004**, *9*, 86–113.

28. Brange, J.; Owens, D.R.; Kang, S.; Vølund, A. Monomeric insulin and their experimental and clinical implications. *Diabetes Care* **1990**, *13*, 923–954.

29. Brange, J.; Havelund, S.; Hougaard, P. Chemical stability of insulin. 2. Formation of higher molecular weight transformation products during storage of pharmaceutical preparations. *Pharm. Res.* **1992**, *9*, 727–734.

30. Robbins, D.C.; Cooper, S.M.; Fineberg, S.E.; Mead, P.M. Antibodies to covalent aggregates of insulin in blood of insulin-using diabetic patients. *Diabetes* **1987**, *36*, 838–841.

31. Ratner, R.E.; Phillips, T.M.; Steiner, M. Persistent cutaneous insulin allergy resulting from high-molecular-weight insulin aggregates. *Diabetes* **1990**, *39*, 728–733.

32. Mansur, H.S.; Oréfice, R.L.; Vasconcelos, W.L.; Lobato, Z.P.; Machado, L.J. Biomaterial with chemically engineered surface for protein immobilization. *J. Mater. Sci. Mater Med.* **2005**, *16*, 333–340.

33. Gander, B.; Wehrli, E.; Alder, R.; Merkle, H.P. Quality improvement of spray-dried, protein-loaded D,L-PLA microspheres by appropriate polymer solvent selection. *J. Microencapsul.* **1995**, *12*, 83–97.

34. Cleland, J.L.; Mac, A.; Boyd, B.; Yang, J.; Duenas, E.T.; Yeung, D.; Brooks, D.; Hsu, C.; Chu, H.; Mukku, V.; *et al.* The stability of recombinant human growth hormone in poly(lactic-co-glycolic acid) (PLGA) microspheres. *Pharm. Res.* **1997**, *14*, 420–425.

35. Petersen, H.; Kunath, K.; Martin, A.L.; Stolnik, S.; Roberts, C.J.; Davies, M.C.; Kissel, T. Star-shaped poly(ethylene glycol)-block-polyethylenimine copolymers enhance DNA condensation of low molecular weight polyethylenimines. *Biomacromolecules* **2002**, *3*, 926–936.

36. Tsaih, M.L.; Chen, R.H. Effect of molecular weight and urea on the conformation of chitosan molecules in dilute solutions. *Int. J. Biol. Macromol.* **1997**, *20*, 233–240.

37. Verma, A.; Verma, A. Polyelectrolyte complex–An overview. *Int. J. Pharm. Sci. Res.* **2013**, *4*, 1684–1691.

38. Borchard, G.; Luessen, H.L.; Boer, A.G.; Verhoef, J.C.; Lehr, C.M.; Junginger, H.E. The potential of mucoadhesive polymers in enhancing intestinal peptide drug absorption .3. Effect of chitosan-glutamate and carbomer on epithelial tight junctions *in vitro*. *J. Control. Release* **1996**, *39*, 131–138.

39. Ma, Z.H.; Yeoh, H.; Lim, L.Y. Formulation pH modulates the interaction of insulin with chitosan nanoparticles. *J. Pharm. Sci.* **2002**, *91*, 1396–1404.

40. Lee, D.W.; Lim, C.; Israelachrili, J.; Hwang, D.S. Strong adhesion and cohesion of chitosan in aqueous solutions. *Langmuir* **2013**, *29*, 14222–14229.

41. Anderson, B.D.; Darrington, R.T. Evidence for a common intermediate in insulin deamidation and covalent dimer formation: Effects of pH and aniline trapping in dilute acidic solutions. *J. Pharm. Sci.* **1995**, *84*, 275–282.

42. Kabanov, V.A. Basic properties of soluble interpolyelectrolyte complexes applied to bioengineering and cell transformation. In *Macromolecular Complexes in Chemistry and Biology*; Dubin, P., Bock, J., Davis, R., Schulz, D.N., Thies, C., Ed.; Springer-Verlag: Berlin, Germany, 1994; pp. 151–174.

43. Wu, Y.; Yang, W.; Wang, C.; Hu, J.; Fu, S. Chitosan nanoparticles as a novel delivery system for ammonium glycyrrhizinate. *Int. J. Pharm.* **2005**, *295*, 235–245.

44. Kasaai, M.R. Calculation of Mark-Houwink-Sakurada (MHS) equation viscometric constants for chitosan in any solvent-temperature system using experimental reported viscometric constant data. *Carbohydr. Polym.* **2007**, *68*, 477–488.

45. Verification of compendial procedures <1226>. In *United States Pharmacopeia*; Unites States Pharmacopeia Convention: Rockville, MD, USA, 2013.

46. *Validation of Analytical Methods*; European Medicine Agency (EMA): London, UK, 1995.

# Chapter III:
# Others

# Bioproduction of Chitooligosaccharides:
# Present and Perspectives

**Woo-Jin Jung and Ro-Dong Park**

**Abstract:** Chitin and chitosan oligosaccharides (COS) have been traditionally obtained by chemical digestion with strong acids. In light of the difficulties associated with these traditional production processes, environmentally compatible and reproducible production alternatives are desirable. Unlike chemical digestion, biodegradation of chitin and chitosan by enzymes or microorganisms does not require the use of toxic chemicals or excessive amounts of wastewater. Enzyme preparations with chitinase, chitosanase, and lysozymeare primarily used to hydrolyze chitin and chitosan. Commercial preparations of cellulase, protease, lipase, and pepsin provide another opportunity for oligosaccharide production. In addition to their hydrolytic activities, the transglycosylation activity of chitinolytic enzymes might be exploited for the synthesis of desired chitin oligomers and their derivatives. Chitin deacetylase is also potentially useful for the preparation of oligosaccharides. Recently, direct production of oligosaccharides from chitin and crab shells by a combination of mechanochemical grinding and enzymatic hydrolysis has been reported. Together with these, other emerging technologies such as direct degradation of chitin from crustacean shells and microbial cell walls, enzymatic synthesis of COS from small building blocks, and protein engineering technology for chitin-related enzymes have been discussed as the most significant challenge for industrial application.

Reprinted from *Mar. Drugs*. Cite as: Jung, W.-J.; Park, R.-D. Bioproduction of Chitooligosaccharides: Present and Perspectives. *Mar. Drugs* **2014**, *12*, 5328-5356.

## 1. Introduction

Chitin and chitosan have numerous applications as functional materials, as these natural polymers have excellent properties such as biocompatibility, biodegradability, non-toxicity, and adsorption. Chitin from crustacean shells is commonly obtained using inorganic acids for demineralization, with strong alkali for deproteinization [1,2]. These chemical processes have several drawbacks, including being a source of pollution [3] and reduction of depolymerization, and thus, chitin quality [4,5].

These chemical processes can be replaced by biotechnological processing with microbes and their metabolites, including organic acids and enzymes, as shown in Figure 1. The strains most frequently applied include *Lactobacillus* sp. and *Serratia marcescens* [6,7]. Biofermentation of crab shell wastes with 10% inoculums of *S. marcescens* FS-3 resulted in 84% deproteinization and 47% demineralization after 7 days of incubation [8]. Co-fermentation of the bacteria *Lactobacillus paracasei* KCTC-3074 and *S. marcescens* FS-3 [6] and the successive two-step fermentation with the two bacteria [7] provided more promising results for the production of chitin from crab shells.

Chitin and chitosan are high molecular-weight polymers with poor solubility at neutral pH values. This property limits their potential uses in the fields of food, health, and agriculture.

However, these limitations may be overcome by the use of their oligomers or monomers. In humans, chitin monomers are precursors of the disaccharide units in glycosaminoglycans (such as hyaluronic acid, chondroitin sulfate, and keratin sulfate), which are necessary to repair and maintain healthy cartilage and joint function. Chitooligosaccharides (oligosaccharides derived mainly from chitin or chitosan, COS) have the potential ability to improve food quality [9–11] and human health [12,13].

COS mixtures can be prepared from chitosan by using different physical methods, like hydrothermal [14], microwave [15], ultra sonication [16] and gamma-rays [17]. Chemical methods using acid [18,19], $H_2O_2$ [20] or $NaNO_2$ [21], can yield COS. Of chemical methods for hydrolysis of chitosan [18–21], acid hydrolysis is probably the best known. Early studies had shown that fully deacetylated chitosan is degradedto COS in concentrated hydrochloric acid [18]. In later studies [19], using a variety of chitosans, the acid-catalyzed degradation rates of chitosans were shown to depend on degree of deacetylation (DD). Acid hydrolysis was found to be highly specific to cleavage of GlcNAc-GlcNAc and GlcNAc-GlcN and A-D glycosidic linkages, with two to three orders of magnitude higher rates than the GlcN-GlcN and GlcN-GlcNAc linkages. In the same study, it was shown that the rate of deacetylation was less than one-tenth of the rate of depolymerization in concentrated acid, whereas the two rates were found to be equal in dilute acid [19]. Even though acid hydrolysis has been commonly used to prepare COS, these chemical and physical methods escape from the scope of this review and will not be dealt with more.

Enzymatic hydrolysis of chitin and chitosan has been proposed as an alternative method during the past few decades. Enzymes with hydrolytic activity on chitin and chitosan include chitinase, chitosanase, lysozyme, cellulase, pectinase, protease, lipase, and pepsin. These chitinolytic and chitosanolytic enzymes all have different modes of action and specificity for substrate size. A flow chart for the bioproduction of chitin, chitosan, and their oligosaccharides from natural resources by using enzymes and microorganisms is shown in Figure 1. Enzymatic hydrolysis seems to be generally preferable to chemical methods because the reaction is performed under more gentle conditions and the MW distribution of the product is more controllable [22,23]. However, production of well-defined COS in terms of length (degree of polymerization, DP), degree of de-N-acetylation (DD), and sequence (pattern of acetylation, PA) by enzymatic conversion processes is not straight forward [24]. The expensive cost of chitinases and chitosanases limits their wide application on an industrial scale, even using immobilized enzymes [22,25,26].

We are primarily concerned with the enzymatic hydrolysis of polysaccharides obtained from crustacean shells for the bioproduction of COS. In this review, we introduce the preparation and bioproduction of COS with enzymes from chitinase- and chitosanase-producing bacteria and fungi. Limitations and challenges in the bioproduction of COS are also discussed.

**Figure 1.** Flow chart for the bioproduction of chitin, chitosan, and their oligosaccharides from biological resources.

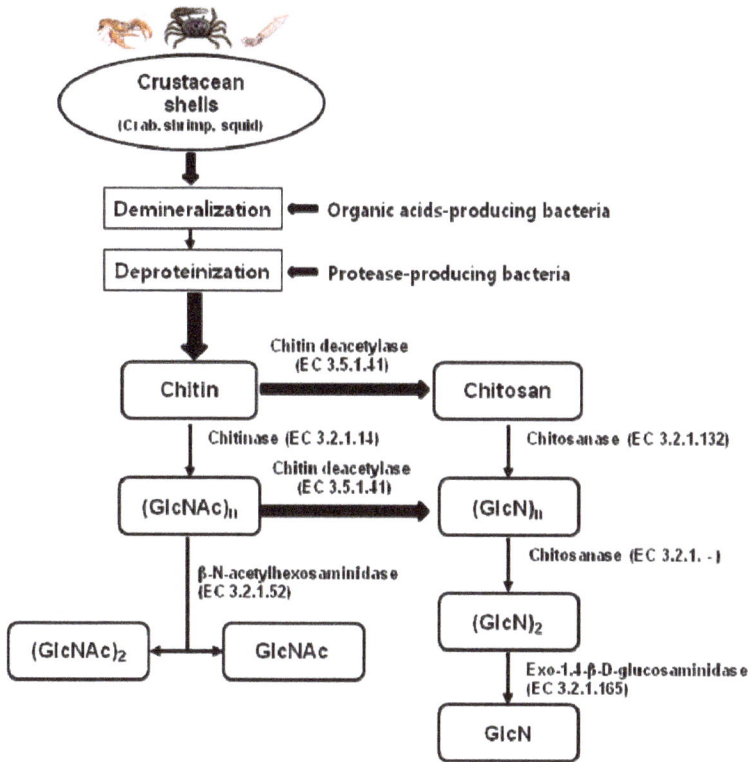

## 2. Bioproduction of Chitin Oligosaccharides and Its Monomer

Chitin oligosaccharides are produced from chitin by using chitinolytic enzymes. These enzymes hydrolyze the glycoside bonds between the sugars and are thus glycoside hydrolases (GH). GHs are classified in the Carbohydrate-Active enZYmes database (CAZy) [27–30]. The CAZy classification is purely based on the amino acid sequence similarity, which gives very useful information since sequence and structure, and hence mechanism, are related. In CAZy system, enzyme properties such as substrate and product activities, exo- *versus* endo-binding, processivity, and the presence of additional modules are not taken into account [27–30]. Chitinases occur in families GH18 and GH19 [31,32]. Chitinases have the unique ability to hydrolyze GlcNAc-GlcNAc bonds and this property discriminates these enzymes from chitosanases.

Chitinases can be classified into two major categories (endochitinases and exochitinases), according to their mode of action. First, endochitinases (EC 3.2.1.14; created 1961) cleave the linkage between GlcNAc-GlcNAc, GlcN-GlcNAc, and GlcNAc-GlcN in chitin chains to release smaller and more soluble chitin oligomers of variable size. Second, β-*N*-acetylhexosaminidase (EC 3.2.1.52; created 1972) includes subcategories of both chitobiase (EC 3.2.1.29; created 1961, deleted 1972) and β-D-acetylglucosaminidase (GlcNAcase, EC 3.2.1.30; created 1961, deleted

1992) [33]. Chitobiase catalyzes the progressive release of chitobiose starting at the nonreducing or reducing end of chitin. GlcNAcase progressively breaks down chitin polymer or chitin oligomers from the non-reducing or reducing end of the molecules, releasing β-D-GlcNAc or α-D-GlcNAc. These enzymes were prepared from bacteria and fungi, as shown in Table 1.

In COS production, it is practical to use crude enzyme preparations, such as microbial culture supernatants and their solid powders. Preparations of cellulase, protease, lipase, pepsin, chitinase, chitosanase, and lysozyme are mainly applied as commercial enzyme sources for the hydrolytic cleavage of chitin and chitosan (Table 1).

Pretreatment is necessary for enzymatic hydrolysis, because the strong crystallinity and insolubility of chitin in an aquatic environment. For example, chitin is normally treated with strong acids, such as hydrochloric acid (for colloidal chitin) [34] or phosphoric acid (for swollen chitin) [35] to break down crystal structure and increase the accessibility of the substrate to the enzyme. In contrast to chitin, chitosan is soluble in dilute mineral acids, thus forming salts with acids.

Enzymatic or chemical hydrolysis of chitin and chitosan results in a mixture of oligomers, not any specific oligomer, even with prolonged reaction time. Several techniques for separation and purification of COS have been reported, like gel filtration [36], ultrafiltration [37], and ion exchange [38] and metal affinity [39] chromatography. Preparative separation of COS is most commonly based on size, through size exclusion chromatography SEC). A SEC system using SuperdexTM 30 (GE Healthcare) columns, coupled in series, allowed separation of COS with similar DP values ranging from DP 2 to DP 20, independently of DD and PA [36]. Separation of COS can be achieved using cation-exchange chromatography, because protonated amino groups on the deacetylated sugars interact with the ion-exchange resin. With this method, COS of identical DP was separated based on the number of deacetylated units [38].

## 2.1. N-Acetyl-β-D-glucosamine

*N*-Acetyl-β-D-glucosamine (GlcNAc) was obtained with 85% yield from β- and α-chitin within 1 and 7 days, respectively, using chitinase from *Burkholderia cepacia* TU09 [40]. GlcNAc and *N,N'*-diacetylchitobiose [(GlcNAc)$_2$] were obtained 75% and 20% yield from β-chitin within 6 days using chitinase from *Bacillus licheniformis* SK-1. In addition, chitinase from SK-1 produced GlcNAc with 41% yield from α-chitin. In most cases, β-chitin from squid pen is a better substrate than α-chitin from crab or shrimp shells.

GlcNAc and *N*-acetyl chitooligosaccharides were produced from colloidal α-chitin using a crude enzyme from *Paenibacillus illinoisensis* KJA-424 [7]. The production rate of monomer GlcNAc increased continuously during incubation, while that of GlcNAc oligomers declined. The maximum production of GlcNAc was 1.71 mg mL$^{-1}$ (yield of 62.2%) after 24 h of incubation. At the same time (GlcNAc)$_2$, tri-*N*-acetylchitotriose [(GlcNAc)$_3$], hepta-*N*-acetylchitoheptaose [(GlcNAc)$_7$] and octa-*N*-acetylchitooctaose [(GlcNAc)$_8$] were 0.13 mg mL$^{-1}$ (yield of 4.9%), 0.03 mg mL$^{-1}$ (1.2%), 0.01 mg mL$^{-1}$ (4.1%), and 0.24 mg mL$^{-1}$ (9.6%), respectively.

Non-chitinase enzymes can be applied to the hydrolysis of chitin. GlcNAc was produced from α-chitin (from crab shell) and β-chitin (from squid pen) using crude cellulase preparations from *Trichoderma viride* (T) and *Acremonium cellulolyticus* (A) [41]. The yield of GlcNAc was enhanced by mixing cellulases T and A. Crystalline chitin (from bee) and α-chitin (from crab shell) were hydrolyzed with the enzymatic preparation Celloviridin G20x from strain *Trichoderma reesei*, which includes cellulases and β-glucanases [42]. After 10 days of incubation in these conditions, the yield of GlcNAc reached 86%.

The mixed enzymes (cellulase: lipase = 9:1) from *Aspergillus niger*, was used in various enzyme concentrations, to investigate the hydrolytic behavior on β-chitin [43]. Increasing substrate concentration while keeping the enzyme concentration constant resulted in higher GlcNAc yield. After 4 days of incubation, the yield of GlcNAc reached 61% from β-chitin (10 mg/mL).

Flake type of chitin together with swollen chitin, colloidal chitin, and powder chitin is also the substrate for the oligosaccharides production. GlcNAc was produced from crab shell α-chitin flake using crude enzyme extract from *Aeromonas hydrophila* H-2330, with 66%–77% yield after 10 days incubation at 17 °C [44].

Exo-type chitinases can use chitin oligosaccharides as a substrate. (GlcNAc)$_2$ was gradually and completely degraded to GlcNAc by exo-type chitinase (*ChiA*71) from *Bacillus thuringiensis* subsp. *pakistani* with time [45] and by *N*-acetyl-β-hexosaminidase (*StmHex*) from *Stenotrophomonas maltophilia* [46]. GlcNAc was produced from (GlcNAc)$_4$ by enzyme purified from *Aeromonas hydrophila* SUWA-9 [47].This kind of trial is not intended for the production of monomers, but for the elucidation of enzyme properties, as oligomers are much more expensive and valuable in application.

There are typical reports on the selective preparation of GlcNAc and (GlcNAc)$_2$ [48]. It was found that α-chitin was effectively hydrolyzed to (GlcNAc) by *Aeromonas* sp. GJ-18 crude enzyme preparation below 45 °C. The enzyme preparation from *Aeromonas* sp. GJ-18 contained GlcNAcase and *N,N*'-diacetylchitobiohydrolase [49]. GlcNAcase was inactive above 50 °C, but *N,N*'-diacetylchitobiohydrolase was stable at this temperature. Therefore, GlcNAc and (GlcNAc)$_2$ were selectively produced from α-chitin at two temperatures. At 45 °C, GlcNAc was the major hydrolytic product with a yield of 74% in 5 days' incubation, while at 55 °C (GlcNAc)$_2$ was the major product with a yield of 35% after 5 days' incubation.

**Table 1.** Bioproduction of chitin oligosaccharides and its monomer by microbial enzymes.

| Chitinsource | Enzyme Source | Enzyme | Mol. Wt. | Condition | Product & Yield | Analysis | Reference |
|---|---|---|---|---|---|---|---|
| Swollen chitin | Aeromonas sp. GJ-18 | Crude enzyme | - | 40 °C, 9 days | GlcNAc 94.9% | HPLC NH2P-50 4E | [48] |
| Swollen chitin | Aeromonas sp. GJ-18 | Crude enzyme | - | 45 °C, 5 days<br>55 °C, 5 days | GlcNAc 74%<br>(GlcNAc)$_2$ 4.8%<br>GlcNAc 3.9%<br>(GlcNAc)$_2$ 34.7% | HPLC NH2P-50 4E | [49] |
| α-Chitin<br>β-Chitin | Aeromonas sp. GJ-18 | Crude enzyme | - | Preincubation<br>(50 °C, 60 min)<br>45 °C, 7 days | (GlcNAc)$_2$ 78.9%<br>(GlcNAc)$_2$ 56.6% | HPLC NH2P-50 4E | [50] |
| α-Chitin<br>(Flake & powder) | A. hydrophila H-2330 | Crude enzyme | - | 17 °C, 10 days | GlcNAc 64~77% | HPLC NH2P-50 | [44] |
| Chitin | A. hydrophila SUWA-9 | Chitinase | - | 37 °C, overnight | (GlcNAc)$_2$-(GlcNAc)$_5$<br>GlcNAc | TLC | [47] |
| Chitosan (60% DD) | Bacillus cereus TKU027 | Chitinase<br>Culture supernatant | 65/63 kDa | 37 °C, 2 h<br>30 °C, 2 days | (GlcNAc/GlcN) DP<br>4~9<br>(GlcNAc/GlcN) DP<br>2~5 | MALDI-TOF MS | [44] |
| β-Chitin | Bacillus cereus TKU022 | Chitosanase | 44 kDa | 37 °C, 2 days | (GlcNAc)$_2$, (GlcNAc)$_4$<br>(GlcNAc)$_5$, (GlcNAc)$_6$ | HPLC | [51] |
| Colloidal chitin | Bacillus thuringiensis subsp. pakistani | Exochitinase | 66/60/47/32 kDa | 37 °C, 24 h | GlcNAc | TLC | [45] |
| α-Chitin<br>β-Chitin | Burkholderia cepacia TU09 | Chitinase | | 37 °C, 7 days<br>37 °C, 1 days | GlcNAc 85%<br>GlcNAc 85% | HPLCNH2P-50 | [40] |
| α-Chitin<br>β-Chitin | Bacillus licheniformis SK-1 | Chitinase | | 37 °C, 6 days | GlcNAc 41%<br>GlcNAc 75% | HPLCNH2P-50 | |

**Table 1.** *Cont.*

| Substrate | Organism | Enzyme | MW | Conditions | Product | Method | Ref. |
|---|---|---|---|---|---|---|---|
| Swollen chitin | *Paenibacillus illinoisensis* KJA-424 | Chitinase | 38/54/63 kDa | 37 °C, 24 h | GlcNAc 62.2% | HPLC | [7] |
| Chitin | *Trichoderma reesei* | Cellulases & β-glucanases | - | 37 °C, 10 days | GlcNAc 86% | TLC/HPLC Separon SGX NH2 | [42] |
| α-Chitin | *Trichoderma viride Acremonium cellulolyticus* | Cellulase | - | 37 °C, 3 days | GlcNAc 16% GlcNAc 22% | HPLC/NMR | [41] |
| β-Chitin | *Aspergillus niger* | Cellulose & lipase | - | 37 °C, 4 days | GlcNAc 61% | HPLC NH2P-50 | [43] |
| Chitin | *Thermococcus kodakaraensis* KOD1 | Chitinase | 90 kDa | 70 °C, 3 h | $(GlcNAc)_2$ | TLC | [52] |
| Chitin | *Vibrio anguillarum* E-383a | Exochitinase | - | - | $(GlcNAc)_2$ 40.3% | HPLC | [47] |
| Chitin Chitosan (80% DD) | *Enterobacter* sp. G1 | Chitosanase | 50 kDa | 35 °C, 5 min | $(GlcNAc)_2$ | TLC/HPLC | [53] |
| Chitin | *Corynebacterium* sp. | Chitobiase | - | 40 °C, 24 h | GlcNAc | HPLC/NMR | [54] |
| Chitin, steam exploded | *Lecanicillium lecanii* | Chitinase | - | 40 °C, 6 days | GlcNAcDP 1–9 | HPLC/ MALDI-TOF MS | [55] |
| $(GlcNAc)_2$, $(GlcNAc)_6$ | *Stenotrophomonas maltophilia* | N-acetyl-β-hexosaminidase & Chitin synthase | - | 40 °C, 60 min | GlcNAc | HPLC | [46] |

*2.2. N,N'-Diacetylchitobiose and Chitin Oligosaccharides*

As mentioned above, (GlcNAc)$_2$ can be obtained as a major hydrolytic product from enzymes by controlling the ratio of GlcNAcase to *N,N'*-diacetylchitobiohydrolase activities in the crude enzyme of *Aeromonas* sp. GJ-18 [50]. After 7 days of incubation, 78.9% and 56.6% of (GlcNAc)$_2$ yields were obtained from swollen α-chitin and powdered β-chitin, respectively, using enzyme preparations that had been pretreated at 50 °C so as to inactivate GlcNAcase.

There are a few more reports on bioproduction of (GlcNAc)$_2$. (GlcNAc)$_2$ was produced from colloidal chitin by chitinase from *Vibrio anguillarum* E-383a, isolated from seawater [56]. The maximum yield of (GlcNAc)$_2$ from chitin was 40.3%. (GlcNAc)$_2$ was produced by shrimp α-chitin (100~200 mesh) from commercial bovine pepsin [57]. The yield of (GlcNAc)$_2$ was 75%, while the yields of GlcNAc and (GlcNAc)$_3$ were 19% and 9.5%, respectively. Tanaka *et al.* [52] also identified (GlcNAc)$_2$ as an end product from colloidal chitin by using chitinase from the hyperthermophilic archaeon *Thermococcus kodakaraensis* KOD1.

The hydrolytic products of chitinase and GlcNAcase are mixtures of hetero-COS (DP 1–15), depending on reaction conditions. Hetero-oligosaccharides [(GlcNAc/GlcN) DP 2~5] were produced from chitosan (60% DD) by culture supernatant obtained from of *Bacillus cereus* TKU027. Chitin oligosaccharides [(GlcNAc/GlcN) DP 4~9] were produced by chitinase (65 and 63 kDa), and oligomers were identified using MALDI-TOF MS [58]. To analysis the distribution of chitin oligosaccharides, chitin oligosaccharides were derivatized with 9-aminopyrene-1,4,6-trisulfonate (APTS) and separated by capillary electrophoresis (CE) with laser-induced fluorescence (LIF) detection [59].

## 3. Bioproduction of Chitosan Oligosaccharides and Its Monomer

The most important tool in the biodegradation of chitosan to its oligosaccharides is chitosanolytic enzymes. The chitosanases have been prepared from various bacteria and fungi, as shown in Table 2. Chitosanases in glycoside hydrolase (GH) families 5, 7, 8, 46, 75, and 80 [27–30], have been classified into subclasses I, II, and III based on their substrate specificities toward chitosan [19,60–63]. Class I chitosanases can hydrolyze both GlcNAc–GlcN and GlcN–GlcN linkages, and class II chitosanases can split only GlcN–GlcN linkages, whereas class III chitosanases can degrade both GlcN–GlcNAc and GlcN–GlcN linkages. Chitosanases can also be classified into two major categories (endochitosanases and exochitosanases), according to their cleavage sites. Endochitosanases (EC 3.2.1.132; created 1990, modified 2004) cleave a partly acetylated chitosan at random and produces COS. Exochitosanases are usually called exo-1,4-β-D-glucosaminidase (GlcNase, EC 3.2.1.165; created 2008), which cleaves β-D-glucosamine (GlcN) residues continuously from the non-reducing end of the substrate ([33].

**Table 2.** Bioproduction of chitosan oligosaccharides and its monomer by microbial enzymes.

| Chitosan Source | Enzyme Source | Enzyme | Mol. Wt. | Condition | Product & Yield | Analysis | Reference |
|---|---|---|---|---|---|---|---|
| Chitosan | *Bacillus* sp. KCTC 0377BP | Chitosanase | 45 kDa | 1700 (unit/mg) | $(GlcN)_3$–$(GlcN)_7$ | TLC/HPLC | [64] |
| Chitosan | *Bacillus cereus* S1 | Chitosanase | 45 kDa | 40 °C, 20 min | $(GlcN)_2$ 27.2% $(GlcN)_3$ 40.6% $(GlcN)_4$ 32.2% | HPLC | [65] |
| Chitosan | *Bacillus* sp. 16 | Chitosanase | - | 37 °C, 30 min | DP 2–9 (DP 5–6) | TLC/HPLC | [66] |
| Chitosan | *Bacillus* sp. KFB-C108 | Chitosanase | 48 kDa | 55 °C, 12 h | $(GlcN)_3$–$(GlcN)_5$ | HPLC | [67] |
| Chitosan | *Bacillus* sp. HW-002 | Chitosanase | 46 kDa | 40 °C, 5 h | $(GlcN)_2$ | HPLC | [68] |
| Chitosan | *Bacillus pumilus* BN-262 | Chitosanase | - | 45 °C, 1 h | $(GlcN)_4$–$(GlcN)_6$ $(GlcN)_5$–$(GlcN)_7$ | HPLC ($NH_2$-60) Bio-Gel P-4gel | [69] |
| Chitosan | *Bacillus megaterium* P1 | Chitosanase (A/B/C) | 43/39.5/22 kDa | 28 °C, 12 h/90 h | $(GlcN)_n$ oligomers | TLC | [70] |
| Chitosan | *Acinetobacter* sp. CHB101 | Chitosanase I (endo) Chitosanase II (endo) | 37 k Da 30 kDa | 37 °C, overnight | $>(GlcN)_5$ | TLC | [71] |
| Chitosan (60% DD) | *Acinetobacter calcoaceticus* TKU024 | Chitosanase (CHSA1) Chitosanase (CHSA2) | 27 kDa 66 kDa | 37 °C, 30min | $(GlcN)_n$ oligomers | - | [72] |
| Chitosan | *Nocardia orientalis* IFO 12806 | Chitosanase (exo) | 97 kDa (70 kDa) | 40 °C, 24 h | GlcN | TLC/HPLC | [73] |
| Chitosan | *Matsuebacter chitosanotabidus* 3001 | Chitosanase | 34 kDa | 30 °C, 10 min | $(GlcN)_2$–$(GlcN)_6$ | TLC | [74] |
| Chitosan | *Aspergillus fumigatus* KH-94 | Chitosanase I (endo) Chitosanase II (exo) | 22.5 kDa 108 kDa | 50 °C, 30 min 50 °C, 5 min | DP 3–6 50% & >DP7 50% GlcN | TLC/HPLC | [75] |
| Chitosan | *Aspergillus fumigates* S-26 | Chitosanase | 104 kDa | 37 °C, 30 min | GlcN $(GlcN)_2$–$(GlcN)_7$ | TLC/HPLC | [76] |
| Chitosan | *Aspergillus oryzae* IAM2660 | Chitosanase(endo) Chitosanase (exo) | 40 kDa 135 kDa | 37 °C, 20 min 40 °C, overnight | >DP 5 GlcN | TLC | [77] |
| Chitosan | *Trichoderma reesei* PC-3-7 | Chitosanase | 93 kDa | 37 °C, 15 h | GlcN | TLC | [78] |
| Chitosan | - | Immobilized papain | - | - | MW < 10,000 49.5% MW 600–2000 11.1% | MALDI-TOF MS | [79] |
| Chitosan(82.8% DD) | - | Novozyme lipase | - | 37 °C, 24 h | DP 1–6 | TLC | [80] |
| Chitosan (76% DD) | Commercial enzymes | Complex (cellulase, α-amylase, proteinase) | - | 40 °C, 40 min | DP 5–17 | MALDI-TOF-MS | [81] |
| Chitosan (95% DD) | *Bacillus cereus* TNU-FC-4 | Chitosanase | 46 kDa | 45 °C, 33 min | >DP 7 | HPLC | [25] |
| *Rhizopus oligosporus* cell wall | *Streptomyces* sp. N174 | Chitosanase | - | 40 °C, 24 h | $(GlcN)_2$, GlcN-GlcNAc, $(GlcN)_2$-GlcNAc | CP/MAS NMR/ MALDI-TOF-MS | [82] |
| Chitosan | *Rhodothermus obamensis* | Branchzyme | 256 kDa | 50 °C, 24 h | DP 2–20 | GC-FID/SEC-HPLC | [83] |
| Chitosan (60% DD) | *Penicillium janthinellum* D4 | Chitosanase | 49 kDa | 50 °C, 60 h | DP 3–9 | MALDI-TOF-MS | [84] |

It is easier and more efficient to cleave the β-1,4-glycosidic linkages in chitosan than in chitin, because of its solubility in weakly acidic solutions. Chitosan, being a base, can be solubilized in both inorganic and organic acids, forming salts with acids. Acetic, lactic, and citric acids have all been used to facilitate enzyme hydrolysis. The solubility of chitosan depends on the molecular weight and degree of N-acetylation of the chitosan, concentration of the acid, and temperature. Homogeneous deacetylation of chitin to chitosan (approximately 50% DD) gives a water-soluble polymer.

The solubilized chitosan salt is a preferred substrate for chitosanases in homogeneous aqueous acids. Thus, chitosan is more rapidly hydrolyzed and gives a higher yield than chitin, which is not soluble and heterogeneous in aqueous environment. The products of the hydrolysis reaction of chitosan salt are accordingly the salt of its oligosaccharides. This means that a desalting process is necessary to obtain a pure oligosaccharide. Desalting is a rather complicated and costly process. In commercial products, the content has been expressed as being the salt of acetic, lactic, and citric acid of the oligosaccharides. Glucosamine is supplied in the marketplace as a dietary supplement in the form of a hydrochloric or sulfuric salt.

## 3.1. β-D-Glucosamine

The hydrolytic products of chitosan are mixtures of COS (DP 1–7), dependent on the reaction conditions, even though the monomer becomes a major end product after prolonged reaction time. Thus, chromatographic separation is necessary to purify each monomer, same as in chitin oligosaccharides. The enzymatic preparation of chitosan oligosaccharides is summarized in Table 2.

Koji mold *Aspergillus oryzae* is a strong producer of two different chitosanolytic enzymes, endochitosanase and exochitosanase (β-GlcNase). β-D-Glucosamine (GlcN) was produced as a final product from chitosan by a 135-kDa exochitosanase purified from *A. oryzae* IAM2660 [77]. In addition, chitosan oligosaccharides over DP 7 were produced from chitosan by a 40-kDa endochitosanase purified from *A. oryzae*. GlcN was produced from soluble chitosan by a 104-kDa exochitosanase purified from *A. fumigates* S-26 [76]. GlcN was produced from chitosan by a 108-kDa exochitosanase II purified from *A. fumigatus* KH-94 [75].

Chitosan oligosaccharides can be applied for chitosanase as a substrate, not for mass production of glucosamine but for elucidation of the reaction mechanism of chitosanase. GlcN resulted from the hydrolysis of chitobiose, chitopentose, and chitosan from the 79-kDa GlcNase of *Nocardia orientalis* IFO 12806 [73]. GlcN was also the final product from $(GlcN)_6$ by the 93-kDa chitosanase purified from *Trichoderma reesei* PC-3-7 [78]. $(GlcN)_6$ appeared to be hydrolyzed to $GlcN_5$ and GlcN at the initial stage of the reaction.

## 3.2. Chitobiose and Chitosan Oligosaccharides

There are a few studies on the bioproduction of chitobiose $(GlcN)_2$. Chitobiosewas produced from chitosan (75%~85% DD) in a mixture by chitosanase from *Bacillus cereus* S1 [65]. The composition of chitobiose, chitotriose, and chitotetraose was 27.2%, 40.6%, and 32.2%, respectively, after a 24-h reaction with a 45-kDa chitosanase. Chitobiose and chitotriose were produced from chitopentose and chitosan by crude proteins from *Acinetobacter* sp. CHB101 [71].

In the case of the 22.5-kDa endochitosanase purified from *Aspergillus fumigatus* KH-94, chitobiose, chitotriose, and chitotetraose were produced from chitohexaose [75]. In addition, chitosan oligomers of DP 3~6 (50% yield) and over DP 7 (50% yield) were produced from chitosan by the 22.5-kDa chitosanase.

These enzyme preparations contained endochitosanase activity. The endo-type activity is responsible for the production of chitosan oligosaccharides. Endo-type chitosanase is a major contributor to decreasing the viscosity of the reaction solution and fouling of the membrane reactor system [69]. The viscosity of high molecular weight material such as chitosan is involved in producing shearing forces in reactors, changes in enzyme-substrate affinity, and the fouling problem. When mixed with endochitosanase, the viscosity of chitosan decreased rapidly in accordance with production of the oligomers.

Thus, a great deal of interest has arisen regarding the reaction pattern of the endochitosanases. The chitosanase from *Bacillus* sp. KCTC 0377BP cleaved $(GlcN)_6$ mainly into $(GlcN)_3$ plus $(GlcN)_3$ and to a lesser extent into $(GlcN)_2$ plus $(GlcN)_4$ [subsequently, $(GlcN)_4 \rightarrow (GlcN)_2 + (GlcN)_2$] [64]. $(GlcN)_7$ was cleaved into $(GlcN)_3$ plus $(GlcN)_4$ [subsequently, $(GlcN)_4 \rightarrow (GlcN)_2 + (GlcN)_2$]. The purified endochitosanase (41-kDa) from *Bacillus cereus* D-11 hydrolyzed chito-oligomers $(GlcN)_{5-7}$ into chitobiose, chitotriose and chitotetraose as the final products [85]. Minimal size of the oligosaccharides for enzymatic hydrolysis was pentamer. To further investigate the cleavage pattern of this enzyme, chitooligosaccharide alcohols (COS with the reducing unit converted into alditol) were prepared and used as substrates. The chitosanase split $(GlcN)_4 GlcNOH$ into $(GlcN)_3 + (GlcN)_1 GlcNOH$, and $(GlcN)_5 GlcNOH$ into $(GlcN)_4 + (GlcN)_1 GlcNOH$ and $(GlcN)_3 + (GlcN)_2 GlcNOH$. The heptamer $(GlcN)_6 GlcNOH$ was split into $(GlcN)_5$ [subsequently, $(GlcN)_5 \rightarrow (GlcN)_3 + (GlcN)_2$] + $(GlcN)_1 GlcNOH$, $(GlcN)_4 + (GlcN)_2 GlcNOH$, and $(GlcN)_3 + (GlcN)_3 GlcNOH$, whereas $(GlcN)_{1-3} GlcNOH$ were not hydrolyzed. The monomer GlcNor GlcNOH was never detected from the enzyme reaction. These results suggest that D-11 chitosanase recognizes three glucosamine residues in minus position and simultaneously two residues in plus position from the cleavage point [85].

Chitobiose as a main end product was produced from chitosan by a 46-kDa chitosanase purified from *Bacillus* sp. HW-002 [68]. A 34-kDa chitosanase purified from *Matsuebacter chitosanotabidus* 3001 was cleaved mainly $(GlcN)_5$ and $(GlcN)_6$ into $(GlcN)_2$ plus $(GlcN)_3$ [74]. Chitosan oligosaccharides $[(GlcN)_{2-6}]$ were produced from chitosan by the purified chitosanase.

Pantaleone *et al.* [86] reported the hydrolytic susceptibility of chitosan to a wide range of enzymes, including glycanases, proteases, and lipases derived from bacterial, fungal, mammalian, and plant sources. These nonspecific enzymes have proven hydrolytic ability on chitosan to produce various chitosan oligomers in immobilized papain [79], lysozyme [87], and pronase [88]. Xie *et al.* [89] reported that chitosan (80% DD) was depolymerized by the cellulase of *Aspergillus niger* to give COS with DP 3–11. Mixture of cellulase, α-amylase and proteinasewas effective in the production of COS (DP 5~17) [81]. This finding presents another opportunity in the industrial scale production of COS, because these enzymes are active enough, commercially available, cheaper than chitosanase, and easy to handle. A commercial lipase was also applied for enzymatic preparation of COS, where COS with DP 1–6 was produced with 93.8% yield for 24 h hydrolysis at 37 °C [80]. Recently, the commercial α-amylase was used to hydrolyze chitosan from *Clanis bilineata* larvae skin under the optimal pH and temperature, thereby affording COS with a DP 2–8 [90].

Most chitosanase-producing bacteria require chitosan as a carbon/nitrogen source and chitosanase-inducer. Thus, one can get COS from the culture supernatant of the microorganism. Reducing COS sugars from shellfish waste were produced in the culture supernatant of *Acinetobacter calcoaceticus* TKU024, including chitosanases (CHSA1 and CHSA2) after 5 days of incubation [72]. Even though the yield of this method is very low, this kind of trial could be considered as a stepping stone to the direct extraction of COS from bio resources.

Intact cells of *Rhizopus oligosporus* NRRL2710were digested with a GH-46 chitosanase from *Streptomyces* sp. N174 [82]. Valuable hetero- and homo-oligosaccharides GlcN–GlcNAc, (GlcN)$_2$–GlcNAc, and (GlcN)$_2$ were produced, functionally, by the enzymatic digestion of the intact cells. The chitosanase digestion of intact fungal cells should be an excellent system for bioconversion of abundant microbial biomass without any environmental impact.

## 4. Chitin Deacetylase and Chitooligosaccharides

The chemical conversion from chitin to chitosan, the most difficult and cost-demanding step, has been done with 50% NaOH and high temperature in industrial applications. In nature, this step occurs at comparatively lower temperatures and neutral pH, by chitin deacetylase (CDA, EC 3.5.1.41; created 1976) [91]. The enzyme hydrolyzes the linkage between the acetyl group and the amine group in *N*-acetyl-D-glucosamine residues of chitin. Thus, bioconversion of chitin oligosaccharides to chitosan oligosaccharides can be achieved by CDA and *vice versa*.

Chitin deacetylase from *Absidia corymbifera* DY-9 was active towards water-soluble chitin (WSCT-50), glycol chitin, chitosan (DD 71%–88%), and chitin oligosaccharides with DP 2~7 [92,93]. CDA displayed little activity on chitin flakes, chitin powder, swollen chitin, or β-chitin powder. Chitin oligosaccharides were a comparatively good substrate because their solubility increased availability and accessibility for the CDA. Deacetylation rate on (GlcNAc)$_{2-6}$ was size-dependent; greater lengths produced a higher rate of activity. These results suggest that solubilization of chitin is a limiting factor for enzymatic bioconversion of chitin to chitosan by CDA. Extracellular CDA from *Mortierella* sp. DY-52 was active on WSCT (DD 50%), glycol chitin and crab chitosan (DD 71%–88%) and also on *N*-acetylglucosamine oligomers (GlcNAc)$_{2-6}$ [94].

Deacetylation by CDA is apparently substrate size-specific. GlcNAc was converted into GlcN by CDA from *Thermococcus kodakaraensis* KOD1, but (GlcNAc)$_2$ was converted into GlcN-GlcNAc, neither GlcNAc-GlcN or GlcN-GlcN [95]. Only the non-reducing residue of (GlcNAc)$_2$ has been deacetylated. CDA from *C. lindemuthianum* ATCC 56676 converted (GlcNAc)$_2$ not into (GlcN)$_2$ but into hetero-disaccharide GlcN-GlcNAc, and transformed (GlcNAc)$_3$ and (GlcNAc)$_4$ into the deacetylated products (GlcN)$_3$ and (GlcN)$_4$, respectively [96]. Alfonso *et al.* [97] found that chitosan oligosaccharides, (GlcN)$_{2-6}$, were produced from chitin by the joint action of endochitinase and CDA from *Aspergillus nidulans*, suggesting that deacetylation mainly occurs after chitin oligosaccharide production by the endochitinase.

A solid natural substrate shrimp chitin could be deacetylated with an 11% deacetylation by CDA from *Saccharomyces cerevisia* [98]. Pre-hydrolysis of crystalline shrimp chitin by grape chitinases increased the deacetylation triggered by CDA and produced COS with a degree of deacetylation of 67% [98]. It is well known that the high crystallinity of chitin microfibril, by the hydrogen bond-stabilized packaging of chitin polymer, greatly impedes the access of the enzyme to the deacetylation reaction site in the chitin molecule. Enzymatic deacetylation is profoundly affected by the physical properties of the substrate, such as crystallinity, degree of deacetylation, particle size, and origin [99]. Pretreatment to destroy the crystalline structure prior to addition of the enzyme seems to be desirable, in order to improve the deacetylation rate and produce novel chitosan polymers and oligomers. The preparation of COS including N-deacetylation and transglycosylation are summarized in Table 3.

Martinou *et al.* [100] investigated the mode of action of CDA from *Mucor rouxii*on fully water-soluble partially N-acetylated chitosans (DP 30) and found that the CDA hydrolyzed acetyl groups according to a multiple attack mechanism, that is, CDA does not preferentially attack any sequences in the chitosan chains. Together with this, a multiple chain mechanism has been suggested in CDA originating from *Colletotrichum lindemuthianum* ATCC 56676 [99].

**Table 3.** Preparation of chitooligosaccharides by N-deacetylation and transglycosylation.

| Product | Reaction Type | Reference |
|---|---|---|
| $(GlcN)_2 \sim (GlcN)_6$ | N-Deacetylation with endochitinase and CDA from *Aspergillus nidulans*; substrates: chitin | [97] |
| GlcN-GlcNAc | N-Deacetylation with CDA from *C. lindemuthianum* ATCC 56676; substrates: $(GlcNAc)_2$ | [96] |
| $(GlcN)_3$ & $(GlcN)_4$ | $(GlcNAc)_3$ and $(GlcNAc)_4$ | |
| Chitosan oligomers | N-Deacetylation with CDA from *Mucor rouxii*; substrates: partially N-acetylated chitosans ($DP_n$, $n = 30$) | [100] |
| GlcN | N-Deacetylation with CDA from *Thermococcus kodakaraensis*KOD1; substrates: GlcNAc | [95] |
| $(GlcN)_2 \sim (GlcN)_7$ | N-Deacetylation with CDA from *Absidia corymbifera* DY-9; substrates: $(GlcNAc)_2 \sim (GlcNAc)_7$ and WSCT-50 | [94] |
| $(GlcN)_2 \sim (GlcN)_7$ | N-Deacetylation with CDA from *Mortierella* sp. DY-52; substrates: $(GlcNAc)_2 \sim (GlcNAc)_7$ | [91] |
| Chitosan (89% DD) & $(GlcN)_2 \sim (GlcN)_4$ | N-Deacetylation with CDA from *Saccharomyces cerevisiae*; substrates: Chitin and $(GlcNAc)_2 \sim (GlcNAc)_4$ | [98] |
| $(GlcNAc)_6 \sim (GlcNAc)_{15}$ | Transglycosylation reaction on $\beta$-1,4-$(GlcNAc)_3$with lysozyme containing $(NH_4)_2SO_4$ (30% w/v) | [101] |
| $\beta$-1,4-$(GlcNAc)_2$ & $\beta$-1,6-$(GlcNAc)_2$ | Transglycosylation reaction on N-acetylchito-oligosaccharides [$\beta$-1,4-$(GlcNAc)_2 \sim \beta$-1,4-$(GlcNAc)_6$] with exo-$\beta$-D-GlcNase from *Alteromonas* sp. OK2607 | [102] |
| n-Butyl $\beta$-D-glucosaminide (C4GlcN) | Transglycosylation reaction on chitosan oligosaccharides & n-butanol with exo-$\beta$-D-GlcNase from *Penicillium funiculosum* KY616 | [103] |

## 5. Transglycosylation and Chitooligosaccharides

In addition to hydrolytic activity, some chitinolytic enzymes possess certain level of transglycosylation ability, that is, the ability to transfer the released oligosaccharide moiety to a suitable acceptor to form a new glycosidic bond. The transglycosylation activity of these chitinolytic enzymes suggests great potential for the synthesis of size- and stereo-specific chitin/chitosan oligomers, or even polymers and their derivatives.

Preparation of higher DP chitin oligosaccharides was achieved by the transglycosylation reaction of glycolytic enzymes including chitinase, chitosanase, and other glycosidases. Chitinase purified from *Trichoderma reesei* KDR-11 was shown to convert (GlcNAc)$_4$ into (GlcNAc)$_2$(55.7%) and (GlcNAc)$_6$(39.6%) by a transglycosylation reaction [104]. Akiyama *et al.* [105] reported that COS with DP 4–12 were successfully synthesized by a lysozyme-catalyzed transglycosylation reaction using $N,N',N''$-tri(monochloro)acetylchitotriose and $N,N',N''$-triacetylchitotriose as substrates followed by a base-catalyzed removal of the $N$-monochloroacetyl groups. Recently, Hattori *et al.* [101] made progress in biopreparation of COS. They tried lysozyme-mediated transglycosylation using β-1,4-(GlcNAc)$_3$ as starting substance and successfully produced chitin oligomers of (GlcNAc)$_6$ to (GlcNAc)$_{15}$ in an aqueous system containing 30% (NH$_4$)$_2$SO$_4$.

When GlcNase purified from *Penicillium funiculosum* KY616 was incubated with a mixture of chitosan oligomers and *n*-butanol, *n*-butyl β-D-glucosaminide (C4GlcN) was synthesized as a product by transglycosylation [103]. Yields of C4GlcN from chitobiose, chitotriose, and chitotetraose were found to be 14%, 23%, and 30%, respectively. The unusual β-1,6-(GlcNAc)$_2$ were synthesized from β-1,4-(GlcNAc)$_{2-6}$ by transglycosylation in chitinase preparation of marine bacterium *Alteromonas* sp. OK2607 [102].

Another example of enzymatic transglycosylation shows its diversity and potential in commercial applications. Fujimoto *et al.* [106] have reported the synthesis of gentiooligosaccharides (DP 3–9) from gentiobiose using a crude enzyme preparation from *P. multicolor.* The transglycosylation was shown to take place in two stages by a combination of β-glucosidase and β-(1-6)-glucanase. In the beginning, β-glucosidase produced gentiotriose from gentiobiose, and then β-(1-6)-glucanase acted on the resulting gentiotriose to produce a series of gentiooligosaccharides (DP 3–9) by transglycosylation. The transglycosylation reaction has high potential in the small-scale preparation of high value glycoside products applicable in medical and industrial fields.

## 6. Chemoenzymatic Glycosylation and Chitooligosaccharides

Chemoenzymatic glycosylation of chitooligosaccharides was intensively reviewed by the Kobayashi group [31,107–109]. *In vitro* synthesis of chitooligosaccharides was first reported by utilizingchitinase (EC 3.2.1.14) from *Bacillus* sp. (classified into glycoside hydrolase family 18; GH18) as catalyst [31,32]. On the basis of the transition state analogue substrate (TSAS) concept [31], the *N,N'*-diacetylchitobiose (GlcNAc-β-(1→4)-GlcNAc) oxazoline monomer was introduced. The enzymatic polymerization of this monomer proceeded via ringopening poly addition under weak alkaline conditions (pH 9.0~11.0), giving a synthetic COS with perfectly controlled stereo- and region selectivity. The DPs were evaluated as 10–20 depending on the reaction conditions [107].

The chitinase-catalyzed glycosylation using the sugar oxazoline substrate was applied to the stepwise elongation of GlcNAc unit by utilizing two enzymes, chitinase for ring-opening polyaddition of N-acetyllactosamine(Gal-β-(1→4)-GlcNAc) oxazoline (Gal = galactose) and β-galactosidase for the removal of the galactose unit from the produced oligosaccharide. [110–114]. The hydrolytic removal affords a new glycosyl acceptor with the GlcNAc unit at the non-reducing end. Repetition of these procedures using the two enzymes enabled the synthesis of chitooligosaccharides with desired chain lengths.

Interestingly, *N*-acetyllactosamine oxazoline was found to bepolymerized by chitinase A1 from *Bacillus circulans* WL-12 catalysis under basic conditions, giving rise to a novel oligosaccharide having the β-(1→4)-β-(1→6)-linked repeating unit in the main chain [115]. The DP of the resulting oligosaccharides was up to 5 based on the disaccharide. This was the first example of enzymatic glycosylation forming β-(1→6)-glycosidic linkage by chitinase catalysis.

The main disadvantage using the chemo-enzymatic approach is poor yield, because the product becomes necessarily a substrate for the enzyme (Table 4). Suppression of the chitinase-catalyzed hydrolysis of the product during the enzymatic polymerization is a challenge for chemoenzymatic glycosylation of COS. Wild-type chitinaseA1 from Bacillus circulans WL-12 has D202 and E204 residues as a DXE (D = Asp, X = any amino acid, E = Glu), a general sequence at the catalytic domain of chitinase [116,117]. A mutant chitinase E204Q (Q = Gln) exhibited less hydrolysis activity of the produced oligosaccharides by the enzymatic glycosylation, probably less protonation ability toward the oxygen of the glycosidic linkage by replacement of COOH in Glu with $CONH_2$ in Gln [118].

**Table 4.** Chemoenzymatic preparation of chitin and chitosan oligosaccharides (COS) and its derivatives.

| Product | Reaction Type | Reference |
|---|---|---|
| *N*-Acetylchitooligosaccharides | Chemoenzymatic elongation of *N*-GlcNAc unit by combined use of chitinase and β-galactosidase | [115] |
| Chitin derivatives with the deacetylated extents ranging from 0% to 50% | Chitinase-catalyzed copolymerization of *N*-acetylchitobiose oxazoline with the *N,N'*-diacetylchitobiose oxazoline | [54] |
| 6-*O*-Carboxymethylated chitotetraose alternatingly | Chitinase-catalyzed chemoenzymatic glycosylation of 6-*O*- and 6'-*O*-carboxymethyled chitobioseoxazolines | [119] |
| 3-*O*-Methylated chitotetraose | Chitinase-catalyzed chemoenzymatic glycosylation with 3-*O*-methyl- and 3'-*O*-methylchitobiose oxazolines | [118] |
| Oligo-*N*-acetyllactosamine derivatives with β-(1→4)-β-(1→6)-linked repeating unit | Chemoenzymatic polymerization by using transition state analogue substrate with chitinase A1 | [116] |
| Alternatingly D-Glcβ-(1→4) *N*-GlcNAc repeating units, a cellulose-chitin hybrid polysaccharide | Chemoenzymatic glycosylation of Glcβ (1→4) GlcN Acoxazoline and GlcNAcβ (1→4) Glc fluoride by chitinase and cellulose, respectively | [103] |
| Alternatingly D-GlcNβ-(1→4) *N*-GlcNAc repeating units, a chitin-chitosan hybrid polysaccharide | Chitinase-catalyzed chemoenzymatic glycosylation of C-2' position modified *N*-acetylchitobiose oxazolines | [55] |
| Fluorinated chitins | Chitinase-catalyzed polymerization C-6, C-6', or both modified *N*-acetylchitobiose oxazolines | [120,121] |

## 7. Perspectives

### 7.1. Direct Degradation and Separation of Chitin from Crustacean Shells or Squid Pens

The direct degradation and separation of α-chitin from crab and shrimp shells, and microbial cell walls poses a significant challenge. In light of the difficulties associated with traditional chitin oligosaccharides' production processes, environmentally compatible and reproducible degradation alternatives are desirable. However, crustacean shells are not soluble in standard aqueous media and their crystallinity is potentially too high to be degraded enzymatically. To solve these problems, pretreatment to break the chitin crystal structure is widely considered.

In this regard, chitin substrates were pretreated with steam explosion prior to enzymatic reaction [122]. A 11.28% reduction of the crystallinity index was observed with steam explosion and a 23.6% yield of chitin oligosaccharides with DP up to 5 was achieved. Interestingly, Nakagawa *et al.* [123] reported a breakthrough in the direct production of oligosaccharides from chitin and crab shells. They introduced a combination protocol of mechanochemical grinding and enzymatic hydrolysis, and produced GlcNAc and (GlcNAc)$_2$ directly from crab shells and chitin. The direct degradation ratio of the chitin in crab shell was close to 100%. For this purpose, they developed a novel "converge" mill [124], a derivative of the medium ball mill. Mechanochemical grinding, with the converge mill, was found to be extremely effective for pretreating chitin and crab shell before enzymatic digestion [125].

Breaking down the chitin crystal structure of biomaterials improves enzymatic degradation, allowing the enzymes to easily access and exert catalytic action. Wu and Miao [126] showed that mechanochemical treatment markedly increases the glucose yield from enzymatic corn flour hydrolysis. Similar results were observed by Fujimoto *et al.* [127] for lignocellulosic biomass. Van Craeyveld *et al.* [128] also showed improvement of extractability and molecular properties of *Psyllium* seed husk arabinoxylan by ball milling.

Mechanochemical grinding also provides an additional advantage. In the case of chitosan oligosaccharide production, salts are inevitably formed from aquatic reaction mixtures. Sometimes the bound salts limit application of COS. Salt production can be circumvented by mechanochemical grinding of the substrate, followed by enzymatic hydrolysis.

### 7.2. New Enzymes with Better Properties

Solubilization has become the first choice for breaking down the chitin crystal structure in chitin and crab shells to improve enzymatic degradation. Solvents are necessary to solvate the substrate, and these are still being studied along with continuing research seeking enzymes that are stable in organic solvents or heterogeneous solvent systems. Enzymes that function in an extreme environment are important for this purpose and their mode of action differ fundamentally from of glycoside hydrolases.

During researches on enzymes capable of efficiently degrading recalcitrant polysaccharides such as cellulose and chitin for biofuels, it has been speculated about the existence of a substrate-disrupting factor that could make the crystalline substrate more accessible to hydrolytic enzymes [129]. Vaaje-Kolstad *et al.* [130] showed that CBP21 (CBP for chitin-binding protein), produced by the chitinolytic bacterium *Serratia marcescens*, is an enzyme that catalyzes cleavage of glycosidic bonds in crystalline chitin, thus opening up the in accessible polysaccharide material for hydrolysis by normal glycoside hydrolases. The products were identified as chitin oligosaccharides with a normal sugar at the non-reducing end and an oxidized sugar, 2-(acetylamino)-2-deoxy-D-gluconic acid (GlcNAcA), at the other end. This is an oxidative enzyme boosting the enzymatic conversion of recalcitrant polysaccharides. This finding helps understand the factors involved in degradation of crystallinechitin and the chitin cycle in nature and provides a stake to more precisely handle the process for COS production from crystalline chitin and even raw materials such as crab and shrimp shells.

Recently, several commercially available hydrolytic enzymes including lysozyme, cellulase, papain, pectinases, and hemicellulase were found to catalyze the cleavage of the glycoside bond in chitin and chitosan [83]. Use of these nonspecific enzymes together with specific chitinase, chotosanase, glycosyltransferase, and CDA certainly opens a possible route to optimize the hydrolysis reactions controlling the production of chitooligosaccharides. Although different nonspecific enzymes have been used to obtain COS from chitin and chitosan, due to the limited capacity of most hydrolytic enzymes there is still interest in finding new enzymes with better properties.

Branchzyme is a relatively inexpensive commercial preparation that contains a branching glycosyltransferase from *Rhodothermus obamensis* expressed in *Bacillus subtilis*. This enzyme catalyzes the transfer of a segment of a 1,4-α-D-glucan chain to a primary hydroxyl group in a similar glucan chain to create 1,6-α-linkages, thereby increasing the number of branch points [131]. Interestingly, Branchzyme was active on chitosan and produced COS with DP 2-20, with a higher concentration having COS with DP 3–8 [132]. Recently, a family 46 chitosanase from *S. coelicolor* A3(2) was employed to degrade both a fully deacetylated chitosan and a 68% deacetylated chitosan for the production of a series of COS and to study in-depth the enzyme's mode of action [133].

## 7.3. Manipulation of the Size-Distribution of Oligomers Produced by Enzymatic Bioconversion

The DD, DP, the molecular weight distribution, and *N*-acetylation pattern (PA) of the resulting COS mixture depend on the starting material (mostly DD of chitin and chitosan) and the specificity of the enzyme used. Product mixtures can be enriched for certain compounds by optimizing the substrate-enzyme combination. This is illustrated by several studies on enzymatic degradation of chitosans [134–140]. The degradation of chitosan by the family 18 chitinases, ChiA, ChiB and ChiC, from *Serratia marcescens* has been studied in detail [36,134,141,142]. The biphasic kinetics of the reaction with ChiB was illustrated, as in the initial rapid phase and the second much slower phase of the reaction [36]. Sorbotten *et al.* [36] showed that the size-distribution of oligomers could be manipulated by varying the DD of the chitosans (DD 87%, 68%, 50%, and 35%) with ChiB; the products get longer as the DD goes up. Very interestingly, Sikorski *et al.* [137,142] have produced a model for the degradation of different chitosans with ChiB, which is capable of predicting the length distributions and yield of the products after extended hydrolysis. These profiles allow for selection of optimal reaction and substrate parameters for efficient production of oligomers with desired lengths. Altogether, this suggests that production of oligomers with desired lengths can be achieved by manipulating the choice of the starting materials with specific DD, and PA, the choice of the enzyme, and the choice of the processing time [130].

*7.4. Genetic Engineering Technology*

Genetic engineering technology is applicable and promising for mass production of recombinant enzymes and understanding mode of action, which is useful for bioproduction of COS and synthesis of structure-specific oligosaccharides. Martinez *et al.* [51] declared that enzymatic synthesis of COS has been a matter of research by exploiting the transglycosylation activity of retaining family 18 chitinases. The mutagenesis of two GH-18 glycoside hydrolase, *B. circulans* WL-12 chitinase A1 (*Bc* ChiA1) and *Trichoderma harzanium* chitinase 42 (*Th* Chit42) abolished the hydrolytic activity of chitin [51]. The mutants D200A and D202A of *Bc* ChiA1, together with D170N of *Th* Chit42 proved to be active for chitinbiose oxazoline polymerization, and also for coupling reaction between Gal ($\beta1\rightarrow4$) chitinbiose oxazoline and chitinpentaose at neutral pH. These mutants have retained the ability to catalyze transglycosylation reaction on natural COS. Such mutants could be considered as chitin transglycosylases.

Chitin synthase, a processive inverting enzyme of glycosyltransferase family 2, transfers GlcNAc from UDP-GlcNAc to preexisting chitin chains in reactions that are typically stimulated by free GlcNAc. This enzyme can be applied for synthesis of chitin oligosaccharides. By using a recombinant *Saccharomyces cerevisiae* chitin synthase with UDP-GlcNAc, $GlcNAc_2$ was obtained as a major reaction product [143]. Formation of both COS and insoluble chitin was stimulated by $GlcNAc_2$ and by *N*-propanoyl-, *N*-butanoyl-, and *N*-glycolyl-glucosamine.

*7.5. Direct Fermentation of Raw Materials such as Crab and Shrimp Shells*

The direct fermentation of raw materials such as crab and shrimp shells presents another opportunity in the production of chitin and COS. Chitin oligosaccharides were directly obtained from 1.5% shrimp head powder after 2 days of fermentation with protease- and chitosanase-producing *Bacillus cereus*TKU022 [144]. $(GlcNAc)_2$, $(GlcNAc)_4$, $(GlcNAc)_5$, and $(GlcNAc)_6$ were all identified in the culture supernatant. Even though the concentration of the products is still very low (0.3–201.5 µg/mL), these findings are meaningful in terms of direct production from raw materials.

*7.6. Reactor Systems*

Finally, the reactor system used should be considered to be a critical factor for efficiency and high yield in bioproduction. There are three types of reactors normally used in the preparation of chitosan oligosaccharides, including batch reactors, column reactors and ultrafiltration reactors [145]. Batch reactors represent the simplest method used for the enzymatic production of COS. This method has a few drawbacks, including limited reuse of reacting enzyme and continuous production of COS, difficulty in controlling molecular weight of COS, low yield and high cost.

Continuous preparation of COS is possible by packing immobilized enzymes into a column reactor that the substrate passes through. Though this method has several advantages over batch reactors, the poorer affinity of immobilized enzymes to chitosan substrate than that of free enzyme limits the activity of enzyme and the usage of column reactors in the commercial preparation of COS.

The ultrafiltration membrane reactor has been applied for overcoming the problems of the reusability of enzymes in batch reactors and the poor affinity of the substrate toward immobilized enzymes in column reactor systems, but suffers from the problem of membrane fouling [25,69]. A dual ultrafiltration membrane reactor system composed of a column reactor packed with immobilized enzymes and an ultrafiltration membrane reactor, has been invented and applied in COS production [146]. Using this reactor, chitosanase from *Bacillus pumilus* BN-262 continuously produced chitosan oligomers of DP 3~6 from chitosan (89% DD), free from any fouling problem.

## 8. Conclusions

Bioproduction of COS with enzymes and microorganismshas been studied for decades. However, the yield of bioproduction is still lower and the cost is higher than traditional chemical methods. Crude rather than pure enzyme preparations of chitinase, chitosanase, lysozyme, cellulase, protease, lipase, and pepsin were preferred for this purpose for the practical production of the oligosaccharides. The transglycosylation activity of chitinolytic enzymes was successfully exploited for the synthesis of desired chitin oligomers and their derivatives. Chitin deacetylase is also applicable to the preparation of oligosaccharides.

The direct degradation and separation of chitin from crab and shrimp shells and microbial cell walls presents a significant challenge in bioproduction of COS. The direct production of oligosaccharides from chitin and crab shells was achieved by using a combination of mechanochemical grinding and enzymatic hydrolysis. In case of chitosan oligosaccharides, salt forms are inevitably formed from aquatic reaction mixtures, which limit the application. However, the mechanochemical grinding of the substrate followed by enzymatic hydrolysis can circumvent this.

Breaking down the crystal structure of chitin and crab shells is necessary to improve enzymatic degradation of the substrate. Solubilization is the first choice for destruction of chitin crystallinity. Once solubilized in organic or heterogeneous solvent systems, the substrate must receive hydrolytic enzymes with special properties. Thus, screening high-potential enzymes that function in extreme environments is an important factor for the optimization of bioproduction.

The direct fermentation of raw biomaterials like crab and shrimp shells presents another opportunity in the production of chitin and COS. Even though the efficiency of this method is still very low, it is significant in terms of the direct production of COS from the row materials.

To overcome these inefficiencies, the optimization of a reactor system appropriate to enzymatic bioproduction is called for. A dual ultrafiltration membrane reactor system has been described that is capable of overcoming the problems of enzyme reusability in batch reactors as well as the poor affinity of the substrate toward immobilized enzymes in standard column reactor systems.

## Acknowledgments

This work was supported by the Korea Science and Engineering Foundation (KOSEF) through the National Research Lab. Program funded by the Ministry of Science and Technology (No. R0A-2003-000-10322-0), and by Bio-industry Technology Development Program, Ministry for Food, Agriculture, Forestry and Fisheries, Republic of Korea.

## Conflicts of Interest

The authors declare no conflict of interest.

## References

1.  No, H.K.; Meyers, S.P.; Lee, K.S. Isolation and characterization of chitin from crawfish shell waste. *J. Agric. Food Chem.* **1989**, *37*, 575–579.

2.  Aye, K.N.; Stevens, W.F. Technical note: Improved chitin production by pre-treatment of shrimp shells. *J. Chem. Technol. Biotechnol.* **2004**, *79*, 421–425.

3.  Allan, G.G.; Fox, J.R.; Kong, N. Marine polymers, part 8. A critical evaluation of the potential sources of chitin and chitosan. In Proceeding of the 1st International Conference on Chitin/Chitosan; Muzzarelli, R.A.A., Pariser, E.R., Eds.; MIT Sea Grant: Cambridge, MA, USA, 1978; pp. 64–78.

4.  Simpson, B.K.; Gagné, N.; Simpson, M.V. Bioprocessing of chitin and chitosan. In *Fisheries Processing: Biotechnological Applications*; Martin, A.M., Ed.; Chapman & Hall: London, UK, 1994; pp. 155–173.

5.  Healy, M.G.; Romo, C.R.; Bustos, R. Bioconversion of marine crustacean shell waste. *Res. Conserv. Recycl.* **1994**, *11*, 139–147.

6.  Jung, W.J.; Jo, G.Y.; Kuk, J.H.; Kim, K.Y.; Park, R.D. Extraction of chitin from red crab shell waste by cofermentation with *Lactobacillus paracasei* subsp. *tolerans* KCTC-3074 and *Serratia marcescens* FS-3. *Appl. Microbiol. Biot.* **2006**, *71*, 234–237.

7.  Jung, W.J.; Jo, G.Y.; Kuk, J.H.; Kim, Y.J.; Oh, K.T.; Park, R.D. Production of chitin from red crab shell waste by successive fermentation with *Lactobacillus paracasei* KCTC-3074 and *Serratia marcescens* FS-3. *Carbohydr. Polym.* **2007**, *68*, 746–750.

8.  Jo, G.H.; Jung, W.J.; Kuk, J.H.; Oh, K.T.; Kim, Y.J.; Park, R.D. Screening of protease-producing *Serratia marcescens* FS-3 and its application to deproteinization of crab shell waste for chitin extraction. *Carbohydr. Polym.* **2008**, *74*, 504–508.

9.  Seyfarth, F.; Schliemann, S.; Elsner, P.; Hipler, U.C. Antifungal effect of high- and low-molecular-weight chitosan hydrochloride, carboxymethyl chitosan, chitosan oligosaccharide and *N*-acetyl-D-glucosamine against *Candida albicans*, *Candida krusei* and *Candida glabrata*. *Int. J. Pharm.* **2008**, *353*, 139–148.

10. Oliveira, E.N., Jr.; El Gueddari, N.E.; Moerschbacher, B.M.; Peter, M.G.; Franco, T.T. Growth of phytopathogenic fungi in the presence of partially acetylated chitooligosaccharides. *Mycopathologia* **2008**, *166*, 163–174.

11. Sasaki, C.; Fukamizo, T. Production of food oligosaccharides by chitinases and chitosanases: Structural biological perspective. *New Food Ind.* **2001**, *43*, 7–14.

12. Lee, H.W.; Park, Y.S.; Choi, J.W.; Yi, S.Y.; Shin, W.S. Antidiabetic effects of chitosan oligosaccharides in neonatal streptozotocin-induced noninsulin-dependent diabetes mellitus in rats. *Biol. Pharm. Bull.* **2003**, *26*, 1100–1103.

13. Xia, W.; Liu, P.; Zhang, J.; Chen, J. Biological activities of chitosan and chitooligosaccharides. *Food Hydrocoll.* **2011**, *25*, 170–179.

14. Sato, K.; Saimoto, H.; Morimoto, M.; Shigemasa, Y. Depolymerization of chitin and chitosan under hydrothermal conditions. *Sen-I Gakkaishi* **2003**, *59*, 104–109.

15. Xing, R.E.; Liu, S.; Yu, H.H.; Guo, Z.Y.; Wang, P.B.; Li, C.P.; Li, Z.; Li, P.C. Salt-assisted acid hydrolysis of chitosan to oligomers under microwave irradiation. *Carbohydr. Res.* **2005**, *340*, 2150–2153.

16. Wu, T.; Zivanovic, S.; Hayes, D.G.; Weiss, J. Efficient reduction of chitosan molecular weight by high-intensity ultrasound: Underlying mechanism and effect of process parameters. *J. Agric. Food Chem.* **2008**, *56*, 5112–5119.

17. Yoksan, R.; Akashi, M.; Miyata, M.; Chirachanchai, S. Optimal gamma-ray dose and irradiation conditions for producing low-molecular-weight chitosan that retains its chemical structure. *Radiat. Res.* **2004**, *161*, 471–480.

18. Domard, A.; Cartier, N. Glucosamine oligomers: 4. Solid state-crystallization and sustained dissolution. *Int. J. Biol. Macromol.* **1992**, *14*, 100–106.

19. Einbu, A.; Vårum, K.M. Depolymerization and de-*N*-acetylation of chitin oligomers in hydrochloric acid. *Biomacromolecules* **2007**, *8*, 309–314.

20. Lin, F.; Jia, X.G.; Lei, W.X.; Li, Z.J.; Zhang, T.Y. Spectra analyses of chitosans degraded by hydrogen peroxide under optimal conditions. *Spectrosc. Spectr. Anal.* **2009**, *29*, 43–47.

21. Morris, V.B.; Neethu, S.; Abraham, T.E.; Pillai, C.K.S.; Sharma, C.P. Studies on the condensation of depolymerized chitosans with DNA for preparing chitosan-DNA nanoparticles for gene delivery applications. *J. Biomed. Mater. Res. Part B* **2009**, *89B*, 282–292.

22. Jeon, Y.J.; Park, P.J.; Kim, S.K. Antimicrobial effect of chitooligosaccharides produced by bioreactor. *Carbohydr. Polym.* **2001**, *44*, 71–76.

23. Qin, C.; Zhou, B.; Zeng, L.; Zhang, Z.; Liu, Y.; Du, Y.; Xiao, L. The physicochemical properties and antitumor activity of cellulase-treated chitosan. *Food Chem.* **2004**, *84*, 107–115.

24. Aam, B.B.; Heggset, E.B.; Norberg, A.L.; Sørlie, M.; Vårum, K.M.; Eijsink, V.G.H. Production of chitooligosaccharides and their potential applications in medicine. *Mar. Drugs* **2010**, *8*, 1482–1517.

25. Lin, Y.W.; Hsiao, Y.C.; Chiang, B.H. Production of high degree polymerized chitooligosaccharides in a membrane reactor using purified chitosanase from *Bacillus cereus*. *Food Res. Int.* **2009**, *42*, 1355–1361.

26. Zeng, H.; Zheng, L.Y. Studies on *Penicillium* sp. ZDZ1 chitosanase immobilized on chitin by cross-linking reaction. *Process Biochem.* **2002**, *38*, 531–535.

27. Cantarel, B.L.; Coutinho, P.M.; Rancurel, C.; Bernard, T.; Lombard, V.; Henrissat, B. The Carbohydrate-Active enZYmes database (CAZy): An expert resource for Glycogenomics. *Nucleic Acids Res.* **2009**, *37*, D233–D238.

28. CAZy. The Carbohydrate-Active enZYmes database. Available online: http://www.cazy.org (accessed on 27 April 2010).

29. Davies, G.; Henrissat, B. Structures and mechanisms of glycosyl hydrolases. *Structure* **1995**, *3*, 853–859.

30. Henrissat, B.; Bairoch, A. Updating the sequence-based classification of glycosyl hydrolases. *Biochem. J.* **1996**, *316*, 695–696.

31. Kobayashi, S.; Kiyosada, T.; Shoda, S. Synthesis of artificial chitin: Irreversible catalytic behavior of a glycosyl hydrolase through a transition state analogue substrate. *J. Am. Chem. Soc.* **1996**, *118*, 13113–13114.

32. Sato, H.; Mizutani, S.; Tsuge, S.; Ohtani, H.; Aoi, K.; Takasu, A.; Okada, M.; Kobayashi, S.; Kiyosada, T.; Shoda, S. Determination of the degree of acetylation of chitin/chitosan by pyrolysis-gas chromatography in the presence of oxalic acid. *Anal. Chem.* **1998**, *70*, 7–12.

33. ExplorEnz—The Enzyme Database. Available online: http://www.enzyme-explorer.org/ (accessed on 27 April 2010).

34. Berger, L.R.; Reynolds, D.M. The chitinase system of a strain of *Streptomyces griseus*. *Biochem. Biophys. Acta* **1958**, *29*, 522–534.

35. Monreal, J.; Reese, E.T. The chitinase of *Serratia marcescens*. *J. Microbiol.* **1969**, *15*, 689–696.

36. Sørbotten, A.; Horn, S.J.; Eijsink, V.G.; Vårum, K.M. Degradation of chitosans with chitinase B from *Serratia marcescens*. Production of chito-oligosaccharides and insight into enzyme processivity. *FEBS J.* **2005**, *272*, 538–549.

37. Lopatin, S.A.; Derbeneva, M.S.; Kulikov, S.N.; Varlamov, V.P.; Shpigun, O.A. Fractionation of chitosan by ultrafiltration. *J. Anal. Chem.* **2009**, *64*, 648–651.

38. Haebel, S.; Bahrke, S.; Peter, M.G. Quantitative sequencing of complex mixtures of heterochitooligosaccharides by MALDI-linear ion trap mass spectrometry. *Anal. Chem.* **2007**, *79*, 5557–5566.

39. Le Dévédec, F.; Bazinet, L.; Furtos, A.; Venne, K.; Brunet, S.; Mateescu, M.A. Separation of chitosan oligomers by immobilized metal affinity chromatography. *J. Chromatogr. A* **2008**, *1194*, 165–171.

40. Pichyangkura, R.; Kudan, S.; Kuttiyawong, K.; Sukwattanasinitt, M.; Aiba, S. Quantitative production of 2-acetamido-2-deoxy-D-glucose from crystalline chitin by bacterial chitinase. *Carbohydr. Res.* **2002**, *337*, 557–559.

41. Sashiwa, H.; Fujishima, S.; Yamano, N.; Kawasaki, N.; Nakayama, A.; Muraki, E.; Sukwattanasinitt, M.; Pichyangkurac, R.; Aiba, S. Enzymatic production of *N*-acetyl-D-glucosamine from chitin. Degradation study of *N*-acetylchitooligosaccharide and the effect of mixing of crude enzymes. *Carbohydr. Polym.* **2003**, *51*, 391–395.

42. Il'ina, A.V.; Zueva, O.Y.; Lopatin, S.A.; Varlamov, V.P. Enzymatic hydrolysis of α-chitin. *Appl. Biochem. Microbiol.* **2004**, *40*, 35–38.

43. Sukwattanasinitt, M.; Zhu, H.; Sashiwa, H.; Aiba, S. Utilization of commercial non-chitinase enzymes from fungi for preparation of 2-acetamido-2-deox-D-glucose from β-chitin. *Carbohydr. Res.* **2002**, *337*, 133–137.

44. Sashiwa, H.; Fujishima, S.; Yamano, N.; Kawasaki, N.; Nakayama, A.; Muraki, E.; Hiraga, K.; Oda, K.; Aiba, S. Production of *N*-acetyl-D-glucosamine from α-chitin by crude enzymes from *Aeromonas hydrophila* H-2330. *Carbohydr. Res.* **2002**, *337*, 761–763.

45. Thamthiankul, S.; Suan-Ngay, S.; Tantimavanich, S.; Panbangred, W. Chitinase from *Bacillus thuringiensis* subsp *pakistani*. *Appl. Microbiol. Biotechnol.* **2001**, *56*, 395–401.

46. Katta, S.; Ankati, S.; Podile, A.R. Chitooligosaccharides are converted to *N*-acetylglucosamine by *N*-acetyl-β-hexosaminidase from *Stenotrophomonas maltophilia*. *FEMS Microbiol. Lett.* **2013**, *348*, 19–25.

47. Lan, X.; Ozawa, N.; Nishiwaki, N.; Kodaira, R.; Okazaki, M.; Shimosaka, M. Purification, cloning, and sequence analysis of β-*N*-acetylglucosaminidase from the chitinolytic bacterium *Aeromonas hydrophila* strain SUWA-9. *Biosci. Biotechnol. Biochem.* **2004**, *68*, 1082–1090.

48. Kuk, J.H.; Jung, W.J.; Jo, G.H.; Ahn, J.S.; Kim, K.Y.; Park, R.D. Selective preparation of *N*-acetyl-D-glucosamine and *N,N'*-diacetylchitobiose from chitin using a crude enzyme preparation from *Aeromonas* sp. *Biotechnol. Lett.* **2005**, *27*, 7–11.

49. Kuk, J.H.; Jung, W.J.; Jo, G.H.; Kim, Y.C.; Kim, K.Y.; Park, R.D. Production of *N*-acetyl-β-D-glucosamine from chitin by *Aeromonas* sp. GJ-18 crude enzyme. *Appl. Microbiol. Biotechnol.* **2005**, *68*, 384–389.

50. Kuk, J.H.; Jung, W.J.; Jo, G.H.; Kim, K.Y.; Park, R.D. Production of *N,N'*-diacetylchitobiose from chitin using temperature-sensitive chitinolytic enzyme preparations of *Aeromonas* sp. GJ-18. *World J. Microbiol. Biotechnol.* **2006**, *22*, 135–139.

51. Martinez, E.A.; Boer, H.; Koivula, A.; Samain, E.; Driguez, H.; Armand, S.; Cottaz, S. Engineering chitinases for the synthesis of chitin oligosaccharides: Catalytic amino acid mutations convert the GH-18 family glycoside hydrolases into transglycosylases. *J. Mol. Catalys. B Enzym.* **2012**, *74*, 89–96.

52. Tanaka, T.; Fukui, T.; Atomi, H.; Imanaka, T. Characterization of an exo-β-D-glucosaminidase involved in a novel chitinolytic pathway from the hyperthermophilic archaeon *Thermococcus kodakaraensis* KOD1. *J. Bact.* **2003**, *185*, 5175–5181.

53. Yamasaki, Y.; Hayashi, I.; Ohta, Y.; Nakagawa, T.; Kawamukai, M.; Matsuda, H. Purification and mode of action of chitosanolytic enzyme from *Enterobacter* sp. G-1. *Biosci. Biotechnol. Biochem.* **1993**, *57*, 444–449.

54. Makino, A.; Sakamoto, J.; Ohmae, M.; Kobayashi, S. Effect of fluorine substituent on the chitinase-catalyzed polymerization of sugar oxazoline derivatives. *Chem. Lett.* **2006**, *35*, 160–161.

55. Makino, A.; Ohmae, M.; Kobayashi, S. Chitinase-catalyzed copolymerization to a chitin derivative having glucosamine unit in controlled proportion. *Polym. J.* **2006**, *38*, 1182–1188.

56. Takiguchi, Y.; Shimahara, K. *N,N*-Diacetylchitobiose production from chitin by *Vibrio anguillarum* strain E-383a. *Lett. Appl. Microbiol.* **1988**, *6*, 129–131.

402

57. Ilankovan, P.; Hein, S.; Ng, C.H.; Trung, T.S.; Stevens, W.F. Production of *N*-acetyl chitobiose from various chitin substrates using commercial enzymes. *Carbohydr. Polym.* **2006**, *63*, 245–250.

58. Wang, S.L.; Liu, C.P.; Liang, T.W. Fermented and enzymatic production of chitin/chitosan oligosaccharides by extracellular chitinases from *Bacillus cereus* TKU027. *Carbohydr. Polym.* **2012**, *90*, 1305–1313.

59. Wang, C.Y.; Hsieh, Y.Z. Analysis of chitin oligosaccharides by capillary electrophoresis with laser-inducedfluorescence. *J. Chromatogr. A* **2002**, *979*, 431–438.

60. Saito, J.; Kita, A.; Higuchi, Y.; Nagata, Y.; Ando, A.; Miki, K. Crystal structure of chitosanase from *Bacillus circulans* MH-K1 at 1.6-angstrom resolution and its substrate recognition mechanism. *J. Biol. Chem.* **1999**, *274*, 30818–30825.

61. Fukamizo, T.; Ohkawa, T.; Ikeda, Y.; Goto, S. Specificity of chitosanase from *Bacillus pumilus*. *Biochim. Biophys. Acta* **1994**, *1205*, 183–188.

62. Cheng, C.Y.; Chang, C.H.; Wu, Y.J.; Li, Y.K. Exploration of glycosyl hydrolase family 75, a chitosanase from *Aspergillus fumigatus*. *J. Biol. Chem.* **2006**, *281*, 3137–3144.

63. Fukamizo, T.; Brzezinski, R. Chitosanase from *Streptomyces* sp. strain N174: A comparative review of its structure and function. *Biochem. Cell Biol.* **1997**, *75*, 687–696.

64. Choi, Y.J.; Kim, E.J.; Piao, Z.; Yun, Y.C.; Shin, Y.C. Purification and characterization of chitosanase from *Bacillus* sp. strain KCTC 0377BP and its application for the production of chitosan oligosaccharides. *Appl. Environ. Microbiol.* **2004**, *70*, 4522–4531.

65. Kurakake, M.; You, S.; Nakagawa, K.; Sugihara, M.; Komaki, T. Properties of chitosanase from *Bacillus cereus* S1. *Curr. Microbiol.* **2000**, *40*, 6–9.

66. Park, R.D.; Rhee, C.O.; Lee, H.C.; Cho, C.S.; Jo, D.H. A comparative study of chitooligosaccharide production from chitosan. *J. Chitin Chitosan* **1999**, *4*, 96–101.

67. Yoon, H.G.; Ha, S.C.; Lim, Y.H.; Cho, H.Y. New thermostable chitosanase from *Bacillus* sp.: Purification and characterization. *J. Microbiol. Biotechnol.* **1998**, *8*, 449–454.

68. Lee, H.W.; Choi, J.W.; Han, D.P.; Park, M.J.; Lee, N.W.; Yi, D.H. Purification and characteristics of chitosanase from *Bacillus* sp. HW-002. *J. Microbiol. Biotechnol.* **1996**, *6*, 19–25.

69. Jeon, Y.J.; Kim, S.K. Production of chitooligosaccharides using ultrafilteration membrane reactor and their antibacterial activity. *Carbohydr. Polym.* **2000**, *41*, 133–144.

70. Pelletier, A.; Sygusch, J. Purification and characterization of three chitosanase activities from *Bacillus megaterium* P1. *Appl. Environ. Microbiol.* **1990**, *56*, 844–848.

71. Shimosaka, M.; Nogawa, M.; Wang, X.Y.; Kumehara, M.; Okazaki, M. Production of two chitosanases from a chitosan-assimilating bacterium, *Acinetobacter* sp. strain CHB101. *Appl. Environ. Microbiol.* **1995**, *61*, 438–442.

72. Wang, S.L.; Tseng, W.N.; Liang, T.W. Biodegradation of shellfish wastes and production of chitosanases by a squid pen-assimilating bacterium, *Acinetobacter calcoaceticus* TKU024. *Biodegradation* **2011**, *22*, 939–948.

73. Nanjo, F.; Katsumi, R.; Sakai, K. Purification and characterization of an exo-β-D-glucosaminidase, a novel type of enzyme, from *Nocardia orientalis. J. Biol. Chem.* **1990**, *265*, 10088–10094.

74. Park, J.K.; Shimono, K.; Ochiai, N.; Shigeru, K.; Kurita, M.; Ohta, Y.; Tanaka, K.; Matsuda, H.; Kawamukai, M. Purification, characterization, and gene analysis of a chitosanase (ChoA) from *Matsuebacter chitosanotabidus* 3001. *J. Bact.* **1999**, *181*, 6642–6649.

75. Kim, S.Y.; Shon, D.H.; Lee, K.H. Purification and characteristics of two types of chitosanases from *Aspergillus fumigatus. J. Microbiol. Biotechnol.* **1998**, *8*, 568–574.

76. Jung, W.J.; Kuk, J.H.; Kim, K.Y.; Jung, K.C.; Park, R.D. Purification and characterization of exo-β-D-glucosaminidase from *Aspergillus fumigatus* S-26. *Protein Expr. Purif.* **2006**, *45*, 125–131.

77. Zhang, X.Y.; Dae, A.L.; Zhang, X.K.; Kuroiwa, K. Purification and characterization of chitosanase and exo-β-D-glucosaminidase from Koji Mold, *Aspergillus oryzae* IAM2660. *Biosci. Biotechnol. Biochem.* **2000**, *64*, 1896–1902.

78. Nogawa, M.; Takahashi, H.; Kasiwagi, A.; Ohshima, K.; Okada, H.; Morikawa, Y. Purification and characterization of exo-β-D-glucosaminidase from a cellulolytic fungus, *Trichoderma reesei* PC-3-7. *Appl. Envoron. Microbiol.* **1998**, *64*, 890–895.

79. Lin, H.; Wang, H.; Xue, C.; Ye, M. Preparation of chitosan oligomers by immobilized papain. *Enzyme Microb. Technol.* **2002**, *31*, 588–592.

80. Lee, D.X.; Xia, W.S.; Zhang, J.L. Enzymatic preparation of chitooligosaccharides by commercial lipase. *Food Chem.* **2008**, *111*, 291–295.

81. Zhang, H.; Du, Y.; Yu, X.; Mitsutomi, M.; Aiba, S. Preparation of chitooligosaccharides from chitosan by acomplex enzyme. *Carbohydr. Res.* **1999**, *320*, 257–260.

82. Mahata, M.; Shinya, S.; Masaki, E.; Yamamoto, T.; Ohnuma, T.; Brzezinski, R.; Mazumder, T.K.; Yamashita, K.; Narihiro, K.; Fukamizo, T. Production of chitooligosaccharides from *Rhizopus oligosporus* NRRL2710 cells by chitosanase digestion. *Carbohydr. Res.* **2014**, *383*, 27–33.

83. Yalpani, M.; Pantaleone, D. An examination of the unusual susceptibility of aminoglycans to enzymatic hydrolysis. *Carbohydr. Res.* **1994**, *256*, 159–175.

84. Nguyen, A.D.; Huang, C.C.; Liang, T.W.; Nguyen, V.B.; Pan, P.S.; Wang, S.L. Production and purification of a fungal chitosanase and chitooligomers from *Penicillium janthinellum* D4 and discovery of the enzyme activators. *Carbohydr. Polym.* **2014**, *108*, 331–337.

85. Gao, X.A.; Jung, W.J.; Kuk, J.H.; Park, R.D. Reaction pattern of *Bacillus cereus* D-11 chitosanase on chito-oligosaccharide alcohols. *J. Microbiol. Biotechnol.* **2009**, *19*, 358–361.

86. Pantaleone, D.; Yalpani, M.; Scollar, M. Unusual susceptibility of chitosan to enzymic hydrolysis. *Carbohydr. Res.* **1992**, *237*, 325–332.

87. Aiba, S.I. Preparation of *N*-acetylchitooligosaccharides from lysozymatic hydroxylate of partially *N*-acetylated chitosans. *Carbohydr. Res.* **1994**, *261*, 297–306.

88. Kumar, A.B.V.; Gowda, L.R.; Tharanathan, R.N. Non-specific depolymerization of chitosan by pronase and characterization of the resultant products. *Eur. J. Biochem.* **2004**, *271*, 713–723.

89. Xie, Y.;Hu, J.; Wei, Y.; Hong, X. Preparation of chitooligosaccharides by the enzymatic hydrolysis of chitosan. *Polym. Degrad. Stab.* **2009**, *94*, 1895–1899.

90. Wu, S. Preparation of chitooligosaccharides from *Clanis bilineata* larvae skin and their antibacterial activity. *Int. J. Biol. Macromol.* **2012**, *51*, 1147–1150.

91. Zhao, Y.; Park, R.D.; Muzzarelli, R.A.A. Chitin deacetylases: Properties and applications. *Mar. Drugs* **2010**, *8*, 24–46.

92. Zhao, Y.; Kim, Y.J.; Oh, K.T.; Nguyen, V.N.; Park, R.D. Production and characterization of extracellular chitin deacetylase from *Absidia corymbifera* DY-9. *J. Korean Soc. Appl. Biol. Chem.* **2010**, *53*, 119–126.

93. Zhao, Y.; Ju, W.T.; Jo, G.H.; Jung, W.J.; Park, R.D. Perspectives of chitin deacetylase research. In *Biotechnology of Biopolymers*; Elnashar, M., Ed.; InTech: Rijeka, Croatia, 2011; pp. 131–144.

94. Kim, Y.J.; Zhao, Y.; Oh, K.T.; Nguyen, V.N.; Park, R.D. Enzymatic deacetylation of chitin by extracellular chitin deacetylase from newly screened *Mortierella* sp. DY-52. *J. Microbiol. Biotechnol.* **2008**, *18*, 759–766.

95. Tanaka, T.; Fukui, T.; Fujiwara, S.; Atomi, H.; Imanaka, T. Concerted action of diacetylchitobiose deacetylase and exo-beta-D-glucosaminidase in a novel Biotechnology of Biopolymers chitinolytic pathway in the hyperthermophilic archaeon *Thermococcus kodakaraensis* KOD1. *J. Biol. Chem.* **2004**, *279*, 30021–30027.

96. Tokuyasu, K.; Ono, H.; Ohnishi-Kameyama, M.; Hayashi, K.; Mori, Y. Deacetylation of chitin oligosaccharides of dp 2-4 by chitin deacetylase from *Colletotrichum lindemuthianum*. *Carbohydr. Res.* **1997**, *303*, 353–358.

97. Alfonso, C.; Nuero, O.M.; Santamarla, F.; Reyes, F. Purification of a heat-stable chitin deacetylase from *Aspergillus nidulans* and its role in cell wall degradation. *Curr. Microbiol.* **1995**, *30*, 49–54.

98. Aguila, E.M.D.; Gomes, L.P.; Andrade, C.T.; Silva, J.T.; Paschoalin, V.M.F. Biocatalytic production of chitosan polymers from shrimp shells, using a recombinant enzyme produced by *Pichia pastoris*. *Am. J. Mol. Biol.* **2012**, *2*, 341–350.

99. Blair, D.E.; Hekmat, O.; Schuttelkopf, A.W.; Shrestha, B.; Tokuyasu, K.; Withers, S.G.; van Aalten, D.M. Structure and mechanism of chitin deacetylase from the fungal pathogen *Colletotrichum lindemuthianum*. *Biochemistry* **2006**, *45*, 9416–9426.

100. Martinou, A.; Bouriotis, V.; Stokke, B.T.; Vårum, K.M. Mode of action of chitin deacetylase from *Mucor rouxii* on partially *N*-acetylated chitosans. *Carbohydr. Res.* **1998**, *311*, 71–78.

101. Hattori, T.; Sakabe, Y.; Ogata, M.; Michishita, K.; Dohra, H.; Kawagishi, H.; Totani, K.; Nikaido, M.; Nakamura, T.; Koshino, H.; Usui, T. Enzymatic synthesis of an α-chitin-like substance via lysozyme-mediated transglycosylation. *Carbohydr. Res.* **2012**, *347*, 16–22.

102. Shimoda, K.; Nakajima, K.; Hiratsuka, Y.; Nishimura, S.I.; Kurita, K. Efficient preparation of β-(1→6)-(GlcNAc)$_2$ by enzymatic conversion of chitin and chito-oligosaccharides. *Carbohydr. Polym.* **1996**, *29*, 149–154.

103. Matsumura, S.; Yao, E.; Toshima, K. One-step preparation of alkyl β-D-glucosaminide by the transglycosylation of chitosan and alcohol using purified exo-β-D-glucosaminidase. *Biotechnol. Lett.* **1999**, *21*, 451–456.

104. Usui, T.; Matsu, H.; Isobe, K. Enzymic synthesis of useful chito-oligosaccharides utilizing transglycosylation by chitinolytic enzymes in a buffer containing ammonium sulfate. *Carbohydr. Res.* **1990**, *203*, 65–77.

105. Akiyama, K.; Kawazu, K.; Kobayashi, A. A novel method for chemo-enzymatic synthesis of elicitor-active chitosan oligomers and partially *N*-acetylated chitin oligomers using *N*-acetylated chitotriose as substrates in a lysozyme-catalyzed transglycosylation reaction system. *Carbohydr. Res.* **1995**, *279*, 151–160.

106. Fujimoto, Y.; Hattori, T.; Uno, S.; Murata, T.; Usui, T. Enzymatic synthesis of gentiooligosaccharides by transglycosylation with β-glycosidases from *Penicillium multicolor. Carbohydr. Res.* **2009**, *344*, 972–978.

107. Kobayashi, S.; Makino, A.; Matsumoto, H.; Kunii, S.; Ohmae, M.; Kiyosada, T.; Makiguchi, K.; Matsumoto, A.; Horie, M.; Shoda, S.I. Enzymatic polymerization to novel polysaccharides having a glucose-N-acetylglucosamine repeating unit, a cellulose-chitin hybrid polysaccharide. *Biomacromolecules* **2006**, *7*, 1644–1656.

108. Kobayashi, S.; Makino, A. Enzymatic polymer synthesis: An opportunity for green polymer chemistry. *Chem. Rev.* **2009**, *109*, 5288–5353

109. Kadokawa, J.I. Precision polysaccharide synthesis catalyzed by enzymes. *Chem. Rev.* **2011**, *111*, 4308–4345.

110. Shoda, S.; Izumi, R.; Fujita, M. Green process in glycotechnology. *Bull. Chem. Soc. Jpn.* **2003**, *76*, 1–13.

111. Kadokawa, J.; Shoda, S.J. New methods for architectures of glyco-materials. *Synthetic Org. Chem. Jpn.* **2003**, *61*, 1207.

112. Misawa, Y.; Lohavisavapanichi, C.; Shoda, S. Chemo-enzymatic synthesis of oligosaccharides having a polymerizable group at the reducing end. *Glycoconj. J.* **1999**, *16*, S122.

113. Shoda, S.; Fujita, M.; Lohavisavapanichi, C.; Misawa, Y.; Ushizaki, K.; Tawata, Y.; Kuriyama, M.; Kohri, M.; Kuwata, H.; Watanabe, T. Efficient method for the elongation of the *N*-acetylglucosamine unit by combined use of chitinase and β-galactosidase. *Helv. Chim. Acta* **2002**, *85*, 3919.

114. Kadokawa, J.; Shoda, S. Enzymatic synthesis of glyco-macromonomers. *Sen'i Gakkaishi* **2003**, *59*, 74–78.

115. Shoda, S.; Misawa, Y.; Nishijima, Y.; Tawata, Y.; Kotake, T.; Noguchi, M.; Kobayashi, A.; Watanabe, T. Chemo-enzymatic synthesis of novel oligo-*N*-acetyllactosamine derivatives having a β(1-4)–β(1-6) repeating unit by using transition state analogue substrate. *Cellulose* **2006**, *13*, 477–484.

116. Watanabe, T.; Kobori, K.; Miyashita, K.; Fujii, T.; Sakai, H.;Uchida, M.; Tanaka, H. Identification of glutamic acid 204 and aspartic acid 200 in chitinase A1 of *Bacillus circulans* WL-12 as essential residues for chitinase activity. *J. Biol. Chem.* **1993**, *268*, 18567–18572.

117. Watanabe, T.; Suzuki, K.; Oyanagi, W.; Ohnishi, K.; Tanaka, H. Gene cloning of chitinase A1 from *Bacillus circulans* WL-12 revealed its evolutionary relationship to Serratia chitinase and to the type III homology units of fibronectin. *J. Biol. Chem.* **1990**, *265*, 15659–15665.

118. Sakamoto, J.; Watanabe, T.; Ariga, Y.; Kobayashi, S. Ring-opening glycosylation of a chitobiose oxazoline catalyzed by a non-chitinolytic mutant of chitinase. *Chem. Lett.* **2001**, *30*, 1180–1181.

119. Ochiai, H.; Ohmae, M.; Kobayashi, S. Enzymatic synthesis of alternatingly 6-*O*-carboxymethylated chitotetraose by selective glycosidation with chitinase catalysis. *Chem. Lett.* **2004**, *33*, 694–695.

120. Ochiai, H.; Ohmae, M.; Kobayashi, S. Enzymatic glycosidation of sugar oxazolines having a carboxylate group catalyzed by chitinase. *Carbohydr. Res.* **2004**, *339*, 2769–2788.

121. Makino, A.; Kurosaki, K.; Ohmae, M.; Kobayashi, S. Chitinase-catalyzed synthesis of alternatingly *N*-Deacetylated chitin: A chitin–chitosan hybrid polysaccharide. *Biomacromolecules* **2006**, *7*, 950–957.

122. Villa-Lerma, G.; Gonzalez-Marquez, H.; Gimeno, M.; Lopez-Luna, A.; Barzana, E.; Shirai, K. Ultrasonication and steam-explosion as chitin pretreatments for chitin oligosaccharide production by chitinases of *Lecanicillium lecanii*. *Biores. Technol.* **2013**, *146*, 794–798.

123. Nakagawa, Y.S.; Oyama, Y.; Kon, N.; Nikaido, M.; Tanno, K.; Kogawa, J.; Inomata, S.; Masui, A.; Yamamura, A.; Kawaguchi, M.; *et al.* Development of innovative technologies to decrease the environmental burdens associated with using chitin as a biomass resource: Mechanochemical grinding and enzymatic degradation. *Carbohydr. Polym.* **2011**, *83*, 1843–1849.

124. Sato, T.; Asada, K.; Takeda, M.; Tanno, K. Mechano-chemical synthesis of compound powders in ZnO–TiO$_2$ system by a new high intensive ball mill. *J. Jpn. Soc. Powder Metall.* **2006**, *53*, 62–67.

125. Takeda, T.; Nikaido, M.; Totani, T.; Obara, M.; Nakano, Y.; Uchimiya, H. Evaluation of high intensive ball mill method for effective saccharification of plant cell wall materials. *J. Appl. Glycosci.* **2009**, *56*, 71–76.

126. Wu, Q.; Miao, Y. Mechanochemical effects of micronization on enzymatic hydrolysis of corn flour. *Carbohydr. Polym.* **2008**, *72*, 398–402.

127. Fujimoto, S.; Inoue, H.; Yano, S.; Sakaki, T.; Minowa, T.; Endo, T. Bioethanol production from lignocellulosic biomass requiring no sulfuric acid: Mechanochemical pretreatment and enzymic saccharification. *J. Jpn. Petrol. Inst.* **2008**, *51*, 264–273.

128. Van Craeyveld, V.; Delcour, J.A.; Courtin, C.M. Ball milling improves extractability and affects molecular properties of Psyllium (*Plantago ovate* Forsk) seed husk arabinoxylan. *J. Agric. Food Chem.* **2008**, *56*, 11306–11311.

129. Reese, E.T.; Siu, R.G.H.; Levinson, H.S. The biological degradation of soluble cellulose derivatives and its relationship to the mechanism of cellulose hydrolysis. *J. Bacteriol.* **1950**, *59*, 485–497.

130. Vaaje-Kolstad, G.; Westereng, B.; Horn, S.J.; Liu, Z.; Zhai, H.; Sørlie, M.; Eijsink, V.G.H. An oxidative enzyme boosting the enzymatic conversion of recalcitrant polysaccharides. *Science* **2010**, *330*, 219–222.

131. Shinohara, M.L.; Ihara, M.; Abo, M.; Hashida, M.; Takagi, S.; Beck, T.C. A novel thermostable branching enzyme from an extremely thermophilic bacterial species, *Rhodothermus obamensis. Appl. Microbiol. Biotechnol.* **2001**, *57*, 653–659.

132. 125. Montilla, A.; Ruiz-Matute, A.I.; Corzo, N.; Cecilia Giacomini, C.; Irazoqui, G. Enzymatic generation of chitooligosaccharides from chitosan using soluble and immobilized glycosyltransferase (Branchzyme). *J. Agric. Food Chem.* **2013**, *61*, 10360–10367.

133. Heggset, E.B.; Dybvik, A.I.; Hoell, I.A.; Norberg, A.L.; Sørlie, M.; Eijsink, V.G.H.; Vårum, K.M. Degradation of chitosans with a family 46 chitosanase from *Streptomyces coelicolor* A3(2). *Biomacromolecules* **2010**, *11*, 2487–2497.

134. Horn, S.J.; Sørbotten, A.; Synstad, B.; Sikorski, P.; Sørlie, M.; Vårum, K.M.; Eijsink, V.G. Endo/exo mechanism and processivity of family 18 chitinases produced by *Serratia marcescens. FEBS J.* **2006**, *273*, 491–503.

135. Fukamizo, T.; Honda, Y.; Goto, S.; Boucher, I.; Brzezinski, R. Reaction mechanism of chitosanase from *Streptomyces* sp. N174. *Biochem. J.* **1995**, *311*, 377–383.

136. Amano, K.; Ito, E. The action of lysozyme on partially deacetylated chitin. *Eur. J. Biochem.* **1978**, *85*, 97–104.

137. Sikorski, P.; Stokke, B.T.; Sørbotten, A.; Vårum, K.M.; Horn, S.J.; Eijsink, V.G. Development and application of a model for chitosan hydrolysis by a family 18 chitinase. *Biopolymers* **2005**, *77*, 273–285.

138. Heggset, E.B.; Hoell, I.A.; Kristoffersen, M.; Eijsink, V.G.; Vårum, K.M. Degradation of chitosans with chitinase G from *Streptomyces coelicolor* A3(2): Production of chito-oligosaccharides and insight into subsite specificities. *Biomacromolecules* **2009**, *10*, 892–899.

139. Mitsutomi, M.; Hata, T.; Kuwahara, T. Purification and characterization of novel chitinases from *Streptomyces griseus* Hut 6037. *J. Ferment. Bioeng.* **1995**, *80*, 153–158.

140. Sasaki, C.; Vårum, K.M.; Itoh, Y.; Tamoi, M.; Fukamizo, T. Rice chitinases: Sugar recognition specificities of the individual subsites. *Glycobiology* **2006**, *16*, 1242–1250.

141. Horn, S.J.; Sikorski, P.; Cederkvist, J.B.; Vaaje-Kolstad, G.; Sørlie, M.; Synstad, B.; Vriend, G.; Vårum, K.M.; Eijsink, V.G.H. Costs and benefits of processivity in enzymatic degradation of recalcitrant polysaccharides. *Proc. Natl. Acad. Sci. USA* **2006**, *103*, 18089–18094.

142. Sikorski, P.; Sørbotten, A.; Horn, S.J.; Eijsink, V.G.; Vårum, K.M. *Serratia marcescens* chitinases with tunnel-shaped substrate-binding grooves show endo activity and different degrees of processivity during enzymatic hydrolysis of chitosan. *Biochemistry* **2006**, *45*, 9566–9574.

143. Gyore, J.; Parameswar, A.R.; Hebbard, C.F.F.; Oh, Y.; Bi, E.; Demchenko, A.V.; Price, N.P.; Orlean, P. 2-Acylamido analogues of *N*-acetylglucosamine prime formation of chitin oligosaccharides by yeast chitin synthase 2. *J. Biol. Chem.* **2014**, *289*, 12835–12841.

144. Liang, T.W.; Hsieh, J.L.; Wang, S.L. Production and purification of a protease, a chitosanase, and chitin oligosaccharides by *Bacillus cereus* TKU022 fermentation. *Carbohydr. Res.* **2012**, *362*, 38–46.

145. Vandanarachchi, J.K.; Kurukulasuriya, M.S.; Kim, S.K. Chitin, chitosan, and their oligosaccharides in food industry. In *Chitin, Chitosan, Oligosaccharides and Their Derivatives*; Kim, S.K., Ed.; CRC Press: Boca Raton, FL, USA, 2011; pp. 543–560.

146. Jeon, Y.J.; Kim, S.K. Continuous production of chitooligosaccharides using a dual reactor system. *Process Biochem.* **2000**, *35*, 623–632.

# Squid Pen Chitin Chitooligomers as Food Colorants Absorbers

**Tzu-Wen Liang, Chih-Ting Huang, Nguyen Anh Dzung and San-Lang Wang**

**Abstract:** One of the most promising applications of chitosanase is the conversion of chitinous biowaste into bioactive chitooligomers (COS). TKU033 chitosanase was induced from squid pen powder (SPP)-containing *Bacillus cereus* TKU033 medium and purified by ammonium sulfate precipitation and column chromatography. The enzyme was relatively more thermostable in the presence of the substrate and had an activity of 93% at 50 °C in a pH 5 buffer solution for 60 min. Furthermore, the enzyme used for the COS preparation was also studied. The enzyme products revealed various mixtures of COS that with different degrees of polymerization (DP), ranging from three to nine. In the culture medium, the fermented SPP was recovered, and it displayed a better adsorption rate (up to 96%) for the disperse dyes than the water-soluble food colorants, Allura Red AC (R40) and Tartrazne (Y4). Fourier transform-infrared spectroscopic (FT-IR) analysis proved that the adsorption of the dyes onto fermented SPP was a physical adsorption. Results also showed that fermented SPP was a favorable adsorber and could be employed as low-cost alternative for dye removal in wastewater treatment.

Reprinted from *Mar. Drugs*. Cite as: Liang, T.-W.; Huang, C.-T.; Dzung, N.A.; Wang, S.-L. Squid Pen Chitin Chitooligomers as Food Colorants Absorbers. *Mar. Drugs* **2015**, *13*, 681-696.

## 1. Introduction

Chitosan is a partially deacetylated derivative of chitin, which consists of *N*-acetyl-D-glucosamine (GlcNAc) and D-glucosamine (GlcN) residues. Chitosanases are enzymes that catalyze the hydrolysis of the β-1,4 glycosidic bonds of chitosan. These enzymes have been found in abundance in a variety of bacteria [1–9]. Although chitosanases are efficient in producing chitosan [2–4,6], chitosan has been produced on an industrial scale mostly by the *N*-deacetylation of chitin using sodium hydroxide [10]. Among the natural chitinous resources, fishery wastes (crustaceans shells and squid pens) have an especially high content of chitin. Therefore, organisms that produce chitosanase with fishery wastes as the sole C/N source not only would solve an environmental problem but also could reduce the production costs of microbial chitosanase.

One of the most important and promising applications of chitosanases is the conversion of chitin-containing fishery waste into bioactive chitooligomers (COS). These oligomers have been shown to have potential to be the important pharmaceutical agents, these include antitumor, antioxidant [11], and antimicrobial activities [12–15]. Because the biological activities of COS are highly dependent on the degrees of polymerization (DP) and/or deacetylation (DD) [13], it is important to produce a well-defined COS mixture for specific uses, and study their structure-function relationship. One of the most important advantages of using chitosanase to produce COS rather than chemical operations (such as acid hydrolysis) is that it is a more environment-friendly process, and it generates a more defined COS mixtures. Therefore, obtaining an efficient mode for chitosanase production and the conversion of chitosan into bioactive COS will be highly beneficial for the chitin biotechnological industry.

In addition, chitin and chitosan have also been used in a wide range of applications, including effluent treatment for dye removal [16–18]. Most commercial systems currently use activated carbon as sorbent because of its excellent adsorption ability, but it is expensive and difficult to regenerate. In recent years, chitosan has been developed as a cheap and effective new alternative for dye removal. Chitosan is also a renewable resource and more environmental friendly than commercial materials. In a previous report, L. paracasei and S. marcescens have been used for the production of chitin from crab shell waste by successive fermentation [19]. Consequently, to decrease the cost of adsorbents for dye removal, the fermented fishery wastes in culture broth should also be able to be recovered for biological applications in dye removal. This idea inspired us to screen chitosanase-producing strains by using fishery wastes and to reclaim the wastes from the medium for dye removal.

A Bacillus cereus strain TKU033 that was capable of utilizing SPP to produce chitosanase was isolated from soil samples. The TKU033 chitosanase was purified, and its biochemical features were also characterized. In addition, the applications of the endo-type TKU033 chitosanase in functional chitooligomer production were also examined. To decrease the cost of adsorbents for dye removal, comparisons of the adsorption rates of the fermented SPP and the unfermented SPP for the disperse dyes (hydrophobic pigments, disperse red 60 (Figure 1a) and disperse yellow 54 (Figure 1b)) and water-soluble food colorants (Allura Red AC, R40 (Figure 1c); and Tartrazne, Y4 (Figure 1d)) were also undertaken.

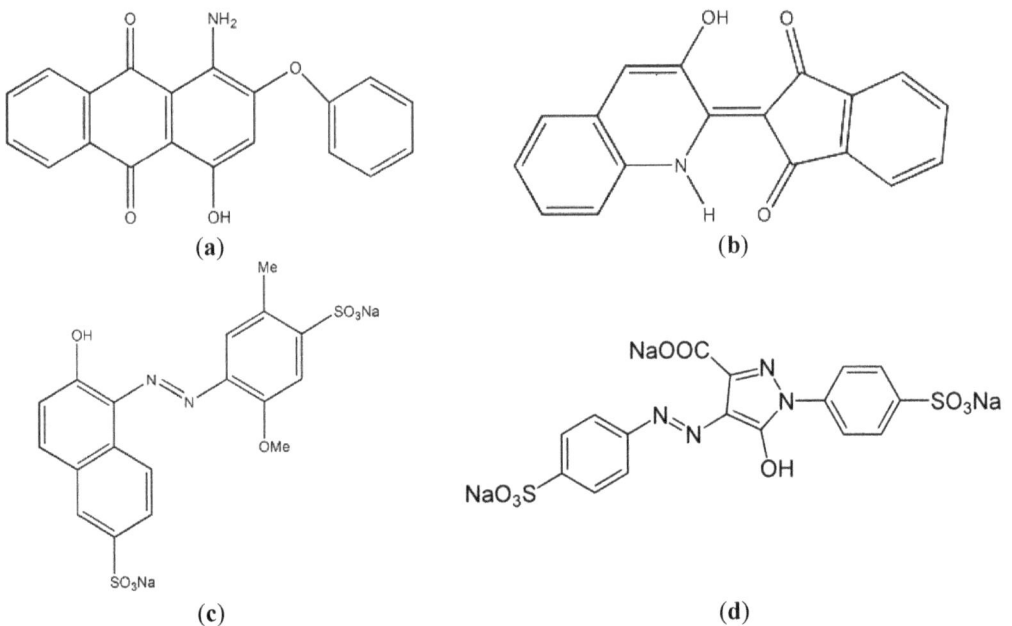

**Figure 1.** Chemical structures of disperse dyes and food colorants. (**a**) disperse red 60; (**b**) disperse yellow 54; (**c**) Allura Red AC; (**d**) Tartrazne.

## 2. Results and Discussion

### 2.1. Isolation and Identification of a Chitosanase-Producing Strain

The microorganisms were isolated from soil samples using the procedure described above. Among over 148 strains that were isolated in the laboratory and screened for chitosanase activity, the TKU033 strain was selected for further study. The TKU033 strain was maintained on nutrient agar and used throughout the study.

Strain TKU033 is a gram-positive and endospore-forming bacillus that contains catalase but not oxidase and is capable of growing in both aerobic and anaerobic environments. According to the results of the 16S rDNA partial nucleotide sequence (approximately 1.5 kbp) analysis, strain TKU033 was the most similar to *Bacillus* sp. According to the API identification, strain TKU033 was the closest to *B. cereus* with a 99.9% similarity. Therefore, the isolate was identified as *B. cereus*.

### 2.2. TKU033 Chitosanase Production and Purification

The production of chitosanase by strain TKU033 was investigated during 5 days of cultivation in the production medium. The 50 mL of basal medium (0.1% $K_2HPO_4$ and 0.05% $MgSO_4 \cdot 7H_2O$, pH 7) containing 1.5% SPP was the most suitable medium for the production of chitosanase by strain TKU033 at 37 °C. It was observed that the culture supernatant exerted strong chitosan degrading activities. Conclusively, the results suggested that the chitosanase from *B. cereus* TKU033 might be secreted extracellularly. Exponential growth of *B. cereus* TKU033 was observed for three days, and the stationary phase was reached after these three days. The highest chitosanase activity of *B. cereus* TKU033 was detected in the culture on the third day of bacterial growth (data not shown).

Extracellular chitosanase was purified from the culture supernatant of *B. cereus* TKU033 using a series of purification procedures. The TKU033 chitosanase was eluted in the DEAE-Sepharose CL-6B chromatography step with a linear gradient of 0–1 M NaCl in the same buffer. The eluted peak fractions were pooled for further purification. After the Macro-prep DEAE chromatography step (data not shown), approximately 5.8 mg of TKU033 chitosanase was obtained (Table 1). A summary of the purification process is presented in Table 1. The purification steps were combined to give approximately an overall 10.4-fold purification of the TKU033 chitosanase. The overall TKU033 chitosanase activity yield was 2% with a specific activity of 0.052 U/mg. The molecular mass of the TKU033 chitosanase was approximately 43 kDa as confirmed by the SDS-PAGE (Figure 2), which corresponded to the gel-filtration chromatography. The molecular mass of the TKU033 chitosanase (43 kDa) was similar to most chitosanases, which have a medium apparent molecular mass within the range of 20–75 kDa [7,20].

**Table 1.** Purification of the chitosanase from *B. cereus* TKU033 [a].

| Step | Total Protein (mg) | Total Activity (U) | Specific Activity (U/mg) | Purification Fold | Yield (%) |
|---|---|---|---|---|---|
| Culture supernatant | 4032.0 | 19.4 | 0.005 | 1.0 | 100 |
| (NH$_4$)$_2$SO$_4$ ppt | 838.4 | 5.9 | 0.007 | 1.4 | 30 |
| DEAE-Sepharose | 46.5 | 1.7 | 0.037 | 7.4 | 9 |
| Macro-prep DEAE | 5.8 | 0.3 | 0.052 | 10.4 | 2 |

[a] *B. cereus* TKU033 was grown in 50 mL of liquid medium in an Erlenmeyer flask (250 mL) containing 1.5% SPP, 0.1% K$_2$HPO$_4$, and 0.05% MgSO$_4$·7H$_2$O in a shaking incubator for 3 days at 37 °C.

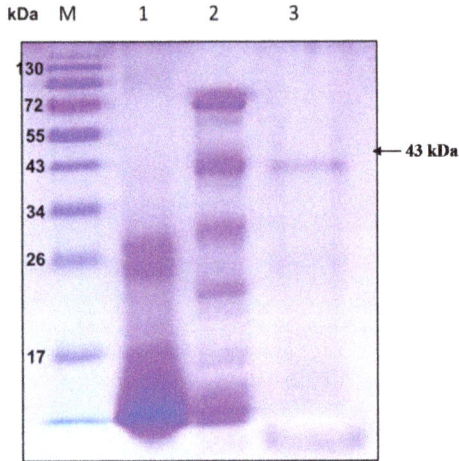

**Figure 2.** Sodium dodecyl sulfate polyacrylamide gel electrophoresis (SDS-PAGE) analysis of the chitosanase produced by *B. cereus* TKU033. Lanes: M, molecular markers (170, 130, 95, 72, 55, 43, 34, 26, 17, and 10 kDa); (1) crude enzyme; (2) adsorbed chitosanase fractions after DEAE-Sepharose CL-6B chromatography; (3) adsorbed chitosanase fractions after Macro-prep DEAE chromatography.

*2.3. Effects of pH and Temperature*

The pH activity profiles of the TKU033 chitosanase revealed maximum activity at pH 5 (Figure 3a). The optimum pH (pH 5) for TKU033 chitosanase activity was similar to that of most bacterial chitosanases, which display optimum activities at acidic pH values in a range from 4.5 to 6.5 [2,3]. The pH stability profiles of the TKU033 chitosanase were determined by measurement of the residual activity at pH 7 after incubation at various pH values at 37 °C for 60 min. The chitosanase was relatively stable at pH 5–9 and retained more than 85% of the initial activity in that range (Figure 3b). The TKU033 chitosanase became more sensitive to pH changes below pH 5 and above pH 9. The decrease of activity at lower and higher pH ranges may be due to the instability of the protein, rather than an acid-base catalytic mechanism, as reported in previous results [3,21].

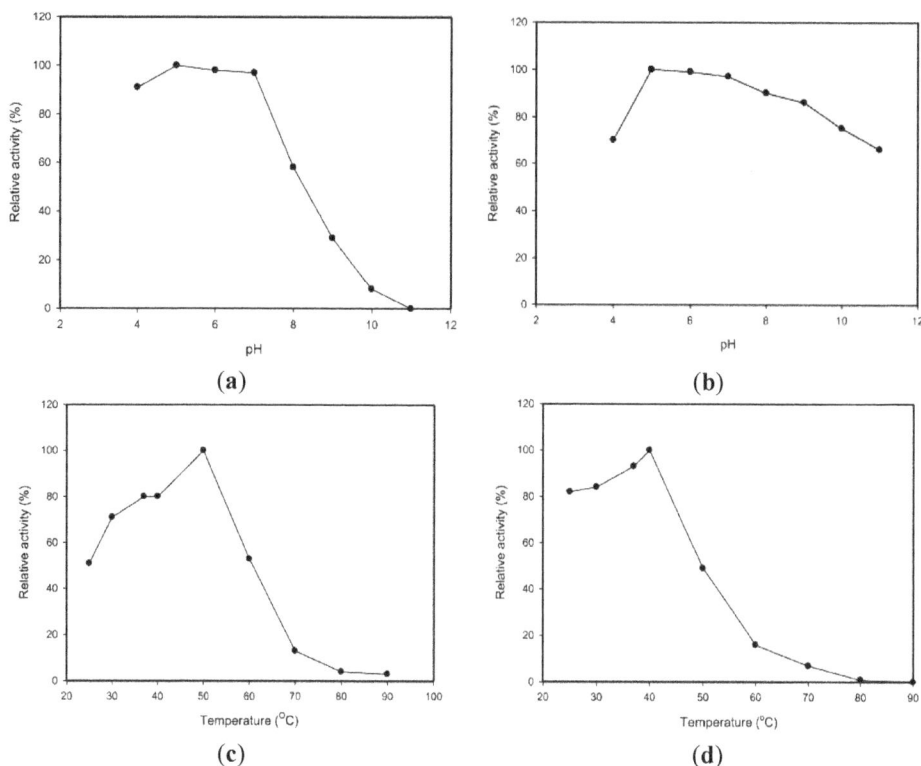

**Figure 3.** Effects of pH and temperature on the activity and stability of the chitosanase from *B. cereus* TKU033. (**a**) optimum pH; (**b**) pH stability; (**c**) optimum temperature; (**d**) thermal stability.

The effect of temperature on the activity of the TKU033 chitosanase was also studied. The optimum temperature for the TKU033 chitosanase was 50 °C (Figure 3c). To examine the thermal stability of the TKU033 chitosanase, the enzyme solution in 50 mM phosphate buffer (pH 7) was allowed to incubate for 60 min at various temperatures; then, the residual activity was measured. Less than 10% of the residual activity could be detected after incubation at 70 °C under the conditions (Figure 3d). The TKU033 chitosanase was relatively stable from 25 to 40 °C and had 50% of its activity at 50 °C, but it was completely inactivated at 80 °C (Figure 3d). However, when the enzyme was incubated for 60 min at 50 °C and pH 5, in the presence of 0.3% (w/v) water-soluble chitosan, the residual activity of the enzyme was 93% (data not shown). These results indicated that the substrate could prevent thermal inactivation of the chitosanase activity. Enhancement of chitosanase thermostability by the substrate has previously been reported for chitosanase of the glycoside hydrolase (GH) family 8 from *Bacillus thuringienesis* [5] and the GH family 46 from *Bacillus subtilis* 168 [6].

## 2.4. Substrate Specificity

For the substrate specificity of the TKU033 chitosanase, chitin and chitosan with DD ranging from 60% to 98% were used as the substrates. The TKU033 chitosanase showed a remarkable specificity toward chitosan with DD ranging from 80% to 98%, although some detectable activity was observed against other substrates (data not shown). The TKU033 chitosanase exhibited no activity on 60% DD chitosan, α-chitin, and colloidal chitin. It has been reported that chitosanase is produced by using various carbon sources, for instance chitosan [2,22,23], wheat bran [1], glucose [4], and shrimp shell [24]. Most chitosanases exhibit a wide range of substrate specificities [25]. In this study, TKU033 chitosanase degraded chitosan specifically and cleaved chitosan with maximal activity on polymers of DD ranging from 80% to 98%. The chitin and highly acetylated chitosans appear to be poor substrates because they contain insufficient glucosamine residues for optimal activity. Further research will be done to determine the structure of the resulting oligo-chitosan terminal units and the site of the enzyme cleavage. In previous reports, most bacterial chitosanases hydrolyze chitosan efficiently and chitin to a lesser extent [3]. These results indicate that the physical form of the substrate affects the rate of hydrolysis. Taken together, these results suggest that the TKU033 chitosanase produced in a specific manner from *B. cereus* TKU033 may be a useful tool for the chitosan biotechnological industry in the production of COS.

## 2.5. Effects of Various Inhibitors and Metal Ions

For the effects of metal ions on enzyme activity, the TKU033 chitosanase activity was measured in response to different metal ions and demonstrated that preincubating the enzyme with 5 mM $Fe^{2+}$, $Zn^{2+}$, $Cu^{2+}$, or $Mn^{2+}$ resulted in 30%, 26%, 82%, and 70% inhibition, respectively (data not shown). In previous reports, $Cu^{2+}$ and $Mn^{2+}$ could activate or inhibit different chitosanases [26–31]; however, both $Cu^{2+}$ and $Mn^{2+}$ inhibited the TKU033 chitosanase at 1–5 mM. The TKU033 chitosanase activity was markedly different from other chitosanases; therefore, we hypothesized that different metal ions might affect the TKU033 chitosanase activity by influencing the protein structure. The TKU033 chitosanase activity was also reduced after the addition of EDTA. However, the TKU033 chitosanase activity was not affected by phenylmethanesulfonyl fluoride (PMSF). Thus, PMSF could be used to control the crude extract serine protease activity and prevent exhaustive protein degradation during downstream processes. Furthermore, the effects of different surfactants (SDS, Tween 20, Tween 40, and Triton X-100) on the stability of the TKU033 chitosanase were also studied. A high stability was observed for the TKU033 chitosanase towards various surfactants (data not shown). Upon incubation with 0.5%–2% of Tween 40, the TKU033 chitosanase activity increased slightly with the concentration of the surfactant. These results may be based on the fact that surface-active reagents might increase the turnover number of chitosanases by increasing the contact frequency between the enzyme active site and the substrate, which is accomplished by lowering the surface tension of the aqueous solution. However, in the presence of 2 mM SDS, the TKU033 chitosanase activity retained 83% of its original activity level. These results suggest that the disulfide bond in the enzyme molecule is associated with its chitosanolytic activity.

## 2.6. COS Preparation and Product Analysis

To determine the applicability of the TKU033 chitosanase for the bioconversion of chitosan into oligosaccharides, the crude enzyme from *B. cereus* TKU033 was used in the experiments. The COS was produced from the water-soluble chitosan with the TKU033 chitosanase. The course of chitosan sample degradation was conveniently studied by measurement of the total and reducing sugars. The results revealed the total sugar and the reducing sugar of the sample as a function of reaction time. The chitosan sample total and reducing sugar values produced a similar pattern (data not shown). The total and reducing sugars increased, and the chitosan sample recovery decreased dramatically in the early reaction stage, which can be attributed to an endo-type degradation process. The TKU033 chitosanase was added into the reaction solution after 24 h and continued hydrolyzing until 48 h, but it did not improve the increase in total and reducing sugar levels (data not shown). Selective precipitation in 90% methanol and acetone solutions was performed to obtain low DP oligomers, as described earlier [13]. A product analysis of the 90% acetone solution precipitation by matrix assisted laser desorption ionization time of flight mass spectrometry (MALDI-TOF) revealed that various COS had DP values up to nine. The higher DP chitooligomers were precipitated as a light yellow powder in the methanol solution. The MALDI-TOF MS of the low DP oligomer fraction revealed pronounced differences among the crude enzyme-generated chitooligomers, as demonstrated for chitosan depolymerization in Figure 4. The hydrolysate ions present in the mass spectra were identified as sodium adducts $[M + Na]^{+}$. Due to the signal interference of matrix (2,5-dihydroxybenzoic acid), DP < 2 oligomers could not be determined by this method. More information about the assigned structure of each signal at different hydrolysis times is given in Table 2. When the hydrolysis time was at 2 h, the hydrolysis products contained (GlcN)$_4$; however, (GlcN)$_4$ could not be observed during 4–48 h, indicating that the TKU033 chitosanase could cleave the GlcN-GlcN links of (GlcN)$_4$ to (GlcN)$_2$ or GlcN. The hydrolysates contained chitooligomers (GlcN-oligomers) and several partial *N*-acetylated forms (Table 2). The TKU033 chitosanase reaction product is a mixture of DP 3–9 hetero-chitooligomers (Table 2). These products were generated by hydrolysis of the water-soluble chitosan with the TKU033 chitosanase and are not a series of fully deacetylated GlcN oligomers. During hydrolysis, the *O*-glycosidic and the *N*-acetyl linkages between the residues can be hydrolyzed. These results indicate that the TKU031 chitosanase might hydrolyze chitosan in an endo-type fashion. From these results, chitosan hydrolysis by the TKU033 chitosanase, combined with a selective methanol precipitation, is a quick and simple method to obtain good chitooligosaccharide yields with DPs up to nine and low molecular weight oligomers.

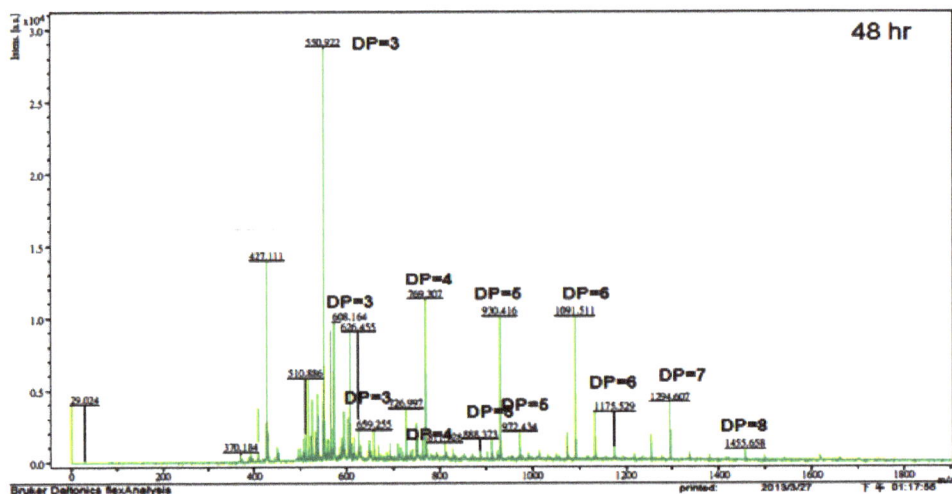

**Figure 4.** Matrix assisted laser desorption ionization time of flight mass spectrometry (MALDI-TOF-MS) of the chitooligomers (COS) mixtures obtained during the water-soluble chitosan hydrolysis for 48 h with the TKU033 crude enzyme. The proportion of low molecular weight oligomers was reduced by precipitation in the 90% methanol soluble/90% acetone insoluble fraction. The identified peaks are labeled with DP, in which DP indicates the degree of polymerisation.

**Table 2.** Ion composition of COS with DP below nine as assigned by the MALDI-TOF-MS spectra, prepared by enzymatic hydrolysis of the TKU033 crude enzyme for the indicated times and fractionated using selective isolation with 90% methanol and acetone.

| m/z | Ion Composition | DP | Hydrolysis Time (h) | | | | | |
|-----|-----------------|-----|------|------|------|------|------|------|
| | | | 2 | 4 | 6 | 12 | 24 | 48 |
| 550 | $(GlcN)_2$-GlcNAc | 3 | + | + | + | + | | + |
| 608 | GlcN-$(GlcNAc)_2$ | 3 | | + | | + | + | + |
| 659 | $(GlcNAc)_3$ | 3 | + | | | + | | + |
| 692 | $(GlcN)_4$ | 4 | + | | | | | |
| 727 | $(GlcN)_3$-GlcNAc | 4 | | + | + | | | |
| 769 | $(GlcN)_2$-$(GlcNAc)_2$ | 4 | + | + | + | + | + | + |
| 811 | GlcN-$(GlcNAc)_3$ | 4 | | + | + | + | | + |
| 888 | $(GlcN)_4$-GlcNAc | 5 | | + | + | | | + |
| 930 | $(GlcN)_3$-$(GlcNAc)_2$ | 5 | + | + | + | + | + | + |
| 972 | $(GlcN)_2$-$(GlcNAc)_3$ | 5 | | + | + | + | + | + |
| 1091 | $(GlcN)_4$-$(GlcNAc)_2$ | 6 | | + | | | + | + |
| 1133 | $(GlcN)_3$-$(GlcNAc)_3$ | 6 | + | | + | + | | |
| 1175 | $(GlcN)_2$-$(GlcNAc)_4$ | 6 | | | | | | + |
| 1294 | $(GlcN)_4$-$(GlcNAc)_3$ | 7 | + | + | + | + | + | + |
| 1455 | $(GlcN)_5$-$(GlcNAc)_3$ | 8 | | + | | + | | + |
| 1616 | $(GlcN)_6$-$(GlcNAc)_3$ | 9 | | + | | + | | |

*2.7. Fermented SPP as a Biosorbent for Dye Removal*

Chitin and chitosan, mostly prepared from shrimp shells, crab shells, and squid pens by chemical treatments, have been used in a wide range of applications, including effluent treatment for dye removal [16–18]. However, the costs of chitin-related preparations were far higher than those of their raw materials, marine chitin-containing byproducts. In this study, we chose SPP as the biosorbent for dye removal. For comparison, the three-day fermented SPP recovered from the culture broth of TKU033 was also analyzed. Appropriate amounts of the reclaimed SPP were added into 2 mL of dye-containing solutions. After shaking at 30 °C for 15 min, the reaction mixtures were centrifuged, and the residual dye in the supernatants was analyzed. The results showed that the color of SPP clearly changed from the colorless original to the color of the dye. The measured adsorption rates for all of the tested dyes also increased with the amounts of the fermented SPP added (data not shown). The maximal adsorption rate of the fermented SPP was 96% for the yellow disperse dye, followed by R40 (90%), the disperse red 60 (87%), and Y4 (68%) (Table 3). For both R40 and Y4 (water-soluble pigments), SPP (the unfermented SPP) showed a better adsorptive effect than that of the fermented SPP. As for the disperse dye (hydrophobic pigments), the fermented SPP exhibited a higher adsorption rate. Similar results were also found in our previous report [18] in which SPP showed a higher adsorption rate for water soluble colorants but a lower adsorption rate for the hydrophobic colorant (prodigiosin) than those of cicada casting and lactobacillus cells. The impact of SPP adsorption for water soluble colorants had been inferred to be related to the protein contained in SPP [18]. In this study, we compared the difference of the dye adsorption between the fermented SPP and the unfermented SPP, in addition to the difference of the protein in the two types of SPP; the difference of chitin structure in them should also be considered. Chitin is an amino polymer and has acetamide groups at the C-2 positions. The fermented SPP might result in a number of amine groups being introduced on the surface of the fermented SPP. The presence of these groups might be highly advantageous in providing distinctive adsorption functions for the disperse dyes.

The fourier transform infrared spectra (FTIR) of the fermented SPP before and after the adsorption of a food colorant (R40 and Y4) are shown in Figure 5. There was no significant change in the spectra at wavenumbers 3289 cm$^{-1}$ (-OH stretching vibration), 3082 cm$^{-1}$ (C-H stretching), 2879 cm$^{-1}$ (-CH$_2$ stretching) and 1647 cm$^{-1}$ (-NH stretching vibration) after the adsorption of the dyes. This implies that the adsorption processes represent a physical adsorption and may not involve a chemical interaction. These results provide a summary of the available information on SPP and its potential as a low-cost sorbent.

**Table 3.** Adsorption effect of squid pen powder (SPP) on the disperse dyes and food colorants.

| Substrate | Adsorption (%) | |
|---|---|---|
| | **Fermented SPP** | **Unfermented SPP** |
| Disperse red 60 | 87 | 70 |
| Disperse yellow 54 | 96 | 80 |
| Food colorant (R40) | 90 | 95 |
| Food colorant (Y4) | 68 | 82 |

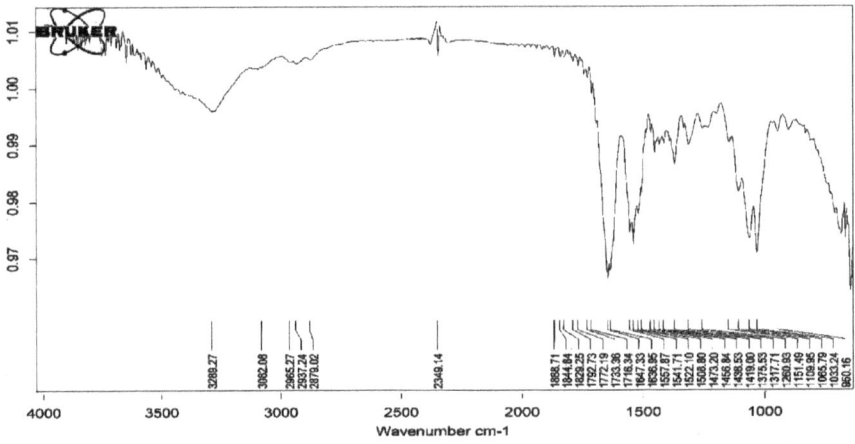

(a)

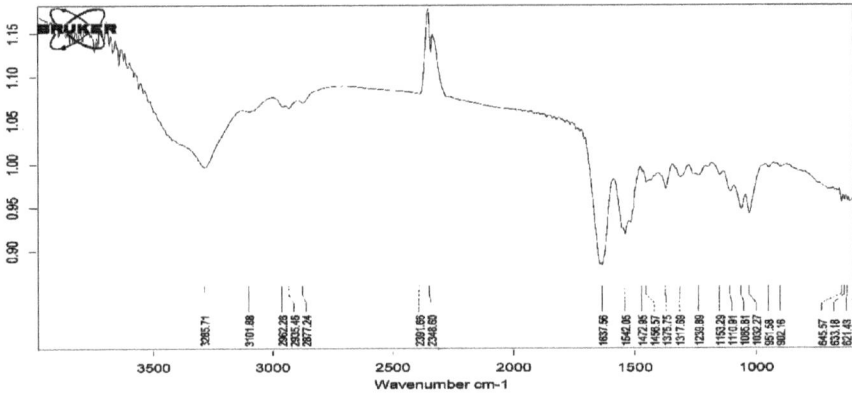

(b)

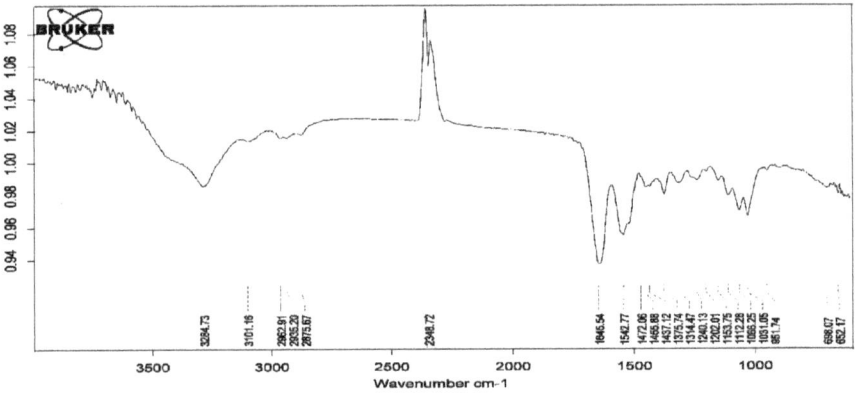

(c)

**Figure 5.** fourier transform infrared spectra (FT-IR) spectra of fermented SPP by *B. cereus* TKU033 before (**a**); and after the adsorption of R40 (**b**); and Y4 (**c**).

## 3. Materials and Methods

### 3.1. Materials

The SPP used in these experiments was prepared as described previously [14]. The squid pens were purchased from Shin-Ma Frozen Food Co. (I-Lan, Taiwan). Diethylaminoethylcellulose (DEAE)-Sepharose CL-6B was purchased from GE healthcare UK Ltd. (Little Chalfont, Buckinghamshire, England). The weak base anion exchange Macro-prep DEAE was obtained from Bio-Rad (Hercules, CA, USA). Water-soluble chitosan with 90% DD was from Charming & Beauty Co., Taipei, Taiwan. Allura Red AC and Tartrazine were obtained from the First Cosmetics Works Company (Taipei, Taiwan). The disperse dyes were obtained from Widetex Biotech Co., Ltd. (Taoyuan, Taiwan). All other reagents used were of the highest grade available.

### 3.2. Screening and Identification of Chitosanase-Producing Strains

The microorganisms were isolated from soil samples collected at different locations in northern Taiwan. One gram of soil was ground in a porcelain mortar, 10 mL of sterile distilled water was then added, and the soil suspension was stirred. The SPP-supplemented media was inoculated with 0.5 mL of the soil suspension and incubated at 30 °C for 2 days. The single strain colonies that appeared were subcultured on agar plates containing 1% SPP, 0.1% $K_2HPO_4$, 0.05% $MgSO_4 \cdot 7H_2O$, and 1.5% agar powder (pH 7). The plates were incubated at 30 °C for 2 days. The organisms obtained from this screening were subcultured in liquid media (containing 1% SPP, 0.1% $K_2HPO_4$, and 0.05% $MgSO_4 \cdot 7H_2O$) in shaking flasks at 30 °C on a rotary shaker (150 rpm, Yih Der LM-570R). After incubation for 2 days, the culture broth was centrifuged (4 °C at 12,000 $g$ for 20 min, Kubota 5922), and the supernatants were collected for the measurement of chitosanase activity using the procedure described below. The TKU033 strain showed the highest chitosanase activity, and it was isolated, maintained on SPP agar, and used throughout the study.

The bacterial strain TKU033 was identified on the basis of morphological, physiological, and biochemical parameters as well as on the basis of a 16S rDNA-based sequence analysis after PCR amplification with primers. The nucleotide bases of the DNA sequence obtained were compiled and compared with sequences in the GenBank databases using the BLAST program. Further identification of the strain TKU033 was performed using the analytical profile index (API).

The strain TKU033 grew on nutrient agar plates. The bacteria that grew on the surface of the agar plates were suspended by gentle mechanical agitation in 2 mL of sterile distilled water. This bacterial suspension was used to inoculate 50 CHB API strips (ATB system, bioMerieux SA, Marcy-I'Etoile, France) following the manufacturer's instructions. The strips were incubated at 30 °C and observed after 16, 24, 40 and 48 h and compared to the API identification index and database.

### 3.3. Preparation of the TKU033 Chitosanase

For the production of the chitosanase, *B. cereus* TKU033 was grown in 50 mL of liquid medium in an Erlenmeyer flask (250 mL) containing 1.5% SPP, 0.1% $K_2HPO_4$, and 0.05% $MgSO_4 \cdot 7H_2O$

(pH 7). One milliliter of the seed culture was transferred into 50 mL of the same medium and grown in an orbital shaking incubator for 3 days at 37 °C and pH 7.2 (the pH after being autoclaved was 7.5). After incubation, the culture broth was centrifuged (4 °C at 12,000 $g$ for 20 min), and the supernatant was used for further purification via chromatography.

### 3.4. Measurement of Chitosanase Activity

The chitosanase enzyme activity was measured by incubating 0.2 mL of the enzyme solution with 1 mL of 0.3% (w/v) water-soluble chitosan (Kiotec Co., Hsinchu, Taiwan; with 60% deacetylation) in 50 mM phosphate buffer, pH 7, at 37 °C for 30 min. The reaction was stopped by heating the reaction mixture to 100 °C for 15 min. The amount of reducing sugar produced was measured with glucosamine as the reference compound [14]; one unit of enzyme activity was defined as the amount of enzyme that produced 1 μmol of reducing sugar per min.

### 3.5. Purification of the TKU033 Chitosanase

Ammonium sulfate (608 g/L) was added to the culture supernatant (450 mL). The resulting mixture was stored at 4 °C overnight, and the precipitate was collected by centrifugation at 4 °C for 20 min at 12,000 $g$. The precipitate was then dissolved in a small amount of 50 mM sodium phosphate buffer (pH 7) and dialyzed against the buffer. The resulting dialysate (the crude enzyme) was loaded onto a DEAE-Sepharose CL-6B column (5 cm × 30 cm) that had been equilibrated with 50 mM sodium phosphate buffer (pH 7). One peak exhibiting chitosanase activity was washed from the column with the same buffer, and the other chitosanase peak was eluted with a linear gradient of 0–1 M NaCl in the same buffer. The fractions of the two peaks containing chitosanase activity were independently pooled and concentrated using ammonium sulfate precipitation. The resultant precipitate was collected by centrifugation and dissolved in 5 mL of 50 mM sodium phosphate buffer (pH 7).

The obtained enzyme solution (the adsorbed chitosanase fractions from the DEAE-Sepharose CL-6B column) was then chromatographed on a Macro-prep DEAE column (12.6 mm × 40 mm) that had been equilibrated with 50 mM sodium phosphate buffer (pH 7). The chitosanase was eluted using a linear 0–1 M NaCl gradient in the same buffer. The fractions containing chitosanase activity were pooled and concentrated using ammonium sulfate precipitation. The pooled enzyme solution fractions were used as a purified preparation.

### 3.6. Protein Determination

The protein content was determined using the Bradford method with a Bio-Rad dye reagent concentrate and bovine serum albumin as the standard. Aromatic amino acids (phenylalanine, tyrosine, and tryptophan) have absorption band between 260 and 280 nm. To recover the protein after purification from the column chromatography, the protein concentration was estimated by comparing the absorbing band at 280 nm of the control tryptophan-containing standard [14].

## 3.7. Determination of Molecular Mass

The molecular mass of the purified chitosanase was determined using sodium dodecyl sulfate-polyacrylamide gel electrophoresis (SDS-PAGE) [14] with 12.5% acrylamide and 2.67% methylene bis acrylamide in a 0.375 M Tris-HCl buffer (pH 8.8) with 0.1% (w/v) SDS. Before electrophoresis, the proteins were exposed overnight to 10 mM phosphate buffer (pH 7) containing β-mercaptoethanol. The electrode buffer was composed of 25 mM Tris, 192 mM glycine and 0.1% (w/v) SDS (pH 8.3). The electrophoresis was performed at a constant current of 70 mA through the stacking gel and 110 mA through the resolving gel. After electrophoresis, the gels were stained with Coomassie Brilliant Blue R-250 in a methanol-acetic acid-water (5:1:5, v/v) solution and decolored in 7% acetic acid. The molecular mass of the purified chitosanase in its native form was determined using a gel filtration method. The sample and the standard proteins were applied to a Sephacryl S-100 column (2.5 cm × 100 cm) equilibrated with 50 mM phosphate buffer (pH 7). Bovine serum albumin (molecular mass: 67 kDa), *Bacillus* sp. α-amylase (50 kDa) and hen egg white lysozymes (14 kDa) were used as the molecular mass markers [14].

## 3.8. Effects of pH and Temperature on Enzyme Activities

The optimum pH values of TKU033 chitosanase were studied by assaying the samples at different pH values. The pH stability of TKU033 chitosanase was determined by measuring the residual activity at pH 7 as described above after the sample had been dialyzed against a 50 mM buffer solution of various pH values (pH 4–11) in seamless cellulose tubing (Daiichi Sankyo, Tokyo, Japan). The buffer systems used were acetate (50 mM, pH 4–5), phosphate (50 mM, pH 6–8) and $Na_2CO_3$-$NaHCO_3$ (50 mM, pH 9–11). To determine the optimum temperatures for TKU033 chitosanase, the activity values of the samples were measured at various temperatures (25–90 °C). The thermal stability of TKU033 chitosanase was studied by incubating the samples at various temperatures for 60 min. The residual activity was measured as described above.

## 3.9. Effects of Various Chemicals and Surfactants on Enzyme Activities

The effects of metal ions (5 mM) were investigated using $Mg^{2+}$, $Cu^{2+}$, $Fe^{2+}$, $Ca^{2+}$, $Zn^{2+}$, $Mn^{2+}$, and $Ba^{2+}$. The effects of enzyme inhibitors were studied using phenylmethylsulfonyl fluoride (PMSF) and ethylenediaminetetraacetic acid (EDTA). The effects of surfactants were also studied using SDS, Tween 20, Tween 40, and Triton X-100. The enzyme was pre-incubated with various chemicals and surfactants for 30 min at 25 °C, and the residual chitosanase activities were then tested.

## 3.10. Measurement of Total Sugars

To evaluate total sugars, the phenol-sulfuric acid method was used [32]. Briefly, 25 μL of 5% phenol was added to 1 mL of sample. After shaking, 2.5 mL of concentrated $H_2SO_4$ was added. The mixture was left to stand for 10 min and absorbance was read at 490 nm. Pure D-glucose was employed as standard.

422

*3.11. Adsorption Effects of SPP and Fermented SPP for Dye Removal*

Two food colorants and two disperse dyes were used as adsorbates. The dyes used in the experiments were Allura Red AC (R40) $\lambda_{max}$ = 504 nm, Tartrazne (Y4) $\lambda_{max}$ = 425 nm, Disperse Red $\lambda_{max}$ = 530 nm and Disperse Yellow $\lambda_{max}$ = 415 nm. Allura Red AC and Tartrazine were obtained from the First Cosmetics Works Company (Taipei, Taiwan). The disperse dyes were obtained from Widetex Biotech Co., Ltd. (Taoyuan, Taiwan). All these dyes were commercial grade and were used directly without further purification. The food colorants (R40 and Y4) and disperse dyes (red and yellow) (0.05%, w/v) were added to different concentrations of the fermented and unfermented SPP, respectively, and incubated at 25 °C on a rotary shaker (150 rpm) for one hour. After centrifugation, the residual pigments in the supernatant were then analyzed with a spectrophotometer.

## 4. Conclusions

In this study, we have succeeded in developing the efficient production procedure of chitosanase by *B. cereus* TKU033 using the cheap medium based on squid pen. This is different from most other reported chitosanase-producing strains which require chitosan as carbon/nitrogen source. The medium for TKU033 is obviously much simpler and cheaper. Besides, enzymatic hydrolysis by TKU033 crude enzyme could obtain the COS with DP 3-9. These results may be useful for biological applications in relation to enzyme and bioactive materials production. The fermented SPP in culture broth could also be recovered from the medium for biological applications in dye removal. It displayed a better adsorption rate for the disperse dyes than the water-soluble food colorants. The adsorptive capacities of fermented SPP on dye may have a potential application in the field of water treatment.

## Acknowledgments

This work was supported in part by a grant from the Ministry of Science and Technology, Taiwan (NSC 102-2313-B-032-001-MY3, NSC 102-2621-M-032-005, and NSC 102-2811-B-032-001).

## Author Contributions

Conceived and designed the experiments: TWL SLW. Performed the experiments: CTH. Analyzed the data: CTH NAD SLW. Wrote the paper: TWL SLW.

## Conflicts of Interest

The authors declare no conflict of interest.

## References

1.  Chiang, C.L.; Chang, C.T.; Sung, H.Y. Purification and properties of chitosanase from a mutant of *Bacillus subtilis* IMR-NK1. *Enzyme Microb. Technol.* **2003**, *32*, 260–267.

2.  Gao, X.A.; Ju, W.T.; Jung, W.J.; Park, R.D. Purification and characterization of chitosanase from *Bacillus cereus* D-11. *Carbohydr. Polym.* **2008**, *72*, 513–520.

3.  Jiang, X.; Chen, D.; Chen, L.; Yang, G.; Zou, S. Purification, characterization, and action mode of a chitosanase from *Streptomyces roseolus* induced by chitin. *Carbohydr. Res.* **2012**, *355*, 40–44.

4.  Kurakake, M.; Yo-U, S.; Nakagawa, K.; Sugihara, M.; Komaki, T. Properties of chitosanase from *Bacillus cereus* S1. *Curr. Microbiol.* **2000**, *40*, 6–9.

5.  Kobayashi, T.; Koide, O.; Deguchi, S.; Horikoshi, K. Characterization of chitosanase of a deep biosphere *Bacillus* strain. *Biosci. Biotechnol. Biochem.* **2011**, *75*, 669–673.

6.  Pechsrichuang, P.; Yoohat, K.; Yamabhai, M. Production of recombinant *Bacillus subtilis* chitosanase, suitable for biosynthesis of chitosan-oligosaccharides. *Bioresour. Technol.* **2013**, *127*, 407–414.

7.  Wang, C.L.; Su, J.W.; Liang, T.W.; Nguyen, A.D.; Wang, S.L. Production, purification and characterization of a chitosanase from *Bacillus cereus*. *Res. Chem. Intermed.* **2014**, *40*, 2237–2248.

8.  Wang, C.L.; Chen C.J.; Nguyen, A.D.; Liang, T.W.; Twu, Y.K.; Huang, S.Y.; Wang, S.L. Environmental chitinous materials as adsorbents for the one-step purification of protease and chitosanase. *Res. Chem. Intermed.* **2014**, *40*, 2363–2370.

9.  Wang, S.L.; Liang, T.W.; Yen, Y.H. Bioconversion of chitin-containing wastes for the production of enzymes and bioactive materials. *Carbohydr. Polym.* **2011**, *84*, 732–742.

10. La Thi, K.N.; Wang, S.L.; Dinh, M.H.; Phung, M.L.; Nguyen, T.V.; Tran, M.D.; Nguyen, A.D. Preparation of chitosan nanoparticles by spray dryer and their antibacterial activity. *Res. Chem. Intermed.* **2014**, *40*, 2165–2176.

11. Wang, S.L.; Liu, K.C.; Liang, T.W.; Kuo, Y.H.; Wang, C.Y. *In vitro* antioxidant activity of liquor and semi-purified fractions from squid pen biowaste by *Serratia ureilytica* TKU013. *Food Chem.* **2010**, *119*, 1380–1385.

12. Busilacchi, A.; Gigante, A.; Mattioli-Belmonte, M.; Manzotti, S.; Muzzarelli, R.A.A. Chitosan stabilizes platelet growth factors and modulates stem cell differentiation toward tissue regeneration. *Carbohydr. Polym.* **2013**, *98*, 665–676.

13. Liang, T.W.; Chen, Y.J.; Yen, Y.H.; Wang, S.L. The antitumor activity of the hydrolysates of chitinous materials hydrolyzed by crude enzyme from *Bacillus amyloliquefaciens* V656. *Process Biochem.* **2007**, *42*, 527–534.

14. Wang, S.L.; Lin, T.Y.; Yen, Y.H.; Liao, H.F.; Chen, Y.J. Bioconversion of shellfish chitin wastes for the production of *Bacillus subtilis* W-118 chitinase. *Carbohydr. Res.* **2006**, *341*, 2507–2515.

15. Wang, S.L.; Lin, H.T.; Liang, T.W.; Chen, Y.J.; Yen, Y.H.; Guo, S.P. Reclamation of chitinous materials by bromelain for the preparation of antitumor and antifungal materials. *Bioresour. Technol.* **2008**, *99*, 4386–4393.

16. Dotto, G.L.; Pinto, L.A.A. Adsorption of food dyes onto chitosan: Optimization process and kinetic. *Carbohydr. Polym.* **2011**, *84*, 231–238.

17. Wan Ngah, W.S.; Ariff, N.F.M.; Hanafiah, M.A.K.M. Preparation, characterization, and environmental application of crosslinked chitosan-coated bentonite for tartrazine adsorption from aqueous solutions. *Water Air Soil Pollut.* **2010**, *206*, 225–236.

18. Wang, S.L.; Chen, S.Y.; Yen, Y.H.; Liang, T.W. Utilization of chitinous materials in pigment adsorption. *Food Chem.* **2012**, *135*, 1134–1140.

19. Jung, W.J.; Jo, G.H.; Kuk, J.H.; Kim, Y.J.; Oh, K.T.; Park, R.D. Production of chitin from red crab shell waste by successive fermentation with *Lactobacillus paracasei* KCTC-3037 and *Serratia marcescens* FS-3. *Carbohydr. Polym.* **2007**, *68*, 746–750.

20. Liang, T.W.; Chen, Y.Y.; Pan, P.S.; Wang, S.L. Purification of chitinase/chitosanase from *Bacillus cereus* and discovery of an enzyme inhibitor. *Int. J. Biol. Macromol.* **2014**, *63*, 8–14.

21. 22. Katsumi, T.; Lacombe-Harvey, M.; Tremblay, H.; Brzezinski, R.; Fukamizo, T. Role of acidic amino acid residues in chitooligosaccharide-binding to *Streptomyces* sp. N174 chitosanase. *Biochem. Biophys. Res. Commun.* **2005**, *338*, 1839–1844.

22. Shimosaka, M.; Nogawa, M.; Wang, X.Y.; Kumehara, M.; Okazaki, M. Production of two chitosanases from a chitosan-assimilating bacterium, *Acinetobacter* sp. Strain CHB101. *Appl. Environ. Microbiol.* **1995**, *61*, 438–442.

23. Chen, X.; Xia, W.; Yu, X. Purification and characterization of two types of chitosanase from *Aspergillus* sp. CJ22–326. *Food Res. Int.* **2005**, *38*, 315–322.

24. Wang, S.L.; Pen, J.H.; Liang, T.W.; Liu, K.C. Purification and characterization of a chitosanase from *Serratia marcescens* TKU011. *Carbohydr. Res.* **2008**, *343*, 1316–1323.

25. Fenton, D.M.; Eveleigh, D.E. Purification and mode of action of a chitosanase from *Penicillium islandicum*. *J. Gen. Microbiol.* **1981**, *126*, 151–165.

26. Alfonos, C.; Martines, M.; Reyes, F. Purification and properties of two endochitosananse from *Mucor rouxii* implication on its cell wall degradation. *FEMS Microbiol. Lett.* **1992**, *95*, 187–194.

27. Cheng, C.Y.; Li, Y. An *Aspergillus* chitosanase with potential for large-scale preparation of chitosan oligosaccharides. *Biotechnol. Appl. Biochem.* **2000**, *32*, 197–203.

28. Nogawa, M.; Takahashi, H.; Kashiwagi, A.; Ohshima, K.; Okada, H.; Morikawa, Y. Purification and characterization of exo-β-D-glucosaminidase from a cellulolytic fungus, *Trichoderma reesei* PC-3-7. *Appl. Environ. Microbiol.* **1998**, *64*, 890–895.

29. Wang, J.; Zhou, W.; Yuan, H.; Wang, Y. Characterization of a novel fungal chitosanase Csn2 from *Gongronella* sp. JG. *Carbohydr. Res.* **2008**, *343*, 2583–2588.

30. Zhang, X.Y.; Dai, A.L.; Zhang, X.K.; Kuroiwa, K.; Kodaira, R.; Shimosaka, M.; Okazaki, M. Purification and characterization of chitosanase and exo-β-D-glucoseaminidase from a koji mold, *Aspergillus oryza* IAM2660. *Biosci. Biotechnol. Biochem.* **2000**, *64*, 1896–1902.

31. Zhou, W.; Yuan, H.; Wang, J.; Yao, J. Production, purification and characterization of chitosanase produced by *Gongronella* sp. JG. *Lett. Appl. Microbiol.* **2008**, *46*, 49.

32. Dubois, M.; Gilles, K.A.; Hamilton, J.K.; Rebers, P.A.; Smith, F. Colorimetric method for determination of sugars and related substances. *Anal. Chem.* **1956**, *28*, 350–356.

# Chitin and Chitosan Preparation from Marine Sources. Structure, Properties and Applications

Islem Younes and Marguerite Rinaudo

**Abstract:** This review describes the most common methods for recovery of chitin from marine organisms. In depth, both enzymatic and chemical treatments for the step of deproteinization are compared, as well as different conditions for demineralization. The conditions of chitosan preparation are also discussed, since they significantly impact the synthesis of chitosan with varying degree of acetylation (DA) and molecular weight (MW). In addition, the main characterization techniques applied for chitin and chitosan are recalled, pointing out the role of their solubility in relation with the chemical structure (mainly the acetyl group distribution along the backbone). Biological activities are also presented, such as: antibacterial, antifungal, antitumor and antioxidant. Interestingly, the relationship between chemical structure and biological activity is demonstrated for chitosan molecules with different DA and MW and homogeneous distribution of acetyl groups for the first time. In the end, several selected pharmaceutical and biomedical applications are presented, in which chitin and chitosan are recognized as new biomaterials taking advantage of their biocompatibility and biodegradability.

Reprinted from *Mar. Drugs*. Cite as: Younes, I.; Rinaudo, M. Chitin and Chitosan Preparation from Marine Sources. Structure, Properties and Applications. *Mar. Drugs* **2015**, *13*, 1133-1174.

## 1. Introduction

Chitin or poly ($\beta$-(1→4)-*N*-acetyl-D-glucosamine) is a natural polysaccharide of major importance, first identified in 1884 (Figure 1). This biopolymer is synthesized by enormous number of living organisms [1] and it belongs to the most abundant natural polymers, after cellulose. In the native state, chitin occurs as ordered crystalline microfibrils which form structural components in the exoskeleton of arthropods or in the cell walls of fungi and yeast. So far, the main commercial sources of chitin are crab and shrimp shells. In industrial processing, chitin is extracted by acid treatment to dissolve the calcium carbonate followed by alkaline solution to dissolve proteins. In addition, a decolorization step is often added in order to remove pigments and obtain a colorless pure chitin. All those treatments must be adapted to chitin source, owing to differences in the ultrastructure of the initial material (the extraction and pre-treatments of chitin will be described later), to produce first a high quality chitin, and then chitosan (after partial deacetylation). Chitin is infusible and sparingly soluble during transformation into different conformations. The question of its solubility is a major problem in the development of both processing and use of chitin as well as its characterization.

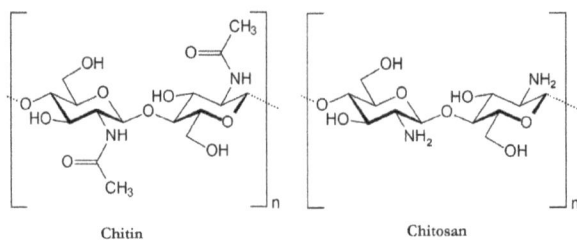

**Figure 1.** Chemical structure of chitin and chitosan

Chitin has more applications while transforming to chitosan (by partial deacetylation under alkaline conditions) [2–4]. Chitosan is a random copolymer with a molar fraction DA (degree of acetylation) of β-(1→4)-N-acetyl-D-glucosamine (Figure 1) and a fraction (1-DA) of β-(1→4)-D-glucosamine (Figure 1). The degree of acetylation of chitosan is characterized by the molar fraction of N-acetylated units (DA) or as a percentage of acetylation (DA%).

This review aims to present the state-of-the-art knowledge on the morphology of chitin and chitosan, the main techniques applied to chitin isolation and chitosan production. Then, the best methods for characterization in solution or solid state are also indicated. It is pointed out that for biomedical products, chitin and chitosan need to be highly purified, since residual proteins and pigments can cause side effects. Finally, the main biological properties will be analyzed in relation with the chemical structure (degree of acetylation and molecular weight of chitosan).

Concerning applications of chitin and chitosan, several examples used for drug release, wound dressing or biofilms are described. It is important to recall that chitin is a natural polymer as well as biocompatible and biodegradable in the body, thus widely used for biomedical and pharmaceutical applications. Additionally, good film forming properties are valuable for wound dressing, artificial skin or packaging.

## 2. Chitin Preparation and Characterization

### 2.1. Morphology of Chitin

Depending on its source, chitin occurs as two allomorphs, namely the α and β forms [5,6], which can be differentiated by infrared and solid-state NMR spectroscopies together with X-ray diffraction. In the solid state, chitin chains are assembled by the H-bonds network which controls the solubility, swelling and reactivity.

α-Chitin isomorph is by far the most abundant; it occurs in fungal and yeast cell walls, in krill, lobster and crab tendons and in shrimp shells, as well as in insect cuticle. In addition to the native chitin, α-chitin is systematically formed by: recrystallization from chitin solution [7,8], by *in vitro* biosynthesis [9,10] or enzymatic polymerization [11] due to high thermodynamical stability of this isomorph.

The rarer β-chitin is found in association with proteins in squid pens [5,12] and in the tubes synthesized by pogonophoran and vestimetiferan worms [13,14]. The crystallographic parameters of the two isomorphs allow us to conclude that there are two antiparallel molecules per unit cell in α-chitin but only one in β-chitin in a parallel arrangement. In these two structures, the chains are organized in sheets and held by intra-sheet hydrogen bonds. In addition, in α-chitin, inter-sheet hydrogen bonds prevent diffusion of small molecules into the crystalline phase. No inter-sheet hydrogen bonds are found in the crystal structure of β-chitin. This may explain its swelling in the presence of polar guest molecules (ranging from water to alcohol and amines) which penetrate the crystal lattice without disturbing the sheet organization and the crystallinity of the sample. The removal of the guest molecule allows us to revert to the original state of anhydrous β-chitin. The reactivity of β-chitin isomorph is larger than the α-isomorph, which is important for enzymatic and chemical transformations of chitin [15]. To conclude, both α and β forms are insoluble in all the common solvents. This insolubility is a major problem in the view of the development of processing and applications of chitin.

## 2.2. Chitin Extraction

The main sources of raw material for the production of chitin are cuticles of various crustaceans, principally crabs and shrimps. In crustaceans or more specifically shellfish, chitin is found as a constituent of a complex network with proteins onto which calcium carbonate deposits to form the rigid shell. The interaction between chitin and protein is very intimate and there is also a small fraction of protein involved in a polysaccharide-protein complex [16]. Thus, chitin isolation from shellfish requires the removal of the two major constituents of the shell, proteins by deproteinization and inorganic calcium carbonate by demineralization, together with small amounts of pigments and lipids that are generally removed during the two previous steps. In some cases, an additional step of decolorization is applied to remove residual pigments. Many methods have been proposed and used over the years to prepare pure chitin; however, no standard method has been adopted. Both deproteinization and demineralization could be carried out using chemical or enzymatic treatments. The order of two steps mentioned before may be reversed with some benefit, especially when enzymatic treatment is considered. Microbial fermentation is also employed; in that case deproteinization and demineralization steps are processed simultaneously.

Regardless to the selected treatment, the isolation of chitin begins with the selection of shells. For example, for lobsters and crabs, the selection has important bearing on the subsequent quality of the final isolated material. Ideally, shells of the same size and species are chosen. In the case of shrimps, the wall of shell is thinner, thus the chitin isolation is easier than from other types of shells. The selected shells are then cleaned, dried and ground into small shell pieces.

### 2.2.1. Chemical Extraction

### 2.2.1.1. Chemical Deproteinization

The deproteinization step is difficulty due to disruption of chemical bonds between chitin and proteins. This is performed heterogeneously using chemicals which also depolymerize the biopolymer. The complete removal of protein is especially important for biomedical applications, as a percentage of the human population is allergic to shellfish, the primary culprit being the protein component.

Chemical methods were the first approach used in deproteinization. A wide range of chemicals have been tested as deproteinization reagents including NaOH, $Na_2CO_3$, $NaHCO_3$, KOH, $K_2CO_3$, $Ca(OH)_2$, $Na_2SO_3$, $NaHSO_3$, $CaHSO_3$, $Na_3PO_4$ and $Na_2S$. Reactions conditions vary considerably in each study. NaOH is the preferential reagent and it is applied at concentration ranging from 0.125 to 5.0 M, at varying temperature (up to 160 °C) and treatment duration (from few minutes up to few days). In addition of deproteinization, the use of NaOH invariably results in partial deacetylation of chitin and hydrolysis of the biopolymer lowering its molecular weight.

## 2.2.1.2. Chemical Demineralization

Demineralization consists in the removal of minerals, primarily calcium carbonate. Demineralization is generally performed by acid treatment using HCl, $HNO_3$, $H_2SO_4$, $CH_3COOH$ and HCOOH [17,18]. Among these acids, the preferential reagent is dilute hydrochloric acid. Demineralization is easily achieved because it involves the decomposition of calcium carbonate into the water-soluble calcium salts with the release of carbon dioxide as shown in the following equation:

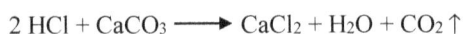

$$2\ HCl + CaCO_3 \longrightarrow CaCl_2 + H_2O + CO_2 \uparrow$$

Most of the other minerals present in the shellfish cuticle react similarly and give soluble salts in presence of acid. Then, salts can be easily separated by filtration of the chitin solid phase followed by washing using deionized water.

Demineralization treatments are often empirical and vary with the mineralization degree of each shell, extraction time, temperature, particle size, acid concentration and solute/solvent ratio. The latter depends on the acid concentration, since it needs two molecules of HCl to convert one molecule of calcium carbonate into calcium chloride. In order to have a complete reaction, acid intake should be equal to the stoichiometric amount of minerals, or even greater. [19,20]. Since, it is difficult to remove all minerals (due to the heterogeneity of the solid), larger volume or more concentrated acid solution is used. Demineralization can be followed by acidimetric titration: the evolution of pH towards neutrality corresponds to acid consumption but the persistence of acidity in the medium indicates the end of the reaction [21].

Several demineralization treatments were previously used, involving various reaction conditions. Conventionally, demineralization is accomplished using dilute hydrochloric acid at different concentrations (up to 10% w/v) at room temperature, during different incubations time (Table 1). Among such methods are those of Muzzarelli *et al.* [22], Hackman [23,24], Anderson *et al.* [25] (Table 1).

Exceptions to the above are seen in the methods of Horowitz *et al.* [26] and Synowiecki *et al.* [27] where demineralization was accomplished with 90% formic acid and 22% HCl, respectively, at room temperature. Most of the aforementioned methods include drastic treatments that may cause modifications, such as depolymerization and deacetylation of native chitin [28]. In order to overcome this problem, other methods have been developed using mild acids (to minimize degradation). For instance, Austin *et al.* [29] used ethylenediaminetetracetic acid (EDTA), Brine and Austin [30] applied acetic acid. Peniston and Johnson [31] studied a sulfurous acid process, *etc.* However, these treatments resulted in chitins with high residual ash content.

Demineralization using HCl usually can be achieved in 2 to 3 h under stirring [19]. However, reaction time varies with preparation methods from 15 min [18] to 48 h as seen in Table 1. Longer demineralization time, even to several days, results in a slight drop in the ash content but also causes polymer degradation [32,33].

Moreover, it was reported that the use of high temperature accelerates the demineralization reaction by promoting the penetration of the solvent into the chitin matrix. Thus, some demineralization reactions were carried out at higher temperature [34]. Furthermore, it was reported that the penetration of solvent into the chitin matrix strongly depends on the particles size. According to Marquis-Duval [35], the decisive factor in the demineralization is related to the contact area between the chitin matrix and the solvent. However, it was reported that high temperatures, longer incubations, high acid concentrations and granulometry affect the final physico-chemical properties of the resulting chitin.

In conclusion, although many experimental conditions can be found in the literature for the removal of minerals, effects on the molecular weight and acetylation degree cannot be avoided. Only Percot *et al.* [18] studied the extraction of chitin from shrimp shells using mild conditions allowing them to obtain chitin with a high DA. The demineralization was performed under the following conditions: at room temperature, in the presence of stoichiometric amount of 0.25 M HCl with regards to the calcium carbonate content, for 15 min incubation time. Deproteinization was later classically processed at 70 °C for 24 h using 1 M NaOH. These conditions well preserve the chitin structure, with a high DA remaining above 95%. Unfortunately, the amount of residual proteins and minerals were not determined and the influence on MW was not studied.

**Table 1.** Comparison of conditions for chitin production according to literature.

| Source | Deproteinization | | | | Demineralization | | | References |
|---|---|---|---|---|---|---|---|---|
| | NaOH Concentration * | Temperature (°C) | Number of Baths | Duration (h) | HCl Concentration * | Temperature (°C) | Duration (h) | |
| 12 species of crustaceous and cephalopods | 0.3 M | 80–85 | From 2 to 7 according to the source | 1 h for each bath | 0.55 M | Room | 15 mn to 1 h by bath repeated 2–5 times according to the source | [21] |
| Shrimp | 0.125 M | 100 | 1 | 0.5 | 1.25 M | Room | 1 | [36] |
| | 0.75 M | 100 | 1 | - | | | | |
| Shrimp | 1.25 M | 100 | 1 | 0.5 | 1.57 M | 20–22 | 1–3 | [37] |
| Crab | 0.5 M | 65 | 1 | 2 | 1.57 M | Room | 5 | [22] |
| Crab | 1 M | 80 | 1 | 3 | 1 M | Room | 12 | [38] |
| Crab | 1 M | 100 | 1 | 36 | 2 M | Room | 48 | [32] |
| Crab | 1 M | 100 | 3 | 72 | 1 M | Room | - | [23] |
| Crab | 1.25 M | 85–90 | 3 | 24 | 1.37 M | Room | 24 | [39] |
| Crab/Lobster | 2.5 M | Room | 3 | 72 | 11 M | -20 | 4 | [40] |
| Krill | 0.875 M | 90–95 | 1 | 2 | 0.6 M | Room | 2 | [25] |
| Lobster | 1 M | 100 | 5 | 12 | 2 M | Room | 5 | [24] |
| Squid | 2 M | Room | 2 | One night | 1 M | Room | One night | [41] |
| | 2 M | 100 | | 4 | | | | |
| Lobster | 10% | 100 | 1 | 2.5 | 10% HCl 90% formic | Room | 18 | [26] |
| Krill | 3.5% | 25 | 1 | 2 | 3.5% | 20 | 1.5 | [42] |
| Lobster | 5% | 80–85 | 2 | 0.5 | 5% | 70 | 4 | [43] |
| Crawfish | 3.5% | 65 | 1 | 2 | 1 M | Room | 0.5 | [44] |
| Crab | 1 M | 50 | 1 | 6 | 1 M | 20 | 3 | [30] |
| Shrimp | 1% | 65 | 1 | 1 | 0.5 M | Room | - | [45] |
| Shrimp | 3% | 100 | 1 | 1 | 1 M | Room | 0.5 | [46] |
| Shrimp | 4% | 100 | 1 | 1 | 5% | Room | - | [47] |

* Reactant concentrations are expressed in molarity or w/v %.

2.2.1.3. Processes Preserving Chitin Structure

To the best of our knowledge, there have been no studies which conduct a production of chitin with the highest DA and MW, free of minerals and proteins.

However, only the partial deacetylation may be controlled (using solid state $^{13}$C-NMR). Furthermore, the chain degradation can be also evaluated by viscometry but after additional treatment, i.e., solubilization of residual chitin in specific solvent, or after conversion to a soluble product (chitosan). Nevertheless, in the last case, the deacetylation process is usually accompanied by polymer degradation. Thus, to estimate the influence of chitin extraction process, only DA is determined as indication of the degree of the chitin degradation. It may be assumed that the higher the DA is obtained for an extracted chitin, the less the polymer is degraded.

Optimized extraction method of pure chitin production with maximum preservation of its structure (MW, DA) allows us to get chitin corresponding to the native chitin in the cuticle structure. This approach was proposed by Tolaimate et al. [21] who used chemical treatments for both demineralization and deproteinization.

In the study of Tolaimate et al. [21], a new approach was proposed using successive baths of lower HCl (0.55 M) and NaOH (0.3 M) concentrations. The number of baths for each step was dependent on the tested animal species. This method has proved a good efficacy on the reduction of proteins and minerals as well as preservation of the native chitin form for 12 different species of crustaceous and cephalopods (Table 2). The DA of the prepared chitins, determined with $^{13}$C-NMR, was varying between 96% and 100% for all the species. For example, for shrimp shells, extracted chitin was 100% acetylated. So far, such high degree of deacetylation has never been mentioned in the literature.

**Table 2.** Comparison of chitin production from different sources according to Tolaimate et al. [48].

| Source | | Number of Deproteinization Baths 0.3 M; NaOH 80 °C; 1 h | Number of Demineralization Baths 0.55 M HCl; 25 °C; 2 h | DA |
|---|---|---|---|---|
| Cirripedia | Anatife | 4 | 2 | 100 |
| Reptantia Brachyura | Red crab | 3 | 5 | 97 |
| | Marbled crab | 3 | 3 | 99 |
| | Spider crab | 3 | 3 | 96 |
| Reptantia Macrura | Lobster | 3 | 3 | - |
| | Crayfish | 7 | 3 | 100 |
| | slipper lobster | 3 | 2 | - |
| | Freshwater crayfish | 3 | 2 | - |
| Natantia | Pink shrimp | 3 | 3 | 100 |
| | Grey Shrimp | 2 | 2 | 100 |
| Stomatopoda | Squilla | 3 | 3 | 100 |
| Cephalopoda | Squid | 2 | 2 | 100 |

## 2.2.2. Biological Extraction of Chitin

The extraction by chemical treatments has many drawbacks: (i) it harms the physico-chemical properties of chitin and leads to MW and DA decrease that negatively affects the intrinsic properties of the purified chitin; (ii) it affects wastewater effluent that contains some chemicals (iii) it increases the cost of chitin purification processes. Furthermore, the development of the green extraction techniques based on the concept of 'Green chemistry' is gaining greater attention, favoring the application of enzymes and microorganisms for chitin extraction. A comparative study was carried out by Khanafari *et al.* [49] for extraction of chitin from shrimp shells by chemical and biological methods. The results indicated that the biological method (using microorganisms) was better than the chemical one because it preserves the structure of chitin. Bustos and Healy [50] also demonstrated that chitin obtained by the deproteinization of shrimp shells with various proteolytic microorganisms has higher molecular weights in comparison with chemically prepared shellfish chitin. The biological extraction of chitin offers high reproducibility in shorter time, simpler manipulation, smaller solvent consumption and lower energy input. However, the biological method is still limited to laboratory scale studies.

Recently, two reviews have reported the most common biological methods used for chitin extraction [51,52], *i.e.*, the use of proteolytic enzymes in order to digest the proteins or a fermentation process using microorganism which allows a digestion of both proteins and minerals.

The use of enzymes in the deproteinization step was first mentioned in the original Rigbv patent from 1934 but there has been a renewed interest in this approach since 1977. This work has led to the lactic acid bacterial fermentation process, studied more extensively later by Guerrero Legarreta *et al.* [53] and Cira *et al.* [54].

## 2.2.2.1. Enzymatic Deproteinization

Chitin extraction requires the use of proteases. Proteolytic enzymes are mainly derived from plant, microbial and animal sources. Many proteases such as alcalase, pepsin, papain, pancreatine, devolvase and trypsin remove proteins from crustacean shells and minimize the deacetylation and depolymerization during chitin isolation. This treatment may be performed either after, or before demineralization step of the solid material, which modifies the accessibility for the reactants.

Both purified and crude extracted proteases are used in the deproteinization step. However, commercially purified enzymes are expensive in contrast to crude proteases, which are not only cheaper but also more efficient due to the presence of coexisting proteases. Crude proteases are mainly derived from bacteria and fish viscera, bacterial proteases being the most common. Marine animals possess the same functional classes of enzymes, which are present in animal tissues and may be recovered in both active and stable forms for commercial use. In several of the major fish producing countries, the by-products represent about 50% of the seafood harvest [55]. These materials are largely underutilized and discarded as waste. Thus, application of these crude enzymes in the chitin extraction process could be interesting in decreasing the costs of this process as well as in preserving the environment.

It must be noted that the efficiency of enzymatic methods is inferior to chemical methods with approximately 5%–10% residual protein typically still associated with the isolated chitin. The final isolated chitin could be then treated with an additional NaOH treatment (under milder conditions and for a shorter time) to increase its purity and preserve the structure of chitin.

Many reports have demonstrated the application of bacterial proteases in deproteinization step. For example, Synowiecki and Al-Khateeb [56] applied enzymatic deproteinization on previously demineralized shrimp waste in order to produce chitin and a nutritionally valuable protein hydrolyzate. Alcalase 2.4 L (Novo Nordisk A/S), a serine endopeptidase obtained from *Bacillus licheniformis*, was used. This enzyme was selected due to its specificity for terminal hydrophobic amino acids, which generally leads to the production of non-bitter hydrolyzate and allows an easy control of the hydrolysis degree. The obtained hydrolyzate is a good source of essential amino acids in food applications. However, the effectiveness of deproteinization was limited by the presence of residual small peptides and amino acids attached to chitin molecules which persist after enzymatic hydrolysis. This method allows the isolation of chitin containing about 4% of protein impurities. Such purity is sufficient for many non-medical applications of chitin. Gilberg and Stenberg [57] also used alcalase 2.4 L for chitin, protein hydrolyzate and asthaxanthin recovery.

Manni *et al.* [58] compared the isolation of chitin from shrimp waste using *Bacillus cereus* SV1 crude alkaline proteases to the use of 1.25 M NaOH. Shrimp shells were demineralized after deproteinization using dilute HCl treatment. The residual protein content was significantly higher in the chitin isolated with the enzymatic deproteinization than that obtained with alkali treatment (10% compared to 6%).

In another study, enzymatic deproteinization was optimized by Younes *et al.* [59] before demineralization. In this study many microbial proteases were compared on the basis of their efficiency in shrimp shells deproteinization. Six alkaline crude microbial proteases from *Bacillus mojavensis* A21, *Bacillus subtilis* A26, *B. licheniformis* NH1, *B. licheniformis* MP1, *Vibrio metschnikovii* J1 and *Aspergillus clavatus* ES1, were used. The highest deproteinization degree was obtained with *B. mojavensis* A21 proteases, being at about 76%. Then, the effect of reaction conditions, *i.e.*, mainly enzyme/substrate ratio, temperature and incubation time, on the deproteinization degree were optimized using response surface methodology to reach 88% deproteinization under the optimized conditions.

Recently many fish and marine invertebrate alkaline crude proteases have been applied for shrimp shell deproteinization. Mukhin and Novikov [60] studied the possibility of using crustacean waste both as a substrate and as a source of proteases. The shell proteins were degraded with crude proteases isolated from the hepatopancreas of crab. The objective was to optimize the protein hydrolyzate yield. However, even under the best conditions, *i.e.*, temperature = 50 °C, time = 12 h, pH = 8.4, Enzyme/Substrate ratio of 6 g/kg, the degree of hydrolysis was never higher than 80%.

Younes *et al.* [61] used alkaline proteases from the red scorpionfish *Scorpaena scrofa* for shrimp waste deproteinized up to 85%. Activities of these crude alkaline proteases are probably related to the fish feeding mainly on crustaceans and mollusks inducing the nature and the specificity of its enzymes.

By contrast, when extraction is carried out by chemical process, the order of two steps (deproteinization and demineralization) does not have significant effect on the quality and the yield of the final chitin [62]. However, if enzymatic deproteinization is applied, the minerals presented in the cuticles may decrease the accessibility of the proteases and affect shrimp shells deproteinization efficiency. Thus, demineralization should be performed firstly.

## 2.2.2.2. Fermentation

The cost of using enzymes can be decreased by performing deproteinization by fermentation process, which can be achieved by endogeneous microorganisms (called auto-fermentation) or by adding selected strains of microorganisms. This latter can be achieved by single-stage fermentation, two-stage fermentation, co-fermentation or successive fermentation.

Many microorganism species were proposed for crustacean shells fermentation as summarized by Arbia *et al.* [51]. Fermentation methods could be separated into two major categories: lactic acid fermentation and non-lactic acid fermentation.

## (a) Lactic Acid Fermentation

Fermentation of crustacean shells can be performed by selected *Lactobacillus* sp. strain as inoculum which produces lactic acid and proteases. Lactic acid is obtained by conversion of glucose resulting in lower pH condition of silage suppressing the growth of spoilage microorganisms. Lactic acid reacts with the calcium carbonate, leading to the formation of a precipitate of calcium lactate separated from lighter shells which are recovered and rinsed with water. This process may be realized either on purified crustaceous shells, or on complete shrimp waste (including heads and viscera). Thus, deproteinization and simultaneous liquefaction of the proteins could occurred by action of proteases produced by added strains, or by gut bacteria present in the intestinal system of the treated shrimps, or by proteases present in the biowaste itself. The efficiency of lactic acid fermentation depends on many factors, mainly the species and quantity of inoculums, carbon source and its concentration, initial pH and pH evolution during fermentation, temperature and the duration of fermentation [63–65].

For example, Choorit *et al.* [66] used response surface methodology to optimize demineralization efficiency in fermented shrimp shells. Following variables were tested: sucrose concentration, initial pH value and soaking time, using *Pediococcus* sp. L1/2. Results showed an increase in demineralization degree (caused by higher sucrose concentration and soaking time) as well as an important effect of the initial pH. Demineralization degree reached at about 83% at pH 7, compared to 68% at pH 6 (sucrose concentration 50 g/L and soaking time 72h).

Otherwise, Rao *et al.* [64] studied the effect of different fermentation parameters (initial pH, initial glucose concentration and inoculation with different quantities of *Lactobacillus*) on deproteinization and demineralization degrees. Combined treatment with *Lactobacillus* and reduction of initial waste pH by addition of acetic acid produced lower deproteinization and higher demineralization degrees than treatment with *Lactobacillus* or acid individually. In addition, inoculation with *Lactobacillus* resulted in a high-quality protein liquor output, whereas autofermented waste (due to the presence of shrimp microflora) gave a strong stinky protein fraction. In the fermentation with lactic acid bacteria, the demineralization efficiency and the quality of the derived product are high, and the addition of commercial proteases may even increase deproteinization.

(b) Non Lactic-Acid Fermentation

In non-lactic acid fermentation, both bacteria and fungi were used for crustacean shells fermentation, for example: *Bacillus* sp. [67–69], *Pseudomonas* sp. [65,70,71] and *Aspergillus* sp. [72].

Ghorbel-Bellaaj *et al.* [69] evaluated six proteolytic *Bacillus* strains on the fermentation of shrimp waste: *Bacillus pumilus* A1, *B. mojavensis* A21, *B. licheniformis* RP1, *B. cereus* SV1, *B. amyloliquefaciens* An6 and *B. subtilis* A26. Results showed that all the *Bacillus* strains were able to deproteinize shrimp waste. The highest deproteinization degree was obtained using *B. cereus* SV1. These authors had also tested the role of additional amount of glucose on fermentation and they concluded that glucose had no significant effect on deproteinization degree and improved demineralization.

Sini *et al.* [68] had studied fermentation of shrimp shells in jaggery broth using *B. subtilis*. About 84% of the proteins and 72% minerals were removed; after this step the residue was treated with 0.8 N HCl and 0.6 N NaOH to reduce residual proteins and minerals to satisfactory level at about 0.8% proteins and 0.8% minerals.

Many factors have been reported to influence the fermentation process and consequently deproteinization and demineralization efficiencies [65,66,73]. Ghorbel-Bellaaj *et al.* [70] used Plackett-Burman factorial design to screen the main factors influencing fermentation efficiency using *P. aeruginosa* A2. This method is thus quite useful in preliminary studies, in which the main objective is to select variables that can be fixed or eliminated in further optimization process. Only four variables were reported to be effective on deproteinization and demineralization degrees: shrimp shell concentration, glucose concentration, inocculum size and incubation time. Under these conditions: initial medium pH, temperature, speed of agitation and volume of culture no effect on fermentation efficiency was observed. Then, from response surface methodology, under optimal conditions for fermented shrimp shells, maximum demineralization was 96%, and deproteinization was 89% [70].

Proteolytic enzymes released from fungus *A. niger* were also tested for their deproteinization and demineralization efficiency of crustacean shells. Teng *et al.* [74] evaluated concurrent production of chitin from shrimp shells and fungi in a one-pot fermentation process where proteases from the fungi hydrolyze proteins into amino acids that in turn act as a nitrogen source for fungal growth. Results showed that residual proteins in the isolated shrimp chitin were below 5%. The protein content in the fungal chitin was higher (10%–15%). They concluded that fungi and shrimp shells supplementation with glucose in a single reactor led to release of protease by the fungi and enhance the deproteinization of shrimp shells. The hydrolyzed proteins in turn were utilized for fungal growth, leading to lower pH of the medium and further demineralization of the shrimp shells.

The various biological methods of chitin extraction by microorganisms are simple, more productive and environmentally friendly when compared to chemical processes. However, microbial fermentation has its drawbacks such as: longer processing time compared to chemical methods, poorer accessibility of proteases (caused by the presence of minerals which lead to high residual proteins). Nevertheless, deproteinization rate could be ameliorated depending on the end use requirements in particular for biomedical applications. This could be achieved by using simultaneous or successive processes such as two-step fermentations or co-fermentation of microorganisms. In order to obtain highly purified chitin, biotechnological process must be completed by further mild chemical treatment to remove the residual protein and minerals.

Recently, Gortani and Hours [52] concluded that a cost-effective, fast, and easily controllable industrial process for producing chitin of high MW and DA still requires further development and optimization of the extraction process, such as: minimization of chitin degradation and decrease the impurity levels to a satisfactory level highly desirable for specific applications.

## 2.3. Chitin Characterization and Solubility

In the solid state, the chains are parallel in β-chitin and antiparallel in α-chitin [75]. Their crystalline structures were reviewed in different papers using X-ray diffraction method [76–79], IR spectroscopy [80–86], and NMR [87–90]. Solid state $^{13}$C-NMR is a commonly used technique for differentiation of the two isomorphs [88], for determination of the deacetylation degree of chitin (DD) and for control of purification conditions. Figure 2 shows typical spectra for α-chitin and chitosans with different acetylation degrees [90].

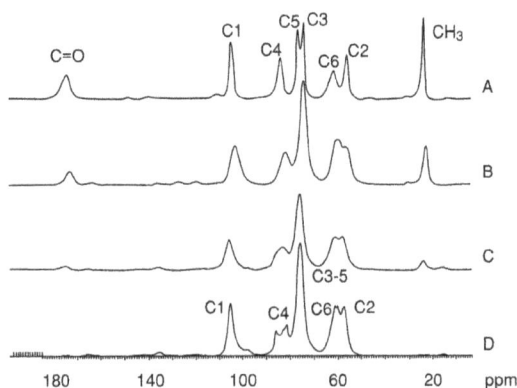

Figure 2. $^{13}$C NMR spectra for (A) chitin and chitosans (B) obtained by homogeneous reacetylation DA = 0.60; (C) commercial chitosan from Pronova DA = 0.2; (D) fully deacetylated chitin. Reproduced with permission from [90]. Copyright 2000 American Chemical Society.

Unfortunately, physical properties of chitin in solution cannot be analyzed correctly due to poor data caused mainly by difficulties in dissolution of this polymer. Dissolution is desired to estimate the molecular weight but also to process chitin (chitin cannot be processed in molten state). Presence of aggregates in solution precludes light scattering measurements and overestimates the molecular weights. Therefore, the most applicable technique here is viscometry where the Mark-Houwink parameters are known under defined thermodynamic conditions used (solvent, temperature). One of the mostly known system is based on complex formation between chitin and LiCl (at 5 wt% in the solvent DMAC) in dimethylacetamide solvent. Experimental values of parameters $K$ and $a$ relating intrinsic viscosity [$\eta$] and molecular weight M for chitin in this solvent are estimated from well-known Mark-Houwink equation according to:

$$[\eta]\ (mL/g) = KM^a \tag{1}$$

with $K = 7.6 \times 10^{-3}$, $a = 0.95$ at 30 °C [91] and $K = 2.4 \times 10^{-1}$, $a = 0.69$ at 25 °C [92].

A review on chitin and chitosan including the question of their solubility was recently published in relation to fiber processing [93]. It has been demonstrated that chitin is able to be processed from solutions. Additionally, chitin, like other polysaccharides derived from cellulose, has good film-forming properties and good stability promoted by the establishment of a hydrogen bond network between extended chains. Chitin gives original properties to the new materials due to its biocompatibility, biodegradability and non-toxicity, with antimicrobial activity and low immunogenicity.

## 3. Chitosan Preparation and Characterization

### 3.1. Chitosan Preparation

The term chitosan usually refers to a family of polymers obtained after chitin deacetylation to varying degrees. In fact, the acetylation degree, which reflects the balance between the two types of residues (Figure 1), differentiates chitin from chitosan. When the DA (expressed as molar percentage) is lower than 50 mol%, the product is named chitosan and becomes soluble in acidic aqueous solutions [94]. During deacetylation, acetyl groups are removed but also depolymerization reaction occurs, indicated by changes in MW of chitosan.

Chitin can be converted to chitosan by enzymatic preparations [95–98] or chemical process [99,100]. Chemical methods are used extensively for commercial purpose of chitosan preparation because of their low cost and suitability to mass production [100].

#### 3.1.1. Chemical Deacetylation

From a chemical point of view, either acids or alkalis can be used to deacetylate chitin. However, glycosidic bonds are very susceptible to acid; therefore, alkali deacetylation is used more frequently [100,101].

The *N*-deacetylation of chitin is either performed heterogeneously [102], or homogeneously [103]. Commonly, in the heterogeneous method, chitin is treated with a hot concentrated solution of NaOH during few hours, and chitosan is produced as an insoluble residue deacetylated up to ~85%–99%. According to the homogeneous method, alkali chitin is prepared after dispersion of chitin in concentrated NaOH (30 g NaOH/45 g $H_2O$/ 3 g Chitin) at 25 °C for 3 h or more, followed by dissolution in crushed ice around 0 °C. This method results in a soluble chitosan with an average degree of acetylation of 48%–55% [99]. This process produces deacetylation with acetyl groups uniformly distributed along the chains, for example chitosan with DA = 10% after 580 h at 25 °C [103].

Rinaudo and Domard [104] reported that the solubility of chitosan can be characterized not only by the fraction of 2-acetamido-2-deoxy-D-glucose units in the molecule but also by the N-acetyl group distribution. Aiba [105] showed that deacetylation reaction performed under heterogeneous conditions gives an irregular distribution of N-acetyl-D-glucosamine and D-glucosamine residues with some blockwise acetyl group distribution along polymeric chains. Thus, solubility and degree of aggregation of chitosan can vary in aqueous solutions leading to changes in their average characteristics. For instance, physico-chemical properties of such chitosans may differ from those of randomly acetylated chitosans obtained under homogeneous conditions.

Furthermore, variations in chitosan preparation may also result in changes of: DA, distribution of acetyl groups along the chains, MW and viscosity in solution [106,107].

In fact, many parameters in the deacetylation reaction can impact the characteristics of the final chitosan [108]. For instance, Rege and Block [109] had investigated the effect of temperature, processing time and mechanical shear on chitosan characteristics, and found that temperature and processing time have a significant effect on DA and MW. Tolaimate et al. [110] reported that chitosan DA is greatly affected by temperature and repetition of alkaline steps. Wu and Bough [45] studied the effects of time and NaOH concentration. Tsaih and Chen [111] also examined the effect of time reaction and temperature. All these studies were conducted using a classical one-variable-at-a-time experimentation. These reports indicate that MW and DA of chitosan are mainly affected by NaOH concentration, reaction time, temperature and repetition of alkaline steps. Additional factors such as reaction reagent, atmosphere, particle size, chitin and solvent ratio, and source of raw material were also tested in others studies [100,102,110,112].

Weska et al. [113] attempted to optimize chitin deacetylation by response surface methodology (controlling MW and/or DA) using temperature and reaction time variables. Hwang et al. [114] studied the effect of temperature, time and NaOH concentration on the deacetylation. Chang et al. [102] reported the influence of NaOH concentration, temperature and solution/chitin ratio and found that chitosan DA was decreasing with increase of temperature and NaOH concentration. Other parameters, such as: the use of alkali successive baths, atmospheric conditions and presence of different additives could influence deacetylation but were not considered previously in optimization studies.

Deacetylation was investigated using seven factors: the alkali reagent, its concentration, temperature, reaction time, the use of successive baths, atmospheric conditions and the use of sodium borohydride, a reducing agent [115]. For that purpose, a fractional factorial design was applied and a mathematical model was established to allow optimizing experimental conditions for chitosan of desired DA. Results clearly revealed a significant effect of temperature and the alkali reagent nature (NaOH treatment is much more efficient than KOH). It has been found that DA is significantly affected by the use of successive baths, reaction time and alkali concentration. By contrast, the atmospheric conditions (nitrogen or air) and the use of a reducing agent ($NaBH_4$) do not have significant effect on the DA of chitosan but MW of chitosan was higher under atmospheric nitrogen and addition of sodium borohydride which prevents polymer degradation. These results are in agreement with previous ones obtained with thiophenol and $NaBH_4$ used as oxygen scavenger and reducing agent, respectively [116].

3.1.2. Enzymatic Deacetylation

Chemical deacetylation has also disadvantages: energy consumption; waste of concentrated alkaline solution, thus an increase of environmental pollution, broad and heterogeneous range of soluble and insoluble products.

In order to overcome these drawbacks in the chitosan preparation, an alternative enzymatic method exploiting chitin deacetylases has been explored. The use of chitin deacetylases for the conversion of chitin to chitosan, in contrast to the currently used chemical procedure, offers the possibility of a controlled, non-degradable process, resulting in the production of novel, well-defined chitosan [117]. This method is specially used to prepare chitosan oligomers.

Chitin deacetylase (EC 3.5.1.41) catalyzes the hydrolysis of *N*-acetamido bonds in chitin to produce chitosan. The presence of this enzyme activity has been reported in several fungi [118–123] and insect species [124]. The mostly well-studied enzymes are those extracted from the fungi *Mucor rouxii* [95,118,119], *Absidia coerulea* [120], *Aspergillus nidulans* [121] and two strains of *Colletotrichum lindemuthianum* [122,123]. All the enzymes are glycoproteins and are secreted either into the periplasmic region or into the culture medium. Furthermore, all enzymes exhibit a remarkable thermal stability at their optimal temperature (50 °C), and exhibit a very strong specificity for β-(1,4)-linked *N*-acetyl-D-glucosamine polymers. However, the enzymes vary significantly in their MW and carbohydrate content and display a wide range of pH optima. It is interesting to notice that chitin deacetylases, produced by *C. lindemuthianum* and *A. nidulans,* are not inhibited by acetate (a product of the deacetylation) which make them suitable for potential biotechnological applications [121–123].

The efficiency of chitin deacetylase, isolated from the fungus *M. rouxii*, on the chitosan preparation was tested using chitin as a substrate (both in its crystalline and amorphous morphology) [125]. Deacetylation degrees remain very low (<10%) indicating that the enzyme is not really effective on insoluble chitins. Similar results were also obtained using chitin deacetylases isolated from other sources [120,122,123]. Thus, pretreatment of chitin substrates before enzyme addition seems to be necessary in order to improve the accessibility of the acetyl groups to the enzyme and therefore to enhance the deacetylation yield. For that purpose, experiments have been performed in homogeneous conditions using chitin deacetylase from *M. rouxii* with partially deacetylated water-soluble chitosans [126]. In selected conditions, the enzyme is able to deacetylate chitosan up to 97% (deacetylation from an initial chitosan with DA = 0.32 and a number-average degree of polymerization of 30) [126].

These findings suggest that the development of a controllable process using the enzymatic deacetylation on chitinous substrates is an attractive alternative process that can result in the preparation of novel chitosan polymers and more interestingly oligomers.

*3.2. Chitosan Characterization and Solubility*

Chitosan obtained from partial deacetylation of chitin becomes soluble in aqueous acidic medium when the average degree of acetylation DA is lower than 0.5. In fact, this limit depends on the distribution of acetyl groups along the chains. At this stage, it is possible to obtain a complete characterization of the polymer but it may differ from the starting material, specially its molecular weight is reduced during deacetylation in strong alkaline medium, as mentioned previously.

The physical properties of chitosan in solution depend strongly on DA and on the acetyl group distribution along the chains. Block-wise distribution of acetyl groups, caused by heterogeneous deacetylation performed on solid state chitin, causes chain association even in dilute solutions and formation of aggregates as well as difficulties in molecular weight determination [127,128]. In addition, fully deacetylated chitosan may be reacetylated in homogeneous phase [129] in order to get samples soluble in acidic conditions up to DA~0.6 in relation with a random distribution of the acetyl groups. Under these conditions, the existence of free -NH$_2$ groups, available on C-2 position of D-glucosamine units along the chains, allows to perform specific reactions in homogeneous conditions [130–136].

The first step in chitosan characterization is the determination of their molecular weights (after dissolution), then DA and eventually the distribution of acetyl group along the chain (by NMR). Additionally, different solvents based on acetic acid have been proposed, for instance: 0.3 M acetic acid added with sodium acetate (up to 0.1 or 0.2 M) in aqueous solution. The presence of an external salt is needed to screen the long-range electrostatic repulsions between the charged chains. Chitosan is also soluble in acetic acid or hydrochloric acid at pH lower than 6 (its intrinsic pK being around 6.5) [1].

The determination of average DA for chitosan may be performed by different techniques: infrared spectroscopy [86], elementary analysis, and potentiometric titration, but [1]H liquid state [89] and solid state [13]C-NMR [90,137,138] are preferred. Infrared spectroscopy has to be used carefully because the result interpretation is related to the difficulty in adopting a convenient base line. This problem was also discussed previously for samples with different DAs [86]. At present, [1]H NMR seems to be the most convenient technique to get the correct DA for soluble samples. An example is given in Figure 3. Additionally, [13]C NMR is also convenient for DA determination in the case of pure chitin up to fully deacetylated chitosan with a good agreement between measurements in solid state and liquid phase (Figure 2) [90].

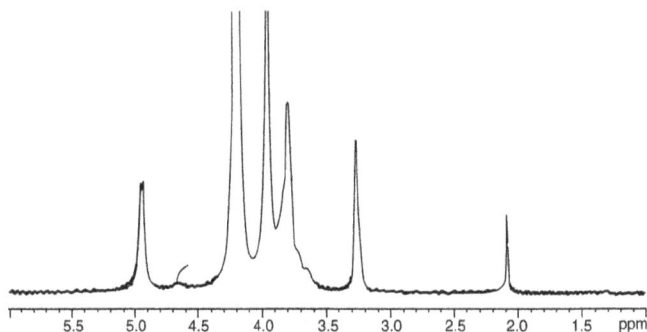

**Figure 3.** [1]H-NMR spectrum of chitosan with DA~0.06 in D$_2$O at pH~4, T = 85 °C and polymer concentration 5 g/L. Signals at 4.9 ppm is for H-1 of D-glucosamine unit, at 4.7 ppm is for H-1 of N-acetyl-D-glucosamine, at 3.2 ppm is for H-2 and at 2.1 ppm is for -CH$_3$ of the acetyl group allowing to get DA.

It is important to recall that high field [13]C-NMR spectroscopy is important to establish the distribution of acetyl groups along the chitosan chains [139,140].

Furthermore, the molecular weight distribution and the average molecular weight as well as the intrinsic viscosity also play a significant role. However, chitosan solution must be free of aggregates, thus the solvent for chitosan must be chosen carefully. The viscometric-average molecular weight has been usually calculated from intrinsic viscosity (lower impact of small fractions of aggregates) using the Mark-Houwink relationship [1]. In order to determine $K$ and $a$ parameters, an absolute MW has to be calculated using light scattering technique; nevertheless, the obtained value is usually overestimated due to high sensitivity to aggregate formation [127,128]. These artifacts may be omitted for instance by the use of 0.3M acetic acid/0.2M sodium acetate (pH = 4.5) solvent which does not form aggregates in this mixture [141]. Under these conditions, the absolute M values were obtained from steric exclusion chromatography (SEC) equipped with viscometer and light scattering detector on line allowing to determine the Mark-Houwink parameters without fractionation and also to obtain the relation between the radius of gyration and the molecular weight [142]. The $K$ (mL/g) and $a$ parameters at 25 °C are $7.9 \times 10^{-2}$ and 0.796 respectively.

The relatively high values obtained for the parameter $a$ are in agreement with the semi-rigid character of this polysaccharide which controls their dimensions, hydrodynamic volume and viscometric contribution. The stiffness is related to the persistence length ($L_t$) of the chain: chitosan in acid medium behaves like a polyelectrolyte, so the actual total persistence length $L_t$ at a given ionic concentration is equal to the intrinsic contribution $L_p$ and the electrostatic contribution $L_e$, calculated following the Odijk treatment [143]. The conformational analysis of chitin with different degrees of deacetylation confirms that chitin and chitosan are semi-rigid polymers characterized by a persistence length which depends moderately on the degree of acetylation of the molecule. From this analysis, chitosan, free of acetyl groups, has an intrinsic persistence length $L_p$ of 9 nm in salt excess [144]. $L_p$ increases when DA increases up to 12.5 nm for DA = 0.6, remaining constant up to pure chitin at 25 °C. These predictions are in agreement with the experimental values obtained by SEC [142].

### 3.3. Processing and Main Properties of Chitosan-Based Materials

Solutions of chitosan prepared in acidic medium are processed to the needed conformation (casted for a film, spun for fibers, freeze dried for sponges, *etc.*), immersed in an alkaline solution (in which they precipitate), washed and dried. The processing of chitosan is easier than that of chitin but the stability of the materials is lower due to the larger hydrophilic character and especially the pH sensitivity. For better stability, chitosan may be crosslinked using reagents such as epichlorohydrin, diisocyanate, 1,4-butanediol diglycidyl ether, or glutaraldehyde [145–147]. Many chitosan hydrogels were obtained by treatment with multivalent anions as oxalic acid [148,149] or citric acid [150–152] or tripolyphosphate [153]. Blends and composites are sometimes produced taking advantage of the polycationic properties of chitosan in acidic conditions.

In fact, chitosan being a polyelectrolyte is able to form interesting electrostatic complexes (hydrogels) with oppositely charged macromolecules. The properties of these complex materials depend on the polymer concentration, temperature, pH and ionic concentration. Electrostatic polyelectrolyte complexes (PEC) are mentioned in the literature involving chitosan complexed with synthetic or natural polymers [4]. Electrostatic interactions between chitosan and lipidic vesicles are also important in the biological and pharmaceutical fields due to bioadhesive and permeabilizer roles of chitosan [154–156]. Coating of liposomes with chitosan also increases their biocompatibility, and stabilizes the composite membrane against pH as well as ionic concentration [155].

Nowadays, these electrostatic interactions are applied for preparation of layer-by-layer polyelectrolyte capsules or films based on charged biocompatible polysaccharides or chitosan/synthetic polyelectrolytes [157–159]. Core-shell phospholipid nanoparticles were stabilized via layer-by-layer self-assembly of anionic alginate and cationic chitosan and were proposed for protein release [157].

Chitosan and alginate electrostatic complexes have been mostly used so far for biological applications [160–162]. Complexes formed between DNA or RNA and chitosan (oligomers or polymers) are actually under further investigation in many laboratories; the charge density and DA of chitosan are essential for the complex stability [163–167].

## 4. Relation between Chemical Structure and Biological Activities

Because chitosan and derivatives possess many beneficially properties such as biocompatibility, biodegradability, safety and also interesting biological activities, much attention has been paid to their applications especially in biomedical, food, biotechnology and pharmaceutical fields [168,169]. Among their attractive biological activities, antimicrobial, antioxidant and antitumor activities will be discussed in detail below. These properties are specially recognized in the field of food preservation and packaging to avoid the use of chemical preservatives and to produce edible antimicrobial films due to the good film forming properties of chitosan. Chitosan, as a polymeric ingredient with a good antimicrobial and antioxidant properties, does not migrate easily out of the protecting film and has better barrier properties. This was previously demonstrated in many studies, such as those of Friedman *et al.* [170], Kardas *et al.* [171] and Alishahi and Aider [172].

Friedman *et al.* [170] studied the antimicrobial activities of chitosan in solution, powders and edible films and coating against foodborne pathogens, spoilage bacteria, and pathogenic viruses and fungi in several food categories. These include fruit juices, eggs and dairy, cereal, meat and seafood products. They suggest that low-molecular-weight chitosans at a pH below 6.0 presents optimal conditions for achieving desirable antimicrobial and antioxidative-preservative effects in liquid and solid foods.

The use of chitosan and derivatives in the food industry was also described in the review of Kardas *et al.* [171]. They demonstrated that these biopolymers offer a wide range of unique applications including preservation of foods from microbial deterioration and formation of biodegradable films.

Alishahi and Aider [172] reported that chitosan films in packaging application tend to exhibit resistance to fat diffusion and selective gas permeability. But, inconvenience comes from their low resistance to water and water vapor transmission. This behavior is due to the strongly hydrophilic character mainly of chitosan, a property that leads to high interaction with water molecules [173]. For this reason, polymer blending or the use of biocomposites and multilayer systems are potential approaches to prepare chitosan-based bioactive coatings.

## 4.1. Antimicrobial Activity

Chitosan was shown to have several advantages over other disinfectants, as it possesses a higher antimicrobial activity, a broader spectrum of activity, a higher kill rate, and lower toxicity towards mammalian cells [174,175]. Many studies have demonstrated that chitosan have an important antimicrobial activity. However, the actual mechanism of inhibition is not yet fully understood. The most feasible hypothesis is a change in cell permeability due to interactions between the positively charged polysaccharide (chitosan at pH lower than 6.5) and the negatively charged membrane. The mechanism underlying the inhibition of bacterial growth should be that the positively charged polymer combines with anionic components such as N-acetylmuramic acid, sialic acid and neuraminic acid, on the cell surface.

Firstly, concerning the antibacterial activity of chitosan, possible actions of chitosan and its derivatives have been proposed. Chitosan (especially low-MW particles) could penetrate cell wall of bacteria, combine with DNA and inhibit synthesis of mRNA and DNA transcription [176]. High MW chitosan could interact with cell surface and consequently alter cell permeability [177], or form an impermeable layer around the cell, thus blocking the transport of essential solutes into the cell [178,179]. Chung et al. [180] confirmed that antibacterial mechanism includes hydrophilicity and the negative charge of cell surface and the adsorption of chitosan onto the bacterial cell. They show that cell wall hydrophilicity and negative charge of the cell surface were higher in gram-negative bacteria compared to gram-positive and that, in addition, the distribution of negative charges on their cell surfaces was quite different from that of gram-positive. Then, the more negatively charged cell surfaces interact more with positively charged chitosan, in acidic conditions. Their results showed a high value of correlation coefficient between adsorbed chitosan and inhibition efficiency. Moreover, many other studies showed that chitosans are more effective for gram-negative bacteria than gram-positive bacteria [181–183].

It was also indicated that adsorbed amounts of chitosan were related to environmental pH values (pH < 6.5) and degree of acetylation of chitosan [183–185]. Chitosan is more absorbed by bacterial cells at lower pH in relation with the increase of the chitosan positive ionic charge in relation with the fraction of deacetylated groups (1 − DA). From literature, it is clearly shown that there is a direct relationship between the antibacterial activity of chitosan and its characteristics especially DA. Effect of DA on chitosan antimicrobial activity has been clearly demonstrated in our previous study [186]. In these data, it is clearly shown that the lower DA, the lower MW and the lower pH give the larger efficiency.

In addition, influence of the MW was introduced by Zheng et al. [187]. They differentiated the effect of chitosan on Staphylococcus aureus (gram-positive) and on Escherichia coli (gram-negative) and demonstrated that, for gram-positive S. aureus, the antimicrobial activity increases with increase of the molecular weight of chitosan. On the opposite, for gram-negative E. coli, they indicate that the antibacterial activity increased with decrease in molecular weight. These authors suggested the two following mechanisms for the antimicrobial activity: in the case of S. aureus, the chitosan on the surface of the cell forms a polymeric membrane, which inhibits nutrients from entering into the cell and, for E. coli, chitosan with a lower molecular weight entered the cell through pervasion.

Effect of MW was also discussed by Benhabiles *et al.* [188] preparing oligomers of chitin and chitosan. Their antimicrobial activities against four gram-positive and seven gram-negative bacteria were compared to initial chitosan and chitin. They conclude that chito-oligomers would have advantages as new antimicrobial agents due to their higher activity and larger water solubility than the native polysaccharides.

Concerning the antifungal activity, it has been reported that chitosan can reduce the infection of *Fusarium oxysporum* f. sp. apii in celery and inhibits the spread of *Sphaerotheca pannosa* var. rosae, *Peronospora sparsa* and *Botrytis cinerea* on roses [189–191]. Treating tomato plants with chitosan solution reduced mycelial growth, sporangial production, release of zoospores and germination of cysts of *Phytophthora infestans* which resulted in significant disease protection [192]. In addition, chitosan seed treatment could reduce *Colletotrichum* sp. infection and improve performance of chilli seedling [193]. Concerning the mechanism, it is suggested that chitosan forms a permeable film at interface [194] and has two functions: direct interference of fungal growth and activation of several defense processes. These defense mechanisms include accumulation of chitinases, synthesis of proteinase inhibitors, lignification and induction of callous synthesis [195].

In fact, dependence of activities on chitosan characteristics was reported to depend on the particular fungal species. For example, it was shown that fungal growth decreased with increasing MW for *F. oxysporum* and with decreasing DA for *Alternaria solani*, but no MW or DA dependences were observed with *A. niger* [186].

## 4.2. Antioxidant Activity

Oxidative stress belongs to the main causes of many diseases, mainly cancer and cardiovascular problems, which significantly increase the worldwide mortality [196–202]. Dietary antioxidants, which inactivate reactive oxygen species and provide protection from oxidative damage [196–202], are considered as important preventive strategic molecules.

Once the lipid oxidation occurs in food products, off-flavors and undesirable chemical compounds are formed and this may be dangerous for health. Therefore, in order to minimize this risk, some antioxidants (like synthetic antioxidants butylated hydroxyanisole (BHA), butylated hydroxytoluene (BHT), t-butylhydroquinone (TBHQ) and propyl gallate) are added to delay the deterioration, caused by lipid oxidation. However, these antioxidants create potential health hazards, and their use has been restricted in some countries. Therefore, there has been a growing interest in natural antioxidants rather than in synthetic ones.

In recent years, much more attention has been paid to study the antioxidant activity of chitosan and its derivatives [203]. It was reported that chitosan and its derivatives act as antioxidants by scavenging oxygen radicals such as hydroxyl, superoxide, alkyl as well as highly stable DPPH radicals tested *in vitro* [204]. Sun and collaborators [205] reported that chitosan and their derivatives act as hydrogen donors to prevent the oxidative sequence.

Furthermore, it was observed that the radical scavenging properties of chitosans depend on their DA and MW. Park *et al.* [204] demonstrated that low-MW chitosans are more active than those with higher MW. Chitosan samples with low MW (1~3 kDa) revealed higher potential to scavenge different radicals. Other examination showed that low-MW chitosans can exhibit more than 80% of superoxide radical scavenging activity at 0.5 mg/mL concentration [206]. The influence of chitosan MW (30, 90, and 120 kDa) on the antioxidant activity in Salmon skin was also studied [207]. The results of this study showed that all chitosans present antioxidant activities, which reduce Salmon lipid oxidation, the 30-kDa chitosan sample having the higher antioxidant activity. In addition, highly deacetylated (90%) chitin are more preferable for scavenging DPPH, hydroxyl, superoxide and carbon-centered radicals [208]. Even though the precise mechanism of radical scavenging activity is not clear, it is attributed to amino and hydroxyl groups (attached to C-2, C-3 and C-6 positions of the pyranose ring) reacting with unstable free radicals, which facilitate formation of stable macromolecule radicals.

## 4.3. Antitumor Activity

Chitosan and its derivatives possess also antitumor activities investigated by both *in vitro* and *in vivo* method [209]. Some *in vivo* studies reported that chitosan inhibits the growth of tumor cells by exerting immunoenhancing effects. They concluded that the observed antitumor activity was not due to a direct killing of tumor cells, but by an increase of lymphokines production resulting in proliferation of cytolytic T-lymphocytes [210]. Chen *et al.* [211] demonstrated that intratumoral administration of a chitosan gel in animals reduces metastatic breast cancer progression. Chitosan also stimulates macrophages maturing into cytotoxic macrophages and suppresses tumor growth in mice [212]. It has been suggested that elevated secretion of IL-1 and IL-2 causes the anti-tumor effect through maturation and infiltration of cytolytic T-lymphocytes [213].

Other studies demonstrated that chitosan also exhibits a direct effect on tumor cells; it inhibits tumor cell proliferation by inducing apoptosis [214]. For instance, Hasegawa *et al.* [215] showed that chitosan may cause apoptotic death of bladder tumor cells via caspase-3 activation. Further studies revealed that chitosan nanoparticles could also induce necrotic death, which had been tested on liver cancer cells via neutralization of cell surface charge, observed as a decrease in mitochondrial membrane potential and induction of lipid peroxidation [216]. Moreover, chitosan may inhibit Ehrlich ascites tumor growth by reduction of glycolysis causing a decrease in glucose uptake and ATP level in the tumor cells [217]. This study also found that chitosan administered orally at a dose of 1 mg kg$^{-1}$ in mice reduces tumor growth by ~62%, without any toxicity to the liver. Thus, chitosan *per se* possesses potential activity against cancer, even when it is administered orally. A similar study, using a chemically-induced tumor model, showed that addition of chitosan to the diet enables to suppress aberrant crypt tumor lesions in the colon of mice [218]. Interestingly, such protection with chitosan additive in feed lasts only up to 6 weeks. This investigation highlighted that chitosan is responsible for an increase in expression of p21/Cip and p27/Kip and consequently a decrease of expression of proliferating cell nuclear antigen in a human gastric cancer cell line. Nevertheless, further studies are required in order to better understand all mechanisms involved in chitosan-based tumor stasis.

Chitosan activity depends not only on the chitosan structural characteristics, such as DA and MW, but also on tumor species. Jeon and Kim [219] studied the antitumor activity of chitosan oligosaccharides with different molecular weights. They found that chitosan oligosaccharides with MW ranging from 1.5 to 5.5 kDa may effectively inhibit the growth of Sarcoma 180 solid (S180) or

Uterine cervix carcinoma No. 14 (U14) tumor in BALB/c mice. Studies on mice examining chitosan samples with different MW revealed significant antimetastatic effects of chitosan against Lewis lung carcinoma. It was shown that the activity increases with decreasing the molecular sizes suggesting an immunostimulating effect which activates peritoneal macrophages and stimulates non-specific host resistance. It was also shown that chitosan samples with higher MW exhibits lower antitumor activity [220]. However, other authors found that decrease of MW of chitosan from 213 to 10 kDa does not affect its *in vitro* cytotoxicity on human lung carcinoma cell line A549 [221]. Additionally, chitosan samples with different MW ranging from 42 to 135 kDa were also evaluated in terms of their cytotoxicity on human bladder cancer RT112 and RT112cp cells and no effect of MW was observed [222]. The same study attempted to examine also the effect of chitosan DA (homogeneous chitosans with DA ranging from 2% to 61%) on cytotoxicity. The results from this experiment indicated that all chitosan samples were active on bladder carcinoma cells, with better activity for samples with higher DA.

It has been shown that chitosan reveals anticancer activity, thus it may be used for encapsulation of anticancer agents. However, before its incorporation into new drugs, pre-tests are required.

## 5. Pharmaceutical and Biomedical Applications of Chitin and Chitosan

The main properties of chitin and chitosan, applied for specific applications, have been already described such as: biocompatibility, renewable origin, non-toxicity [223], non-allergenicity and biodegradability in the body [224]. In addition, due to their attractive biological activities (antifungal, antibacterial, antitumor, immunoadjuvant, antithrombogenic, anticholesteremic agent) and bioadhesivity (especially of chitosan and its derivatives [225]), they are widely used as absorption promoters and hydrating agents, as well as for film production and wound healing [1–4,226]. Chitin and more easily chitosan may be processed, depending on the intended application, into different conformations such as fibers, powders, films, sponges, beads, solutions, gels and capsules [171]. Consequently, chitosan may be used in oral, nasal as well as ocular routes, for drug delivery in both implantable and injectable forms. Chitin and chitosan in fiber or film state, are mainly applied for tissue engineering and wound care dressing [227–229]. Additionally, transmucosal absorption promoter effect of chitosan is especially important for nasal and oral delivery of polar drugs to administrate peptides and proteins and for vaccine delivery [230,231]. Cationic chitosan may affect transport of ions through an interaction with the cell surface (inducing perturbation of membrane phospholipids bilayers). Chitin is also used as excipient and drug carrier in film, gel or powder form for applications involving mucoadhesivity [52]. Actually, the main promising developments are aimed to pharmaceutical and biomedical domains [232–245]. Several selected applications for chitin and chitosan will be described below and summarized in Table 3.

Applications of chitin are less developed compared to those of chitosan due to its large insolubility and difficulties in processing. Therefore, chitin is very often combined with chitosan which gives in fact similar applications.

Chitin accelerates wound-healing in spray, gel and gauze [246–249]. It is used as support of medicaments or to control drug release [238] taking into account the biodegradability, low toxicity, physiological inertness, antibacterial properties, hydrophilic character, gel forming properties, affinity for proteins and mucoadhesivity [250].

Great attention had been paid to a composite material made of hydroxyapatite-chitin-chitosan which may be used as bone filling material for guided tissue regeneration (treatment of periodontal bony defects). This composite forms a self-hardening paste [251–261]. Chitin was also used for enzymes and whole cells immobilization [262] as well as for tissue engineering [263,264].

Chitosan (the only pseudo-natural polycationic substance) and its electrostatic complexes formed with synthetic or natural polymers (as alginate) are used as antithrombogenic materials for: controlled release, drugs encapsulation, enzymes and cells immobilization and also as gene carriers. Advantage of chitosan-based materials is related to their biodegradability, antibacterial activity, hydrophilic property, as well as presence of polar groups which are able to form secondary interaction with other polymers (-OH and -NH$_2$ groups involved in hydrogen bonds and the N-acetyl groups in hydrophobic interactions).

Materials for wound dressing and tissue engineering are important but still under development [274–282]. New adhesives were also proposed [283,284]. The Az-chitosan derivative is non-toxic, cytocompatible and mechanically suitable for peripheral surgeries [285]. Chitosan films, like many other polysaccharide-based films, exhibit resistance to fat diffusion and selective gas permeability but they are relatively poor in terms of resistance to the transmission of water and water vapor. This behavior is observed due to their hydrophilic character leading to high interaction with water molecules [173]. In order to overcome this problem, polymer blending or biocomposites and multilayer systems are used for preparation of chitosan-based bioactive and stable coatings.

Mucoadhesivity of chitosan and its cationic derivatives is recognized and proved to enhance the adsorption of drugs especially at neutral pH. N-trimethyl chitosan chloride interacts with the negatively charged cell membranes [286]. N-lauryl-carboxymethylchitosan being an amphiphilic polymer forms micelles solubilizing taxol which becomes more efficient. This type of chitosan derivative is safe in terms of membrane toxicity and it could be useful as carrier for hydrophobic cancer drugs [287,288]. Chitosan or its derivatives were used for gene transfection. It was shown for N-alkylated chitosan that transfection efficiency increases upon elongation of the alkyl side chains up to eight carbons in the side chain [289]. Quaternized chitosan was also used for the same purpose [290]. Porous chitosan (and derivatives) microspheres were prepared in order to deliver antigens in a controlled way [291]. This type of particles was loaded with Newcastle disease virus vaccine and tested *in vitro* and *in vivo* [291,292].

An interesting application of the chitosan- calcium phosphate cement was found. Chitosan or chitosan glycerophosphate was mixed with calcium phosphate and citric acid and an attractive injectable self-hardening system for bone repair or filling indications was formed [253–255].

At the end, several examples of applications for drug delivery are mentioned [265,293–296]. Chitosan may be processed more easily than chitin to different forms: in sponge, capsule or nanoparticle depending on the tested system and the goal of its administration.

**Table 3.** Main applications of chitin and chitosan in pharmaceutical and biomedical domains.

| Forms | Applications |
|---|---|
| Beads | Drug delivery [266] |
| Microspheres [265] | Enzyme immobilization |
| | Gene delivery vehicle [267] |
| Nanoparticles | Encapsulation of sensitive drugs [172] |
| Coatings | Surface modification |
| | Textile finishes |
| Fibers | Medical textiles |
| | Suture |
| Nanofibers [268] | Guided bone regeneration |
| | Scaffold for nerve tissue regeneration |
| Nonwonen bioactive fibers [269] | Wound healing |
| | Wound care |
| Films | Dialysis membrane |
| | Antitumoral [270] |
| | Semi-permeable film for wound dressing [271] |
| | Adsorbent for pharmaceutical and medical devices |
| Powder | Surgical glove powder |
| | Enzyme immobilization |
| | Mucosomal hemostatic dressing |
| | Wound dressing |
| Sponge [272] | Drug delivery [272] |
| | Enzyme entrapment |
| | Artificial skin [271] |
| Shaped objects | Orthopedics |
| | Contact lenses |
| | Cosmetics |
| | Bacteriostatic agent |
| | Hemostatic agent |
| Solutions | Anticoagulants |
| | Antitumor agent |
| | Gene delivery [267] |
| | Spermicide [245] |
| | Delivery vehicle |
| Gels | Implants, coating |
| | Tissue engineering |
| | Wound dressing for wet treatment [271] |
| | Compressed diluent |
| Tablets | Disintegrating agent |
| | Excipient [273] |
| Capsules | Delivery vehicle |

## 6. Conclusions

In this review, the characteristics of chitin and chitosan are described. This was followed by a discussion on the solubilization required to process the polysaccharides to obtain new materials. Their fiber and film-forming abilities are recognized on the basis of the H-bonds network formation in the solid state which may be useful for new potential applications.

However, the most important applications come from their hydrophilic character and antimicrobial properties, especially desired for production of new biomaterials.

Chitosan in comparison with chitin is soluble in acidic media, which is applied for improvement of processing methods. In fact, chitosan may be easily processed as fiber, film, sponge, bead, gel or solution. Additionally, its cationic charge provides the possibility to form electrostatic complexes and/or multilayer structures. The presence of free -NH$_2$ groups along chitin and chitosan chains allows to perform specific modifications (performed on the C-2 position of the D-glucosamine unit) under pretty mild conditions (even in aqueous conditions with chitosan). Furthermore, chitin and chitosan can be blended with synthetic or natural polymers (proteins, DNA, alginate, hyaluronan, *etc.*).

## Acknowledgments

The authors would like to thank Anna Wolnik for her valuable contribution to ameliorate the English language of this manuscript.

## Author Contributions

This work was performed in strong cooperation between the two co-authors.

## Conflicts of Interest

The authors declare no conflict of interest.

## References

1. Rinaudo, M. Chitin and chitosan: Properties and applications. *Prog. Polym. Sci.* **2006**, *31*, 603–632.
2. Rinaudo, M. Main properties and current applications of some polysaccharides as biomaterials, *Polym. Int.* **2008**, *57*, 397–430.
3. Rinaudo, M. Physical properties of chitosan and derivatives in sol and gel states. In *Chitosan-Based Systems for Biopharmaceuticals: Delivery, Targeting and Polymer Therapeutics*; Sarmento, B., das Neves, J., Eds.; John Wiley & Sons: Chichester, UK, 2012; pp. 23–44.
4. Rinaudo, M. Materials based on chitin and chitosan. In *Bio-Based Plastics: Materials and Applications*; Kabasci, S., Ed.; John Wiley & Sons: Chichester, UK, 2014; pp. 63–80.
5. Rudall, K.M.; Kenchington, W. The chitin system. *Biol. Rev.* **1973**, *40*, 597–636.
6. Blackwell, J. Chitin. In *Biopolymers*; Walton, A.G., Blackwell, J., Eds.; Academic Press: New York, NY, USA, 1973; pp. 474–489.

7.  Persson, J.E.; Domard, A.; Chanzy, H. Single crystals of a-chitin. *Int. J. Biol. Macromol.* **1990**, *13*, 221–224.

8.  Helbert, W.; Sugiyama, J. High-resolution electron microscopy on cellulose II and α-chitin single crystals. *Cellulose* **1998**, *5*, 113–122.

9.  Ruiz-Herrera, J.; Sing, V.O.; van der Woude, W.J.; Bartnicki-Garcia, S. Microfibril assembly by granules of chitin synthetase. *Proc. Natl. Acad. Sci. USA* **1975**, *72*, 2706–2710.

10. Bartnicki-Garcia, S.; Persson, J.; Chanzy, H. An electron microscope and electron diffraction study of the effect of calcofluor and congo red on the biosynthesis of chitin *in vitro*. *Arch. Biochem. Biophys.* **1994**, *310*, 6–15.

11. Sakamoto, J.; Sugiyama, J.; Kimura, S.; Imai, T.; Itoh, T.; Watanabe, T.; Kobayashi, S. Artificial chitin spherulites composed of single crystalline ribbons of α-chitin via enzymatic polymerization. *Macromolecules* **2000**, *33*, 4155–4160.

12. Rudall, K.M. Chitin and its association with other molecules. *J. Polym. Sci. Part C* **1969**, *28*, 83–102.

13. Blackwell, J.; Parker, K.D.; Rudall, K.M. Chitin in pogonophore tubes. *J. Mar. Biol. Assoc. UK* **1965**, *45*, 659–661.

14. Gaill, F.; Persson, J.; Sugiyama, P.; Vuong, R.; Chanzy, H. The chitin system in the tubes of deep sea hydrothermal vent worms. *J. Struct. Biol.* **1992**, *109*, 116–128.

15. Kurita, K.; Tomita, K.; Ishi, S.; Nishimura, S-I.; Shimoda, K. β-chitin as a convenient starting material for acetolysis for efficient preparation of *N*-acetylchitooligosaccharides. *J. Polym. Sci. A Polym. Chem.* **1993**, *31*, 2393–2395.

16. Horst, M.N.; Walker, A.N.; Klar, E. The pathway of crustacean chitin synthesis. In *The Crustacean Integument: Morphology and Biochemistry*; Horst, M.N., Freeman, J.A., Eds.; CRC: Boca Raton, FL, USA, 1993; pp. 113–149.

17. No, H.K.; Hur, E.Y. Control of foam formation by antifoam during demineralization of crustacean shell in preparation of chitin. *J. Agric. Food. Chem.* **1998**, *46*, 3844–3846.

18. Percot, A.; Viton, C.; Domard, A. Characterization of shrimp shell deproteinization. *Biomacromolecules* **2003**, *4*, 1380–1385.

19. Johnson, E.L.; Peniston, Q.P. Utilization of shellfish waste for chitin and chitosan production. In *Chemistry & Biochemistry of Marine Food Products*; Martin, R.E., Flick, G.J., Hebard, C.E., Ward, D.R., Eds.; AVI Publishing Co.: Westport, CT, USA, 1982; Chapter 19, p. 415.

20. Shahidi, F.; Synowiecki, J. Isolation and characterization of nutrients and value-added products from snow crab *(Chifroeceles opilio)* and shrimp *(Panda- 111sb orealis)* processing discards. *J. Agric. Food Chem.* **1991**, *39*, 1527–1532.

21. Tolaimate, A.; Desbrieres, J.; Rhazi, M.; Alagui, A. Contribution to the preparation of chitins and chitosans with controlled physico-chemical properties. *Polymer* **2003**, *44*, 7939–7952.

22. Muzzarelli, R.A.A.; Tanfani, F.; Emanuelli, M.; Gentile, S. The chelation of cupric ions by chitosan membranes [*Callinectes sapidus*, blue crab shell]. *J. Appl. Biochem.* **1980**, *2*, 380–389.

23. Hackman, R.H. Studies on chitin. I. Enzymatic degradation of chitin and chitin esters. *Aust. J. Biol. Sci.* **1954**, *7*, 168–178.

24. Hakman, R.H.; Goldberg, M. Light-scattering and infrared-spectrophotometric studies of chitin and chitin derivatives. *Carbohydr. Res.* **1974**, *38*, 35–45.

25. Anderson, G.G.; de Pablo, N.; Romo, C. Antartic krill (*Euphausia superba*) as a source of chitin and chitosan. In *Proceedings of First International Conference on Chitin and Chitosan*; Muzzarelli, R.A.A., Priser, E.R., Eds.; Mit Sea Grant Program: Cambridge, MA, USA, 1978; pp. 54–63.

26. Horowitz, S.T.; Roseman, S.; Blumental, H.J. Preparation of glucosamine oligosaccharides. 1. Separation. *J. Am. Chem. Soc.* **1957**, *79*, 5046–5049.

27. Synowiecki, J.; Sikorski, Z.E.; Naczk, M. Immobilization of invertase on krill chitin. *Biotechnol. Bioeng.* **1981**, *23*, 231–233.

28. Foster, A.B.; Webber, J.M. Chitin. *Adv. Carbohydr. Chem.* **1960**, *15*, 371–393.

29. Austin, P.R.; Brine, C.J.; Castle, J.E.; Zikakis, J.P. Chitin: New facets of research. *Science* **1981**, *212*, 749–753.

30. Brine, C.J.; Austin, P.R. Chitin variability with species and method of preparation. *Comp. Biochem. Physiol.* **1981**, *69B*, 283–286.

31. Peniston, Q.P.; Lohnson, E.L. Process for Demineralization of Crustacea Shells. *U.S. Patent 4,066,735*, 3 January 1978.

32. Shimahara, K.; Ohkouchi, K.; Ikeda, M. In *Chitin Chemistry*; Roberts, G.A.F., Ed.; Macmillan Press: London, UK, 1992; p. 56.

33. Okafor, N. Isolation of chitin from the shell of the cuttlefish, Sepia oficirralis L. *Biochim. Biophys. Acta* **1965**, *101*, 193–200.

34. Truong, T.; Hausler, R.; Monette, F.; Niquette, P. Fishery industrial waste valorization for the transformation of chitosan by hydrothermo-chemical method. *Rev. Sci. Eau* **2007**, *20*, 253–262.

35. Marquis-Duval, F.O. Isolation et valorisation des constituants de la carapace de la crevette nordique. Ph.D. Dissertation, Laval University, Quebec, Canada, 2008.

36. Madhavan, P.; Nair, K.G.R. Utilisation of prawn waste-isolation of chitin and its conversion to chitosan. *Fish. Technol.* **1974**, *11*, 50–53.

37. Moorjani, M.N.; Achutha, V.; Khasim, D.I. Parameters affecting the viscosity of chitosan from prawn waste. *J. Food Sci. Technol.* **1975**, *12*, 187–189.

38. Mima, S.; Miya, M.; Iwamoto, R.; Yoshikawa, S. Highly deacetylated chitosan and its properties. *J. Appl. Polym. Sci.* **1983**, *28*, 1909–1917.

39. Broussignac, P. Un haut polymère naturel peu connu dans l'industrie, Le chitosane. *Chim. Ind. Genie Chim.* **1968**, *99*, 1241–1247.

40. BeMiller, J.N.; Whistler, R.L. Alkaline degradation of amino sugars. *J. Org. Chem.* **1963**, *27*, 1161–1164.

41. Kurita, K.; Tomita, K.; Tada, T.; Ishii, S.; Nishimura, S.I.; Shimoda, K. Squid chitin as a potential alternative chitin source: Deacetylation behavior and characteristic properties. *J. Polym. Sci. Pol. Chem.* **1993**, *31*, 485–491.

42. Brzeski, M.M. Concept of chitin chitosan isolation from Antartic Krill *(Euphausia superba)* shells on *a* technical scale. In *Proceedings of the Second International Conference on Chitin and Chitosan*; Hirano, S., Tokura, S., Eds.; The Japan Society of Chitin and Chitosan: Sapporo, Japan, 1982; pp. 15–29.

43. Blumberg, R.; Southall, C.L.; van Rensburg, N.J.; Volckman, O.B. South African fish products. XXXII—The rock lobster: A study of chitin production from processing wastes. *J. Sci. Food Agric.* **1951**, *2*, 571–576.

44. No, H.K.; Meyers, S.P.; Lee, K.S. Isolation and characterization of chitin from crawfish shell waste. *J. Agric. Food Chem.* **1989**, *37*, 575–579.

45. Wu, A.C.M.; Bough, W.A. A study of variables in the chitosan manufacturing process in relation to molecular-weight distribution, chemical characteristics and waste-treatment effectiveness. In Proceedings of the 1st International Conference on Chitin/Chitosan, Boston, USA, 11–13 April 1977; Muzzarelli, R.A.A., Pariser, E.R., Eds.; MIT Sea Grant Program, Massachusetts Institute of Technology: Cambridge, MA, USA, 1978; pp. 88–102.

46. Bough, W.A.; Salter, W.L.; Wu, A.C.M.; Perkins, B.E. Influence of manufacturing variables on the characteristics and effectiveness of chitosan products 1. Chemical composition, viscosity, and molecular-weight distribution of chitosan products. *Biotechnol. Bioeng.* **1978**, *20*, 1931–1943.

47. Sluyanarayana Rao, S.V.; Yashodha, K.P.; Mahendrakar, N.S. Puttarajappa. Deacetylation of chitin at low temperature by a novel alkali impregnation technique. *Indian J. Technol.* **1987**, *25*, 194–196.

48. Tolaimate, A. Exploration des gisements chitineux de la faune marine marocaine. Procédé d'extraction de chitines fortement acétylées. Préparation de chitosanes à caractéristiques contrôlées. Ph.D. Dissertation, Cadi Ayyad University, Marrakech, Maroc, 2000.

49. Khanafari, A.; Marandi, R.; Sanatei, S. Recovery of chitin and chitosan from shrimp waste by chemical and microbial methods. *Iran. J. Environ. Health Sci. Eng.* **2008**, *5*, 1–24.

50. Bustos, R.O.; Healy, M.G. Microbial deproteinization of waste prawn shell. In *Proceedings of the Second International Symposium on Environmental Biotechnology*; Biotechnology' 94: Brighton, UK, 1994; pp. 15–25.

51. Arbia, W.; Arbia, L.; Adour, L.; Amrane, A. Chitin extraction from crustacean shells using biological methods—A review. *Food Technol. Biotech.* **2013**, *51*, 12–25.

52. Gortari, M.C.; Hours, R.A. Biotechnological processes for chitin recovery out of crustacean waste: A mini-review. *Electron. J. Biotechnol.* **2013**, *16*, 14–14.

53. Guerrero Legarreta, I.; Zakaria, Z.; Hall, G.M. Lactic fermentation of prawn waste: Comparison of commercial and isolated starter cultures. In *Advances in Chitin Science*; Domard, A., Jeuniaux, C., Muzzarelli, R., Roberts, G., Eds.; Jacques Andre publishers: Lyon, France, 1996; Volume I, pp. 399–406.

54. Cira, L.A.; Huerta, S.; Guerrero, I.; Rosas, R.; Shirai, K. Scaling up of lactic acid fermentation of prawn wastes in packed-bed column reactor for chitin recovery. In *Advances in Chitin Science*; Peter, M.G., Domard, A., Muzzarelli, R.A.A., Eds.; Potsdam University: Postdam, Germany, 2000; Volume IV, pp. 2–27.

55. Rao, M.B.; Tanksale, A.M.; Ghatge, M.S.; Deshpande, V.V. Molecular and biotechnological aspects of microbial proteases. *Microbiol. Mol. Biol. Rev.* **1998**, *62*, 597–635.

56. Synowiecki, J.; Al-Khateeb, N.A.A.Q. The recovery of protein hydrolysate during enzymatic isolation of chitin from shrimp Crangon crangon processing discards. *Food Chem.* **2000**, *68*, 147–152.

57. Gildberg, A.; Stenberg, E. A new process for advanced utilisation of shrimp waste. *Process Biochem.* **2001**, *36*, 809–812.

58. Manni, L.; Ghorbel-Bellaaj, O.; Jellouli, K.; Younes, I.; Nasri, M. Extraction and characterization of chitin, chitosan, and protein hydrolysates prepared from shrimp waste by treatment with crude protease from Bacillus cereus SV1. *Appl. Biochem. Biotechnol.* **2010**, *162*, 345–357.

59. Younes, I.; Ghorbel-Bellaaj, O.; Nasri, R.; Chaabouni, M.; Rinaudo, M.; Nasri, M. Chitin and chitosan preparation from shrimp shells using optimized enzymatic deproteinization. *Process Biochem.* **2012**, *47*, 2032–2039.

60. Mukhin, V.A.; Novikov, V.Y. Enzymatic hydrolysis of proteins from crustaceans of the Barents Sea. *Appl. Biochem. Micro+* **2001**, *37*, 538–542.

61. Younes, I.; Nasri, R.; Bkahiria, I.; Jellouli, K.; Nasri, M. New proteases extracted from red scorpionfish (*Scorpaena scrofa*) viscera: Characterization and application as a detergent additive and for shrimp waste deproteinization. *Food Bioprod. Process.* **2014**, doi:10.1016/j.fbp.2014.06.003.

62. Kaur, S.; Dhillon, G.S. Recent trends in biological extraction of chitin from marine shell wastes: A review. *Crit. Rev. Biotechnol.* **2015**, *35*, 44–61.

63. Prameela, K.; Murali Mohan, C.; Smitha, P.V.; Hemablatha, K.P.J. Bioremediation of shrimp biowaste by using natural probiotic for chitin and carotenoid production an alternative method to hazardous chemical method. *Int. J. Appl. Biol. Pharm. Technol.* **2010**, *1*, 903–910.

64. Rao, M.S.; Muñoz, J.; Stevens, W.F. Critical factors in chitin production by fermentation of shrimp biowaste. *Appl. Microbiol. Biotechnol.* **2000**, *54*, 808–813.

65. Oh, K.T.; Kim, Y.J.; Nguyen, V.N.; Jung, W.J.; Park, R.D. Demineralization of crab shell waste by Pseudomonas aeruginosa F722. *Process Biochem.* **2007**, *42*, 1069–1074.

66. Choorit, W.; Patthanamanee, W.; Manurakchinakorn, S. Use of response surface method for the determination of demineralization efficiency in fermented shrimp shells. *Bioresour. Technol.* **2008**, *99*, 6168–6173.

67. Yang, J.K.; Shih, I.L.; Tzeng, Y.M.; Wang, S.L. Production and purification of protease from a *Bacillus subtilis* that can deproteinize crustacean wastes. *Enzyme Microb. Technol.* **2000**, *26*, 406–413.

68. Sini, T.K.; Santhosh, S.; Mathew, P.T. Study on the production of chitin and chitosan from shrimp shell by using Bacillus subtilis fermentation. *Carbohydr. Res.* **2007**, *342*, 2423–2429.

69. Ghorbel-Bellaaj, O.; Younes, I.; Maalej, H.; Hajji, S.; Nasri, M. Chitin extraction from shrimp shell waste using Bacillus bacteria. *Int. J. Biol. Macromol.* **2012**, *51*, 1196–1201.

70. Ghorbel-Bellaaj, O.; Jellouli, K.; Younes, I.; Manni, L.; Ouled Salem, M.; Nasri, M. A solvent-stable metalloprotease produced by Pseudomonas aeruginosa A2 grown on shrimp shell waste and its application in chitin extraction. *Appl. Biochem. Biotechnol.* **2011**, *164*, 410–425.

71. Wang, S.L.; Chio, S.H. Deproteination of shrimp and crab shell with the protease of Pseudomonas aeruginosa K-1*Enzy. Microb. Technol.* **1998**, *22*, 629–633.

72. Mahmoud, N.S.; Ghaly, A.E.; Arab, F. Unconventional approach for demineralization of deproteinized crustacean shells for chitin production. *Am. J. Biochem. Biotechnol.* **2007**, *3*, 1–9.

73. Jung, W.J.; Kuk, J.H.; Kim, K.Y.; Park, R.D. Demineralization of red crab shell waste by lactic acid fermentation. *Appl. Microbiol. Biotechnol.* **2005**, *67*, 851–854.

74. Teng, W.L.; Khor, E.; Tan, T.K.; Lim, L.Y.; Tan, S.C. Concurrent production of chitin from shrimp shells and fungi. *Carbohydr. Res.* **2001**, *332*, 305–316.

75. Atkins, E.D.T. Conformation in polysaccharides and complex carbohydrates. *J. Biosci.* **1985**, *8*, 375–387.

76. Gonell, H.W. Roëtgenographische studien an chitin. *Z. Physiol. Chem.* **1926**, *152*, 18–30.

77. Clark, G.L.; Smith, A.F. X-ray studies of chitin, chitosan, and derivatives. *J. Phys. Chem.* **1936**, *40*, 863–879.

78. Gardner, K.H.; Blackwell, J. Refinement of the structure of β-chitin. *Biopolymers* **1975**, *14*, 1581–1595.

79. Minke, R.; Blackwell, J. The structure of α-chitin. *J. Mol. Biol.* **1978**, *120*, 167–181.

80. Darmon, S.E.; Rudall, K.M. Infra-red and X-ray studies of chitin. *Disc. Faraday. Soc.* **1950**, *9*, 251–260.

81. Pearson, F.G.; Marchessault, R.H.; Liang, C.Y. Infrared spectra of crystalline polysaccharides. V. Chitin. *J. Polym. Sci.* **1960**, *13*, 101–116.

82. Falk, M.; Smith, D.G.; McLachlan, J.; McInnes, A.G. Studies on chitin (b-(1–4)-linked 2-acetamido-2-deoxy-D-glucan) fibers of the diatom Thalassiosira fluviatilis Hustedt. II.Proton magnetic resonance, infrared and X-ray studies. *Can. J. Chem.* **1966**, *44*, 2269–2281.

83. Galat, A.; Koput, J.; Popowicz, J. Analyses of infrared amide bands of chitin. *Acta Biochim. Pol.* **1979**, *26*, 303–308.

84. Iwamoto, R.; Miya, M.; Mima, S. Vibrational polarization spectra of α-type chitin. In *Chitin and Chitosan*, Proceedings of the Second International Conference on Chitin and Chitosan, Sapporo, Japan, 12–14 July 1982; Hirano, S., Tokura, S., Eds.; The Japanese Society of Chitin and Chitosan:Tottori, Japan, 1982; pp. 82–86.

85. Focher, B.; Naggi, A.; Torri, G.; Cosani, A.; Terbojevich, M. Structural differences between chitin polymorphs and their precipitates from solutions-evidence from CP-MAS 13CNMR, FT-IR and FT-Raman spectroscopy. *Carbohydr. Polym.* **1992**, *17*, 97–102.

86. Brugnerotto, J.; Lizardi, J.; Goycoolea, F.M.; Arguelles-Monal, W.; Desbrieres, J.; Rinaudo, M. An infrared investigation in relation with chitin and chitosan characterization. *Polymer* **2001**, *42*, 3569–3580.

87. Saito, H.; Tabeta, R.; Hirano, S. Conformation of chitin and N-acyl chitosans in solid state as revealed by 13C cross polarization/magic angle spinning (CP/MAS) NMR spectroscopy. *Chem. Lett.* **1981**, *10*, 1479–1482.

88. Tanner, S.F.; Chanzy, H.; Vincendon, M.; Roux, J.C.; Gaill, F. High resolution solid-state carbon-13 nuclear magnetic resonance study of chitin. *Macromolecules* **1990**, *23*, 3576–3583.

89. Kono, H. Two-dimensional magic angle spinning NMR investigation of naturally occurring chitins: Precise $^1$H and $^{13}$C resonance assignment of α- and β-chitin. *Biopolymers* **2004**, *75*, 255–263.

90. Heux, L.; Brugnerotto, J.; Desbrieres, J.; Versali, M.F.; Rinaudo, M. Solid state NMR for determination of degree of acetylation of chitin and chitosan. *Biomacromolecules* **2000**, *1*, 746–751.

91. Poirier, M.; Charlet, G. Chitin fractionation and characterization in N, N-dimethylacetamide/ lithium chloride solvent system. *Carbohydr. Polym.* **2002**, *50*, 363–370.

92. Terbojevich, M.; Carraro, C.; Cosani, A. Solution studies of the chitin-lithium chloride-N, N-dimethylacetamide system. *Carbohydr. Res.* **1988**, *180*, 73–86.

93. Pillai, C.K.S.; Paul, W.; Sharma, C.P. Chitin and chitosan polymers: Chemistry, solubility and fiber formation. *Prog. Polym. Sci.* **2009**, *34*, 641–678.

94. Roberts, G.A.F. Structure of chitin and chitosan. In *Chitin Chemistry*; Roberts, G.A.E., Ed.; Palgrave Macmillan: London, UK, 1992; pp. 85–91.

95. Kafetzopoulos, D.; Martinou, A.; Bouriotis, V. Bioconversion of chitin to chitosan: Purification and characterization of chitin deacetylase from Mucor rouxii. *Proc. Natl. Acad. Sci. USA* **1993**, *90*, 2564–2568.

96. Aiba, S.I. Preparation of N-acetylchitooligosaccharides by hydrolysis of chitosan with chitinase followed by N-acetylation. *Carbohyd. Res.* **1994**, *265*, 323–328.

97. Ilyina, A.V.; Tatarinova, N.Y.; Varlamov, V.P. The preparation of low-molecular-weight chitosan using chitinolytic complex from Streptomyces kurssanovii. *Process Biochem.* **1999**, *34*, 875–878.

98. Tokuyasu, K.; Mitsutomi, M.; Yamaguchi, I.; Hayashi, K.; Mori, Y. Recognition of chitooligosaccharides and their N-acetyl groups by putative subsites of chitin deacetylase from a deuteromycete, Colletotrichum lindemuthianum. *Biochemistry* **2000**, *39*, 8837–8843.

99. Kurita, K.; Sannan, T.; Iwakura, Y. Studies on chitin, 4: Evidence for formation of block and random copolymers of N-acetyl-D-glucosamine and D-glucosamine by hetero- and homogeneous hydrolyses. *Makromol. Chem.* **1977**, *178*, 3197–3202.

100. No, H.K.; Meyers, S.P. Preparation and characterization of chitin and chitosan—A review. *J. Aquat. Food Prod. Technol.* **1995**, *2*, 27–52.

101. Hajji, S.; Younes, I.; Ghorbel-Bellaaj, O.; Hajji, R.; Rinaudo, M.; Nasri, M.; Jellouli, K. Structural differences between chitin and chitosan extracted from three different marine sources. *Int. J. Biol. Macromol.* **2014**, *65*, 298–306.

102. Chang, K.L.B.; Tsai, G.; Lee, J.; Fu, W.R. Heterogeneous N-deacetylation of chitin in alkaline solution. *Carbohyd. Res.* **1997**, *303*, 327–332.

103. Sannan, T.; Kurita, K.; Iwakura, Y. Studies on chitin, 2. Effect of deacetylation on solubility. *Makromol. Chem.* **1976**, *177*, 3589–3600.

456

104. Rinaudo M.; Domard, A. Solution properties of chitosan. In *Chitin and Chitosan*; Skjak-Bræk, G., Anthonsen, T., Stanford, P., Eds.; Kluwer Academic Publisher: Dordrecht, The Netherlands, 1989; pp. 71–86.

105. Aiba, S.I. Studies on chitosan: 3. evidence for the presence of random and block copolymer structures in partially *N*-acetylated chitosans. *Int. J. Biol. Macromol.* **1991**, *13*, 40–44.

106. Berger, J.; Reist, M.; Chenite, A.; Felt-Baeyens, O.; Mayer, J.M.; Gurny, R. Erratum to Pseudo-thermosetting chitosan hydrogels for biomedical application. *Int. J. Pharm.* **2005**, *28*, 197–206.

107. Rong, H.C.; Hwa, H.D. Effect of molecular weight of chitosan with the same degree of deacetylation on the thermal, mechanical, and permeability properties of the prepared membrane. *Carbohydr. Polym.* **1996**, *29*, 353–358.

108. Li, Q.; Dunn, E.T.; Grandmaison, E.W.; Goosen, M.F.A. Applications and properties of chitosan. *J. Bioact. Compat. Pol.* **1992**, *7*, 370–397.

109. Rege, P.R.; Block, L.H. Chitosan processing: Influence of process parameters during acidic and alkaline hydrolysis and effect of the processing sequence on the resultant chitosan's properties. *Carbohydr. Res.* **1999**, *321*, 235–245.

110. Tolaimate, A.; Desbrieres, J.; Rhazi, M.; Alagui, A.; Vincendon, M.; Vottero, P. On the influence of deacetylation process on the physicochemical characteristics of chitosan from squid chitin. *Polymer* **2000**, *41*, 2463–2469.

111. Tsaih, M.L.; Chen, R.H. The effect of reaction time and temperature during heterogenous alkali deacetylation on degree of deacetylation and molecular weight of resulting chitosan. *J. Appl. Polym. Sci.* **2003**, *88*, 2917–2923.

112. Sannan, T.; Kurita, K.; Iwakura, Y. Studies on chitin. V. Kinetics of deacetylation reaction. *Polym. J.* **1977**, *9*, 649–651.

113. Weska, R.F.; Moura, J.M.; Batista, L.M.; Rizzi, J.; Pinto, L.A.A. Optimization of deacetylation in the production of chitosan from shrimp wastes: Use of response surface methodology. *J. Food Eng.* **2007**, *80*, 749–753.

114. Hwang, K.T.; Jung, S.T.; Lee, G.D.; Chinnan, M.S.; Park, Y.S.; Park, H.J. Controlling molecular weight and degree of deacetylation of chitosan by response surface methodology. *J. Agr. Food Chem.* **2002**, *50*, 1876–1882.

115. Younes, I.; Ghorbel-Bellaaj, O.; Chaabouni, M.; Rinaudo, M.; Souard, F.; Vanhaverbeke, C.; Nasri, M. Use of a fractional factorial design to study the effects of experimental factors on the chitin deacetylation. *Int. J. Biol. Macromol.* **2014**, *70*, 385–390.

116. Le Dung, P.; Milas, M.; Rinaudo, M.; Desbrières, J. Water soluble derivatives obtained by controlled chemical modifications of chitosan. *Carbohydr. Polym.* **1994**, *24*, 209–214.

117. Tsigos, I.; Martinou, A.; Kafetzopoulos, D.; Bouriotis, V. Chitin deacetylases: New, versatile tools in biotechnology. *Trends Biotechnol.* **2000**, *18*, 305–312.

118. Araki, Y.; Ito. E. A pathway of chitosan formation in Mucor rouxii: Enzymatic deacetylation of chitin. *Eur. J. Biochem.* **1975**, *189*, 249–253.

119. Martinou, A.; Kafetzopoulos, D.; Bouriotis, V. Isolation of chitin deacetylase from Mucor rouxii by immunoaffinity chromatography. *J. Chromatogr.* **1993**, *644*, 35–41.

120. Gao, X.D.; Katsumoto, T.; Onodera, K. Purification and characterization of chitin deacetylase from Absidia coerulea. *J. Biochem.* **1995**, *117*, 257–263.

121. Alfonso, C.; Nuero, O.M.; Santamaría, F.; Reyes, F. Purification of a heat stable chitin deacetylase from Aspergillus nidulans and its role in cell wall degradation. *Curr. Microbiol.* **1995**, *30*, 49–54.

122. Tsigos, I.; Bouriotis, V. Purification and characterization of chitin deacetylase from Colletotrichum lindemuthianum. *J. Biol. Chem.* **1995**, *270*, 26286–26291.

123. Tokuyasu, K.; Kameyama, M.O.; Hiyashi, K. Purification and characterization of extracellular chitin deacetylase from Colletotrichum lindemuthianum. *Biosci. Biotechnol. Biochem.* **1996**, *60*, 1598–1603.

124. Sundara, R.*G.;* Aruchami, M.; Gowri, N. Natural deacetylation of chitin to chitosan in the abdominal cuticle of the physogastric queen of Macrotermes estherae. In Proceeding Second International Conference Chitin/Chitosan, Sapporo, Japan, 12–14 July 1982; Tokura S., Hirano, S., Eds.; Japanese Soc. Chitin: Tottori, Japan, 1982.

125. Martinou, A.; Kafetzopoulos, D.; Bouriotis, V. Chitin deacetylation by enzymatic means: Monitoring of deacetylation processes. *Carbohydr. Res.* **1995**, *273*, 235–242.

126. Martinou, A.; Bouriotis, V.; Stokke, B.T.; Vårum, K.M. Mode of action of chitin deacetylase from M. rouxii on partially *N*-acetylated chitosans. *Carbohydr. Res.* **1998**, *311*, 71–78.

127. Philippova, O.E.; Volkov, E.V.; Sitnikova, N.L.; Khokhlov, A.; Desbrières, J.; Rinaudo, M. Two types of hydrophobic aggregates in aqueous solutions of chitosan and its hydrophobic derivative. *Biomacromolecules* **2001**, *2*, 483–490.

128. Philippova, O.E.; Korchagina, E.V.; Volkov, E.V.; Smirnov, V.A.; Khokhlov, A.R.; Rinaudo, M. Aggregation of some water-soluble derivatives of chitin in aqueous solutions: Role of the degree of acetylation and effect of hydrogen bond breaker. *Carbohydr. Polym.* **2012**, *87*, 687–694.

129. Maghami, G.G.; Roberts, G.A.F. Evaluation of the viscometric constants for chitosan. *Makromol. Chem.* **1988**, *189*, 195–200.

130. Auzely, R.; Rinaudo, M. Controlled chemical modifications of chitosan characterization and investigation of original properties. *Macromol. Biosci.* **2003**, *3*, 562–565.

131. Rinaudo, M.; le Dung. P.; Milas, M. A new and simple method of synthesis of carboxymethyl chitosans, In *Advances in Chitin and Chitosan*; Brine, C.J., Sanford, P.A., Zitakis, J.P., Eds.; Elsevier: London, UK, 1992; pp. 516–525.

132. Desbrieres, J.; Martinez, C.; Rinaudo, M. Hydrophobic derivatives of chitosan: Characterization and rheological behaviour. *Int. J. Biol. Macromol.* **1996**, *19*, 21–28.

133. Rinaudo, M.; Auzely, R.; Vallin, C.; Mullagaliev, I. Specific interactions in modified chitosan systems. *Biomacromolecules* **2005**, *6*, 2396–2407.

134. Auzely-Velty, R.; Rinaudo, M. New supramolecular assemblies of a cyclodextrin grafted chitosan through specific complexation. *Macromolecules* **2002**, *35*, 7955–7962.

135. Recillas, M.; Silva, L.L.; Peniche, C.; Goycoolea, F.M.; Rinaudo, M.; Argelles-Monal, W.M. Thermoresponsive behavior of chitosan-g-*N*-isopropylacrylamide copolymer solutions. *Biomacromolecules* **2009**, *10*, 1633–1641.

136. Rinaudo, M. New way to crosslink chitosan in aqueous solution. *Eur. Polym. J.* **2010**, *46*, 1537–1544.

137. Saito, H.; Tabeta, R.; Ogawa, K. High-resolution solid-state [13]C-NMR study of chitosan and its salts with acids: Conformational characterization of polymorphs and helical structures as viewed from the conformation-dependent [13]C chemical shifts. *Macromolecules* **1987**, *20*, 2424–2430.

138. Raymond, L.; Morin, F.G.; Marchessault, R.H. Degree of deacetylation of chitosan using conductometric titration and solid-state NMR. *Carbohydr. Res.* **1993**, *246*, 331–336.

139. Varum, K.M.; Anthonsen, M.W.; Grasdalen, H.; Smisrød, O. Determination of the degree of *N*-acetylation and the distribution of *N*-acetyl groups in partially N-deacetylated chitins (chitosans) by high-field n.m.r. spectroscopy. *Carbohydr. Res.* **1991**, *211*, 17–23.

140. Varum, K.M.; Anthonsen, M.W.; Grasdalen, H.; Smisrød, O. 13 C-NMR studies of the acetylation sequences in partially N-deacetylated chitins (chitosans). *Carbohydr. Res.* **1991**, *217*, 19–27.

141. Rinaudo, M.; Milas, M.; le Dung, P. Characterization of chitosan. Influence of ionic strength and degree of acetylation on chain expansion. *Int. J. Biol. Macromol.* **1993**, *15*, 281–285.

142. Brugnerotto, J.; Desbrieres, J.; Roberts, G.; Rinaudo, M. Characterization of chitosan by steric exclusion chromatography. *Polymer* **2001**, *42*, 9921–9927.

143. Odijk, T. On the ionic-strength dependence of the intrinsic viscosity of DNA. *Biopolymers* **1979**, *18*, 3111–3113.

144. Mazeau, K.; Perez, S.; Rinaudo, M. Predicted influence of *N*-acetyl group content on the conformational extension of chitin and chitosan chains. *J. Carbohydr. Chem.* **2000**, *19*, 1269–1284.

145. Wei, Y.C.; Hudson, S.M.; Mayer, J.M.; Kaplan, D.L. The crosslinking of chitosan fibers. *J. Polym. Sci. Part A Polym. Chem.* **1992**, *30*, 2187–2193.

146. Welsh, E.R.; Price, R.R. Chitosan cross-linking with a water-soluble, blocked diisocyanate. 2. Solvates and hydrogels. *Biomacromolecules* **2003**, *4*, 1357–1361.

147. Arguelles-Monal, W.; Goycoolea, F.M.; Peniche, C.; Higuera-Ciapara, I. Rheological study of the chitosan/glutaraldehyde chemical gel system. *Polym. Gels Netw.* **1998**, *6*, 429–440.

148. Hirano, S.; Yamaguchi, R.; Fukui, N.; Iwata, M. A chitosan oxalate gel: Its conversion to an *N*-acetylchitosan gel via a chitosan gel. *Carbohydr. Res.* **1990**, *201*, 145–149.

149. Yamaguchi, R.; Hirano, S.; Arai, Y.; Ito, T. Chitosan salt gels thermally reversible gelation of chitosan. *Agric. Biol. Chem.* **1978**, *42*, 1981–1982.

150. Yokoyama, A.; Yamamoto, S.; Kawasaki, T.; Kohgo, T.; Nakasu, M. Development of calcium phosphate cement using chitosan and citric acid for bone substitute materials. *Biomaterials* **2002**, *23*, 1091–1101.

151. Shen, X.; Tong, H.; Jiang, T.; Zhu, Z.; Wan, P.; Hu, J. Homogeneous chitosan/carbonate apatite/citric acid nanocomposites prepared through a novel *in situ* precipitation. *Compos. Sci. Technol.* **2007**, *67*, 2238–2245.

152. Hsieh, S.H.; Chen, W.H.; Wei, L.L. A spectroscopic analysis of the reaction mechanism of polycarboxylic acid crosslinking with chitosan and cotton fabric. *Cellul. Chem. Technol.* **2003**, *37*, 359–369.

153. Desai, K.G.H.; Park, H.J. Encapsulation of vitamine C in tripolyphosphate cross-linked chitosan microspheres by spray drying, *J. Microencapsul.* **2005**, *22*, 179–192.

154. Quemeneur, F.; Rinaudo, M.; Maret, G.; Pepin-Donat, B. Decoration of lipid vesicles by polyelectrolytes: Mechanism and structure. *Soft Matter* **2010**, *6*, 4471–4481.

155. Rinaudo, M.; Quemeneur, F.; Pepin-Donat, B. Stabilization of liposomes against stress using polyelectrolytes: Interaction mechanisms, influence of pH, molecular weight, and polyelectrolyte structure. *Int. J. Polym. Anal. Charact.* **2009**, *14*, 667–677.

156. Bordi, F.; Sennato, S.; Truzzolillo, D. Polyelectrolyte-induced aggregation of liposomes: A new cluster phase with interesting applications. *J. Phys. Condens. Matter* **2009**, *21*, 203102:1–203102:26.

157. Haidar, Z.S.; Hamdy, R.C.; Tabrizian, M. Protein release kinetics for core-shell hybrid nanoparticles based on the layer-by-layer assembly of alginate and chitosan on liposomes. *Biomaterials* **2008**, *29*, 1207–1215.

158. Boddohi, S.; Killingsworth, C.E.; Kipper, M.J. Polyelectrolyte multilayer assembly as a function of pH and ionic strength using the polysaccharides chitosan and heparin. *Biomacromolecules* **2008**, *9*, 2021–2028.

159. Hillberg, A.L.; Tabrizian, M. Biorecognition through layer-by-layer polyelectrolyte assembly: *In situ* hybridation on living cells. *Biomacromolecules* **2006**, *7*, 2742–2750.

160. Majima, T.; Funakosi, T.; Iwasaki, N.; Yamane, S.T.; Harada, K.; Nonaka, S.; Minami, A.; Nishimura, S.I. Alginate and chitosan polyion complex hybrid fibers for scaffolds in ligament and tendon tissue engineering. *J. Orthopaedic. Sci.* **2005**, *10*, 302–307.

161. Iwasaki, N.; Yamane, S.T.; Majima, T.; Kasahara, Y.; Minami, A.; Harada, K.; Nanaka, S.; Maekawa, N.; Tamura, H.; Tokura, S.; *et al.* Feasibility of polysaccharide hybrid materials for scaffolds in cartilage tissue engineering: Evaluation of chondrocyte adhesion to polyion complex fibers prepared from alginate and chitosan. *Biomacromolecules* **2004**, *5*, 828–823.

162. Chung, T.W.; Yang, J.; Akaike, T.; Cho, K.Y.; Nah, J.W.; Kim, S.I.; Cho, C.S. Preparation of alginate/galactosylated chitosan scaffold for hepatocyte attachment. *Biomaterials* **2002**, *23*, 282–283.

163. Lavertu, M.; Méthot, S.; Tran-Khanh, N.; Buschmann, M.D. High efficiency gene transfer using chitosan/DNA nanoparticles with specific combinations of molecular weight and degree of deacetylation. *Biomaterials* **2006**, *27*, 4815–4824.

164. Jean, M.; Smaoui, F.; Lavertu, M.; Méthot, S.; Bouhdoud, L.; Buschmann, M.D.; Merzouki, A. Chitosan-plasmid nanoparticle formulations for IM and SC delivery of recombinant FGF-2 and PDGF-BB or generation of antibodies. *Gene Ther.* **2009**, *16*, 1097–1110.

165. Alameh, M.Z.; Jean, M.; Dejesus, D.; Buschmann, M.D.; Merzouki, A. Chitosanase-based method for RNA isolation from cells transfected with chitosan/siRNA nanocomplexes for real-time RT-PCR in gene delivery. *Int. J. Nanomedecine* **2010**, *5*, 473–481.

166. Thibault, M.; Nimesh, S.; Lavertu, M.; Buschmann, M. Intracellular trafficking and decondensation kinetics of chitosan-pDNA polyplexes. *Mol. Ther.* **2010**, *18*, 1787–1795.

167. Strand, S.P.; Danielsen, S.; Christensen, B.E.; Varum, K.M. Influence of chitosan structure on the formation and stability of DNA-Chitosan polyelectrolyte complexes. *Biomacromolecules* **2005**, *6*, 3357–3366.

168. Farkas, V. Fungal cell walls: Their structure, biosynthesis and biotechnological aspects. *Acta Biotechnol.* **1990**, *10*, 225–238.

169. Fleet, G.H.; Phaff, H.J. Fungal glucans-structure and metabolism. *Encycl. Plant Physiol. N S* **1981**, *13B*, 416–440.

170. Friedman, M.; Juneja, V.K. Review of Antimicrobial and Antioxidative Activities of Chitosans in Food. *J. Food Protect.* **2010**, *73*, 1737–1761.

171. Kardas, I.; Struszczyk, M.H.; Kucharska, M.; van den Broek, L.A.M.; van Dam, J.E.G.; Ciechańska, D. Chitin and chitosan as functional biopolymers for industrial applications. In *The European Polysaccharide Network of Excellence (EPNOE). Research Initiatives and Results*; Narvard. P., Ed.; Springer-Verlag: Wien, Austria, 2012; pp. 329–374.

172. Alishahi, A.; Aïder, M. Applications of chitosan in the seafood industry and aquaculture: A review. *Food Bioprocess Technol.* **2012**, *5*, 817–830.

173. Bordenave, N.; Grelier, S.; Cama, V. Water and moisture susceptibility of chitosan and paper-based materials: Structure-property relationships. *J. Agric. Food Chem.* **2007**, *55*, 9479–9488.

174. Franklin, T.J.; Snow, G.A. *Biochemistry of Antimicrobial Action;* 3rd ed.; Chapman and Hall: London, UK, 1981; p. 217.

175. Synowiecki, J.; Al-khatteb, N.A.A. Production, properties and some new applications of chitin and its derivatives. *Crit. Rev. Food Sci. Nut.* **2003**, *43*, 144-171.

176. Sudarshan, N.R.; Hoover, D.G.; Knorr, D. Antibacterial action of chitosan. *Food Biotechnol.* **1992**, *6*, 257–272.

177. Leuba, S.; Stossel, P. Chitosan and other polyamines: Antifungal activity and interaction with biological membranes. In *Chitin in Nature and Technology*; Muzzarelli, R.A.A., Jeuniaux, C., Gooday, C., Eds.; Plenum Press: New York, NY, USA, 1985; p. 217.

178. Choi, B.K.; Kim, K.Y.; Yoo, Y.J.; Oh, S.J.; Choi, J.H.; Kim. C.Y. *In vitro* antimicrobial activity of a chitooligosaccharide mixture against *Actinobacillus actinomycetemcomitans* and *Streptococcus mutans. Int. J. Antimicrob. Agent* **2001**, *18*, 553–557.

179. Eaton, P.; Fernandes, J.C.; Pereira, E.; Pintado, M.E.; Malcata. F.X. Atomic force microscopy study of the antibacterial effects of chitosans on *Escherichia coli* and *Staphylococcus aureus*. *Ultramicroscopy* **2008**, *108*, 1128–1134.

180. Chung, Y.C.; Su, Y.P.; Chen, C.C.; Jia, G.; Wang, H.L.; Wu, J.G.; Lin, J.G. Relationship between antibacterial activity of chitosan and surface characteristics of cell wall. *Acta Pharm. Sin.* **2004**, *25*, 932–936.

181. Jeon, Y.J.; Park, P.J.; Kim, S.K. Antimicrobial effect of chitooligosaccharides produced by bioreactor. *Carbohydr. Polym.* **2001**, *44*, 71–76.

182. Muzzarelli, R.; Tarsi, R.; Filippini, O.; Giovanetti, E.; Biagini, G.; Varaldo, P.E. *Antimicrob. Agents Chemother.* **1990**, *34*, 2019–2023.

183. Rhoades, J.; Roller, S. Antimicrobial actions of degraded and native chitosan against spoilage organisms in laboratory media and foods. *Appl. Environ. Microbiol.* **2000**, *66*, 80–86.

184. Helander, I.M.; Nurmiaho-Lassila, E.L.; Ahvenainen, R.; Rhoades, J.; Roller. S. Chitosan disrupts the barrier properties of the outer membrane of Gram-negative bacteria. *Int. J. Food Microbiol.* **2001**, *71*, 235–244.

185. No, H.K.; Young Park, N.; ho Lee, S.; Meyers. S.P. Antibacterial activity of chitosans and chitosan oligomers with different molecular weights. *Int. J. Food Microbiol.* **2002**, *74*, 65–72.

186. Younes, I.; Sellimi, S.; Rinaudo, M.; Jellouli, K.; Nasri, M. Influence of acetylation degree and molecular weight of homogeneous chitosans on antibacterial and antifungal activities. *Int. J. Food Microbiol.* **2014**, *185*, 57–63.

187. Zheng, L.Y.; Zhu. J.F. Study on antimicrobial activity of chitosan with different molecular weights. *Carbohydr. Polym.* **2003**, *54*, 527–530.

188. Benhabiles, M.S.; Salah, R.; Lounici, H.; Drouiche, N.; Goosen, M.F.A.; Mameri, N. Antibacterial activity of chitin, chitosan and its oligomers prepared from shrimp shell waste. *Food Hydrocolloid.* **2012**, *29*, 48–56.

189. Bell, A.A.; Hubbard, J.C.; Liu, L.; Davis, R.M.; Subbarao, K.V. Effects of chitin and chitosan on the incidence and severity of *Fusarium* yellows of celery. *Plant Dis.* **1998**, *82*, 322–328.

190. Ben-Shalom, N.; Ardi, R.; Pinto, R.; Aki, C.; Fallik. E. Controlling gray mould caused by *Botrytis cinerea* in cucumber plants by means of chitosan. *Crop. Prot.* **2003**, *22*, 285–290.

191. Wojdyła. A.T. Chitosan (Biochikol 020 PC) in the control of some ornamental foliage diseases. *Commun. Agric. Appl. Biol. Sci.* **2004**, *69*, 705–715.

192. Atia, M.M.M.; Buchenauer, H.; Aly, A.Z.; Abou-Zaid, M.I. Antifungal activity of chitosan against *Phytophthora* infestans and activation of defence mechanisms in tomato to late blight. *Biol. Agric. Hortic.* **2005**, *23*, 175–197.

193. Photchanachai, S.; Singkaew, J.; Thamthong, J. Effects of chitosan seed treatment on *Colletotrichum* sp. and seedling growth of chili cv. "jinda". In *ISHS Acta Horticulturae 712*, Proceedings of the IV International Conference on Managing Quality in Chains-The Integrated View on Fruits and Vegetables Quality, Bangkok, Thailand, 30 June 2006; Purvis, A.C., McGlasson, W.B., Kanlayanarat, S., Eds.; International Society for Horticultural Science: Leuven, Belgium, 2006; pp. 585–590.

194. Bai, R.K.; Huang, M.Y.; Jiang, Y.Y. Selective permeabilities of chitosan-acetic acid complex membrane and chitosan-polymer complex membranes for oxygen and carbon dioxide. *Polym. Bull.* **1988**, *20*, 83–88.

195. El-Ghaouth, A.; Arul, J.; Asselin, A.; Benhamou, N. Antifungal activity of chitosan on two postharvest pathogens of strawberry fruits. *Phytopathology* **1992**, *82*, 398–402.

196. Ames, B.N.; Gold, L.S.; Willet, W.C. Causes and prevention of cancer. *Proc. Nat. Acad. Sci. USA* **1995**, *92*, 5258–5265.

197. Pincernail, J. Free radicals and antioxidants in human disease. In *Analysis of Free Radicals in Biological Systems*; Favier, A.E., Cadet, J., Kalyanaraman, B., Fontecave, M., Pierre, J.L., Eds.; Birkhauser: Basel, Switzerland, 1995; pp. 83–98.

198. Stadtman, E.R. Protein oxidation and aging. *Science* **1992**, *257*, 1220–1224.

199. Witztum, J.L. The oxidation hypothesis of atherosclerosis. *Lancet* **1994**, *344*, 793–795.

200. Ames, B.N.; Shigenaga, M.K.; Hagan, T.M. Oxidants, antioxidants and the degenerative diseases of aging. *Proc. Natl. Acad. Sci. USA* **1993**, *90*, 7915–7922.

201. Halliwell, B.; Murcia, M.A.; Chirico, S.; Aruoma, O.I. Free radicals and antioxidants in food and *in vivo*: What they do and how they work. *Crit. Rev. Food Sci. Nutr.* **1995**, *35*, 7–20.

202. Halliwell, B. Free radicals, antioxidants and human disease: Curiosity, cause or consequence. *Lancet* **1994**, *344*, 721–724.

203. Chiang, M.T.; Yao, H.T.; Chen, H.C. Effect of dietary chitosans with different viscosity on plasma lipids and lipid peroxidation in rats fed on a diet enriched with cholesterol *Biosci. Biotech. Bioch.* **2000**, *5*, 965–971.

204. Park, P.J.; Je, J.Y.; Kim S.K. Free radical scavenging activity of chitooligosaccharides by electron spin resonance spectrometry *J. Agric. Food Chem.* **2003**, *51*, 4624–4627.

205. Sun, T.; Xie, W.; Xu, P. Antioxidant activity of graft chitosan derivatives. *Macromol. Biosci.* **2003**, *3*, 320–323.

206. Yin, X.Q.; Lin, Q.; Zhang, Q.; Yang. L.C. $O_2^-$ scavenging activity of chitosan and its metal complexes. *Chin. J. Appl. Chem.* **2002**, *19*, 325–328.

207. Kim, K.W.; Thomas, R.L. Antioxidative activity of chitosans with varying molecular weights. *Food Chem.* **2007**, *101*, 308–313.

208. Je, J.Y.; Park, P.J.; Kim, S.K. Free radical scavenging properties of hetero-chitooligosaccharides using an ESR spectroscopy. *Food Chem. Toxicol.* **2004**, *42*, 381–387.

209. Qi, L.; Xu, Z. *In vivo* antitumor activity of chitosan nanoparticles. *Bioorg. Med. Chem. Lett.* **2006**, *16*, 4243–4245.

210. Dass, C.R.; Choong, P.F. The use of chitosan formulations in cancer therapy. *J. Microencapsul.* **2008**, *25*, 275–279.

211. Chen, W.R.; Adams, R.L.; Carubelli, R.; Nordquist, R.E. Laser-photosensitizer assisted immunotherapy: A novel modality for cancer treatment. *Cancer Lett.* **1997**, *115*, 25–30.

212. Nishimura, K.; Nishimura, S.; Nishi, N.; Saiki, I.; Tokura, S.; Azuma, I. Immunological activity of chitin and its derivatives. *Vaccine* **1984**, *2*, 93–99.

213. Tokoro, A.; Tatewaki, N.; Suzuki, K.; Mikami, T.; Suzuki, S.; Suzuki, M. Growth inhibitory effect of hexa-*N*-acetylchitohexaose and chitohexaos and Meth-A solid tumor. *Chem. Pharm. Bull. (Tokyo)* **1998**, *36*, 784–790.

214. Murata, J.; Saiki, I.; Nishimura, S.; Nishi, N.; Tokura, S.; Azuma, I. Inhibitory effect of chitin heparinoids on the lung metastasis of B16-BL6 melanoma. *Jpn. J. Cancer Res.* **1989**, *80*, 866–872.

215. Hasegawa, M.; Yagi, K.; Iwakawa, S.; Hirai, M. Chitosan induces apoptosis via caspase-3 activation in bladder tumor cells. *Jpn. J. Cancer Res.* **2001**, *92*, 459–466.

216. Qi, L.; Xu, Z.; Chen, M. *In vitro* and *in vivo* suppression of hepatocellular carcinoma growth by chitosan nanoparticles. *Eur. J. Cancer* **2007**, *43*, 184–193.

217. Guminska, M.; Ignacak, J.; Wojcik, E. *In vitro* inhibitory effect of chitosan and its degradation products on energy metabolism in Ehrlich ascites tumour cells (EAT). *Polish J. Pharmacol.* **1996**, *48*, 495–501.

218. Lin, S.Y.; Chan, H.Y.; Shen, F.H.; Chen, M.H.; Wang, Y.J.; Yu, C.K. Chitosan prevents the development of AOM-induced aberrant crypt foci in mice and suppressed the proliferation of AGS cells by inhibiting DNA synthesis. *J. Cell Biochem.* **2007**, *100*, 1573–1580.

219. Jeon, Y.J.; Kim. S.K. Antitumor activity of chitosan oligosaccharides produced in an ultra filtration membrane reactor system. *J. Microbiol. Biotechn.* **2002**, *12*, 503–507.

220. Suzuki, K.; Mikami, T.; Okawa, Y.; Tokoro, A.; Suzuki, S.; Suzuki, M. Antitumor effect of hexa-*N*-acetylchitohexaose and chitohexaose. *Carbohydr. Res.* **1986**, *151*, 403–408.

221. Huang, M.; Khor, E.; Lim, L.Y. Uptake and cytotoxicity of chitosan molecules and nanoparticles: Effects of molecular weight and degree of deacetylation. *Pharm. Res.* **2004**, *21*, 344–353.

222. Younes, I.; Frachet, V.; Rinaudo, M.; Jellouli, K.; Nasri, M. Sfax University, Sfax, Tunisia. Cytotoxicity of homogeneous chitosans with different acetylation degrees and molecular weight on bladder carcinoma cells. 2015, Unpublished work.

223. Ravi Kumar, M.N.V.; Muzzarelli, R.A.A.; Muzzarelli, C.; Sashiwa, H.; Domb, A.J. Chitosan Chemistry and Pharmaceutical Perspectives. *React. Funct. Polym.* **2000**, *46*, 1–27.

224. Patil, R.S.; Ghormade, V.; Deshpande, M.V. Chitinolytic enzymes: An exploration. *Enzym. Microb. Technol.* **2000**, *26*, 473–483.

225. Venter, J.P.; Kotze, A.F; Auzely-Velty, R.; Rinaudo, M. Synthesis and evaluation of the mucoadhesivity of a CD-chitosan derivative. *Int. J. Pharm.* **2006**, *313*, 36–42.

226. Khor, E. Chitin: A biomaterial in waiting. *Curr. Opin. Solid State Mater. Sci.* **2002**, *6*, 313–317.

227. Maeda, Y.; Jayakumar, R.; Nagahama, H.; Furuike, T.; Tamura, H. Synthesis, characterization and bioactivity studies of novel b-chitin scaffolds for tissue-engineering applications, *Int. J. Biol. Macromol.* **2008**, *42*, 463–467.

228. Nagahama, H.; Nwe, N.; Jayakumar, R.; Koiwa, S.; Furuike, T.; Tamura, H. Novel biodegradable chitin membranes for tissue engineering applications. *Carbohydr. Polym.* **2008**, *73*, 295–302.

229. Yang, T.L. Chitin-based materials in tissue engineering: Applications in soft tissue and epithelial organ. *Int. J. Mol. Sci.* **2011**, *12*, 1936–1963.

230. Mi, F.L.; Lin, Y.M.; Wu, Y.B.; Shyu, S.S.; Tsai, Y.H. Chitin/PLGA blend microspheres as a biodegradable drug-delivery system: Phase-separation, degradation and release behavior. *Biomaterials* **2002**, *23*, 3257–3267.

231. Illum, L.; Davis, S. Chitosan as a delivery system for the transmucosal administration of drugs. In *Polysaccharides. Structural Diversity and Functional Versatility*, 2nd ed.; Dumitriu, S., Ed.; Marcel Dekker Publisher: New York, NY, USA, 2005; pp. 643–660.

232. Kumirska, J.; Weinhold, M.X.; Thöming, J.; Stepnowski, P. Biomedical Activity of Chitin/Chitosan Based Materials—Influence of Physicochemical Properties Apart from Molecular Weight and Degree of *N*-Acetylation. *Polymers* **2011**, *3*, 1875–1901.

233. Jayakumar, R.; Menon, D.; Manzoor, K.; Nair, S.V.; Tamura, H. Biomedical applications of chitin and chitosan based nanomaterials-A short review. *Carbohydr. Polym.* **2011**, *82*, 227–232.

*234.* Aranaz, I.; Mengíbar, M.; Harris, R.; Paños, I.; Miralles, B.; Acosta, N.; Galed, G.; Heras, A. Functional Characterization of Chitin and Chitosan. *Curr. Chem. Biol.* **2009**, *3*, 203–230.

235. Dutta, P.K.; Dutta, J.; Tripathi, V.S. Chitin and chitosan: Chemistry, properties and applications. *J. Sci. Ind. Res. India* **2004**, *63*, 20–31.

236. Park, B.K.; Kim, M-M. Applications of chitin and its derivatives in biological medicine. *Int. J. Mol. Sci.* **2010**, *11*, 5152–5164.

237. Cheba, B.A. Chitin and Chitosan: Marine Biopolymers with Unique Properties and Versatile Applications. *Glob. J. Biotechnol. Biochem.* **2011**, *6*, 149–153.

238. De Alvarenga, E.S. Characterization and properties of chitosan. In *Biotechnology of Biopolymers*; Elnashar, M., Ed.; In Tech: Rijeka, Croatia, 2011; pp. 91–108.

239. Kim, S.K. *Chitin and Chitosan Derivatives: Advances in Drug Discovery and Developments*; Kim, S.K., Ed.; CRC Press: Boca Raton, FL, USA, 2013.

240. Sarmento, B.; Das Neves, J. *Chitosan-Based Systems for Biopharmaceuticals: Delivery, Targeting and Polymer Therapeutics*; Wiley & Sons: Hoboken, NJ, USA, 2012.

241. Park, B.K.; Kim, M.M. Applications of Chitin and Its Derivatives in Biological Medicine. *Int. J. Mol. Sci.* **2010**, *11*, 5152–5164.

242. Dash, M.; Chiellini, F.; Ottenbrite, R.M.; Chiellini, E. Chitosan—A versatile semi-synthetic polymer in biomedical applications. *Prog. Polym. Sci.* **2011**, *36*, 981–1014.

243. Kanke, M.; Katayama, H.; Tsuzuki, S.; Kuramoto, H. Application of chitin and chitosan to pharmaceutical preparations. *Chem. Pharm. Bull.* **1989**, *37*, 523–525.

244. Kato, Y.; Onishi, H.; Machida, Y. Application of chitin and chitosan derivatives in the pharmaceutical field. *Curr. Pharm. Biotechnol.* **2003**, *4*, 303–309.

245. Felse, P.A.; Panda, T. Studies on applications of chitin and its derivatives. *Bioprocess Eng.* **1999**, *20*, 505–512.

246. Yusof, N.L.; Wee, A.; Lim, L.Y.; Khor, E. Flexible chitin films as potential wound-dressing materials: Wound model studies. *J. Biomed. Mater. Res. Part A* **2003**, *66A*, 224–232.

247. Liu, J.; Zhu, L. Method for preparing chitin composite artificial skin that can be used as woundplast. *Faming Zhuanli Shenqing CN 101411897 A 20090422*, 2009.

248. Wongpanit, P.; Sanchavanakit, N.; Pavasant, P.; Supaphol, P.; Tokura, S.; Rujiravanit, R. Preparation and characterization of microwave-treated carboxymethylchitin and carboxymethylchitosan films for potential use in wound care application. *Macromol. Biosci.* **2005**, *5*, 1001–1012.

249. Muzzarelli, R.A.A.; Morganti, G.; Palombo, P.; Biagini, G.; Mattioli Belmonte, M.; Giantomassi, F.; Orlandi, F.; Muzzarelli, C. Chitin nanofibrils/chitosan glycolate composites as wound medicaments. *Carbohydr. Polym.* **2007**, *70*, 274–284.

250. Bernkop-Schnurch, A. Mucoadhesive polymers. *In Polymeric Biomaterials*; Dumitriu, S., Ed., Marcel Dekker: New York, NY, USA, 2002; pp. 147–165.

251. Ito, M. *In vitro* properties of a chitosan-bonded hydroxyapatite bone-filling paste. *Biomaterials* **1991**, *12*, 41–45.

252. Swetha, M.; Sahithi, K.; Moorthi, A.; Srinivasan, N.; Ramasamy, K.; Selvamurugan, N. Biocomposites containing natural polymers and hydroxyapatite for bone tissue engineering. *Int. J. Biol. Macromol.* **2010**, *47*, 1–4.

253. Khor, E.; Lim, L.Y. Implantable applications of chitin and chitosan. *Biomaterials* **2003**, *24*, 2339–2349.

254. Vankatesan, J.; Kim, S.K. Chitosan composites for bone tissue engineering—An overview. *Mar. Drugs* **2010**, *8*, 2252–2266.

255. El Zein, A.R.; Dabbarh, F.; Chaput, C. Injectable self-setting calcium phosphate cement. In *Chitosan in Pharmacy and Chemistry*; Muzzarelli, R.A.A., Muzzarelli, C., Eds.; ATEC: Grottammare, Italy, 2002; pp. 365–370.

256. Yi, H.; Wu, L.Q.; Bentley, W.E.; Ghadssi, R.; Rubloff, G.W.; Culver, J.N.; Payne, G.F. Biofabrication with chitosan. *Biomacromolecules* **2005**, *6*, 2881–2894.

257. Saravanan, S.; Nethala, S.; Pattnaik, S.; Tripathi, A.; Moorthi, A.; Selvamurugan, N. Preparation, characterization and antimicrobial activity of a bio-composite scaffold containing chitosan/nano-hydroxyapatite/nano-silver for bone tissue engineering. *Int. J. Biol. Macromol.* **2011**, *49*, 188–193.

258. Venkatesan, J.; Kim, S.K. Chitosan Composites for Bone Tissue Engineering—An Overview. *Mar. Drugs* **2010**, *8*, 2252–2266.

259. Teng, S.; Lee, E.; Yoon, B.; Shin, D.; Kim, H.; Oh, J. Chitosan/nanohydroxyapatite composite membranes via dynamic filtration for guided bone regeneration. *J. Biomed. Mater. Res. Part A* **2009**, *88*, 569–580.

260. Bin, J.; Feng, Y.; Zhi-kun, L. Basic fibroblast growth factor combined with nano-hydroxyapatite/chitosan composites for repair of radial bone defects in rabbits. *Chin. J. Tissue Eng. Res.* **2012**, *16*, 6343–6348.

261. Costa-Pinto, A.R.; Reis, R.L.; Neves, N.M. Scaffolds based bone tissue engineering: The role of chitosan. *Tissue Eng. Part B Rev.* **2011**, *17*, 331–347.

262. Krajewska, B. Application of chitin- and chitosan-based materials for enzyme immobilizations: A review. *Enzym. Microb. Technol.* **2004**, *35*, 126–139.

263. Freier, T.; Montenegro, R.; Koh, S.; Shoichet, M.S. Chitin tubes for tissue engineering in the nervous system. *Biomaterials* **2005**, *26*, 4624–4632.

264. Yang, T.L. Chitin-based Materials in Tissue Engineering: Applications in Soft Tissue and Epithelial Organ. *Int. J. Mol. Sci.* **2011**, *12*, 1936–1963.

265. Kuo, S.M.; Niu, G.C.; Chang, S.J.; Kuo, C.H.; Bair, M.S. A one‐step method for fabricating chitosan microspheres. *J. Appl. Polym. Sci.* **2004**, *94*, 2150–2157.

266. Honarkar, H.; Barikani, M. Applications of biopolymers I: Chitosan. *Monatsh. Chem.* **2009**, *140*, 1403–1420.

267. Özbas-Turan, S.; Aral, C.; Kabasakal, L.; Keyer-Uysal, M.; Akbuga, J. Co-encapsulation of two plasmids in chitosan microspheres as a non-viral gene delivery vehicle. *J. Pharm. Pharmaceut. Sci.* **2003**, *6*, 27–32.

268. Ohkawa, K.; Minato, K.I.; Kumagai, G.; Hayashi, S.; Yamamoto, H. Chitosan nanofiber. *Biomacromolecules* **2006**, *7*, 3291–3294.

269. Kucharska, M.; Niekraszewicz, A.; Lebioda, J.; Malczewska-Brzoza, K.; Wesołowska, E. Bioactive Composite Materials In *Progress on Chemistry and Application of Chitin and Its Derivatives*; Jaworska, M.M., Ed.; Polish Chitin Society: Lodz, Poland, 2007; Volume 12, pp. 131–138.

270. Dhanikula, A.B.; Panchagnula, R. Development and characterization of biodegradable chitosan films for local delivery of paclitaxel. *AAPS J.* **2004**, *6*, 88–89.

271. Kucharska, M.; Struszczyk, M.H.; Cichecka, M.; Brzoza, K. Preliminary studies on the usable properties of innovative wound dressings. In *Progress on Chemistry and Application of Chitin and Its Derivatives*; Jaworska, M.M., Ed.; Polish chitin Society: Lotz, Poland, 2011; Volume 16, pp. 131–137.

272. Pereira, A.O.; Cartucho, D.J.; Duarte, A.S.; Gil, M.H.; Cabrita, A.; Patricio, J.A.; Barros, M.M. Immobilisation of cardosin A in chitosan sponges as a novel implant for drug delivery. *Curr. Drug Discov. Technol.* **2005**, *2*, 231–238.

273. Illum, L. Chitosan and its use as a pharmaceutical excipient. *Pharm. Res.* **1998**, *15*, 1326–1331.

274. Dai, T.; Tanaka, M.; Huang, Y.Y.; Hamblin, M.R. Chitosan preparations for wounds and burns: Antimicrobial and wound-healing effects. *Expert Rev. Anti. Infect. Ther.* **2011**, *9*, 857–879.

275. Jayakumar, R.; Prabaharan, M.; Sudheesh Kumar, P.T.; Nair, S.V.; Tamura, H. Biomaterials based on chitin and chitosan in wound dressing applications. *Biotechnol. Adv.* **2011**, *29*, 322–337.

276. Loke, W.K.; Lau, S.K; Yong, L.L.; Khor, E.; Sum, C.K. Wound dressing with sustained anti-microbial capability. *J. Biomed. Mater. Res.* **2000**, *53*, 8–17.

277. Kumari, R.; Dutta, P.K. Physicochemical and biological activity study of genipin-crosslinked chitosan scaffolds prepared by using supercritical carbon dioxide for tissue engineering applications. *Int. J. Biol. Macromol.* **2010**, *46*, 261–266.

278. Luna-barcenas, G.; Prokhorov, E.; Elizalde-pena, E.; Nuno-licona, A.; Sanchez, I.C. *Chitosan-Based Hydrogels for Tissue Engineering Applications, Biotechnology in Agriculture, Industry and Medicine Series*; Nova Science Publisher: New York, NY, USA, 2011.

279. Croisier, F.; Jérôme, C. Chitosan-based biomaterials for tissue engineering. *Eur. Polym. J.* **2013**, *49*, 780–792.

280. Riva, R.; Ragelle, H.; des Rieux, A.; Duhem, N.; Jérôme, C.; Préat, V. Chitosan and chitosan derivatives in drug delivery and tissue engineering. In *Chitosan for Biomaterials II*; Jayakumar, R., Prabaharan, M., Muzzarelli, R.A.A., Eds.; Springer: Berlin-Heidelberg, Germany, 2011; pp. 19–44.

281. Suh, J.K.F.; Matthew, H.W.T. Application of chitosan-based polysaccharide biomaterials in cartilage tissue engineering: A review. *Biomaterials* **2000**, *21*, 2589–2598.

282. Shi, C.; Zhu, Y.; Ran, X.; Wang, M.; Su, Y.; Cheng, T. Therapeutic potential of chitosan and its derivatives in regenerative medicine. *J. Surg. Res.* **2006**, *133*, 185–192.

283. Farzaneh, N.H.; Soheila, S.K.; Faramarz, A.T.; Zahra, A. Novel Topical Biocompatible Tissue Adhesive Based on Chitosan-modified Urethane Pre- S polymer. *Iran Polym. J.* **2011**, *20*, 671–680.

284. Kotzé, A.F.; Hamman, J.H.; Snyman, D.; Jonker, C.; Stander, M. Mucoadhesive and absorption enhancing properties of *N*-trimethyl chitosan chloride. In *Chitosan in Pharmacy and Chemistry*; Muzzarelli, R.A.A., Muzzarelli, C., Eds.; ATEC: Grottammare, Italy, 2002; pp. 31–40.

285. Rickett, T.A.; Amoozgar, Z.; Tuchek, C.A.; Park, J.; Yeo, Y.; Shi, R. Rapidly photo-cross-linkable chitosan hydrogel for peripheral neurosurgeries. *Biomacromolecules* **2011**, *12*, 57–65.

286. Hamman, J.H.; Kotzé, A.F. Paracellular absorption enhancement across intestinal epithelia by *N*-trimethyl chitosan chloride. In *Chitosan in Pharmacy and Chemistry*; Muzzarelli, R.A.A., Muzzarelli, C., Eds.; ATEC: Grottammare, Italy, 2002; pp. 41–50.

287. Miwa, A.; Ishibe, A.; Nakano, M.; Yamahira, T.; Itai, S.; Jinno, S.; Kawahara, H. Development of novel chitosan derivatives as micellar carriers of taxol. *Pharm. Res.* **1998**, *15*, 1844–1850.

288. Liu, W.; Sun, S.J.; Zhang, X.; de Yao, K. Self-aggregation behaviour of alkylated chitosan and its effect on the release of a hydrophobic drug. *J. Biomater. Sci. Polym. Edn.* **2003**, *14*, 851–859.

289. Liu, W.; Zang, X.; Sun, S.J.; Sun, G.J.; Yao, K.D.; Liang, D.C.; Guo, G.; Zhang, J.Y. *N*-alkylated chitosan as a potential nonviral vector for gene transfection. *Bioconjug. Chem.* **2003**, *14*, 782–789.

290. Ouchi, T.; Murata, J.I.; Ohya, Y. Gene delivery by quaternary chitosan with antennary galactose residues. In *Polysaccharide Applications: Cosmetics and Pharmaceuticals*; El-Nokaly, M.A., Soini, H.A., Eds.; American Chemical Society: Washington, DC, USA, 1999; pp. 15–23.

291. Mi, F.L.; Shyu, S.S.; Chen, C.T.; Schoung, J.Y. Porous chitosan microspheres suitable for controlling the antigen release of Newcastle disease vaccine: Preparation of antigen-adsorbed microsphere and *in vitro* release. *Biomaterials* **1999**, *20*, 1603–1612.

292. Park, I.K.; Jiang, H.L.; Yun, C.H.; Choi, Y.J.; Kim, S.J.; Akaike, T.; Kim, S.I.; Cho, C.S. Release of Newcastle disease virus vaccine from chitosan microspheres *in vitro* and *in vivo*. *Asian-Aust. J. Anim. Sci.* **2004**, *17*, 543–547.

293. Foda, N.H.; El-Iaithy, M.; Tadros, I. Implantable biodegradable sponges: Effect of interpolymer complex formation of chitosan with gelatin on the release behavior of tramadol hydrochloride. *Drug Dev. Ind. Pharm.* **2007**, *33*, 7–17.

294. Dhanaraj, S.A.; Selvadurai, M.; Santhi, K.; Hui, A.L.S.; Wen, C.J.; Teng, H.C. Targeted drug delivery system:-formulation and evaluation of chitosan nanospheres containing doxorubicin hydrochloride. *Int. J. Drug Deliv.* **2014**, *6*, 186–193.

295. Makhlof, A.; Tozuka, Y.; Takeuchi, H. Design and evaluation of novel pH-sensitive chitosan nanoparticles for oral insulin delivery. *Eur. J. Pharm. Sci.* **2011**, *42*, 445–451.

296. Cheng, S.Y.; Yuen, M.C.; Lam, P.L.; Gambari, R.; Wong, R.S.; Cheng, G.Y.; Lai, P.B.; Tong, S.W.; Chan, K.W.; Lau, F.Y.; *et al.* Synthesis, characterization and preliminary analysis of *in vivo* biological activity of chitosan/celecoxib microcapsules. *Bioorg. Med. Chem. Lett.* **2010**, *20*, 4147–4151.

MDPI AG
Klybeckstrasse 64
4057 Basel, Switzerland
Tel. +41 61 683 77 34
Fax +41 61 302 89 18
http://www.mdpi.com/

*Marine Drugs* Editorial Office
E-mail: marinedrugs@mdpi.com
http://www.mdpi.com/journal/marinedrugs

www.ingramcontent.com/pod-product-compliance
Lightning Source LLC
Chambersburg PA
CBHW051926190326
41458CB00026B/6422